Nutrigenetics and Nutrigenomics

Nutrigenetics and Nutrigenomics

Editor: Arthur Willis

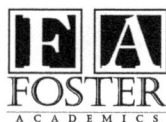

FA
FOSTER
ACADEMICS

www.fosteracademics.com

www.fosteracademics.com

FA FOSTER
ACADEMICS

Cataloging-in-Publication Data

Nutrigenetics and nutrigenomics / edited by Arthur Willis.
    p. cm.
Includes bibliographical references and index.
ISBN 978-1-63242-937-7
1. Nutrition--Genetic aspects. 2. Nutrient interactions. 3. Genomics.
4. Nutritionally induced diseases--Genetic aspects. 5. Diet in disease. I. Willis, Arthur.
QP144.G45 N88 2020
612.3--dc23

Foster Academics,
118-35 Queens Blvd., Suite 400,
Forest Hills, NY 11375, USA

ISBN 978-1-63242-937-7 (Hardback)

Contents

Preface

Food nutrients can have a consequence on human health through epigenetic modifications. This can occur due to DNA methylation and histone modification. Diet can directly have an impact on methylation patterns and gene expression. This is due to the dependence of DNA methylation mechanism on compounds derived from dietary sources, such as choline and folate. Further, dietary components can influence epigenetic events and alter gene expression, thereby disrupting functions such as metabolic balance, appetite control and fuel utilization. Different organs have their unique developmental stages. Any compromise in their development can predispose individuals to certain diseases. The prenatal and perinatal periods are believed to be important stages where nutrition is most vital. However, nutritional intake during adulthood can also significantly affect the epigenome. Cancer is a disease that is most commonly associated with adult nutrition. There has been rapid progress in the understanding of the association between genes and nutrition in recent years. From theories to research to practical applications, case studies related to all contemporary topics of relevance to this domain have been included in this book. It is a complete source of knowledge on the present status of nutrigenomics.

The information contained in this book is the result of intensive hard work done by researchers in this field. All due efforts have been made to make this book serve as a complete guiding source for students and researchers. The topics in this book have been comprehensively explained to help readers understand the growing trends in the field.

I would like to thank the entire group of writers who made sincere efforts in this book and my family who supported me in my efforts of working on this book. I take this opportunity to thank all those who have been a guiding force throughout my life.

Editor

Betaine reduces β-amyloid-induced paralysis through activation of cystathionine-β-synthase in an Alzheimer model of *Caenorhabditis elegans*

Anne Leiteritz, Benjamin Dilberger, Uwe Wenzel and Elena Fitzenberger[*] ⓘ

Abstract

Background: The neurodegenerative disorder Alzheimer's disease is caused by the accumulation of toxic aggregates of β-amyloid in the human brain. On the one hand, hyperhomocysteinemia has been shown to be a risk factor for cognitive decline in Alzheimer's disease. On the other hand, betaine has been demonstrated to attenuate Alzheimer-like pathological changes induced by homocysteine. It is reasonable to conclude that this is due to triggering the remethylation pathway mediated by betaine-homocysteine-methyltransferase. In the present study, we used the transgenic *Caenorhabditis elegans* strain CL2006, to test whether betaine is able to reduce β-amyloid-induced paralysis in *C. elegans*. This model expresses human β-amyloid 1–42 under control of a muscle-specific promoter that leads to progressive, age-dependent paralysis in the nematodes.

Results: Betaine at a concentration of 100 μM was able to reduce homocysteine levels in the presence and absence of 1 mM homocysteine. Simultaneously, betaine both reduced normal paralysis rates in the absence of homocysteine and increased paralysis rates triggered by addition of homocysteine. Knockdown of cystathionine-β-synthase using RNA interference both increased homocysteine levels and paralysis. Additionally, it prevented the reducing effects of betaine on homocysteine levels and paralysis.

Conclusion: Our studies show that betaine is able to reduce homocysteine levels and β-amyloid-induced toxicity in a *C. elegans* model for Alzheimer's disease. This effect is independent of the remethylation pathway but requires the transsulfuration pathway mediated by cystathionine-β-synthase.

Keywords: Alzheimer's disease, β-Amyloid, *Caenorhabditis elegans*, Hyperhomocysteinemia, Betaine

Background

Alzheimer's disease (AD) is the most common age-related neurodegenerative disorder caused by the accumulation of aggregated β-amyloid (Aβ) as senile plaques in the human brain [1, 2]. These deposits are associated with synaptotoxicity that leads to the characteristic cognitive decline [3]. Moderately elevated plasma homocysteine (Hcy) levels were identified as a strong risk factor not only for vascular dementia but also for AD [4]. Several mechanisms underlying the noxious effect of Hcy in the brain have been proposed. These include DNA damage [5], activation of N-methyl-D-aspartate receptors [6], and the alteration of the amyloid precursor protein (APP) metabolic pathway by hypomethylation [7]. Slightly increased homocysteine levels can be due to single nucleotide polymorphisms in the gene encoding 5,10-methylene-tetrahydrofolate-reductase (MTHFR) [8]. It has been shown that in such cases folic acid supplementation reduces Hcy levels [9]. Alternatively, remethylation of Hcy to methionine and S-adenosylmethionine (SAM) can also be achieved by supplementing betaine as a methyl donor [10]. Indeed, in hyperhomocysteinemic rats betaine supplementation was shown to ameliorate Hcy-induced AD-like pathological changes and memory deficits [11]. In

* Correspondence: elena.fitzenberger@ernaehrung.uni-giessen.de
Molecular Nutrition Research, Interdisciplinary Research Center,
Justus-Liebig-University of Giessen, Heinrich-Buff-Ring 26-32, 35392 Giessen,
Germany

the nematode *Caenorhabditis elegans*, however, effects of betaine on remethylation of Hcy can be excluded since the nematode has no orthologue of betaine-Hcy-methyltransferase (BHMT), encoding the relevant enzyme for betaine mediated remethylation [12]. Another biochemical pathway, through which Hcy can be detoxified, is transsulfuration of Hcy to cystathionine by the vitamin B6-dependent enzyme cystathionin-β-synthase (CBS).

In the present study, we used the transgenic *C. elegans* strain CL2006, which expresses the human Aβ under the control of the muscle-specific *unc-54* promotor and displays progressive paralysis [13], in order to test the effects of betaine supplementation on the AD phenotype. To explore the contribution of CBS on the measured effects, RNA interference was used. Moreover, the effects of betaine intervention and CBS knockdown on Hcy levels were estimated by ELISA.

Methods

Strains
The transgenic nematode strain CL2006 (($dvIs2$[p-CL12(*unc-54*/human Aβ$_{1-42}$ minigene) + pRF4]) was obtained from the *C. elegans* Genetics Center, CGC (University of Minnesota, MN, USA). CL2006 expresses human Aβ$_{1-42}$ under the control of the muscle-specific promoter *unc-54*, leading to progressive, adult-onset paralysis [13]. *E. coli* HT115 RNAi clones were purchased from Source Bioscience (Cambridge, UK) and included a negative control (empty L4440 vector), *cbs-1* (ZC373.1), *gcs-1* (F37B12.2), and *metr-1* (R03D7.1).

C. elegans maintenance
The maintenance and experimental procedures were conducted according to standard protocols. The nematodes were cultivated at 20 °C on nematode growth medium (NGM) agar plates that contained an *E. coli* OP50 lawn as the major food source [14]. For the experiments, synchronous populations of larvae were used, which were obtained by bleaching egg-laying adults with a hypochlorite solution [15].

RNA interference
RNA interference (RNAi) was performed by using the feeding method. As described elsewhere, it was conducted in liquid cultures, which were enriched with RNAi bacteria [16, 17]. In brief, in the RNAse III-deficient *E. coli* strain HT115 gene-specific dsRNA expression was induced by incubation with 1 mM isopropyl-β-D-thiogalactopyranoside for 4 h at 37 °C. Subsequently, the bacteria were centrifuged and resuspended in NGM, containing 50 µg/ml kanamycin to inactivate bacterial growth. This suspension was applied to each well of a 96-well plate together with a volume of 10 µl M9 buffer containing 10–15 synchronized L1 larvae. The volume of the NGM-bacteria-suspension varied between 44 and 46 µl, depending on the number of effectors, which were added later. That is, in case of betaine supplementation only, 44 µl NGM-bacteria suspension were used, and if Hcy and betaine were applied together, 46 µl NGM were added.

Treatment of *C. elegans* with Hcy and betaine
To young adult CL2006 nematodes, which are characterized by the ability to lay eggs, a volume of 6 µl betaine or 7 µl of both betaine and homocysteine were added. Effector solutions were prepared in M9 buffer and contained tenfold enriched concentrations compared to the final concentration in the experiment. Control nematodes were always treated with the identical volumes of M9 buffer only. Treatments were performed for 48 h before heat-shock was applied.

Measurement of paralysis
The expression and aggregation of Aβ$_{1-42}$ in *C. elegans* results in the paralyzation phenotype, which is described as a movement that is restricted to waving of the head without translocation of the animal [18].

Before scoring paralysis, the nematodes were heat-shocked for 1.5 h at 35 °C in order to accelerate the paralyzation process and to generate a paralyzation rate in the control population of about 50%. After heat shock, the individual nematodes were transferred with M9/Tween 20®- buffer on NGM agar plates. The paralysis phenotype was examined by visual analysis of 25 nematodes per treatment group. Each nematode was tapped with a bent platinum wire, and subsequently, its moving ability was scored.

Hcy-ELISA
For determination of Hcy concentrations, a quantitative, competitive human Hcy-ELISA Kit (NeoScientific, Cambridge; USA) was employed. To this end, nematodes were treated with lysis buffer (HEPES 50 mM, NaCl 150 mM, EDTA 5 mM, DTT 2 mM) and frozen at – 80 °C to extract proteins. After thawing on ice, worms were homogenized with Peqlab Precellys 24-Dual (VWR, Erlangen, Germany). Subsequently, the concentration of extracted protein was determined by using the Bio-Rad Protein Assay. The measurement of the Hcy concentration was set up according to the instruction manual. In brief, the protein solution and a Hcy-HRP conjugate were added to the wells of the ELISA plate, which were coated with a Hcy-specific antibody. Hcy in the samples competes with the conjugate for binding to the plate-bound antibody. Higher Hcy concentrations in the probes lead to decreased Hcy-HRP conjugate binding. By using a HRP substrate, the amount of captured Hcy-HRP can be quantified colorimetrically. The OD of the probes was compared to a

standard curve, which was generated by using the included calibration standards.

Calculations and statistics

For statistical analyses, GraphPad Prism 5.0 software (GraphPad, La Jolla, CA, USA) was used. Analysis of variance (ANOVA) and Bonferroni-Holm multiple comparison test as well as 2-way ANOVA were performed for multiple group comparisons. Differences between two groups were examined with Student's t test. The results shown are representatives of at least three independent experiments and are presented as means ± SD. Significance levels were assumed as $p < 0.05$ (*), $p < 0.01$ (**), and $p < 0.001$ (***).

Results

Knockdown of cbs-1 increases Hcy levels and paralysis in CL2006

In order to test whether one-carbon metabolism is functional in *C. elegans*, we knocked down the genes for *cbs-1* and and 5-methyltetrahydrofolate-methyltransferase *metr-1*, which is synonymous for methionine synthase. Knockdown of either gene caused an increase of Hcy levels (Fig. 1a). These results suggest that, with regard to Hcy remethylation and transsulfuration, both enzymes possess the same functional role in *C. elegans* and in humans.

Moreover, both knockdowns significantly increased the paralysis rate in CL2006 (Fig. 1b).

Hcy levels are directly associated with the paralysis phenotype in CL2006

Next, we assessed whether the observed paralysis under knockdown of *cbs-1* and *metr-1* are indeed due to the increased Hcy levels. To this end, 100 µM betaine was applied in the absence or presence of 1 mM exogenous Hcy. Although the reduction of Hcy levels by betaine treatment was not significant, betaine was able to significantly reduce Hcy levels after application of 1 mM exogenous Hcy (Fig. 2a). Significant interactions of homocysteine and betaine were observed (p < 0.001). Moreover, paralysis rate decreased upon betaine treatment both in the absence of exogenous Hcy and when paralysis was first increased by addition of Hcy to the nematodes (Fig. 2b).

Betaine does no longer affect paralysis under cbs-1 RNAi

In order to find out whether the paralysis-reducing effects of betaine depend on the activity of CBS, we knocked down the corresponding gene again. RNAi for *cbs-1* completely prevented the reducing effect of betaine on Hcy levels (Fig. 3a) and paralysis (Fig. 3b). These findings suggest that, on the one hand, betaine acts via

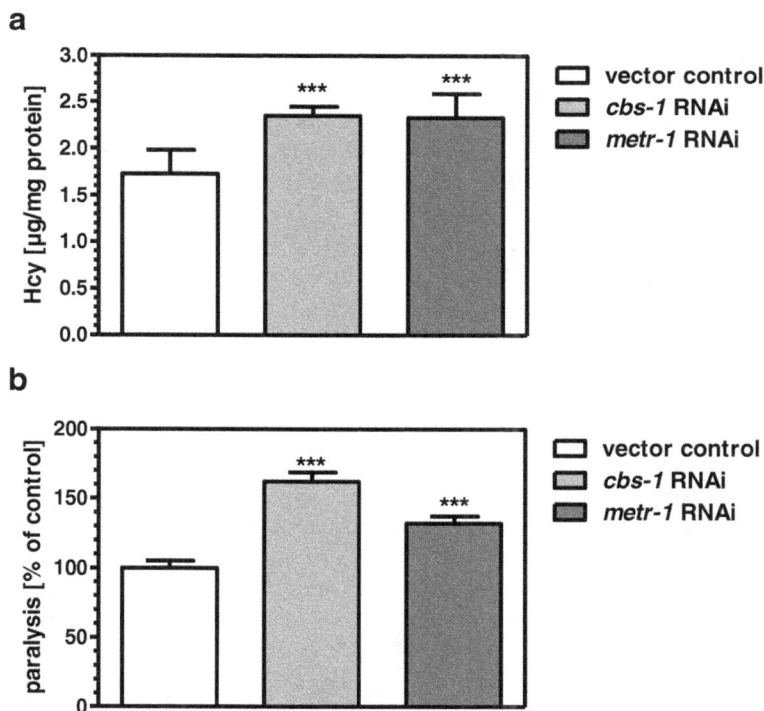

Fig. 1 Knockdown of *cbs-1* and *metr-1* via RNAi increase Hcy level and paralysis rate in CL2006. Hcy concentration was determined with the Human Hcy-ELISA Kit 48 h after nematodes had reached the young adult stage (**a**). At the same, stage paralysis in CL2006 was assessed subsequent to a heat-shock for 1.5 h at 35 °C by tapping the nematodes with a bent platinum wire and subsequent scoring of their moving ability (**b**). ***p < 0.001 versus the vector control

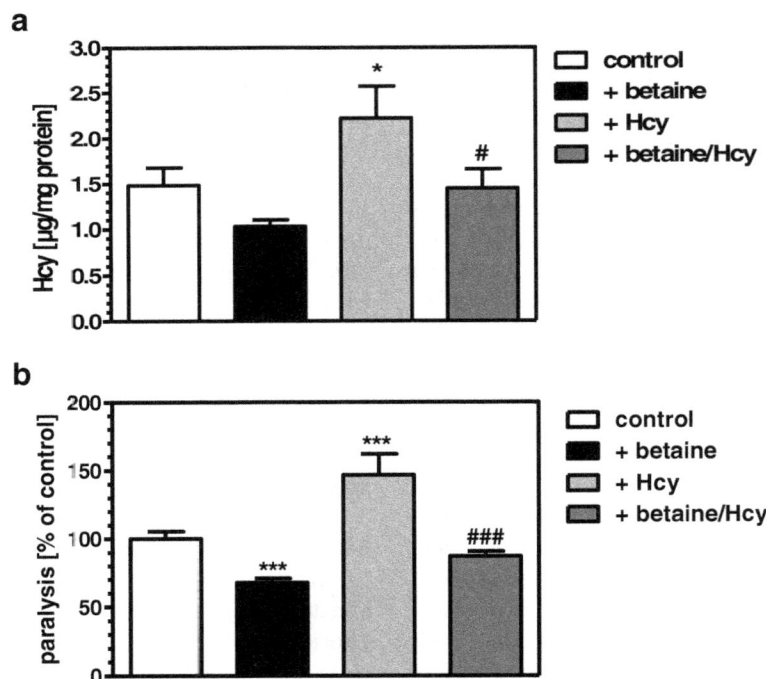

Fig. 2 Betaine reduces Hcy level and paralysis rate in the absence and presence of exogenous Hcy. Hcy level was determined either in control nematodes or those treated with 1 mM Hcy. Moreover, in an additional experiment, both groups were exposed to 100 μM betaine also (**a**). Paralysis was determined under identical conditions as described for Hcy measurements (**b**). *$p < 0.05$, ***$p < 0.001$ versus the control; ###$p < 0.001$ versus worms treated with Hcy

triggering the transsulfuration pathway. On the other hand, increased transsulfuration of Hcy would provide more cysteine, which could serve as a substrate for glutathione synthesis. This could be of special importance in preventing the AD-phenotype, since AD is frequently shown to be associated with increased oxidative stress. However, when we knocked down gcs-1 (γ-glutamyl-cysteine-synthetase), encoding the key enzyme for glutathione synthesis, we did not observe any influence on the paralysis rate. Moreover, betaine was still able to reduce paralysis in CL2006 to the same extent as in the presence of GCS-1 (Fig. 3c).

Discussion

Senile plaques consisting of Aβ are a hallmark of AD and are considered as responsible for neuronal damage [19]. It is suggested that Aβ oligomers are neurotoxic because they lead to increased oxidative stress [20], mitochondrial dysfunction [21], disturbed metal ion homeostasis [22], and apoptosis [23]. Hyperhomocysteinemia has been shown to be associated with AD and represents a factor which is influenced genetically and environmentally [24]. The impact of genetic impairments of one-carbon metabolism, as is case by MTHFR C677T polymorphism, prevails especially under insufficient folate, vitamin B6, and/or vitamin B12 levels [24]. Increased Hcy

levels, as a consequence of insufficient remethylation and/or transsulfuration, have been described to increase the production of reactive oxygen species via autoxidation of homocysteine [25]. In addition, homocysteine and the oxidized metabolite homocysteic acid are described as potent neurotoxins because of its property to be an endogenous NMDA (N-methyl-D-aspartate) receptor agonists [6]. High levels of homocysteine also are associated with DNA damage because the amino acid impairs the DNA repair, supporting neuronal cell death [5]. These processes increase indirectly the vulnerability of neurons to get damaged by Aβ [26, 27]. There is, moreover, also a direct effect of increased Hcy concentrations on Aβ toxicity, which is due to the enhanced aggregation propensity of Aβ$_{1-42}$ via the homocysteinylation of lysine residues leading to stabilized soluble oligomeric intermediates [28].

Nutritional factors able to decrease Hcy levels and to cause slowing of cognitive decline and of atrophy in critical brain regions, consistent with modification of the AD process at least in high risk subjects with baseline vitamin B status, are folate, vitamin B6, and vitamin B12 [4]. Whereas vitamin B6 could increase the synthesis of cystathionine from Hcy and serine by CBS, folate as cofactor for MTHFR and B12 for methionine-synthase might increase under those conditions remethylation of Hcy, betaine could serve also as methyl group donor for

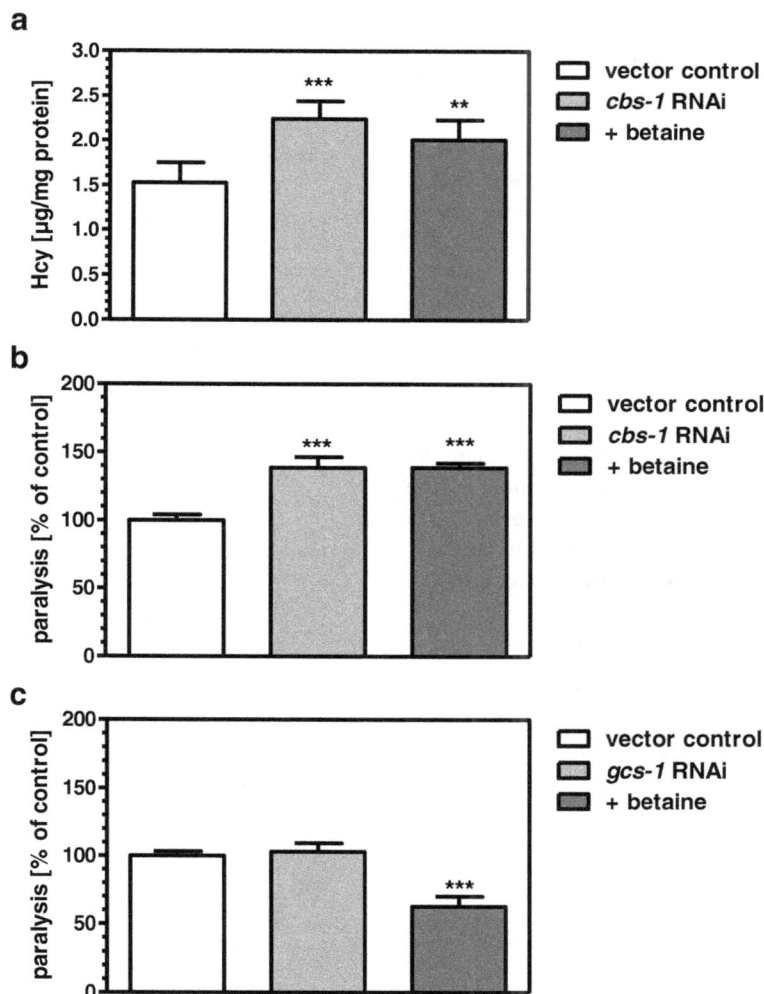

Fig. 3 The glutathione synthesis is not involved in the paralysis reducing effects of betaine. Under *cbs-1* RNAi, betaine was no longer able to reduce Hcy level significantly (**a**) nor to diminish paralysis (**b**). Knockdown of *gcs-1*, encoding the key enzyme for glutathione synthesis, did neither affect paralysis nor prevent the paralysis reducing effects of betaine (**c**). ******$p < 0.01$, *******$p < 0.001$ versus vector control

Hcy as mediated by BHMT. Indeed betaine has been shown in this context to arrest Hcy-induced AD-like pathological changes and memory deficits more efficient than supplementation of folate [11]. In *C. elegans*, however, BHMT is not present due to genetic loss [12]. Accordingly, *C. elegans* represents the perfect model to investigate whether there are effects of betaine on AD-like phenotypes which are independent on the remethylation of Hcy.

In *C. elegans* CL2006, expressing a transgene for human Aβ, inhibition of remethylation by *metr-1* RNA, or transsulfuration by *cbs-1* RNAi both increased Hcy levels and paralysis. This demonstrates that one-carbon metabolism is functional also in *C. elegans* as has been observed previously with regard to adaptive responses to dietary restriction [29]. Moreover, the results suggest

that Hcy levels are directly associated with the paralytic phenotype in CL2006. The latter was substantiated by the findings that increased Hcy levels by addition of exogenous Hcy lead to increased paralysis whereas lowering of Hcy levels in the presence or absence of exogenous Hcy reduces the paralysis rate to a similar extent at the same dose. Although it might be concluded that lowering of Hcy levels by betaine could be due to activation of MTHFR and methionine-synthase. We did not perceive it as rationale to follow this possibility since enhanced levels of SAM would allosterically activate CBS [30]. We therefore focused on CBS as a target for the observed betaine effects. Indeed betaine was no longer able to reduce Hcy levels or paralysis when increased by *cbs-1* RNAi. We finally postulated that increased Hcy detoxification under betaine exposure by increased cystathionine synthesis could, through cleavage by cystathionase, deliver more cysteine for glutathione synthesis. As described above, enhanced generation of reactive oxygen species is a typical phenomenon of AD and has been attributed to decreased levels of the brain antioxidant, glutathione [31]. Moreover, lowered cortical glutathione levels were found as a biomarker of early Alzheimer disease pathogenesis [32]. However, in CL2006, the knockdown of *gcs-1*, encoding the rate-limiting enzyme for glutathione synthesis, did neither affect the paralysis rate nor did it prevent betaine from being active in diminishing paralysis.

Conclusions

In conclusion, our study shows that betaine reduces the Aβ-induced degeneration in an Alzheimer model of the nematode *C. elegans* by lowering the Hcy levels. CBS was, moreover, identified as the target enzyme through which betaine exerts its degeneration preventing effects.

Abbreviations
AD: Alzheimer's disease; Aβ: β-Amyloid; BHMT: Betaine-homocysteine-methyltransferase; CBS: Cystathionine-β-synthase; GCS: γ-Glutamyl-cysteine-synthetase; Hcy: Homocysteine; HRP: Horseradish peroxidase; METR: 5-Methyltetrahydrofolate-homocysteine-methyltransferase: MTHFR: 5,10-Methylene-tetrahydrofolate-reductase; SAM: S-Adenosylmethionine

Acknowledgements
Some strains were provided by the CGC, which is funded by NIH Office of Research Infrastructure Programs (P40 OD010440).

Authors' contributions
AL made substantial contributions to acquisition, analysis, and interpretation of data. BD contributed to data acquisition. AL drafted the manuscript. UW made substantial contributions to conception and design as well as interpretation of data and manuscript revision. EF contributed to the data analysis and interpretation as well as manuscript revision. All authors read and approved the final manuscript.

Competing interests
The authors declare that they have no competing interests.

References
1. LaFerla FM, Green KN, Oddo S. Intracellular amyloid-beta in Alzheimer's disease. Nat Rev Neurosci. 2007;8(7):499–509.
2. Glenner GG, Wong CW. Alzheimer's disease. Biochem Biophys Res Commun. 2012;425(3):534–9.
3. Selkoe DJ. Alzheimer's disease. Cold Spring Harb Perspect Biol. 2011;3(7): a004577
4. Smith AD, Refsum H. Homocysteine, B vitamins, and cognitive impairment. Annu Rev Nutr. 2016;36:211–39.
5. Vanzin CS, Manfredini V, Marinho AE, et al. Homocysteine contribution to DNA damage in cystathionine β-synthase-deficient patients. Gene. 2014; 539(2):270–4.
6. Sibarov DA, Abushik PA, Giniatullin R, Antonov SM. GluN2A subunit-containing NMDA receptors are the preferential neuronal targets of homocysteine. Front Cell Neurosci. 2016;10:246.
7. Lin H-C, Hsieh H-M, Chen Y-H, Hu M-L. S-Adenosylhomocysteine increases beta-amyloid formation in BV-2 microglial cells by increased expressions of beta-amyloid precursor protein and presenilin 1 and by hypomethylation of these gene promoters. Neurotoxicology. 2009;30(4):622–7.
8. Masud R, Baqai HZ. The communal relation of MTHFR, MTR, ACE gene polymorphisms and hyperhomocysteinemia as conceivable risk of coronary artery disease. Appl Physiol Nutr Metab. 2017;42(10):1009–14.
9. Liew SC, Gupta ED. Methylenetetrahydrofolate reductase (MTHFR) C677T polymorphism: epidemiology, metabolism and the associated diseases. Eur J Med Genet. 2015;58(1):1–10.
10. McBreairty LE, Robinson JL, Harding SV, et al. Betaine is as effective as folate at re-synthesizing methionine for protein synthesis during moderate methionine deficiency in piglets. Eur J Nutr. 2016;55(8):2423–30.
11. Chai GS, Jiang X, Ni ZF, et al. Betaine attenuates Alzheimer-like pathological changes and memory deficits induced by homocysteine. J Neurochem. 2013;124(3):388–96.
12. Bito T, Watanabe F. Biochemistry, function, and deficiency of vitamin B12 in Caenorhabditis elegans. Exp Biol Med. 2016;241(15):1663–8.
13. Link CD. Expression of human beta-amyloid peptide in transgenic Caenorhabditis elegans. Proc Natl Acad Sci U S A. 1995;92(20):9368–72.
14. Brenner S. The genetics of Caenorhabditis elegans. Genetics Dev. 1974;77(1): 71–94.
15. Stiernagle T. Maintenance of C. elegans, WormBook the online review of C. elegans biology, ed. The C. elegans Research Community. 2006:1–11. http://www.wormbook.org.
16. Lehner B, Tischler J, Fraser AG. RNAi screens in Caenorhabditis elegans in a 96-well liquid format and their application to the systematic identification of genetic interactions. Nat Protoc. 2006;1(3):1617–20.
17. Timmons L, Court DL, Fire A. Ingestion of bacterially expressed dsRNAs can produce specific and potent genetic interference in Caenorhabditis elegans. Gene. 2001;263(1–2):103–12.
18. Link C, Taft A, Kapulkin V, et al. Gene expression analysis in a transgenic Caenorhabditis elegans Alzheimer's disease model. Neurobiol Aging. 2003; 24(3):397–413.
19. Haass C, Selkoe DJ. Soluble protein oligomers in neurodegeneration: lessons from the Alzheimer's amyloid beta-peptide. Nat Rev Mol Cell Biol. 2007;8(2):101–12.
20. Tamagno E, Bardini P, Guglielmotto M, et al. The various aggregation states of beta-amyloid 1-42 mediate different effects on oxidative stress, neurodegeneration, and BACE-1 expression. Free Radic Biol Med. 2006; 41(2):202–12.
21. Lin M, Beal MF. Mitochondrial dysfunction and neurodegenerative diseases. Biochim Biophys Acta. 1998;1366(1–2):211–23.
22. Demuro A, Mina E, Kayed R, et al. Calcium dysregulation and membrane disruption as a ubiquitous neurotoxic mechanism of soluble amyloid oligomers. J Biol Chem. 2005;280(17):17294–300.
23. Guglielmotto M, Monteleone D, Piras A, et al. Aβ1-42 monomers or oligomers have different effects on autophagy and apoptosis. Autophagy. 2014;10(10):1827–43.
24. Troesch B, Weber P, Mohajeri MH. Potential links between impaired one-carbon metabolism due to polymorphisms, inadequate B-vitamin status, and the development of Alzheimer's disease. Nutrients. 2016;8(12)
25. Zou CG, Banerjee R. Homocysteine and redox signaling. Antioxid Redox Signal. 2005;7(5–6):547–59.
26. Ho PI, Collins SC, Dhitavat S, et al. Homocysteine potentiates beta-amyloid neurotoxicity: role of oxidative stress. J Neurochem. 2001;78(2): 249–53.
27. Kruman II, Kumaravel TS, Lohani A, et al. Folic acid deficiency and homocysteine impair DNA repair in hippocampal neurons and sensitize them to amyloid toxicity in experimental models of Alzheimer's disease. J Neurosci. 2002;22(5):1752–62.
28. Khodadadi S, Riazi GH, Ahmadian S, et al. Effect of N-homocysteinylation on physicochemical and cytotoxic properties of amyloid β-peptide. FEBS Lett. 2012;586(2):127–31.
29. Klapper M, Findeis D, Koefeler H, Döring F. Methyl group donors abrogate adaptive responses to dietary restriction in C. Elegans. Genes Nutr. 2016;11:4.
30. Ereño-Orbea J, Majtan T, Oyenarte I, et al. Structural insight into the molecular mechanism of allosteric activation of human cystathionine β-synthase by S-adenosylmethionine. Proc Natl Acad Sci U S A. 2014;111(37): E3845–52.

Transcriptomic responses of the liver and adipose tissues to altered carbohydrate-fat ratio in diet

Mitsuru Tanaka[1], Akihito Yasuoka[2], Manae Shimizu[3], Yoshikazu Saito[4], Kei Kumakura[3], Tomiko Asakura[4] and Toshitada Nagai[3]*

Abstract

Background: To elucidate the effects of altered dietary carbohydrate and fat balance on liver and adipose tissue transcriptomes, 3-week-old rats were fed three kinds of diets: low-, moderate-, and high-fat diets (L, M, and H) containing a different ratio of carbohydrate-fat (C-F) (65:15, 60:20, and 35:45 in energy percent, respectively).

Methods: The rats consumed the diets for 9 weeks and were subjected to biochemical and DNA microarray analyses.

Results: The rats in the H-group exhibited lower serum triacylglycerol (TG) levels but higher liver TG and cholesterol content than rats in the L-group. The analysis of differentially expressed genes (DEGs) between each group (L vs M, M vs H, and L vs H) in the liver revealed about 35% of L vs H DEGs that were regulated in the same way as M vs H DEGs, and most of the others were L- vs H-specific. Gene ontology analysis of these L vs H DEGs indicated that those related to fatty acid synthesis and circadian rhythm were enriched. Interestingly, about 30% of L vs M DEGs were regulated in a reverse way compared with L vs H and M vs H DEGs. These reversed liver DEGs included M-up/H-down genes (*Sds* for gluconeogenesis from amino acids) and M-down/H-up genes (*Gpd2* for gluconeogenesis from glycerol, *Agpat9* for TG synthesis, and *Acot1* for beta-oxidation). We also analyzed L vs H DEGs in white (WAT) and brown (BAT) adipose tissues and found that both oxidation and synthesis of fatty acids were inhibited in these tissues.

Conclusions: These results indicate that the alteration of dietary C-F balance differentially affects the transcriptomes of metabolizing and energy-storing tissues.

Keywords: Transcriptome, Carbohydrate-fat ratio, Liver, White adipose tissue, Brown adipose tissue

Background

Availability of body carbohydrate (C) and fat (F) for energy production varies depending on the animal's circumstances. Fat is mainly consumed during resting conditions at about 90% of total energy; however, this ratio can be rapidly decreased to nearly 10% through acute bouts of exercise and substituted by the energy supply from aerobic or anaerobic respiration of C [7, 38]. Under fasting conditions, carbohydrate is depleted within a day, and about four fifths of basal metabolic rate is maintained by fat and the rest by amino acids for several days [4]. These metabolic switches of energy source between C and F are more interchangeable than protein (P) or amino acids because of the metabolic linkage mediated by the key organic substances: glycerol-3-phosphate both as the product of triacylglycerol (TG) hydrolysis and as the substrate for gluconeogenesis, NADP(H) both as the hydrogen acceptor of the pentose phosphate pathway and as the hydrogen donor for fatty acid (FA) synthesis, and acetyl-CoA as the activated substrate of the TCA cycle and of FA synthesis. Thus, dietary C to F ratio (C-F ratio) has a considerable effect on the energy homeostasis of animals.

* Correspondence: tnagai@takasaki-u.ac.jp
[3]Department of Health and Nutrition, Takasaki University of Health and Welfare, 37-1 Nakaorui-machi, Takasaki, Gunma 370-0033, Japan
Full list of author information is available at the end of the article

Generally, experimental rodents accept diets composed of energetic C-F ranging from 50:30 to 70:10 to provide a constant energy ratio of 20% P [39]. In rodents, AIN93G (C:F:P = 64:16:20) during rapid growth, pregnancy, and lactation and AIN93M (C:F:P = 76:9:15) during maintenance were often used for standard diets [28]. Keeping this P energy ratio over 15% is critical for normal growth of adolescent animals [13, 23, 29]. But effects of an altered C-F on metabolic parameters differ depending on dietary fat species such as soybean and corn oils of plant origin, and beef tallow and lard of animal origin. It was shown that a high-fat diet (HFD, C:F:P = 30:40:20) made of lard was more deleterious to insulin resistance and hepatic steatosis than an HFD made of soybean oil in comparison with a low-fat diet (LFD, C:F:P = 14:64:22) [45, 50]. Deol et al. reported that an HFD (C:F:P = 43:40:16) containing soybean oil and hydrogenated coconut oil at 1:1 ratio was more obesogenic than an HFD mainly containing hydrogenated coconut oil [10]. These differences were considered to be caused by the lipid composition of the dietary fat [1, 8, 12, 17, 32, 34]. Polyunsaturated FAs (PUFAs) are the main contributors to the physiological activity of dietary fat; soybean oil contains 15% saturated FAs and 55% PUFAs, while lard contains 40% saturated FAs and 10% PUFAs. Duivenvoorde et al. showed that an HFD with predominantly saturated FAs increased ectopic fat storage, liver damage, and adipocyte size as compared to an HFD with predominantly PUFAs and reduced response flexibility to fast re-feeding and oxygen restriction [11]. Especially, eicosapentaenoic (EPA) and docosahexaenoic acid (DHA) were reported to reduce insulin resistance and hepatic steatosis [26, 31]. Though small in percentage, sterols are critical factors for animal lipid homeostasis; the soybean oil used in our study contained 0.0024% cholesterol and 0.33% phytosterols, while the lard contained 0.086% cholesterol and no phytosterols. Specifically, phytosterols have been shown to exert beneficial effects on lipid homeostasis under metabolically stressed conditions such as an HFD containing predominantly saturated FAs [5, 6, 16, 27, 36]. However, there are few studies on the transcriptomic effects of a gradual change in the C-F under more moderate conditions, such as the use of diets containing natural plant oils or restricted feeding [30, 37]. In the present study, we conducted an isoenergetic study using a soybean oil-rich diet and found fewer deleterious effects on tissue metabolism but a drastic change in the tissue transcriptome.

Methods
Animals
Three-week-old male Wistar rats (Charles River Laboratories Japan, Kanagawa, Japan) were housed in a temperature- and humidity-controlled room with a 12-h light-dark cycle (light 06:30–18:30, dark 18:30–06:30).

All animal experimental protocols were approved by the Animal Use Committee of the Takasaki University of Health and Welfare.

Experimental procedure
The rats were acclimated to the laboratory environment for a week with chow diets (MF, Oriental yeast, Tokyo, Japan). The animals were divided into three groups so that the average body weights of each group were equal to each other before being given diets with different C-F energy ratios: low (L) 65:15, moderate (M) 60:20, and high (H) 35:45 fat diet groups. The rats were fed diets ad libitum for a week. Then, the L-group was fed ad libitum and the other groups were fed isoenergetically compared with the L-group for 9 weeks. The diets were purchased from Research Diets, Inc. (New Brunswick, NJ, USA). Detailed compositions of each diet are shown in Additional file 1. Diets were removed 17 h before dissection, and the rats were sacrificed to collect the blood, liver, white adipose tissue (WAT), and brown adipose tissue (BAT). Because an obviously decreased dietary intake was observed for two rats belonging to the M- or H-groups (M_7 and H_11 in identical number), the use of these two rats were not included in all analyses to achieve consistency in the isoenergetic study (n = 4–5 in each group). Serum and plasma were extracted using standard methods and separated from whole blood. Small hepatic pieces were immersed into RNAlater (Qiagen, Tokyo, Japan). The rest hepatic pieces, WAT, and BAT were frozen immediately after extirpation using liquid nitrogen. All samples were stored at −80 or −150 °C until analysis.

Measurement of blood biochemical parameters
All blood biochemical parameters, except insulin, listed in Table 1, were analyzed by Nagahama Life Science (Shiga, Japan). Plasma was used to measure glucose, pyruvic acid, total lipids, phospholipids, and total ketone bodies. Other parameters were assayed using the serum. Serum insulin levels were measured by using the rat insulin ELISA kit (Morinaga Institute of Biological Science, Kanagawa, Japan).

Measurement of hepatic lipids
Hepatic lipids were extracted according to a previous method [14]. Briefly, 100 mg of frozen hepatic pieces were homogenized in 2 mL of cooled chloroform-methanol solution (2:1) using a multibead shocker (Yasui Kikai Corporation, Osaka, Japan). Filtered samples were adjusted to 4 mL with chloroform-methanol solution and were washed with 0.8 mL of purified water. Subsequent washes were performed by adding 3.75 mL of chloroform-methanol-water solution (2:1:0.75), and the resulting extracts were dried by evaporation. Extracted lipids were resolved with 1 mL of isopropanol.

Table 1 Blood and liver biochemical analysis

		L-group	M-group	H-group
Blood	Aspartate Aminotransferase (IU / L)	128±16	126±5	154±22
	Alanine Aminotransferase (IU / L)	25±2 [a]	23±4 [a]	52±13 [b]
	Alkaline Phosphatase (IU / L)	232±43	194±52	247±39
	Lactate Dehydrogenase (IU / L)	2136±375	2183±310	1866±228
	Leucine Aminopeptidase (IU / L)	71±4	71±5	79±5
	Choline Esterase (IU / L)	13±2	13±2	14±3
	Total Bilirubin (mg / dL)	0.07±0.02	0.07±0.01	0.07±0.02
	Glucose (mg / dL)	154±17	160±20	160±14
	Pyruvic Acid (mg / dL)	2.37±1.07	1.68±1.50	2.45±1.61
	Total Lipid (mg / dL)	259±45 [a]	193±31 [ab]	172±35 [b]
	Triacylglycerol (mg / dL)	76±19 [a]	58±21 [ab]	28±14 [b]
	Phospholipid (mg / dL)	120±11 [a]	101±7 [b]	93±8 [b]
	Non-esterified Fatty Acid (μEq / L)	435±104	364±121	275±40
	Total Cholesterol (mg / dL)	76±10 [a]	58±4 [b]	65±9 [ab]
	LDL-Cholesterol (mg / dL)	7±1	6±1	5±1
	HDL-Cholesterol (mg / dL)	22±1 [a]	18±2 [b]	19±1 [b]
	Total Ketone Body (μmol / L)	1131±249	923±398	1068±374
	Total Bile Acid (μmol / L)	8±4	5±3	7±5
	Insulin (ng / mL)	0.946±0.547	1.278±0.277	0.843±0.458
Liver	Triacylglycerol (mg / g-tissue)	11.0±2.7 [a]	14.5±1.3 [ab]	18.6±3.1 [b]
	Total Cholesterol (mg / g-tissue)	1.97±0.18 [a]	2.53±0.22 [ab]	2.81±0.56 [b]
	Total Bile Acid (nmol / g-tissue)	13.8±1.7 [a]	17.4±3.4 [a]	25.6±2.3 [b]

[b] shaded cell entries: significant difference detected by Tukey-Kramer comparison ($p < 0.05$)
[a,ab] no significant difference compared with L-group

Hepatic TG, total cholesterol, and total bile acids were measured using Cholestest TG, Cholestest CHO (Sekisui Medical, Tokyo, Japan), and total bile acids assay kits (Diazyme Laboratories, Poway, CA, USA), respectively.

DNA microarray assay

Total RNA was isolated from each immersed hepatic piece, WAT, and BAT by TRIzol reagent (Invitrogen Japan, Tokyo, Japan) and purified using RNeasy mini kits (Qiagen). Anti-sense RNA was synthesized from 100 or 200 ng of purified total RNA, and biotinylated complementary RNA (cRNA) was obtained using a GeneChip 3′IVT Express Kit (Affymetrix, Santa Clara, CA, USA). The cRNA was fragmented and hybridized to a GeneChip Rat Genome 230 2.0 Array (Affymetrix) for 16 h at 45 °C. The arrays were washed and stained with phycoerythrin using the GeneChip Fluidics Station 450 (Affymetrix) and submitted to scanning on an Affymetrix GeneChip Scanner 3000 7G. The Affymetrix GeneChip Command Console Software was used to make CEL files.

DNA microarray data analysis

The CEL files derived from the liver, WAT, and BAT were quantified using robust multi-array average (RMA), factor analysis for robust microarray summarization (quantile normalization, qFARMS), and GCRMA, respectively [19, 22, 46], using the statistical language R (2.7.1) (http://www.r-project.org/) (R [35]), and Bioconductor (2.2) (http://www.bioconductor.org/) [15]. Hierarchical clustering was performed using the pvclust function in R [41]. The rank products (RP) method was used to identify differentially expressed gene probe sets of the quantified data [3]. The probe sets with a false discovery rate (FDR) <0.05 were considered to be differentially expressed between each group (L vs M, M vs H, and L vs H).

The up- and downregulated probe sets picked out at FDR < 0.05 were functionally classified by the Biological Process in Gene Ontology (GO) with the Functional Annotation Tool of the Database for Annotation, Visualization, and Integrated Discovery (DAVID) [9, 21] and Quick GO (http://www.ebi.ac.uk/QuickGO/) [20]. In analysis of the liver, EASE scores, which are modified Fisher's exact test p values were used to extract statistically overrepresented GO terms, and GO terms with p values <0.01 were regarded as significantly enriched. In analysis of WAT and BAT, Benjamini-Hochberg correction p values were used to extract statistically overrepresented GO terms, and GO terms with p values <0.05 were regarded as significantly enriched.

Predicted upstream regulators among liver and adipose tissue transcriptomes were analyzed using Qiagen's Ingenuity Pathway Analysis (IPA, Qiagen, https://www.qiagenbioinformatics.com/products/ingenuity-pathway-analysis/). Activation z-scores were calculated as a measure of upstream regulators analysis. An absolute z-score ≥ 2.5 was judged as significantly activated or inhibited. Common upstream regulators that were predicted to be activated or inhibited in the liver, WAT, and BAT were picked out from a list of all upstream regulators.

Statistical analysis

The results are shown as the means $\pm$ SDs. One-way ANOVA was used to assess the differences among three groups, and Tukey-Kramer comparison was used for pairwise comparisons between multiple groups. Differences at $p \leq 0.05$ were considered to be significant.

Results

Characterization of hepatic genes affected by the altered balance of carbohydrate and fat in the diet

Rats were fed three kinds of diets containing different ratios of C-F in constant total energy (L, M, and H, Additional file 1). In our preliminary experiment of feeding ad libitum, energy intakes (Kcal/g-BW) were almost the same among the three groups from week 2 to week 4. Therefore, rats were pair-fed to keep by isoenergetic conditions, and dietary restriction derived from pair-feeding has not been occurred. During the experimental period of 9 weeks, the rats in each group showed no between-group differences in body weight (Additional file 2a, b). Also, the liver and the WAT weights showed no differences among groups (Additional file 2b). Biochemical analysis of the blood revealed differences in several markers among experimental groups (Table 1). The H-group showed higher levels of alanine aminotransferase (ALT) and lower levels of TG, phospholipid, and HDL cholesterol (HDL-Chl). The M-group showed lower levels of phospholipids, total Chl, and HDL-Chl. In addition, the liver biochemical analysis indicated increases in TG, total Chl, and total bile acid (BA) in the H-group. Serum insulin levels did not change among the three groups (Table 1).

The liver transcriptomes of the H-group were segregated from those in the L- and M-groups in the cluster dendrogram (Fig. 1). To dissect this overall difference in transcriptomes at a single gene level, we analyzed the coincidence of differentially expressed genes (DEGs) estimated from the comparison among L-, M-, and H-groups (Fig. 2a). The DEGs were termed according to the experimental groups and the number of members. For example, LM43 + 83 formed the smallest population among MH131 + 106 and LH206 + 230, and shared about half of the members (15 + 5 and 40 + 1) with LH206 + 230.

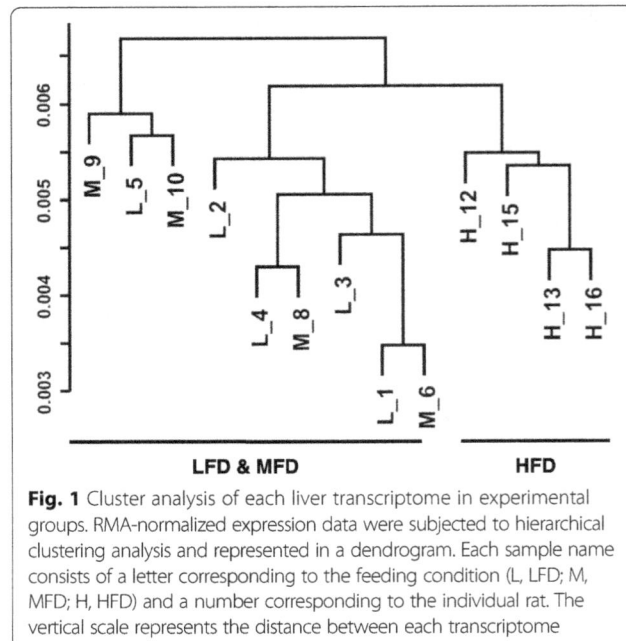

Fig. 1 Cluster analysis of each liver transcriptome in experimental groups. RMA-normalized expression data were subjected to hierarchical clustering analysis and represented in a dendrogram. Each sample name consists of a letter corresponding to the feeding condition (L, LFD; M, MFD; H, HFD) and a number corresponding to the individual rat. The vertical scale represents the distance between each transcriptome

In contrast, about one third of LH206 + 230 members were included by MH131 + 106. This indicates that the transcriptomic change from L to H is more similar to the change from M to H than the change from L to M.

Then, we examined the function of the DEGs specific to the L vs H change (LH186 + 189 probe sets, Fig. 2a shaded area) using GO enrichment analysis [9, 21]. As a result, 53 genes were attributed to the nine GO terms located at the lowest position in the hierarchy (Table 2). Among these GO terms, four terms were related to lipid metabolism (GO0019216, 0006633, 0008203, and 0033189). The enriched genes included 5 + 3 metabolic enzyme genes. *Fads1*, *Msmo1*, *Cyp7b1*, *Idi1*, and *Sqle* were upregulated and *Cyp4a1*, *Elovl5*, and *Scd1* were downregulated in the H-group (Additional file 3, shaded cell entries), suggesting down- or upregulation of PUFA synthesis and upregulation of Chl/BA synthesis. In addition, *Apoa4*, a key regulator of enteric and hepatic TG transportation was downregulated in the H-group. Other members of this category were mostly regulatory protein genes such as *Prkaa1* (protein kinase, AMP-activated, alpha 1) and 2, *Srebf1* (sterol regulatory element-binding transcription factor 1), *Il1a* (interleukin-1 alpha), glucocorticoid receptor, *Lepr* (leptin receptor), and *Dusp1* (MAPK phosphatase); among these, only Srebf1 was upregulated and the others were downregulated in the H-group. There were 6 genes that belong to the GO term, circadian rhythm (GO0007623). Upregulation of *Arntl/Clock*, *Npas2/Clock* paralog, and *Egfr* (epidermal growth factor receptor) as day genes and downregulation of *Prf1*(perforin 1), *Per* (period circadian clock) *1* and *2* as night genes in the H-group was

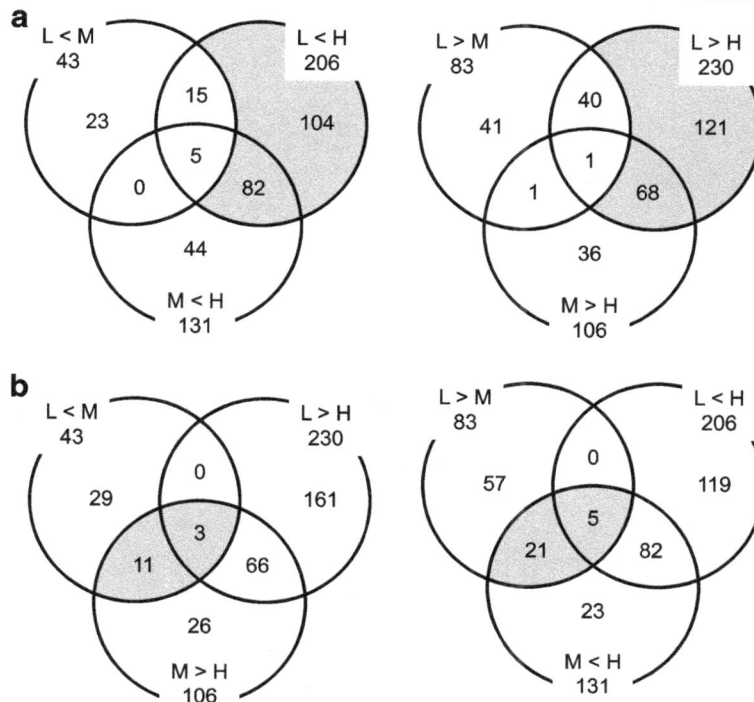

Fig. 2 Number of liver probe sets that were differentially expressed between experimental groups. **a** Coincidence of DEGs among experimental groups. The subsets of DEGs specific to the L vs H change are indicated by *shaded areas*. **b** Oppositely regulated DEGs (*shaded areas*)

consistent with the reversed expression pattern of these genes at the time point of tissue sampling (zeitgeber time 3) [2]. Fourteen genes were identified as those related to RNA polymerase II-dependent transcription (GO0045944 and 0000122); among these, only *Ppargc1b* (*Pgc1b*) was upregulated, and the others were downregulated in the H-group.

Besides the significant enrichment of LH186 + 189 genes to the GO terms related to lipid metabolism, LM43 + 83 genes were hard to analyze in this way

because of the small population. We then dissected these genes with reference to the regulation of M vs H or L vs H DEGs (Fig. 2b). It was revealed that 14 + 26 probe sets were reversely regulated compared with L vs H or M vs H DEGs (Table 3). These sets included 11 metabolic enzyme genes (shaded cell entries): *Sds* (serine dehydratase) for utilization of glycogenic amino acids; *Acot1* (acyl-CoA thioesterase 1) for negative regulation of beta-oxidation; *Acsm2* (acyl-CoA synthetase medium-chain family member 2) for positive regulation of FA

Table 2 Significantly enriched GO terms found in liver LH186 + 189 genes

GO-ID	Term	*p* value	Gene count
	Biological process		
0007623	─── Circadian rhythm	1.82E-03	7
0007568	─── Aging	5.77E-03	10
0009991	─── Response to extracellular stimulus	5.66E-04	17
0031667	└── Response to nutrient levels	2.20E-03	15
0033189	└── Response to vitamin A	4.30E-02	9
0016525	─── Negative regulation of angiogenesis	9.58E-03	4
0006882	─── Cellular zinc ion homeostasis	9.78E-03	3
0019216	─── Regulation of lipid metabolic process	4.72E-03	9
0016053	─── Organic acid biosynthetic process	3.59E-04	12
0046394	└── Carboxylic acid biosynthetic process	3.59E-04	12
0006633	└── Fatty acid biosynthetic process	4.39E-03	7
0006631	└── Fatty acid metabolic process	1.49E-04	14
0008610	─── Lipid biosynthetic process	9.86E-03	13
0008203	─── Cholesterol metabolic process	7.85E-04	8
0008202	─── Steroid metabolic process	7.11E-04	12
0016125	└── Sterol metabolic process	2.15E-04	9
0051254	└── Positive regulation of RNA metabolic process	7.84E-03	18
0045893	└── Positive regulation of transcription, DNA-dependent	7.11E-03	18
0045944	└── Positive regulation of transcription from RNA polymerase II promoter	7.29E-03	16

Shaded cell entries indicate GO terms at the lowest hierarchy

Table 3 The list of the reversely regulated liver LM43 + 83 genes

Expression pattern		Probe ID	Gene symbol	Description
		1369268_at	Atf3	activating transcription factor 3
	L > H	1370988_at	Cyp2b1	cytochrome P450, family 2, subfamily b, polypeptide 1
		1393510_at	Golsyn	Golgi-localized protein
		1382451_at	Hebp2	heme binding protein 2
		1382284_at	LOC685440, Nek3	similar to NIMA (never in mitosis gene a)-related expressed kinase 5, NIMA (never in mitosis gene a)-related kinase 3
		1397745_at	Mib1	mindbomb homolog 1
14 probe sets		1369202_at	Mx2	myxovirus (influenza virus) resistance 2
L < M and M > H	L > H	1389990_at	RGD15637	similar to Gene model 609
		1383956_at	RGD1565709	similar to ovostatin-2
		1397859_x_at	RT1-A3	RT1 class I, locus A3
	L > H	1369864_a_at	Sds	serine dehydratase
		1373740_at	---	---
		1382517_at	---	---
		1392860_at	---	---
	L < H	1398250_at	Acot1	acyl-CoA thioesterase 1
		1370436_at	Acsm2	acyl-CoA synthetase medium-chain family member 2
	L < H	1374610_at	Agpat9	1-acylglycerol-3-phosphate O-acyltransferase 9.
		1368121_at	Akr7a3	aldo-keto reductase family 7, member A3 (aflatoxin aldehyde reductase)
		1383242_a_at	Cebpa	CCAAT/enhancer binding protein (C/EBP), alpha
		1389625_at	Chchd4	coiled-coil-helix-coiled-coil-helix domain containing 4
		1384392_at	Cyp26b1	cytochrome P450, family 26, subfamily b, polypeptide 1
		1368607_at	Cyp4a8	cytochrome P450, family 4, subfamily a, polypeptide 8
		1388342_at	Etv3	Ets variant 3
		1387670_at	Gpd2	glycerol-3-phosphate dehydrogenase 2, mitochondrial
26 probe sets	L < H	1371942_at	Gstt3	glutathione S-transferase, theta 3
L > M and M < H		1370912_at, 1368247_at	Hspa1a, Hspa1b	heat shock 70kD protein 1A, heat shock 70kD protein 1B (mapped)
		1389251_at	Nudt7	nudix (nucleoside diphosphate linked moiety X)-type motif 7
		1397164_at	Pola2	polymerase (DNA directed), alpha 2
		1392854_at	RGD1564560	Similar to RCK
		1373777_at	Rgs16	regulator of G-protein signaling 16
	L < H	1371143_at	Serpina7	serine (or cysteine) peptidase inhibitor, clade A (alpha-1 antiproteinase, antitrypsin), member 7
	L < H	1389142_at	Sqrdl	sulfide quinone reductase-like (yeast)
		1393160_at	Tbx3	T-box 3
		1374924_at	Upf3b	UPF3 regulator of nonsense transcripts homolog B (yeast) (predicted)
		1380306_at, 1381553_at, 1392613_at	Zbtb16	zinc finger and BTB domain containing 16
		1393192_at	---	---
		1397225_at	---	---

Shaded cell entries: metabolic enzyme genes related to lipid

synthesis; *Agpat9* (1-acylglycerol-3-phosphate *O*-acyltransferase 9) for TG synthesis; *Gpd2* (glycerol-3-phosphate dehydrogenase 2, mitochondrial) for gluconeogenesis from glycerol; and *Cyp2b1*, *Akr7a3*, *Cyp26b1*, *Cyp4a8*, *Gstt3*, and *Sqrdl* for detoxication. The other genes were involved in more diversified functions. This result indicates that the M-group is situated in a nutritional condition that controls the regulatory switching of these metabolic genes.

Response of the adipose tissue transcriptomes to the increased ratio of fat to carbohydrate

Because the hepatic transcriptome response as described above suggested some change in energetic interaction with other tissues such as adipose tissues, we analyzed the transcriptomes of WAT and BAT in each experimental condition (Table 4). The L vs H DEGs of these tissues were subjected to GO term enrichment analysis as in the case of the liver. WAT LH235 + 336 DEGs showed marked enrichment to the terms related to lipid metabolism (42 genes to GO0008610, 0006635, and 0045444)

(Table 5), and most of the metabolic enzyme genes were downregulated in the H-group (Additional file 4). It is possible that both lipid synthesis and beta-oxidation were suppressed in this condition. Other characteristics of WAT LH235 + 336 DEGs were the high frequency of regulatory protein genes in the GO terms related to glucose metabolism (GO006006) (*Pik3r1*, *Lep*, *Il6st*, *Igf2*, *Atf3*, *Crem*, *Pdk1*, and *Ppp1r1a*, totally 8 genes/another 13 genes), and insulin signaling (GO0032868) (*Lyn*, *Foxo1*, *Acvr1c*, *Pde3b*, and *Shc1*, totally 5 genes/another 9 genes). Most of these genes were downregulated in the H-group except *Lep* encoding satiety hormone leptin,

Table 4 Differentially expressed genes in the liver and in the adipose tissues

Tissue	L < H	L > H
Liver	206	230
WAT	235	336
BAT	212	405

Table 5 Significantly enriched GO terms found in WAT LH235 + 336 genes

GO-ID	Term	p value	Count
	Biological process		
0008610	Lipid biosynthetic process	6.17E-06	25
0045444	Fat cell differentiation	1.96E-04	10
0001503	Ossification	2.57E-04	13
0060348	Bone development	4.80E-05	15
0005996	Monosaccharide metabolic process	4.41E-06	21
0019318	Hexose metabolic process	8.08E-06	19
0006006	Glucose metabolic process	1.18E-05	17
0009991	Response to extracellular stimulus	1.43E-06	28
0031667	Response to nutrient levels	1.20E-05	25
0007584	Response to nutrient	2.84E-04	18
0009719	Response to endogenous stimulus	1.89E-08	47
0009725	Response to hormone	1.25E-07	42
0043434	Response to peptide hormone	1.59E-04	20
0032868	Response to insulin	4.31E-04	14
0010033	Response to organic substance	4.50E-09	65
0016042	Lipid catabolic process	3.15E-04	14
0044242	Cellular lipid catabolic process	1.33E-04	11
0009062	Fatty acid catabolic process	2.42E-05	9
0006635	Fatty acid beta-oxidation	2.70E-05	8
0046395	Carboxylic acid catabolic process	1.17E-05	14
0016054	Organic acid catabolic process	1.17E-05	14
0006631	Fatty acid metabolic process	3.43E-08	24
0019395	Fatty acid oxidation	3.85E-04	8
0034440	Lipid oxidation	3.85E-04	8
0055114	Oxidation-reduction process	1.62E-04	34

Shaded cell entries indicate GO terms at the lowest hierarchy

Il6st encoding IL-6 inflammatory signal transducer, and *Lyn* encoding tyrosine kinase. There were 12 genes attributed to the GO terms related to bone formation (GO0060348 and GO0001503).

BAT LH212 + 405 DEGs exhibited a regulatory pattern similar to that of WAT DEGs (Table 6), where all of the enzyme genes related to lipid metabolism were downregulated in the H-group (24 genes in GO0006631 and 0006695, shaded cell entries in Additional file 5). The other 23 enzyme genes were in the oxidation-reduction category (GO0055114) of which 15 genes were downregulated in the H-group. BAT DEGs also contained another 46 genes classified as organic substance responsive components (GO0010033) that encode regulatory proteins, transcription factors (SREBF2, glucagon receptor), and transporters. The remainder was 12 genes for muscle contraction (GO0006936) such as *actin, myosin,* and *troponin* genes.

Search for upstream regulators common among the liver and adipose tissues

Given the results of GO analysis that the H-diet generally induced the upregulation of FA unsaturation and Chl synthesis in the liver (Additional file 3) and the downregulation of FA synthesis in the adipose tissues

(Additional files 4 and 5), we assessed whether these gene regulations were caused by some biological signals common among these tissues using the Ingenuity Pathway Analysis (IPA). Table 7 lists the IPA upstream regulators that were predicted to be activated or repressed (absolute z-score > 2.5) from the input of L vs H DEGs (Table 4). Relatively high z-scores were observed with LY294002 (PI3 kinase inhibitor) in WAT (3.07) and BAT (2.73) [44], suggesting the inhibition of insulin signaling in the H-group. This is consistent with the result that two well-known components of insulin downstream signaling (SREBF1 for FA synthesis and SREBF2 for Chl synthesis) were inactivated (negative z-scores) both in WAT (−3.68 and −4.18) and BAT (−3.52 and −4.17). It is also notable that INSIG (insulin-induced gene protein) 1 and 2, which play roles as repressors of SREBF [48, 49], seemed to be activated in BAT (3.61 and 2.93). In addition, pirinixic acid, a specific agonist of PPAR (peroxisome proliferator-activated receptor) alpha, was detected as a WAT/BAT common upstream regulator. The negative z-scores for pirinixic acid (−3.07 in WAT and −2.99 in BAT) suggest the repression of this process. The liver transcriptome showed relatively low absolute z-scores except for peptidylprolyl isomerase F (PPIF or cyclophilin D) (z-score = 2.83).

Table 6 Significantly enriched GO terms found in BAT LH212 + 405 genes

GO-ID	Term	*p* value	Count
	Biological process		
0055114	Oxidation-reduction process	4.18E-06	41
0010033	Response to organic substance	6.50E-06	61
0006631	Fatty acid metabolic process	4.40E-05	20
0003012	Muscle system process	1.43E-05	15
0006936	Muscle contraction	8.02E-05	13
0008610	Lipid biosynthetic process	2.59E-11	36
0006694	Steroid biosynthetic process	6.54E-05	12
0016126	Sterol biosynthetic procell	4.38E-08	11
0006695	Cholesterol biosynthetic process	7.52E-09	11
0008203	Cholesterol metabolic process	3.75E-08	16
0016125	Sterol metabolic process	1.01E-07	16
0008202	Steroid metabolic process	7.84E-06	20

Shaded cell entries indicate GO terms at the lowest hierarchy

Discussion

We have analyzed the transcriptomic responses of the liver and adipose tissues to an increased ratio of F to C under isoenergetic conditions. In this study, three types of diets were adjusted with soybean oil to construct the C-F ratios, since it is the major oil in human diets. Soybean oil has some beneficial effects [45, 50], and hepatic transcriptomes can be influenced by oil and fat profiles [18]. Although the fatty acid profile was different among three diets because of identical quantities of lard rich in saturated FA, it is crucial that the main energy resource was changed from C to F. The rats showed no between-group differences in body weight or in relative tissue weight (Additional file 2b); however, higher serum ALT levels were observed in the H-group compared with the L- and M-groups (Table 1). Because no significant fluctuations were observed among the other damage markers, the liver damage in the H-group seems to be limited in extent. This is in accordance with the fact that no significant enrichment of DEGs detected in GO terms related to liver damage, such as inflammation or fibrosis [25].

Interestingly, H-group rats exhibited a significant biochemical characteristic relevant to lipid homeostasis: lower TG and HDL-Chl levels in the sera and higher TG, total Chl, and total BA content in the liver than in

Table 7 Comparison of IPA upstream regulators among the liver and the adipose tissue transcriptomes

	Upstream Regulator	Activation z-score		
Abbreviation	Description	Liver	WAT	BAT
LY294002	PI3 kinase inhibitor	-0.756	3.07	2.73
SREBF1	Sterol regulatory element-binding transcription factor 1	1.27	-3.68	-4.18
SREBF2	Sterol regulatory element-binding transcription factor 2	1.12	-3.52	-4.17
INSIG1	Insulin induced gene 1	-2.15	1.61	3.61
INSIG2	insulin induced gene 2	-	2.39	2.93
PPARG	peroxisome proliferator-activated receptor (PPAR) gamma	-1.01	-2.73	-2.15
gemfibrozil	PPAR alpha activator	-1.57	-2.21	-2.80
pirinixic acid	PPAR alpha activator	-1.79	-3.07	-2.99
CREB1	cAMP responsive element binding protein 1	0.751	-3.17	-2.14
IL4	interleukin 4	0.789	-2.64	-2.41
MLXIPL	MLX interacting protein-like, Carbohydrate-responsive element-binding protein	-	-2.41	-2.61
CD38	CD38 molecule	-0.269	-2.28	-3.41
paclitaxel	taxol	1.19	-2.19	-2.66
PPIF	peptidylprolyl isomerase F, cyclophilin D	2.83	0.200	2.00

The absolute Z-scores of larger than 2.5 are represented by the shaded cell entries. -; no significant Z-score
Upstream Regulators are classified according to their relevance to each other

the L-group (Table 1). Our transcriptomic analysis suggested the upregulation of Chl/BA synthesis in the liver (Table 2 and Additional file 3), the downregulation of lipid synthesis and beta-oxidation in WAT (Table 5 and Additional file 4), and the downregulation of Chl biosynthesis in BAT (Table 6 and Additional file 5). The former liver transcriptomic response may facilitate acetyl-CoA consumption via Chl synthesis and BA secretion (Fig. 3) [43]. Moreover, the downregulation of *Scd1* and *Elovl5* indicates suppression of de novo synthesis and elongation of monounsaturated FAs, while the upregulation of *Fads1* implies facilitation of C20 PUFAs (precursors of bioactive eicosanoids) synthesis from 18:2 n-6 linoleic acid, rich in H-diet, with the help of *Fads2* [24]. These results suggest that the hepatic transcriptome was regulated not only by the C-F ratios but also by the fatty acid profiles of the diets. The downregulation of *Apoa4* may inhibit export of TG from the liver leading to the decrease in serum TG level and the increase in liver TG content (Fig. 3) [42]. The latter responses of adipose tissues may suppress FA release to the sera.

A comparison of L vs M transcriptomes in liver showed 126 (43 + 83) genes as differentially expressed (Fig. 2); this was less than the number of differentially expressed genes as compared to M vs H (131 + 106 genes) and L vs H (206 + 230 genes). This means that the transcriptome of the L-group was more closely related to that of the M-group than H-group (Fig. 1). Then, we analyzed LM43 + 83 DEGs to clarify C-F ratio dependency of hepatic transcriptome and we found 32 reversely regulated genes (i.e., upregulated in M-condition and downregulated in H-condition, or vice versa) (listed in Table 3). These reversely regulated liver DEGs can exert potential effects on lipid homeostasis; the upregulation of *Acot1*, *Acsm2*, and *Agpat9* in the H-group may increase TG accumulation in the liver. Also, the role of LM43 + 83 DEGs in macronutrient conversion (e.g., amino acid to C and F to C) should be emphasized because our study was conducted under the isoenergetic conditions. In this context, the downregulation of *Sds* in the H-group may reduce utilization of amino acids for gluconeogenesis, and the upregulation of *Gpd2* in the H-group may increase gluconeogenesis from glycerol produced by TG hydrolysis. Because the expression pattern of these genes was biphasic, the regulation of these metabolisms may have a balancing point close to the M-condition. As we used outbred Wistar rats, transcriptomic difference among the L-group and the M-group could be influenced by genetic or epigenetic differences between animals. Further indirect calorimetric studies with altered C-F ratios or animal strains are needed to clarify this metabolic regulation switching.

A question arising is whether these transcriptomic regulations are governed by any cellular signals common among these tissues. We computationally detected the downregulation of both insulin-PI3K-SREBF and PPAR alpha signals in the adipose tissues but not in the liver (Table 7). This suggests that both the anabolic signal of insulin (i.e., FA synthesis) and the catabolic signal of PPAR alpha (i.e., FA oxidation) are inhibited in adipose tissues. Because the rats in the H-group showed a growth rate (Additional file 2b) and serum insulin levels almost the same as in the L- and M-groups (Table 1), the suppression of insulin signals may be intrinsic to

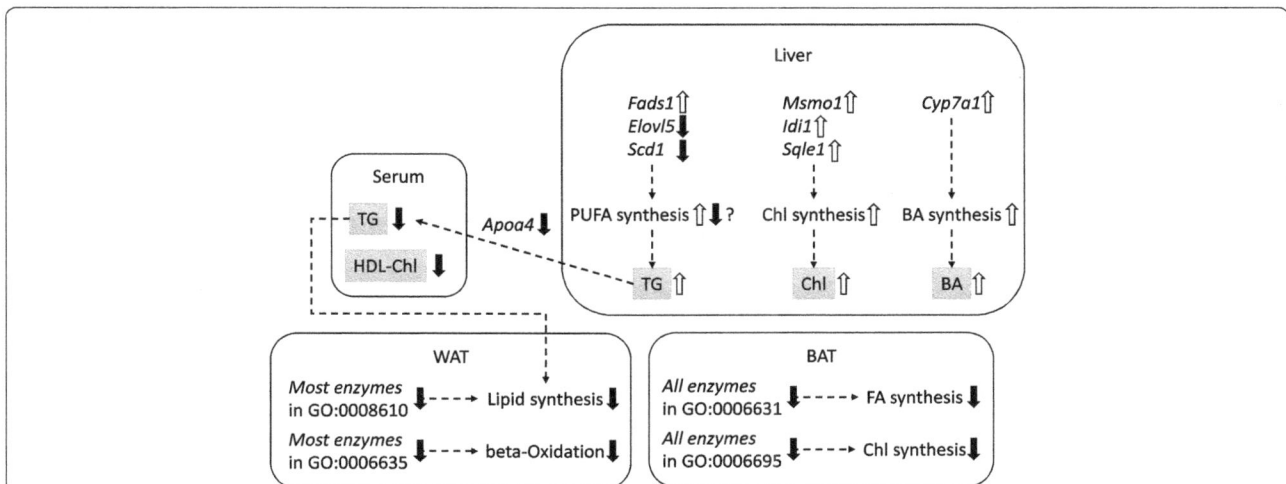

Fig. 3 Transcriptomic and metabolic changes in H-condition compared to L-condition. *Shaded molecules* indicate the metabolites, and others indicate the transcripts specific to L vs H change (liver LH186 + 189, WAT LH235 + 336, and BAT LH212 + 405). *Upward arrows* indicate the H-up genes (*italics*) or predicted pathways compared to L-condition, and vice versa. *TG* triacylglycerol, *Chl* cholesterol, *BA* bile acid, *FA* fatty acid, *PUFA* polyunsaturated fatty acid

adipose tissues [33, 40, 47]. In the case of PPAR alpha signal, the low level of serum TG in the H-group might affect the concentration of FA in adipose tissues.

Conclusions

To investigate the effects of altered dietary C-F ratio, we compared with L vs M and L vs H DEGs. We found that hepatic genes for gluconeogenesis and lipid metabolism were reversely regulated, indicating that a turning point for gene expression switching from C to F as energy source may exist in the M-condition (C:F = 60:20) or a C-F ratio around M.

L vs H analyses revealed that high-fat diet upregulated Chl/BA synthesis in the liver and downregulated lipid synthesis in WAT and BAT. Also, our computational search for upstream regulators in these tissues suggested that insulin and PPAR alpha signals were downregulated both in WAT and BAT in the H-group.

In conclusion, the liver and adipose tissues differentially adapts to altered C-F by changing their gene expressions and not by merely responding to endocrine signals.

Additional files

Additional file 1: Composition of diets.

Additional file 2: Physical parameters of the animals a, Energy intake during the experimental period. The intakes of the rats in the M- and H-groups were restricted to the average intake of the rats in the L-group. Data for the M- and H-groups after day 0 were omitted. b, Body and tissue weights. The *inset* represents the relative tissue weights (percent to body weight) at the time of sacrifice (week 9). Values are represented as means ± SD (n = 4–5).

Additional file 3: The list of liver LH186 + 189 genes that belongs to the GO terms located at the lowest level of hierarchy.

Additional file 4: The list of WAT LH235 + 336 genes that belong to the GO terms located at the lowest level of hierarchy.

Additional file 5: The list of BAT LH212 + 405 genes that belong to the GO terms located at the lowest level of hierarchy.

Abbreviations

Experimental conditions
C: Carbohydrate; F: Fat; P: Protein, LFD or L: Low-fat diet; MFD or M: Moderate-fat diet; HFD or H: High-fat diet
Methods and biochemical terms
ALT: Alanine aminotransferase; BA: Bile acid; BAT: Brown adipose tissues; Chl: Cholesterol; DEGs: Differentially expressed genes; FA: Fatty acid; FDR: False discovery rate; GO: Gene ontology; HDL: High-density lipoprotein; INSIG: Insulin-induced gene protein; IPA: Ingenuity Pathway Analysis; PPAR: Peroxisome proliferator-activated receptor; PPIF: Peptidylprolyl isomerase F (cyclophilin D); PUFA: Polyunsaturated fatty acid; SREBF: Sterol regulatory element-binding transcription factor; TG: Triacylglycerol; WAT: White adipose tissues

Genes
Acot1: Acyl-CoA thioesterase 1; *Acsm2*: Acyl-CoA synthetase medium-chain family member 2; *Acvr1c*: Activin A receptor, type IC; *Agpat9*: 1-Acylglycerol-3-phosphate O-acyltransferase 9; *Akr7a3*: Aldo-keto reductase family 7, member A3 (aflatoxin aldehyde reductase); *Apoa4*: Apolipoprotein A-IV; *Arntl/Clock*: Aryl hydrocarbon receptor nuclear translocator-like; *Atf3*: Activating transcription factor 3; *Crem*: cAMP responsive element modulator; *Cyp*: Cytochrome P450; *Dusp1*: Dual specificity phosphatase 1; *Egfr*: Epidermal

growth factor receptor; *Elovl5*: ELOVL fatty acid elongase 5; *Fads1*: Fatty acid desaturase 1; *Foxo1*: Forkhead box O1A; *Gpd2*: Glycerol-3-phosphate dehydrogenase 2, mitochondrial; *Gstt3*: Glutathione S-transferase, theta 3; *Idi1*: Isopentenyl-diphosphate delta isomerase 1; *Igf2*: Insulin-like growth factor 2; *Il1a*: Interleukin 1 alpha; *Il6st*: Interleukin 6 signal transducer; *Lep*: Leptin; *Lepr*: Leptin receptor; *Lyn*: LYN proto-oncogene, Src family tyrosine kinase; *Msmo1*: Methylsterol monooxygenase 1; *Npas2*: Neuronal PAS domain protein 2; *Pde3b*: Phosphodiesterase 3B, cGMP-inhibited; *Pdk1*: Pyruvate dehydrogenase kinase, isozyme 1; *Per*: Period circadian clock; *Pik3r1*: Phosphoinositide-3-kinase; *Ppargc1b/Pgc1b*: Peroxisome proliferator-activated receptor gamma coactivator 1 beta; *Ppp1r1a*: Protein phosphatase 1, regulatory (inhibitor) subunit 1A; *Prf1*: Perforin 1 (pore-forming protein); *Prkaa*: Protein kinase, AMP-activated, alpha; *Scd1*: Stearoyl-coenzyme A desaturase 1; *Sds*: Serine dehydratase; *Shc1*: SHC (Src homology 2 domain containing) transforming protein 1; *Srebf1*: Sterol regulatory element-binding transcription factor 1; *Sqle*: Squalene epoxidase; *Sqrdl*: Sulfide quinone reductase-like

Acknowledgements
The authors thank the Cross-ministerial Strategic Innovation Promotion Program (SIP) (Grant No. 14532924) in Japan for their support.

Funding
This research was supported by the Cross-ministerial Strategic Innovation Promotion Program (SIP) (Grant No. 14532924) in Japan. The funders had no role in the study design, data collection and analysis, decision to publish, or preparation of the manuscript.

Authors' contributions
The experimental design was constructed and supervised by MT and TN. The animal experiments and biochemical analysis were performed by MS, KK, and YS. MT, YS, and TA worked on the DNA microarray assay. The manuscript was drafted and written by AY, TN, and MT. All authors read and approved the final manuscript.

Competing interests
The authors declare that they have no conflict of interests.

Author details
[1]Nissin Global Innovation Center, Nissin Foods Holdings, 2100 Tobukimachi, Hachioji-shi, Tokyo 192-0001, Japan. [2]Project on Health and Anti-Aging, Kanagawa Academy of Science and Technology, Life Science and Environment Research Center (LiSE) 4F C-4, 3-25-13 Tonomachi, Kawasaki-ku, Kawasaki, Kanagawa 210-0821, Japan. [3]Department of Health and Nutrition, Takasaki University of Health and Welfare, 37-1 Nakaorui-machi, Takasaki, Gunma 370-0033, Japan. [4]Department of Applied Biological Chemistry, Graduate School of Agricultural and Life Sciences, The University of Tokyo, 1-1-1 Yayoi, Bunkyo-ku, Tokyo 113-8657, Japan.

References
1. Aguila MB, Pinheiro Ada R, Parente LB, Mandarim-de-Lacerda CA. Dietary effect of different high-fat diet on rat liver stereology. Liver Int. 2003;23:363–70.
2. Bell-Pedersen D, Cassone VM, Earnest DJ, Golden SS, Hardin PE, Thomas TL, Zoran MJ. Circadian rhythms from multiple oscillators: lessons from diverse organisms. Nat Rev Genet. 2005;6:544–56. doi:10.1038/nrg1633.
3. Breitling R, Armengaud P, Amtmann A, Herzyk P. Rank products: a simple, yet powerful, new method to detect differentially regulated genes in replicated microarray experiments. FEBS Lett. 2004;573:83–92. doi:10.1016/j.febslet.2004.07.055.
4. Cahill Jr GF. Starvation in man. Clin Endocrinol Metab. 1976;5:397–415.
5. Carter BA, Taylor OA, Prendergast DR, Zimmerman TL, Von Furstenberg R, Moore DD, Karpen SJ. Stigmasterol, a soy lipid-derived phytosterol, is an antagonist of the bile acid nuclear receptor. FXR Pediatr Res. 2007;62:301–6. doi:10.1203/PDR.0b013e3181256492.
6. Chai JW, Lim SL, Kanthimathi MS, Kuppusamy UR. Gene regulation in beta-sitosterol-mediated stimulation of adipogenesis, glucose uptake, and lipid mobilization in rat primary adipocytes. Genes Nutr. 2011;6:181–8. doi:10.1007/s12263-010-0196-4.
7. Coyle EF. Substrate utilization during exercise in active people. Am J Clin Nutr. 1995;61:968s–79s.

8. Crescenzo R, Bianco F, Mazzoli A, et al. Fat quality influences the obesogenic effect of high fat diets. Nutrients. 2015;7:9475–91. doi:10.3390/nu7115480.

9. Dennis Jr G, Sherman BT, Hosack DA, Yang J, Gao W, Lane HC, Lempicki RA. DAVID: Database for Annotation, Visualization, and Integrated Discovery. Genome Biol. 2003;4:3.

10. Deol P, Evans JR, Dhahbi J, Chellappa K, Han DS, Spindler S, Sladek FM. Soybean oil is more obesogenic and diabetogenic than coconut oil and fructose in mouse: potential role for the liver. PLoS One. 2015;10:e0132672. doi:10.1371/journal.pone.0132672.

11. Duivenvoorde LP, van Schothorst EM, Swarts HM, Kuda O, Steenbergh E, Termeulen S, Kopecky J, Keijer J. A difference in fatty acid composition of isocaloric high-fat diets alters metabolic flexibility in male C57BL/6JOlaHsd Mice. PLoS One. 2015;10:e0128515. doi:10.1371/journal.pone.0128515.

12. Enns JE, Hanke D, Park A, Zahradka P, Taylor CG. Diets high in monounsaturated and polyunsaturated fatty acids decrease fatty acid synthase protein levels in adipose tissue but do not alter other markers of adipose function and inflammation in diet-induced obese rats. Prostaglandins Leukot Essent Fatty Acids. 2014;90:77–84. doi:10.1016/j.plefa.2013.12.002.

13. Even PC, Bertin E, Gangnerau MN, Roseau S, Tome D, Portha B. Energy restriction with protein restriction increases basal metabolism and meal-induced thermogenesis in rats. Am J Physiol Regul Integr Comp Physiol. 2003;284:R751–759. doi:10.1152/ajpregu.00268.2002.

14. Folch J, Lees M, Sloane Stanley GH. A simple method for the isolation and purification of total lipides from animal tissues. J Biol Chem. 1957;226:497–509.

15. Gentleman RC, Carey VJ, Bates DM, et al. Bioconductor: open software development for computational biology and bioinformatics. Genome Biol. 2004;5:R80. doi:10.1186/gb-2004-5-10-r80.

16. Grattan Jr BJ. Plant sterols as anticancer nutrients: evidence for their role in breast cancer. Nutrients. 2013;5:359–87. doi:10.3390/nu5020359.

17. Hanke D, Zahradka P, Mohankumar SK, Clark JL, Taylor CG. A diet high in alpha-linolenic acid and monounsaturated fatty acids attenuates hepatic steatosis and alters hepatic phospholipid fatty acid profile in diet-induced obese rats. Prostaglandins Leukot Essent Fatty Acids. 2013;89:391–401. doi:10.1016/j.plefa.2013.09.009.

18. Hashimoto Y, Yamada K, Tsushima H, et al. Three dissimilar high fat diets differentially regulate lipid and glucose metabolism in obesity-resistant Slc: Wistar/ST rats. Lipids. 2013;48:803–15. doi:10.1007/s11745-013-3805-3.

19. Hochreiter S, Clevert DA, Obermayer K. A new summarization method for Affymetrix probe level data. Bioinformatics. 2006;22:943–9. doi:10.1093/bioinformatics/btl033.

20. Hosack DA, Dennis Jr G, Sherman BT, Lane HC, Lempicki RA. Identifying biological themes within lists of genes with EASE. Genome Biol. 2003;4:R70. doi:10.1186/gb-2003-4-10-r70.

21. Huang da W, Sherman BT, Zheng X, Yang J, Imamichi T, Stephens R, Lempicki RA. Extracting biological meaning from large gene lists with DAVID. Curr Protoc Bioinformatics. 2009;Chapter 13(Unit 13):11. doi:10.1002/0471250953.bi1311s27.

22. Irizarry RA, Hobbs B, Collin F, Beazer-Barclay YD, Antonellis KJ, Scherf U, Speed TP. Exploration, normalization, and summaries of high density oligonucleotide array probe level data. Biostatistics. 2003;4:249–64. doi:10.1093/biostatistics/4.2.249.

23. Itoh H, Kaneko M, Ohshima S, Shumiya S, Sakaguchi E. Effect of low protein and low energy diet on physiological status and digestibility of F344 rats. Exp Anim. 2002;51:485–91.

24. Jump DB. Fatty acid regulation of hepatic lipid metabolism. Curr Opin Clin Nutr Metab Care. 2011;14:115–20. doi:10.1097/MCO.0b013e328342991c.

25. Kamei A, Watanabe Y, Shinozaki F, Yasuoka A, Kondo T, Ishijima T, Toyoda T, Arai S, Abe K. Administration of a maple syrup extract to mitigate their hepatic inflammation induced by a high-fat diet: a transcriptome analysis. Biosci Biotechnol Biochem. 2015;79:1893–7. doi:10.1080/09168451.2015.1042833.

26. Kuda O, Jelenik T, Jilkova Z, et al. n-3 fatty acids and rosiglitazone improve insulin sensitivity through additive stimulatory effects on muscle glycogen synthesis in mice fed a high-fat diet. Diabetologia. 2009;52:941–51. doi:10.1007/s00125-009-1305-z.

27. Laos S, Caimari A, Crescenti A, Lakkis J, Puiggros F, Arola L, del Bas JM. Long-term intake of soyabean phytosterols lowers serum TAG and NEFA concentrations, increases bile acid synthesis and protects against fatty liver development in dyslipidaemic hamsters. Br J Nutr. 2014;112:663–73. doi:10.1017/s0007114514001342.

28. Lien EL, Boyle FG, Wrenn JM, Perry RW, Thompson CA, Borzelleca JF. Comparison of AIN-76A and AIN-93G diets: a 13-week study in rats. Food Chem Toxicol. 2001;39:385–92.

29. Minana-Solis Mdel C, Escobar C. Post-weaning protein malnutrition in the rat produces short and long term metabolic impairment, in contrast to earlier and later periods. Int J Biol Sci. 2008;4:422–32.

30. Nyima T, Müller M, Hooiveld GJ, Morine MJ, Scotti M. Nonlinear transcriptomic response to dietary fat intake in the small intestine of C57BL/6J mice. BMC Genomics. 2016;17:106. doi:10.1186/s12864-016-2424-9.

31. Pavlisova J, Bardova K, Stankova B, Tvrzicka E, Kopecky J, Rossmeisl M. Corn oil versus lard: metabolic effects of omega-3 fatty acids in mice fed obesogenic diets with different fatty acid composition. Biochimie. 2016;124:150–62. doi:10.1016/j.biochi.2015.07.001.

32. Pimentel GD, Dornellas AP, Rosa JC, et al. High-fat diets rich in soy or fish oil distinctly alter hypothalamic insulin signaling in rats. J Nutr Biochem. 2012;23:822–8. doi:10.1016/j.jnutbio.2011.04.006.

33. Poletto AC, Anhê GF, Eichler P, et al. Soybean and sunflower oil-induced insulin resistance correlates with impaired GLUT4 protein expression and translocation specifically in white adipose tissue. Cell Biochem Funct. 2010; 28:114–21. doi:10.1002/cbf.1628.

34. Portillo MP, Chavarri M, Duran D, Rodriguez VM, Macarulla MT. Differential effects of diets that provide different lipid sources on hepatic lipogenic activities in rats under ad libitum or restricted feeding. Nutrition. 2001;17:467–73.

35. R Development Core Team. R: a language and environment for statistical computing. Vienna: R Foundation for Statistical Computing; 2006.

36. Racette SB, Spearie CA, Phillips KM, Lin X, Ma L, Ostlund Jr RE. Phytosterol-deficient and high-phytosterol diets developed for controlled feeding studies. J Am Diet Assoc. 2009;109:2043–51. doi:10.1016/j.jada.2009.09.009.

37. Renaud HJ, Cui JY, Lu H, Klaassen CD. Effect of diet on expression of genes involved in lipid metabolism, oxidative stress, and inflammation in mouse liver-insights into mechanisms of hepatic steatosis. PLoS One. 2014;9:e88584. doi:10.1371/journal.pone.0088584.

38. Romijn JA, Coyle EF, Sidossis LS, Gastaldelli A, Horowitz JF, Endert E, Wolfe RR. Regulation of endogenous fat and carbohydrate metabolism in relation to exercise intensity and duration. Am J Physiol. 1993;265:E380–391.

39. Shahkhalili Y, Mace K, Moulin J, Zbinden I, Acheson KJ. The fat:carbohydrate energy ratio of the weaning diet programs later susceptibility to obesity in male sprague dawley rats. J Nutr. 2011;141:81–6. doi:10.3945/jn.110.126557.

40. Shankar K, Harrell A, Kang P, Singhal R, Ronis MJ, Badger TM. Carbohydrate-responsive gene expression in the adipose tissue of rats. Endocrinology. 2010;151:153–64. doi:10.1210/en.2009-0840.

41. Suzuki R, Shimodaira H. Pvclust: an R package for assessing the uncertainty in hierarchical clustering. Bioinformatics. 2006;22:1540–2. doi:10.1093/bioinformatics/btl117.

42. VerHague MA, Cheng D, Weinberg RB, Shelness GS. Apolipoprotein A-IV expression in mouse liver enhances triglyceride secretion and reduces hepatic lipid content by promoting very low density lipoprotein particle expansion. Arterioscler Thromb Vasc Biol. 2013;33:2501–8. doi:10.1161/atvbaha.113.301948.

43. Vidon C, Boucher P, Cachefo A, Peroni O, Diraison F, Beylot M. Effects of isoenergetic high-carbohydrate compared with high-fat diets on human cholesterol synthesis and expression of key regulatory genes of cholesterol metabolism. Am J Clin Nutr. 2001;73:878–84.

44. Vlahos CJ, Matter WF, Hui KY, Brown RF. A specific inhibitor of phosphatidylinositol 3-kinase, 2-(4-morpholinyl)-8-phenyl-4H-1-benzopyran-4-one (LY294002). J Biol Chem. 1994;269:5241–8.

45. Wang X, Cheng M, Zhao M, et al. Differential effects of high-fat-diet rich in lard oil or soybean oil on osteopontin expression and inflammation of adipose tissue in diet-induced obese rats. Eur J Nutr. 2013;52:1181–9. doi:10.1007/s00394-012-0428-z.

46. Wu Z, Irizarry RA, Gentleman R, Martinez-Murillo F, Spencer F. A model-based background adjustment for oligonucleotide expression arrays. J Am Stat Assoc. 2004;99:909–17. doi:10.1198/016214504000000683.

47. Xue B, Nie J, Wang X, DuBois DC, Jusko WJ, Almon RR. Effects of high fat feeding on adipose tissue gene expression in diabetic goto-kakizaki rats. Gene Regul Syst Bio. 2015;9:15–26. doi:10.4137/grsb.s25172.

48. Yabe D, Brown MS, Goldstein JL. Insig-2, a second endoplasmic reticulum protein that binds SCAP and blocks export of sterol regulatory element-binding proteins. Proc Natl Acad Sci U S A. 2002;99:12753–8. doi:10.1073/pnas.162488899.

3

Genetic susceptibility to dyslipidemia and incidence of cardiovascular disease depending on a diet quality index in the Malmö Diet and Cancer cohort

Sophie Hellstrand[1][*] , Ulrika Ericson[1], Christina-Alexandra Schulz[1], Isabel Drake[1], Bo Gullberg[2], Bo Hedblad[3], Gunnar Engström[3], Marju Orho-Melander[1] and Emily Sonestedt[1]

Abstract

Background: By taking diet quality into account, we may clarify the relationship between genetically elevated triglycerides (TG) and low-density lipoprotein-cholesterol (LDL-C), and better understand the inconsistent results regarding genetically elevated high-density lipoprotein-cholesterol (HDL-C), and cardiovascular disease (CVD) risk.

Methods: We included 24,799 participants (62 % women, age 44–74 years) from the Malmö Diet and Cancer cohort. During a mean follow-up time of 15 years, 3068 incident CVD cases (1814 coronary and 1254 ischemic stroke) were identified. Genetic risk scores (GRSs) were constructed by combining 80 validated genetic variants associated with higher TG and LDL-C or lower HDL-C. The participants' dietary intake, assessed by a modified diet history method, was ranked according to a diet quality index that included six dietary components: saturated fat, polyunsaturated fat, fish, fiber, fruit and vegetables, and sucrose.

Results: The GRS_{LDL-C} ($P = 5 \times 10^{-6}$) and GRS_{HDL-C} ($P = 0.02$) but not GRS_{TG} ($P = 0.08$) were significantly associated with CVD risk. No significant interaction between the GRSs and diet quality was observed on CVD risk ($P > 0.39$). A high compared to a low diet quality attenuated the association between GRS_{LDL-C} and the risk of incident ischemic stroke (P interaction = 0.01).

Conclusion: We found some evidence of an interaction between diet quality and GRS_{LDL-C} on ischemic stroke.

Keywords: Cholesterol, Epidemiology, Lipoproteins, Nutrition, Triglycerides

Background

Plasma concentrations of low-density lipoprotein-cholesterol (LDL-C) and high-density lipoprotein-cholesterol (HDL-C) are well-established prognostic factors for cardiovascular disease (CVD), in particular coronary heart disease (CHD) [12]. Lifestyle changes to reduce LDL-C and increase HDL-C, such as dietary modification and increased physical activity, are widely used in the primary prevention of CVD [29, 39]. Plasma LDL-C and triglycerides (TG) have been confirmed to be causally linked to CHD in Mendelian randomization studies [7, 15, 42]; however, so

* Correspondence: sophie.hellstrand@med.lu.se
[1]Diabetes and Cardiovascular Disease—Genetic Epidemiology, Department of Clinical Sciences Malmö, Lund University, Jan Waldenströms gata 35, SE-20502 Malmö, Sweden
Full list of author information is available at the end of the article

far, evidence regarding the causal relevance of HDL-C is lacking [2, 7, 15, 42]. For example, a recent Mendelian randomization study by Voight et al. found that a genetic score of 13 LDL-C-increasing alleles increased the risk of CHD, whereas a genetic score of 14 HDL-C-increasing alleles did not decrease the risk of CHD [42]. The authors concluded that some genetic mechanisms that increase HDL-C do not automatically reduce the risk of CHD. Several randomized clinical trials have evaluated the benefit of reducing LDL-C and increasing HDL-C concentrations in the tertiary prevention of CHD [2, 5]. However, none of these studies have successfully demonstrated that increasing HDL-C has a protective effect on CVD. On the other hand, studies and trials on patients with hypercholesterolemia strongly indicate that LDL-C-lowering therapies reduce the risk of CHD [1, 4], which is in line with the results from observational studies [11].

A high diet quality based on the Swedish nutrition recommendations and the Swedish dietary guidelines has been shown to reduce the risk of CVD compared to a low diet quality index [14]. The diet quality index was constructed by combining six dietary components: saturated fat, polyunsaturated fat (PUFA), fish and shellfish, dietary fiber, fruit and vegetables, and sucrose [8]. The diet quality index was associated with CVD more strongly than the individual dietary components [14], illustrating the importance of examining the whole diet with regard to disease risk. Additionally, a high diet quality was associated with decreased risk of all-cause and CVD mortality, particularly among men [9], reduced systemic inflammation [6], and lower risk of developing high TG and high LDL-C during 16 years of follow-up compared with a low diet quality [35]. However, a high diet quality index was not associated with lower incidence of type 2 diabetes in the MDC cohort [20]. We hypothesize that by taking diet quality into account, we may clarify the relationship between genetically elevated TG and LDL-C and better understand the results regarding genetically elevated HDL-C and the risk of CVD. Therefore, we examine the association between genetic susceptibility to dyslipidemia and the incidence of CVD, including coronary events and ischemic stroke, and assess whether these associations differ depending on diet quality.

Methods
Study population
The Malmö Diet and Cancer (MDC) study is a population-based prospective cohort including 30,447 participants, with baseline data collection conducted throughout the years 1991–1996 [3]. The study population includes individuals born during 1923–1950 [22] living in the southern part of Sweden in the third largest city, Malmö. The participants were invited via personal letters and advertisements in the local newspapers and public places. The participation rate was approximately 40 % [21], and limited Swedish language skills and mental incapacity were the only exclusion criteria. In this study, we included 28,098 participants (11,063 men and 17,035 women) with complete dietary information and anthropometric measures. After excluding individuals with a history of coronary events or stroke ($n = 855$), self-reported diabetes or glucose-lowering medication ($n = 798$), and successful genotyping of less than 60 % of the single-nucleotide polymorphisms (SNP) ($n = 1,646$), 24,799 participants (62 % women, age 44–74 years) remained and formed the study sample. All individuals provided written informed consent, and the ethics committee of Lund University approved the MDC study protocols (LU 51–90).

Case definition and follow-up
In total, 3068 (1759 men and 1309 women) CVD cases were identified during 369,996 person-years of follow-up. Of these, 1814 had a coronary event and 1254 had an ischemic stroke as the first event. The mean follow-up time was 15 years (range 0–20 years). Information regarding prevalent and incident CVD was retrieved from the national Swedish Hospital Discharge register [13], the Cause-of-Death register [33], and the local stroke register in Malmö (STROMA) [17, 30, 43]. A coronary event was defined on the basis of codes 410–414 (fatal or non-fatal myocardial infarction or death due to ischemic heart disease) in the International Classification of Diseases, 9th Revision (ICD-9). Ischemic stroke was defined on the basis of code 434 (ICD-9) and diagnosed when computed tomography, magnetic resonance imaging, or autopsy could verify the infarction and/or exclude hemorrhage and non-vascular disease. A stroke was classified as unspecified if neither imaging nor autopsy was performed. Hemorrhagic or non-specific stroke cases (ICD-9 codes 430, 431, and 436) do not have the same underlying risk factors as ischemic stroke and were therefore excluded. The National Tax Board provided information on vital status and emigration. The participants contributed person-time from their date of enrollment until their first CVD event, death, emigration from Sweden, or the end of follow-up (i.e., 31 December 2010).

Genotyping and the construction of genetic risk scores
Susceptibility to dyslipidemia was estimated by combining the validated genetic variants reported in the genome-wide association study (GWAS) meta-analysis by Teslovich et al. [38]. All SNPs ($n = 91$) that reached the GWAS significance level (i.e., $P < 5 \times 10^{-8}$) for TG, LDL-C, or HDL-C were genotyped except *LPA* rs1084651, *JMJD1C* rs10761731, and *NPC1L1* rs217386 because of difficulties in genotyping or a lack of proxies available. Genotyping was performed using Sequenom MassARRAY (Sequenom, San Diego, CA, USA) or Taqman allelic discrimination on an ABI 7900 (Applied Biosystems, Foster City, CA, USA) at the Clinical Research Center, Malmö, Sweden. Thereafter, the SNPs with a success rate of less than 90 % (i.e., *COBLL1* rs10195252, *KLF14* rs4731702, *PLEC1* rs11136341, and *ABCA8* rs4148008) and those with Hardy-Weinberg equilibrium P values less than 0.00057 (0.05/87) (i.e., *ANGPTL3* rs2131925, *TYW1B* rs13238203, *SCARB1* rs838880, *OSBPL7* rs7206971, *LILRA3* rs386000, *PLTP* rs6065906, and *MOSC1* rs2642442) were excluded. Weighted genetic risk scores (GRSs) were constructed using PLINK (version 1.07) for TG (26 SNPs), HDL-C (41 SNPs), and LDL-C (32 SNPs) (Additional file 1) by multiplying the effect size (i.e., β-coefficients) found in the meta-analysis [38] by the number of risk alleles and then summing the products. The respective GRSs

explained 7.3 % of the variance in LDL-C, 5.7 % of the variance in HDL-C, and 4.7 % of the variance in TG.

Dietary information

Dietary intake was measured by a modified diet history methodology specifically designed for the MDC study by combining a 168-item dietary questionnaire (i.e., "habitual" diet information), a 7-day menu book (i.e., "current" diet information), and a 1-h diet history interview [31, 41]. The dietary questionnaire covered food items regularly consumed during the past year. The 7-day menu book covered cooked lunch and dinner meals, cold beverages (including alcoholic beverages), medications, natural remedies, and dietary supplements used by the participants. During the interview, the menu book and questionnaire were checked for notably high reported intakes and overlapping information and the participants were asked about their food choices, food preparation practices, and portion sizes of the food reported in the menu book. The relative validity of a slightly different methodology (130-item questionnaire and 2-week food records without the interview was compared with a reference method of 18 days weighted food records with three consecutive days every second month during 1 year) in the Malmö population has been published earlier [10, 31]. The energy-adjusted correlation coefficients between the modified diet history method and the reference method were for saturated fat (0.56 and 0.68 for men and women, respectively), PUFA (0.26; 0.64), fish (0.35; 0.70), fiber (0.74; 0.69), fruit (0.60; 0.77), vegetables (0.65; 0.53), and sugar (0.60; 0.74) [10, 31].

We also noted the season of the dietary interview: winter (Jan–Mar), spring (Apr–Jun), summer (Jul–Sept), or autumn (Oct–Dec). The routines for coding dietary data were slightly altered in September 1994 to shorten the interview time, and a diet assessment method version variable was constructed to indicate whether the data were collected before or after the 1 September 1994. This change did not appear to have any major influence on the ranking of individuals [41]. The average daily intake (i.e., grams per day) of food and supplements was calculated based on the information from the menu book, interview, and questionnaire and converted into nutrient and energy intakes using the MDC Food and Nutrient Database, developed from the PC KOST-93 of the Swedish National Food Administration.

The diet quality index was developed to assess diet quality based on the Swedish nutrition recommendations issued in 2005 and has been described previously [8]. The diet quality index includes six dietary components: contribution to non-alcohol energy percentage (E%) from saturated fat, E% from PUFA, intake of fish and shellfish (g/week), dietary fiber (g/MJ), fruit and vegetables (g/day), and E% from sucrose. The following cutoffs were used: saturated fat ≤14 E%, PUFA 5-10 E%, fish and shellfish ≥300 g/week, fiber ≥2.4 g/MJ, fruit and vegetables ≥400 g/day, and sucrose ≤10 E%. The revised version of the Nordic nutrition recommendations from 2012 would not have influenced the cutoffs used. Because only 2 % of the participants had an intake below the recommended level (≤10 E%) for saturated fat, the cutoff for saturated fat was increased to ≤14 E% (i.e., one standard deviation (SD) increase). One point was given to the participants for each dietary component that reached the recommended intake level, and zero points were given if they were not within the recommended range. A total score was created by summing the points and divided into three categories: low (0–1 point), medium (2–4 points), and high (5–6 points).

Information regarding dietary change in the past (yes/no) was based on the question "Have you substantially changed your eating habits because of illness or for other reasons?". The dietary habits of participants reporting dietary changes may reflect only a short period of their lives and may therefore have less influence on the development of chronic disease. Potential misreports of energy intake were identified by comparing reported energy intake with total energy expenditure (i.e., estimated from a calculated basal metabolic rate and self-reports of leisure time physical activity, work activity, household work, and sleep hours). Individuals with reported energy intake outside the 95 % confidence interval (CI) for total energy expenditure were categorized as "misreporters", as is further explained elsewhere [23].

Other variables

Age and sex were identified from each individual's civil registration number. Body mass index (BMI) (kg/m^2) was calculated from a direct measurement of weight and height, wearing light clothes and no shoes, conducted by a nurse. A self-administered questionnaire was used to determine lifestyle and socioeconomic factors including smoking habits, alcohol habits, physical activity habits, and educational level, current medication, diet supplement use, and history of diseases. Three categories of smoking habits were used: current (including irregular smoking), former, and never smokers. Individuals were divided into five categories based on their alcohol habits. Individuals reporting no alcohol consumption during the last year in the questionnaire, who were also zero reporters of alcohol in the 7-day menu book, were categorized as zero consumers of alcohol. We divided the other study participants into categories (low, moderate, high, and very high) based on their alcohol consumption (grams per day) with different cutoffs according to gender. The cutoff levels for females were 5, 10, and 20 g of alcohol per day, and the cutoff levels for males were 10, 20, and 40 g of alcohol per day. Educational level was categorized based on the highest level of education attained: elementary or less, primary and secondary, upper secondary, further education without a degree, and university degree. Physical activity levels during leisure time were calculated from a list of 17 different activities in the questionnaire. The time spent on each activity was multiplied with an intensity factor, creating a leisure time physical activity score [19]. The leisure time physical activity score was then divided into quintiles with the same cutoffs for both genders because of similar scores in men and women. Separate categories for smoking habits, alcohol habits, educational level, and leisure time physical activity were constructed for the participants with missing data.

Statistical analyses

Statistical Package of the Social Science (SPSS, version 22.0; IBM Corporation, Armonk, NY, USA) was used for statistical analyses. Differences in baseline characteristics across the diet quality categories (i.e., low, medium, and high) and GRSs per SD were tested in men and women separately using chi^2-test for categorical variables and general linear model adjusted for age for continuous variables. All continuous variables except age were logarithmically (Ln) transformed to achieve a normal distribution when testing for trends across the diet quality index (0–6) and GRSs (continuous); before transformation, a very small amount (i.e., 0.001 g) was added to fish and shellfish and fruit and vegetables, intakes to handle zero intakes. Additionally, differences in the number of diet changers and non-diet changers between tertiles of GRSs were tested using chi^2-test. Linear regression was used to examine the association between the GRSs and TG and HDL-C and LDL-C concentrations at baseline. For analyses of the P for trend and variance explained, we used Ln-transformed TG, LDL-C, and HDL-C. Cox proportional hazard regression was used to examine associations between GRSs and incident CVD, coronary events, and ischemic stroke, adjusted for age and sex and with years of follow-up as the underlying time variable. We also added dietary fiber in this model because it is a known risk factor for CVD and for being associated with all three GRSs in this study. Additionally, we examined these associations in strata of diet quality categories (i.e., low, medium, and high) adjusted for age and sex and both with and without BMI because BMI can be regarded as a mediating factor. The combined diet index was the main dietary variable, but we also examined the associations between the GRSs and CVD with adherence to each component separately. The interactions between the diet quality index and the three GRSs on CVD were examined by introducing multiplicative factors of GRSs and diet quality index as continuous variables, in addition to the main factors as separate

variables, in a multivariable model adjusted for age, sex, dietary assessment method version, season, total energy intake, smoking habits, alcohol habits, leisure time physical activity, educational level, and BMI. These variables were selected from the literature for being known risk factors for CVD [26, 29] and for being associated with dietary intakes in this study. Because many of the SNPs included in the GRSs have pleiotropic effects, the analyses for each GRS were adjusted for the other two GRSs. To further interpret the statistically significant interactions between GRSs and the diet quality index on CVD risk, we examined associations with diet quality index (both as a continuous and categorical variable) in tertiles of GRSs. The lowest diet quality index category was used as the reference. All analyses were also carried out separately in men and women due to gender differences in food selection and reporting, as well as biological differences. Formal tests for interactions by sex were also performed. In sensitivity analyses, we excluded individuals reporting dietary changes in the past, because they may have unstable food habits, and potential "misreporters" of energy intake.

Results

Baseline characteristics

Baseline characteristics across the diet quality categories are shown in Additional file 2. GRSs were composed of 26 SNPs for TG, 32 SNPs for LDL-C, and 41 SNPs for HDL-C (Additional file 1). The GRSs explained 4.7, 7.3, and 5.7 %, respectively, of the variance in the traits (Additional file 3). We observed several statistically significant associations between baseline characteristics and the GRSs; for example, all the GRSs were associated with higher dietary fiber intakes and lower saturated fat intakes (Additional file 4). These associations were in the same direction in men and women. In addition, we observed a significantly higher frequency of diet changers in the highest tertile of GRS$_{LDL-C}$ compared to the lowest tertile (23 and 20 % P (chi^2-test) = 6 × 10^{-5}). Similar tendencies were observed for GRS$_{HDL-C}$ ($P = 0.06$) and GRS$_{TG}$ ($P = 0.09$) (Additional file 4). The associations between dietary intakes and GRSs were attenuated when excluding diet changers in the past and potential misreporters of energy.

Genetic risk for dyslipidemia and CVD

GRS$_{LDL-C}$ was significantly associated with an increased risk of CVD ($P = 5 × 10^{-6}$), coronary events ($P = 1.5 × 10^{-4}$), and ischemic stroke ($P = 0.02$) after adjusting for age and sex (Table 1). GRS$_{HDL-C}$ was significantly associated with an increased risk of CVD ($P = 0.02$) and ischemic stroke ($P = 0.04$) but not with an increased risk of coronary events ($P = 0.18$). GRS$_{TG}$ was significantly associated with an increased risk of coronary events ($P = 0.01$) but not

Table 1 HR of incident CVD, coronary event, and ischemic stroke per 1 SD increase of GRS

GRSs	Total CVD		Coronary event		Ischemic stroke	
	Cases n_{men} = 1759/n_{women} = 1309		Cases n_{men} = 1129/n_{women} = 685		Cases n_{men} = 630/n_{women} = 624	
	Model 1[a]	Model 2[b]	Model 1	Model 2	Model 1	Model 2
GRS$_{LDL-C}$						
All	1.09 (1.05–1.13)	1.08 (1.04–1.12)	1.09 (1.04–1.15)	1.08 (1.03–1.14)	1.07 (1.01–1.13)	1.07 (1.01–1.14)
Men	1.08 (1.03–1.13)	1.07 (1.02–1.12)	1.08 (1.02–1.14)	1.07 (1.01–1.14)	1.07 (0.99–1.16)	1.07 (0.99–1.16)
Women	1.10 (1.04–1.16)	1.09 (1.03–1.15)	1.13 (1.05–1.22)	1.11 (1.03–1.20)	1.07 (0.99–1.16)	1.07 (0.99–1.16)
GRS$_{HDL-C}$						
All	1.05 (1.01–1.08)	1.03 (1.00–1.07)	1.03 (0.99–1.08)	1.00 (0.95–1.05)	1.06 (1.00–1.12)	1.08 (1.01–1.14)
Men	1.03 (0.98–1.08)	1.01 (0.96–1.06)	1.01 (0.95–1.07)	0.97 (0.91–1.04)	1.06 (0.98–1.15)	1.08 (0.99–1.18)
Women	1.07 (1.01–1.13)	1.06 (1.00–1.13)	1.08 (1.00–1.16)	1.05 (0.97–1.14)	1.06 (0.98–1.14)	1.07 (0.98–1.17)
GRS$_{TG}$						
All	1.03 (1.00–1.07)	1.00 (0.96–1.04)	1.07 (1.02–1.12)	1.05 (1.00–1.10)	0.99 (0.93–1.04)	0.94 (0.88–1.00)
Men	1.03 (0.99–1.08)	1.02 (0.96–1.07)	1.06 (1.00–1.13)	1.06 (1.00–1.14)	0.98 (0.91–1.06)	0.94 (0.86–1.02)
Women	1.03 (0.98–1.09)	0.98 (0.93–1.04)	1.07 (0.99–1.15)	1.02 (0.94–1.11)	0.99 (0.91–1.07)	0.94 (0.86–1.03)

Cox proportional hazard regression model was used to calculate HRs (95 % CI), among 9383 men and 15,416 women in the Malmö Diet and Cancer cohort
[a]Model 1 is adjusted for age and sex
[b]Model 2 is adjusted for age, sex, and the two GRSs simultaneously

with an increased risk of CVD ($P = 0.08$) and ischemic stroke ($P = 0.59$).

When we adjusted for pleiotrophy (i.e., adding the other two GRSs to the statistical model), the estimated risk was slightly changed, especially the associations with GRS$_{HDL-C}$ and GRS$_{TG}$ (Table 1). Adding dietary fiber to this model did not markedly change the results (data not shown).

Interaction with diet quality index

No significant interaction between the GRSs and diet quality was observed for the incidence of CVD (GRS$_{LDL-C}$ $P = 0.39$, GRS$_{HDL-C}$ $P = 0.85$, and GRS$_{TG}$ $P = 0.86$) (Table 2). When coronary and ischemic stroke events were examined separately, we observed a significant interaction between GRS$_{LDL-C}$ and diet quality index on ischemic stroke incidence ($P = 0.01$). When the analysis was

Table 2 HR in strata of diet quality index on incident CVD, coronary event, and ischemic stroke

	Diet quality index			P interaction[a]
	Low	Medium	High	
	n = 3360	n = 15,538	n = 2833	
	HR (95 % CI)	HR (95 % CI)	HR (95 % CI)	
Total CVD	530 cases	2186 cases	352 cases	
GRS$_{LDL-C}$	1.11 (1.02–1.21)	1.09 (1.04–1.14)	1.07 (0.96–1.19)	0.39 (0.86)[b]
GRS$_{HDL-C}$	1.08 (0.99–1.18)	1.03 (0.99–1.07)	1.10 (0.99–1.22)	0.85 (0.58)
GRS$_{TG}$	1.02 (0.93–1.11)	1.03 (0.99–1.08)	1.05 (0.95–1.17)	0.86 (0.20)
Coronary event	Cases n = 313	Cases n = 1285	Cases n = 216	
GRS$_{LDL-C}$	1.13 (1.01–1.26)	1.08 (1.02–1.14)	1.15 (1.01–1.32)	0.33 (0.08)
GRS$_{HDL-C}$	1.02 (0.91–1.14)	1.03 (0.97–1.08)	1.11 (0.97–1.27)	0.35 (0.78)
GRS$_{TG}$	1.06 (0.95–1.19)	1.06 (1.01–1.12)	1.09 (0.95–1.25)	0.78 (0.23)
Ischemic stroke	Cases n = 217	Cases n = 901	Cases n = 136	
GRS$_{LDL-C}$	1.08 (0.95–1.24)	1.10 (1.03–1.17)	0.93 (0.79–1.10)	0.01 (0.07)
GRS$_{HDL-C}$	1.16 (1.02–1.33)	1.04 (0.97–1.11)	1.07 (0.91–1.26)	0.18 (0.21)
GRS$_{TG}$	0.96 (0.84–1.10)	0.99 (0.93–1.06)	0.99 (0.83–1.17)	0.98 (0.59)

Cox proportional hazard regression was used to calculate HRs (95 % CI) per 1 SD increase of the GRSs, $P < 0.05$, adjusted for age and sex among 24,799 participants in the Malmö Diet and Cancer cohort
[a]P interactions (GRSs × diet quality index as continuous variables) adjusted for age, sex, BMI, diet assessment method version, season, total energy intake, alcohol habits, leisure time physical activity, educational level, and smoking habits
[b]P values in parentheses are sensitivity analyses excluding those reporting dietary changes in the past and potential energy misreporters, n = 16,030

stratified by diet quality categories, a high compared to a low diet quality attenuated the association between GRS_{LDL-C} and the increased risk of incident ischemic stroke (hazard ratio (HR) per SD, HR_{low} = 1.08 (0.95–1.24), P = 0.26; HR_{medium} = 1.10 (1.03–1.17), P = 0.01; HR_{high} = 0.93 (0.79–1.10), P = 0.40 (Table 2)). This association became significant when we combined the low and medium diet quality group ($HR_{low+medium}$ = 1.09; 95 % CI, 1.03–1.16; P = 0.004). When we examined the association between the diet quality index and the incidence of ischemic stroke in tertiles of GRS_{LDL-C}, we observed only a significant inverse association between the diet quality index and the incidence of ischemic stroke among the participants in the highest tertile of GRS_{LDL-C} (HR for highest vs. lowest diet quality = 0.64 (0.44–0.95), P trend = 0.001) (Fig. 1). Adding BMI to the statistical model did not markedly change the results. Thereafter, we examined the interaction between the GRSs and each diet index component on the incidence of CVD, coronary events, and ischemic stroke. There was no significant interaction between any of the diet index components and the GRS_{LDL-C} ($P_{lowest\ for\ PUFA}$ = 0.22 to $P_{highest\ for\ fish\ and\ shellfish}$ = 0.95), GRS_{HDL-C} ($P_{lowest\ for\ fish\ and\ shellfish}$ = 0.18 to $P_{highest\ for\ PUFA}$ = 0.81), and GRS_{TG} ($P_{lowest\ for\ sucrose}$ = 0.09 to $P_{highest\ for\ PUFA}$ = 0.96) on the incidence of CVD (Additional file 5). However, we observed a significant interaction between GRS_{LDL-C} and fruit and vegetable intake (P = 0.01) on ischemic stroke incidence. The association between GRS_{LDL-C} and increased risk of ischemic stroke was attenuated among the participants with high intake of fruit and vegetables (>400 g/day). No significant interactions were observed between the GRSs and diet quality

index components on the incidence of coronary events (Additional file 5).

Furthermore, we preformed all analyses separately in men and women. There were no three-way statistical interactions (i.e., sex*diet quality index*GRS) on CVD (P > 0.48), coronary events (P > 0.36), or ischemic stroke (P > 0.38). However, the interaction between GRS_{LDL-C} and the diet quality index on ischemic stroke was statistically significant in women (P = 0.03) but not in men (P = 0.12) (Additional file 6). This interaction was mainly driven by fruit and vegetable intakes (P = 1 × 10^{-3}) in men and saturated fat (P = 0.02) and PUFA (P = 0.06) in women (Additional file 5). There was only a significant association between GRS_{LDL-C} and increased risk of ischemic stroke among men with low fruit and vegetable intake (≤400 g/day). In women, a significant association between GRS_{LDL-C} and increased risk of ischemic stroke was observed only among those with high intake of saturated fat (≥14 E%) and outside the recommended range of PUFA (5–10 E%).

In sensitivity analyses, we excluded participants reporting dietary changes in the past and those with suspected misreporting of energy (n = 8,769; 35 % of the study sample). In line with the results reported above, no significant interactions between the GRSs and diet quality index on the incidence of CVD were observed (GRS_{LDL-C} P = 0.86, GRS_{HDL-C} P = 0.58, and GRS_{TG} P = 0.20). The interaction between GRS_{LDL-C} and the diet quality index on ischemic stroke was somewhat attenuated in this reduced study sample (P = 0.07). The interaction between GRS_{LDL-C} and fruit and vegetable intake on ischemic stroke remained statistically significant (P = 0.049). Overall, the results did not markedly change when adding the two GRSs simultaneously to the statistical model.

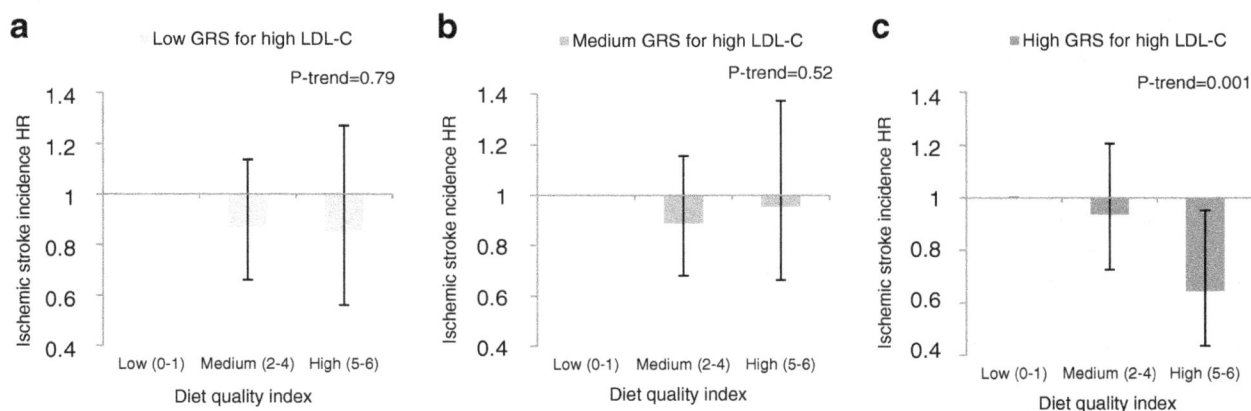

Fig. 1 Association between the diet quality index and incidence of ischemic stroke according to tertiles of GRS_{LDL-C}, low (**a**), medium (**b**) and high (**c**) among 24,799 participants in the Malmö Diet and Cancer cohort. A Cox proportional hazard regression was used to calculate HR for each diet quality category with the lowest category as a reference. Multivariable models were adjusted for age, sex, BMI, diet assessment method version, season, total energy intake, alcohol habits, leisure time physical activity, educational level, and smoking habits. In tertiles of GRS_{LDL-C} (non-cases/cases) of ischemic stroke; low n = 7293/395; medium n = 7272/415; high n = 7166/444

Discussion

In this study, we examined the association between genetic susceptibility to dyslipidemia and the risk of CVD by combining 80 validated genetic variants associated with blood lipids and lipoproteins. These variants have been suggested to account for approximately 25–30 % of the genetic variance of blood lipid and lipoprotein concentrations [38] and can therefore be used as a marker of genetic susceptibility to dyslipidemia in Caucasians.

We found some evidence of an interaction between diet quality and GRS_{LDL-C} affecting the risk of ischemic stroke but not CVD or coronary events. A high compared to a low diet quality attenuated the genetic susceptibility of high LDL-C on the risk of ischemic stroke incidence.

The GRS_{LDL-C} was significantly associated with an increased risk of CVD and coronary events. This is in line with a number of Mendelian randomization studies [7, 15, 42]. Additionally, numerous potential genetic risk alleles for stroke have been reported; however, the evidence is so far not conclusive [16], and studies examining the association between GRS_{LDL-C} and stroke are missing. In the present study, a high compared to low diet quality attenuated the association between GRS_{LDL-C} and the increased risk of incident ischemic stroke. Although GRS_{LDL-C} tended to be associated with increased risk in the low and medium diet quality groups, no such tendency was observed in the high diet quality group. However, the non-significant trend among the participants in the high and low diet quality groups might, at least in part, be explained by a lower number of individuals in these groups (n_{low} = 3890, n_{medium} = 17,724, and n_{high} = 3185). When we divided the GRS_{LDL-C} into tertiles, we observed that a high diet quality was inversely associated with ischemic stroke incidence among individuals in the highest tertile of GRS_{LDL-C}. The observed interaction between GRS_{LDL-C} and the diet quality index on ischemic stroke seems to mainly be driven by fruit and vegetable intakes in men and fat quality (i.e., saturated fat and PUFA) in women, although no significant heterogeneities regarding these interactions were observed between the sexes.

The included genetic variants are located in or near genes that are involved in various and, in many cases, unknown mechanisms and pathways of lipid and lipoprotein metabolism, which may attenuate the interactions when they are combined into GRSs. It may therefore be important to examine genetic variants affecting specific mechanisms and pathways separately to address whether genetic susceptibility affecting such specific mechanisms or pathways would modify the associations. In addition, several of the SNPs included in the GRSs have pleiotropic effects associated with several lipid traits, which could bias our results. We chose to include these SNPs to avoid weakening the effects of the GRSs and corrected for pleiotropic associations in the statistical models. In addition, it is important to note the small overlap between variants identified in GWAS for cardio-metabolic traits and variants showing indication of gene-environment interaction [27]. Genetic variants under genetic pressure may be more prone to interaction with environmental factors [28].

The GRSs are composed of common genetic variants (<0.05 minor allele frequency). Low-frequency missense variants have been associated with larger differences in lipid and lipoprotein concentrations and with coronary artery disease [4, 18, 24, 32]. For example, carriers of loss-of-function mutations in *ANGPTL4* had 35 % lower TG concentrations than non-carriers; these mutations were also associated with protection from coronary artery disease [24]. Since these low-frequency variants markedly affect TG concentrations, they may be useful to include when examining interactions with diet on CVD incidence; however to conduct these kind of studies, the study material has to be extremely large.

In this type of population-based studies, the participants are often healthier than the general population. This may contribute to fewer cases of CVD and also narrow the range of dietary intakes among the participants. This may decrease the likelihood of observing differences in genetic risk for dyslipidemia and CVD depending on diet quality. The significant associations between several baseline characteristics, (e.g., higher dietary fiber and lower saturated fat intakes) and high GRSs, are not easy to explain. It may, however, indicate that those individuals with high genetic risk for dyslipidemia are more likely to be aware of their dietary habits. An explanation may be that these individuals have experienced different health problems previously and may therefore have changed their food habits. This hypothesis is supported by our observation of significantly higher frequency of diet changers in the highest tertile of GRS_{LDL-C} compared to the lowest tertile. Similar tendencies were observed for GRS_{HDL-C} and GRS_{TG}. However, the associations between these baseline characteristics and GRSs were in the same direction, but attenuated, when excluding diet changers in the past and potential misreporters of energy. Unfortunately, we have dietary data only from the baseline examination, and therefore, we do not have any information regarding changes of exposure that might have occurred during the 15 years of follow-up. However, diet changers are most likely prone to unstable food habits [34, 37]. In addition, studies on long-term reproducibility have indicated that single measurements of dietary intakes can be used as proxies of long-term exposures [25, 40], and because the participants in the MDC study were middle-aged at the baseline examinations during the 90s, they are more likely to have well-established food habits than a younger population.

The strengths of this study are the prospective design, large sample size, and detailed information on dietary intakes based on a 168-item dietary questionnaire, a 7-day record, and a 1-h interview. Other major strengths of this study are the almost complete follow-up of participants through registers and the detailed ascertainment and verification of CVD diagnosis [13, 17, 30, 43].

The dietary assessment method used in the MDC study was specifically designed to measure intakes of vegetables, fiber, and fat [3], and the relative validity of the method is generally high. The high validity may contribute to the ability to observe significant interactions between GRS_{LDL-C} and fruit and vegetable intakes affecting ischemic stroke incidence. However, the relative validity is rather low for fish and PUFA intake in men. Because fish consumed at main meals was registered only during seven consecutive days and fish is likely to be consumed relatively infrequently, misclassification might be a problem. The high relative validity of PUFA intakes in women (0.64) compared to men (0.26) might explain why we observed a nominal interaction between GRS_{LDL-C} and PUFA intake affecting ischemic stroke in women but not in men.

The diet quality index itself could be a limitation and is only one of several ways to examine associations between diet quality and disease risk. The diet quality index has previously been shown to reflect overall diet quality and sufficiently rank participants in the MDC cohort into low, medium, and high diet quality on the basis of their intake of a wide range of foods and nutrients and may thus be more predictive of disease risk than individual foods or nutrients. However, reducing dietary habits, which are very complex, into a diet quality index constructed by adding a few dichotomous diet variables may be a disadvantage. Additionally, there may be individual dietary components that interact more strongly with GRSs [35, 36]. Dietary patterns are likely to vary according to social and cultural backgrounds; therefore, it is necessary to replicate our results in other populations. Although we adjusted for potential confounders, the diet quality index might correlate with other factors important for CVD risk; thus, residual confounding can still occur.

Conclusions

In conclusion, we found no convincing evidence that dietary quality modifies the association between the GRSs for TG, LDL-C, and HDL-C and CVD risk. Further studies may need to consider different mechanisms and pathways for genetic variants associated with dyslipidemia separately to clarify the interaction between GRSs and diet quality on CVD risk. Finally, we performed multiple tests; thus, some of the observed significant associations and interactions could be due to chance and need to be replicated. In addition, to examine the modifying effect of diet quality, further studies are needed to examine whether any specific dietary factors may modify the associations between genetic susceptibility to dyslipidemia and the incidence of CVD.

Additional files

Additional file 1: Characteristics of the included single nucleotide polymorphisms.

Additional file 2: Baseline characteristics among 9383 men and 15,416 women in the Malmö Diet and Cancer cohort according to the diet quality index.

Additional file 3: Association between the genetic risk scores and LDL-C, HDL-C, and TG in the Malmö Diet and Cancer cohort.

Additional file 4: Association (P values and directions) between baseline characteristics and the genetic risk scores among 24,799 participants in the Malmö Diet and Cancer cohort.

Additional file 5: Interaction (P value) between the genetic risk scores and the diet index components on incidence of total cardiovascular disease, coronary event, and ischemic stroke among 24,799 participants in the Malmö Diet and Cancer cohort.

Additional file 6: Hazard ratios for per 1 SD increase of the genetic risk scores in strata of diet quality index on incidence of total cardiovascular disease, coronary event, and ischemic stroke among 9383 men and 15,416 women in the Malmö Diet and Cancer cohort.

Abbreviations
BMI, body mass index; CHD, coronary heart disease; CI, confidence interval; CVD, cardiovascular disease; E%, energy percentage; GRS, genetic risk score; GWAS, genome-wide association study; HR, hazard ratio; ICD-9, International Classification of Diseases, 9th revision; MAF, minor allele frequency; MDC, Malmö Diet and Cancer; PUFA, polyunsaturated fat; SD, standard deviation; SE, standard error; SNP, single-nucleotide polymorphism; STROMA, stroke register in Malmö

Acknowledgements
We would like to thank all the participants in the MDC study who made this study possible. We are also very grateful to Malin Svensson for excellent technical assistance.

Funding
This study was founded by the Swedish Research Council (K2012-99X-220018-01-3), The Påhlsson Foundation, and the Swedish Heart and Lung Foundation (20130598; 20140783).

Authors' contributions
SH designed the research, performed the statistical analyses, wrote the first manuscript draft, and had primary responsibility for the final content. ES designed the research, helped to draft the manuscript, and had primary responsibility for the final content. MOM designed the research and was responsible for the genotyping. UE provided critical review. CAS constructed the genetic risk scores and provided critical review. ID constructed the diet index score and provided critical review. BG provided help with the statistical analyses and provided critical review. BH and GE provided critical review. All authors read and approved the final manuscript.

Competing interests
The authors declare that they have no competing interests.

Author details

[1]Diabetes and Cardiovascular Disease—Genetic Epidemiology, Department of Clinical Sciences Malmö, Lund University, Jan Waldenströms gata 35, SE-20502 Malmö, Sweden. [2]Nutritional Epidemiology, Department of Clinical Sciences Malmö, Lund University, Jan Waldenströms gata 35, SE-20502 Malmö, Sweden. [3]Cardiovascular Epidemiology, Department of Clinical Sciences Malmö, Lund University, Jan Waldenströms gata 35, SE-20502 Malmö, Sweden.

References

1. Baigent C et al. Efficacy and safety of cholesterol-lowering treatment: prospective meta-analysis of data from 90,056 participants in 14 randomised trials of statins. Lancet. 2005;366:1267–78. doi:10.1016/S0140-6736(05)67394-1.
2. Barter PJ et al. Effects of torcetrapib in patients at high risk for coronary events. N Engl J Med. 2007;357:2109–22. doi:10.1056/NEJMoa0706628.
3. Berglund G, Elmstahl S, Janzon L, Larsson SA. The Malmo Diet and Cancer Study. Design and feasibility. J Intern Med. 1993;233:45–51.
4. Cohen JC, Boerwinkle E, Mosley Jr TH, Hobbs HH. Sequence variations in PCSK9, low LDL, and protection against coronary heart disease. N Engl J Med. 2006;354:1264–72. doi:10.1056/NEJMoa054013.
5. Constance C et al. Atorvastatin 10 mg plus ezetimibe versus titration to atorvastatin 40 mg: attainment of European and Canadian guideline lipid targets in high-risk subjects >/=65 years. Lipids Health Dis. 2014;13:13. doi:10.1186/1476-511X-13-13.
6. Dias JA et al. A high quality diet is associated with reduced systemic inflammation in middle-aged individuals. Atherosclerosis. 2015;238:38–44. doi:10.1016/j.atherosclerosis.2014.11.006.
7. Do R et al. Common variants associated with plasma triglycerides and risk for coronary artery disease. Nat Genet. 2013;45:1345–52. doi:10.1038/ng.2795.
8. Drake I et al. Development of a diet quality index assessing adherence to the Swedish nutrition recommendations and dietary guidelines in the Malmo Diet and Cancer cohort. Public Health Nutr. 2011;14:835–45. doi:10.1017/S1368980010003848.
9. Drake I et al. Scoring models of a diet quality index and the predictive capability of mortality in a population-based cohort of Swedish men and women. Public Health Nutr. 2013;16:468–78. doi:10.1017/S1368980012002789.
10. Elmstahl S, Riboli E, Lindgarde F, Gullberg B, Saracci R. The Malmo Food Study: the relative validity of a modified diet history method and an extensive food frequency questionnaire for measuring food intake. Eur J Clin Nutr. 1996;50:143–51.
11. Emerging Risk Factors C et al. Major lipids, apolipoproteins, and risk of vascular disease. JAMA. 2009;302:1993–2000. doi:10.1001/jama.2009.1619.
12. Expert Panel on Detection E, Treatment of High Blood Cholesterol in Adults. Executive Summary of The Third Report of The National Cholesterol Education Program (NCEP) Expert Panel on Detection, Evaluation, And Treatment of High Blood Cholesterol in Adults (Adult Treatment Panel III). JAMA. 2001;285:2486–97.
13. Hammar N, Alfredsson L, Rosen M, Spetz CL, Kahan T, Ysberg AS. A national record linkage to study acute myocardial infarction incidence and case fatality in Sweden. Int J Epidemiol. 2001;30 Suppl 1:S30–34.
14. Hlebowicz J et al. A high diet quality is associated with lower incidence of cardiovascular events in the Malmo diet and cancer cohort. PLoS One. 2013;8:e71095. doi:10.1371/journal.pone.0071095.
15. Holmes MV et al. Mendelian randomization of blood lipids for coronary heart disease. Eur Heart J. 2014. doi:10.1093/eurheartj/eht571.
16. Huang HD et al. Genetic predisposition of stroke: understanding the evolving landscape through meta-analysis. Int J Clin Exp Med. 2015;8:1315–23.
17. Jerntorp P, Berglund G. Stroke registry in Malmo, Sweden. Stroke. 1992;23:357–61.
18. Kathiresan S. A PCSK9 missense variant associated with a reduced risk of early-onset myocardial infarction. N Engl J Med. 2008;358:2299–300. doi:10.1056/NEJMc0707445.
19. Li C, Aronsson CA, Hedblad B, Gullberg B, Wirfalt E, Berglund G. Ability of physical activity measurements to assess health-related risks. Eur J Clin Nutr. 2009;63:1448–51. doi:10.1038/ejcn.2009.69.
20. Mandalazi E, Drake I, Wirfält E, Orho-Melander M, Sonestedt E. A high diet quality based on dietary recommendations is not associated with lower incidence of type 2 diabetes in the Malmö Diet and Cancer Cohort. Int J Mol Sci. 2016;17:901. doi:10.3390/ijms17060901.
21. Manjer J et al. The Malmo Diet and Cancer Study: representativity, cancer incidence and mortality in participants and non-participants. Eur J Cancer Prev. 2001;10:489–99.
22. Manjer J, Elmstahl S, Janzon L, Berglund G. Invitation to a population-based cohort study: differences between subjects recruited using various strategies. Scand J Public Health. 2002;30:103–12. doi:10.1080/14034940210133771.
23. Mattisson I, Wirfalt E, Aronsson CA, Wallstrom P, Sonestedt E, Gullberg B, et al. Misreporting of energy: prevalence, characteristics of misreporters and influence on observed risk estimates in the Malmo Diet and Cancer cohort. Br J Nutr. 2005;94:832–42.
24. Myocardial Infarction G, Investigators CAEC. Coding variation in ANGPTL4, LPL, and SVEP1 and the risk of coronary disease. N Engl J Med. 2016;374:1134–44. doi:10.1056/NEJMoa1507652.
25. Nagel G, Zoller D, Ruf T, Rohrmann S, Linseisen J. Long-term reproducibility of a food-frequency questionnaire and dietary changes in the European Prospective Investigation into Cancer and Nutrition (EPIC)-Heidelberg cohort. Br J Nutr. 2007;98:194–200. doi:10.1017/S0007114507691636.
26. National Cholesterol Education Program Expert Panel on Detection E, Treatment of High Blood Cholesterol in A. Third Report of the National Cholesterol Education Program (NCEP) Expert Panel on Detection, Evaluation, and Treatment of High Blood Cholesterol in Adults (Adult Treatment Panel III) final report. Circulation. 2002;106:3143–421.
27. Parnell LD et al. CardioGxE, a catalog of gene-environment interactions for cardiometabolic traits. BioData Min. 2014;7:21. doi:10.1186/1756-0381-7-21.
28. Parnell LD, Lee YC, Lai CQ. Adaptive genetic variation and heart disease risk. Curr Opin Lipidol. 2010;21:116–22. doi:10.1097/MOL.0b013e3283378e42.
29. Perk J et al. European Guidelines on cardiovascular disease prevention in clinical practice (version 2012). The Fifth Joint Task Force of the European Society of Cardiology and Other Societies on Cardiovascular Disease Prevention in Clinical Practice (constituted by representatives of nine societies and by invited experts). Eur Heart J. 2012;33:1635–701. doi:10.1093/eurheartj/ehs092.
30. Pessah-Rasmussen H, Engstrom G, Jerntorp I, Janzon L. Increasing stroke incidence and decreasing case fatality, 1989-1998: a study from the stroke register in Malmo, Sweden. Stroke. 2003;34:913–8. doi:10.1161/01.STR.0000063365.10841.43.
31. Riboli E, Elmstahl S, Saracci R, Gullberg B, Lindgarde F. The Malmo Food Study: validity of two dietary assessment methods for measuring nutrient intake. Int J Epidemiol. 1997;26:161–73.
32. Romeo S, Pennacchio LA, Fu Y, Boerwinkle E, Tybjaerg-Hansen A, Hobbs HH, et al. Population-based resequencing of ANGPTL4 uncovers variations that reduce triglycerides and increase HDL. Nat Genet. 2007;39:513–6. doi:10.1038/ng1984.
33. Socialstyrelsen. Evaluation of diagnostic quality for acute myocardial infarction in patient register 1987 to 1995 (Värdering av diagnoskvaliteten för akut hjärtinfarkt i patientregistret 1987 och 1995). Stockholm: Socialstyrelsen; 2000.
34. Sonestedt E, Gullberg B, Wirfalt E. Both food habit change in the past and obesity status may influence the association between dietary factors and postmenopausal breast cancer. Public Health Nutr. 2007;10:769–79. doi:10.1017/S1368980007246646.
35. Sonestedt E, et al. Diet quality and change in blood lipids during 16 years of follow-up and their interaction with genetic risk for dyslipidemia. Nutrients. 2016;8. doi:10.3390/nu8050274.
36. Sonestedt E et al. The association between carbohydrate-rich foods and risk of cardiovascular disease is not modified by genetic susceptibility to dyslipidemia as determined by 80 validated variants. PLoS One. 2015;10:e0126104. doi:10.1371/journal.pone.0126104.
37. Sonestedt E, Wirfalt E, Gullberg B, Berglund G. Past food habit change is related to obesity, lifestyle and socio-economic factors in the Malmo Diet and Cancer Cohort. Public Health Nutr. 2005;8:876–85.
38. Teslovich TM et al. Biological, clinical and population relevance of 95 loci for blood lipids. Nature. 2010;466:707–13.
39. WHO. Prevention of cardiovascular disease: guidelines for assessment and management of total cardiovascular risk. 2007.

40. Willett W, Lenart E. Nutritional epidemiology. 3rd ed. New York: Oxford University Press; 2013.

41. Wirfalt E, Mattisson I, Johansson U, Gullberg B, Wallstrom P, Berglund G. A methodological report from the Malmo Diet and Cancer study: development and evaluation of altered routines in dietary data processing. Nutr J. 2002;1:3.

42. Voight BF et al. Plasma HDL cholesterol and risk of myocardial infarction: a mendelian randomisation study. Lancet. 2012;380:572–80. doi:10.1016/S0140-6736(12)60312-2.

43. Zia E, Hedblad B, Pessah-Rasmussen H, Berglund G, Janzon L, Engstrom G. Blood pressure in relation to the incidence of cerebral infarction and intracerebral hemorrhage. Hypertensive hemorrhage: debated nomenclature is still relevant. Stroke. 2007;38:2681–5. doi:10.1161/STROKEAHA.106.479725.

4

Effect of diets supplemented with different conjugated linoleic acid (CLA) isomers on protein expression in C57/BL6 mice

L. Della Casa[1], E. Rossi[1], C. Romanelli[1], L. Gibellini[2] and A. Iannone[1]*

Abstract

Background: The individual genetic variations, as a response to diet, have recently caught the attention of several researchers. In addition, there is also a trend to assume food containing beneficial substances, or to supplement food with specific compounds. Among these, there is the conjugated linoleic acid (CLA), which has been demonstrated to reduce fat mass and to increase lean mass, even though its mechanism of action is still not known. We investigated the effect of CLA isomers (CLA c9,t11 and CLA t10,c12) on the proteomic profile of liver, adipose tissue, and muscle of mouse, with the aim of verifying the presence of a modification in fat and lean mass, and to explore the mechanism of action.

Methods: C57/BL6 mice were fed for 2 months with different diets: (1) standard chow, (2) CLA c9,t11 diet, (3) CLA t10,c11 diet, (4) CLA isomers mixture diet, and (5) linoleic acid diet. The proteomic profile of liver, white adipose tissue, and muscle was investigated. Statistical significance of the spots with an intensity higher than twofold in expression compared to the control was tested using student's t test (two-tail).

Results: We found that both isomers modulate the proteomic profiles of liver, adipose tissue, and muscle by different mechanisms of action. Liver steatosis is mostly due to the isomer CLA t10,c12, since it alters the expression of lipogenetic proteins; it acts also reducing the adipose tissue and increasing fatty acid oxidation in muscle. Conversely, CLA c9,t11 has no relevant effects on liver and adipose tissue, but acts mostly on muscle, where it enhances muscular cell differentiation.

Conclusions: Administration of CLA in humans has to be carefully personalized, since even considering the presence of a species-specific effect, adverse effects might occur on long-term supplementation. Here we demonstrated that, in mouse, CLA is effective in reducing fat mass, but it also induces liver steatosis. The increase of lean mass is linked to an induction of cell proliferation, which, on long-term supplementation, might also lead to adverse effects.

Background

The individual genetic variations, as a response to diet, have recently caught the attention of several researchers leading to an impressive growth of the nutrigenomic field. The term nutrigenomic, in fact, refers to the associations between specific nutrients and genetic factor and in particular the way in which foods and food ingredients can influence the response to diet. The

study of these food-induced modifications may be at the level of single nucleotide polymorphisms rather than at the gene level [6].

In the last 10 years, there is a trend to assume food directly containing beneficial substances or to supplement food with specific compounds that naturally occur in milk and meat and, among these, conjugated linoleic acid (CLA) plays an important role. CLA is a mixture of positional and geometrical isomers of linoleic acid, with two conjugated unsaturated double bonds at various carbon positions in the fatty acid (FA) chain. Two major forms of CLA are CLA c9,t11 and CLA t10,c12, and a mixture of them has been used in most of the published

* Correspondence: anna.iannone@unimore.it
[1]"ProteoWork Lab", Dipartimento di Medicina Diagnostica, Clinica e di Sanità Pubblica, Università di Modena e Reggio Emilia, via Campi 287, 41125 Modena, Italy
Full list of author information is available at the end of the article

studies. CLA occurs naturally in many foods; however, the most important dietary sources are dairy products and other foods derived from ruminants animals [7]. In fact, CLA originates from two sources: one source is CLA formed during ruminal biohydrogenation of linoleic acid; the other source is CLA synthesized by the animal's tissues from vaccenic acid, another intermediate in the biohydrogenation of unsaturated fatty acids.

Nowadays, CLA is supplemented in ruminants fodder, not to improve meat quality but to obtain a milk rich in CLA, optimizing the presence of bio-active substances in the lipid fraction. Recently, CLA is also used in gyms as a supplement, in order to quickly obtain a good shape, since it is known that CLA is able to reduce fat body mass, significantly increasing the capacity of resistance to physical effort.

It has been already demonstrated that diet containing CLA reduced the amount of adipose fat in several species including rat, pig, hamster, chicken, and mouse [16]. Several studies suggest that CLA t10,c12 supplementation is able to reduce fat mass in mice and this is associated to a several-fold increase in the amount of fat stored in liver [8, 26].

In the present study, we, as well as others, have found that CLA had a steatosic effect in mice fed with different diets, containing 1 % CLA t10,c12 isomer, 1 % CLA c9,t11 isomer, and a 50:50 mixture of them. None of the published reports has used the proteomic approach to investigate the mechanism of action involved in such lipogenetic/lipolitic effect. We have simultaneously explored the proteome of liver and white adipose tissue (WAT), in order to consider the possibility that a CLA-containing diet may alter lipid metabolism through a modulation of proteins expression.

Methods
Animals and feeding protocols
For this study, 25 adult male C57/BL6 mice (Harlan Italy S.r.l., Udine, Italy), weighing 100–120 g, were kept in air-conditioned colony room (temperature 21 ± 1 °C, humidity 50 %) on a natural light-dark cycle and allowed diet and water ad libitum. Housing conditions and experiments were approved by the local Ethical Committee and by the Italian Ministry of Health (prot. # 121, followed by a modification, prot. # 38). The animals were acclimatized to our housing conditions for a week before being fed with different diets. For this purpose, they were divided into five groups receiving the following diets: control group (5 mice) fed with a repelletted purified complete 4RF21 chow; CLA c9,t11 group (5 mice) fed with a 1 % CLA c9,t11 isomer; CLA t10,c12 group (5 mice) fed with a 1 % CLA t10,c12 isomer; CLA mix group (5 mice) fed with a 1 % of a CLA isomer mixture of c9,t11 and t10,c12 (approx. 50:50); and

linoleic acid group (5 mice) fed with a 1 % linoleic acid. The dietary treatments were carried out for a 60-day period. All diets were purchased from Mucedola S.r.l., Settimo Milanese, Italy; CLA and CLA isomers were from NV-CHEK-PREP, INC (Elysian, MN, USA). The animals were kept in fasting conditions until the sacrifice. The mice were anesthetized by diethyl ether inhalation and after beheading, liver, muscle, and WAT were collected and immediately frozen in liquid nitrogen for proteomic and western blotting analysis. Additionally, hematoxylin and eosin staining was used to investigate the liver histopathology.

Proteomic analysis
Proteomic analysis has been performed on liver, muscle, and WAT of all the animals, and each sample was analyzed twice. Tissues (about 150 mg) were crushed to frozen powder by using a pestle under cooling in liquid nitrogen. The powder was incubated for 30 min. at 4 °C in 300 ml of extraction buffer (6 M urea, 2 M thiourea, 4 % CHAPS, 25 mM DTT, 0.2 % ampholytes), containing a protease inhibitor cocktail (Roche Complete EDTA-free, Roche Diagnostic, Milan). Samples were sonicated at 4 °C in rehydratation buffer (10 s/cycle, 3 cycles) for improving cell lysis and then centrifuged at 13,000×g for 1 h at 4 °C. The supernatant was collected, and sample concentration was estimated by Bio-Rad Protein Assay (Bio Rad, Hercules, CA, USA).

For isoelectric focusing (IEF), a total of 120 mg of proteins in rehydratation buffer with a final volume of 300 ml and trace of BPB were used in each IPG strips (17 cm, pH 3–10 NL). The strip rehydratation was performed for 12 h at 20 °C with a constant voltage (50 V) in Protean IEF Cell from Bio-Rad, and the isoelectric focusing was carried out by rapidly increasing the voltage until 250 V for 15 min, then linearly increasing the voltage from 250 to 10,000 V for the next 3 h; after that, focusing was continued at 10,000 V until 75,000 V/h and the temperature was maintained at 20 °C. After IEF, the IPG strips were equilibrated in a buffer containing 1 % m/v DTT by gentle shaking for 15 min. The proceedings were repeated with equilibration buffer containing 2.5 % m/v iodoacetamide (IAA).

The strips were applied on 12.5 % polyacrylamide gels, and SDS-PAGE was performed in a Protean Plus Dodeca Cell (Bio Rad, Hercules, CA, USA), that guarantees the reliability of data and reduces experimental variation. Indeed, this analysis has been performed in duplicate for each sample type and by the use of a electrophoretic dodeca cell, which allows to run simultaneously 12 gels under identical conditions, reducing the number of run variables and improving reproducibility. The electrophoresis was performed in TGS running buffer (250 mM Tris, 1.92 M glycine, 1 % SDS, pH 8.3) and was carried out with a constant current of 40 mA/gel for 30 min, followed by constant 500 V at 10 °C until BPB dye marker had reached the bottom of the gels. Proteins were visualized with a silver-staining modified protocol compatible with protein digestion and MS analysis (Bellei et al., [3]).

Image capture and analysis

All stained gel images were captured with a calibrated densitometer GS-800 (Bio Rad, Hercules, CA, USA) and then analyzed with PDQuest 7.3.1, 2D Image Analysis software program (BioRad, Hercules, CA, USA). The quantity of protein in each spot was normalized by the total valid spot intensity according to the manufacturer's instruction. Only the spots clearly showing a greater than twofold change in expression compared with controls were selected.

Statistical analysis

Spots with an intensity change higher than twofold in expression compared to the control were undergoing to statistical analysis. Statistical significance was tested using student's t test (two-tail) and the level selected was set at $P < 0.05$. Significantly varied protein spots were purified and sent to *CIGS* (*Centro Interdipartimentale Grandi Strumenti-University of Modena and Reggio Emilia*) for mass spectrometry analysis. Student's t test

was also used to evaluate the statistical significance of western blot data.

Tryptic in-gel digestion of proteins

Spots were excised from gels with a cut end pipette tip and transferred into a microcentrifuge tube (0.5 ml). Briefly, the gel pieces were incubated with 200 ml of 1:1 v/v solution 30 mM potassium hexacyano-ferrate (III) and 100 mM sodium thiosulphate in order to destain the spots. After two washes with 100 ml of water for 15 min, 100 ml of 100 % acetonitrile was added to restrict the gels. Proteins were reduced and alkylated adding sequentially 50 ml of a DTT solution (10 mM DTT in 25 mM ammonium bicarbonate) and 50 ml of a iodoacetamide solution (55 mM iodoacetamide in 25 mM ammonium bicarbonate). After 15 min in a Savant SpeedVac® concentrator (Thermo Fisher Scientific, USA), a volume of 30 ml trypsin (Promega, Madison WI, USA) solution (12.5 ng/μl in 25 mM ammonium bicarbonate) was added to the spots and the gel pieces were incubated at 4 °C for 30 min. After tryptic digestion, the solution was removed and the samples were incubated at 37 °C o/n in the same solution, without trypsin. Resulting supernatants, representing peptide solution, were recovered and dried in a SpeedVac® concentrator. Finally, 15 ml of a 5 % formic

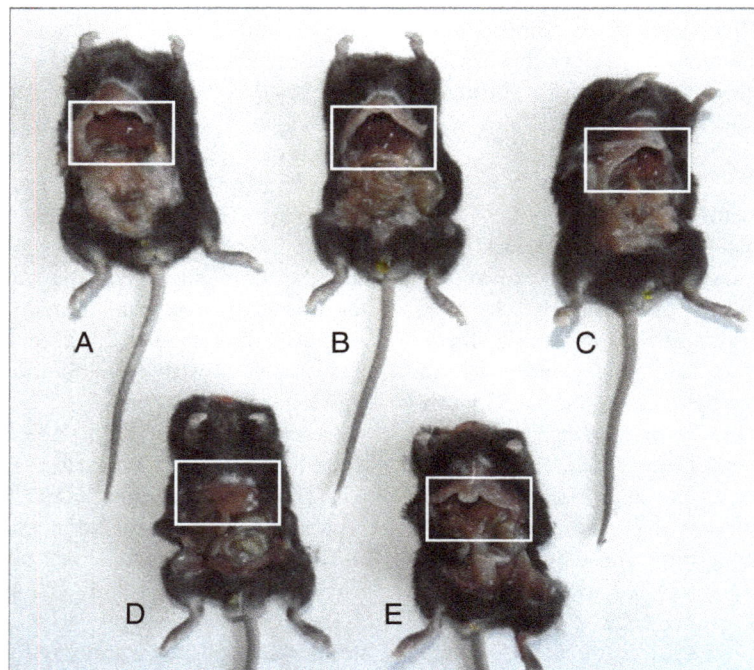

Fig. 1 Necroscopic analysis from mice fed with different diets. **a** Control mice. **b** Linoleic acid treated mice. **c** CLA c9,t11 treated mice. **d** CLA t10, c12 treated mice. **e** CLA mix (50:50) treated mice

acid solution was added and the mass spectrometry analysis of peptides was performed.

Mass spectrometry analysis and MS data processing

The spectrometer was an ESI-CHIP 6520 accurate mass Q-TOF-LC/MS (Agilent). Mass spectrometry (MS) data were automatically registered in PKL file format, analyzed, and searched with a mammalian public protein/genome database using MASCOT MS/MS ion search program version 2.2.06 (Matrix Science, http://www.matrixscience.com). Search parameters were set as follows: species rodents; enzyme trypsin; allowance of one missed cleavage site; carbamidomethylation as fixed modification; peptide tolerance ±0.8 Da; MS/MS tolerance error of ±0.4 Da; monoisotopic mass values and protein mass unrestricted. The score cut-off for 95 % protein identification was set to 37. Protein identification was repeated at least once using spots from different

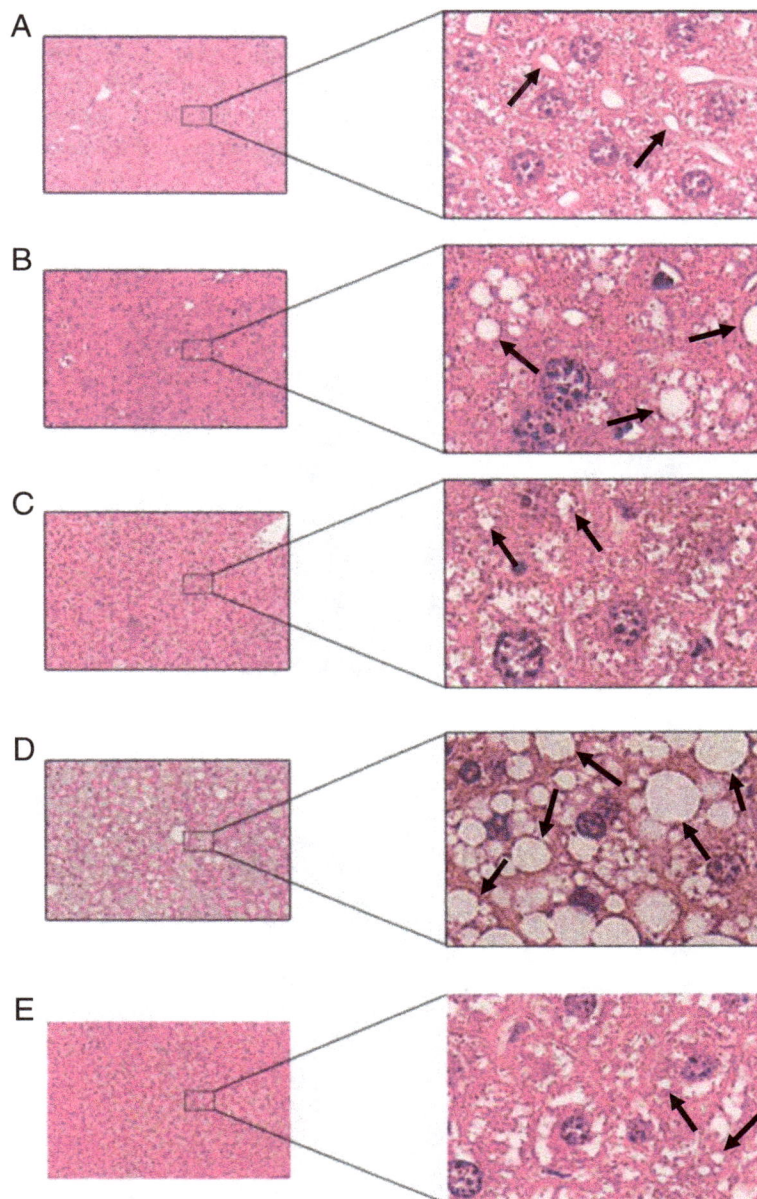

Fig. 2 Mice liver sections stained with Ehrlich's hematoxylin and eosin (H&E). The results of staining were viewed with ×4 and ×40 magnifications. *Arrows* indicate some lipid droplets. Control group fed with a repelletted standard chow (**a**). CLA mix group fed with a 1 % by weight of a mixture of CLA c9,t11 and CLA t10, c12 isomers (**b**). CLA c9,t11 group fed with a 1 % by weight of CLA c9,t11 isomer (**c**). CLA t10, c12 group fed with a 1 % by weight of CLA t10, c12 isomer (**d**). Linoleic acid group fed with a 1 % by weight of linoleic acid (**e**)

gels. The highest score hits among MASCOT search results were selected. The Micromass software (MassLynx™; version 4.1—2005) allows for the automated selection of peptides for fragmentation (and therefore primary structure determination) when peptide ions above a certain detection level are recorded. Since ESI normally produces multiply charged peptide ions, parameters were chosen so that only multiply charged ions were selected for sequencing by MS/MS. The database searched was the SwissProt 2012_07 version (536789 sequences; 190518892 residues).

Western blot analysis

Equivalent amounts (150 mg) of liver, muscle, and WAT were pulverized using a mortar in liquid nitrogen. The powder was dissolved in 300 ml of extraction buffer

(50 mM Tris pH 7.6, 150 mM NaCl, 1 % Triton X-100, 0,1 % SDS, 1 M PMSF) containing a protease inhibitor cocktail (Roche Complete EDTA-free, Roche Diagnostic, Milan) and incubated for 30 min at 4 °C. In order to improve cell lysis, samples were sonicated at 4 °C (10 s/cycle, 3 cycles) and then centrifuged at 13,000×g for 1 h at 4 °C. Protein concentration was calculated using Bio-Rad Protein Assay (Bio Rad, Hercules, CA, USA).

A total of 120 mg of proteins in loading buffer 1× (62.5 mM Tris–HCl pH 6.8, 2 % SDS, 10 % glycerol, 0.002 % bromophenol blue) was loaded on 13 % SDS-polyacrylamide gel, and electrophoresis was performed in TGS buffer. After electroblotting, performed at 200 mA for 2 h at 4 °C in transfer buffer 1× (25 mM Tris pH 8.8, 192 mM glycine, 20 % methanol), the proteins were transferred to a nitrocellulose membrane (Trans-Blot Transfer

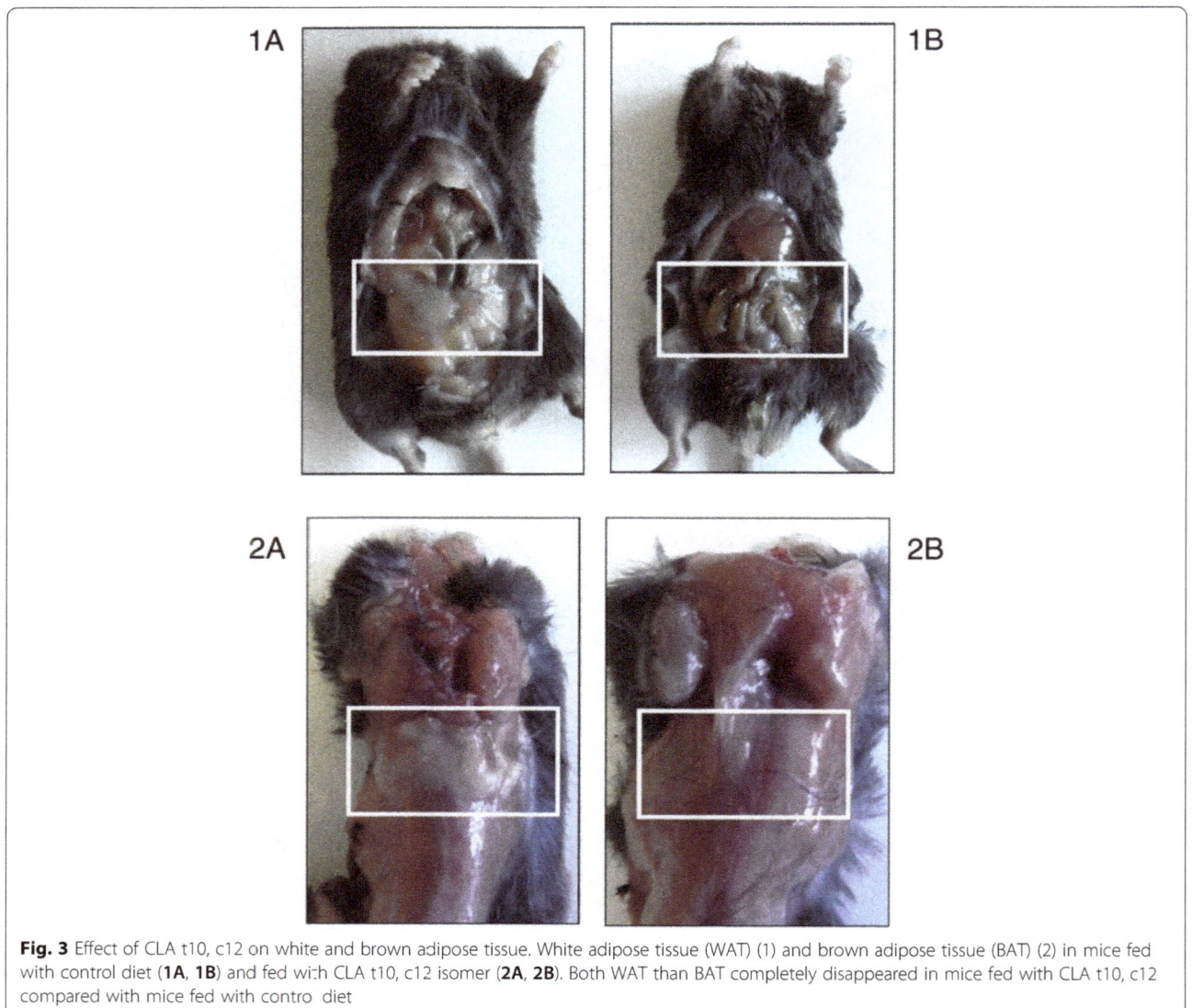

Fig. 3 Effect of CLA t10, c12 on white and brown adipose tissue. White adipose tissue (WAT) (1) and brown adipose tissue (BAT) (2) in mice fed with control diet (**1A**, **1B**) and fed with CLA t10, c12 isomer (**2A**, **2B**). Both WAT than BAT completely disappeared in mice fed with CLA t10, c12 compared with mice fed with control diet

Medium, Bio-Rad). Thus, the membranes were washed in 1× TBST (0.05 M Tris–HCl pH 7.4, 0.15 M NaCl, 0.1 % Tween 20) and blocked in blocking solution (5 % milk in 1 % TBST) for 1 h at room temperature. The proteins blocked on membrane support were then incubated with specific antibodies: polyclonal anti-peroxisomal acyl-coenzime A oxidase 1 (1:1000 dilution o/n, 4 °C, Abcam ab59964), polyclonal anti-ketohexokinase (1:100 diluition for 1 h, 4 °C, Abcam ab38281), polyclonal anti-galectin-3 (1: 300 dilution o/n, 4 °C, Santa Cruz sc-19283), and monoclonal anti-β actin (1:5000 dilution for 2 h, room temperature, Santa Cruz sc-47778) followed by 1 h incubation at room temperature with a secondary specific anti-goat, anti-rabbit, and anti-mouse conjugated to horseradish peroxidase. Anti-peroxisomal acyl-coenzime A oxidase 1 and anti-ketohexokinase were purchased from Abcam (Cambridge, UK), while anti-β actin and anti-galectin-3 were from Santa Cruz Biotechnology (Santa Cruz, CA, USA). Detection was carried out using chemiluminescence

blotting substrate (ECL Plus kit, Amersham Bioscences) following the manufacturer's instructions.

The autoradiographic slabs were captured with a calibrated densitometer GS-800 (Bio Rad, Hercules, CA, USA) and then analyzed with Quantity One software (Bio Rad, Hercules, CA, USA) for densitometric analysis.

Histological analysis

The liver tissue from different mice group was fixed in 4 % formalin, embedded in paraffin, and cut into 5-micron sections. The sections were stained with Ehrlich's hematoxylin and eosin (H&E). The results of staining were viewed and photographed with an Nikon Eclips 50i microscope (Nikon. Tokyo, Japan) using a Plan Fluor X lens and a Nikon Digital Sight DS-L1 camera with ×4 and ×40 magnifications. In order to evaluate the steatosis grade, a four-grade semi-quantitative method was used: grade 0, no or minimal steatosis (<5 %); grade 1, ≥5 % but <25 % mild steatosis; grade 2, ≥25 % but <50 % moderate steatosis; and grade 3, ≥50 % severe steatosis.

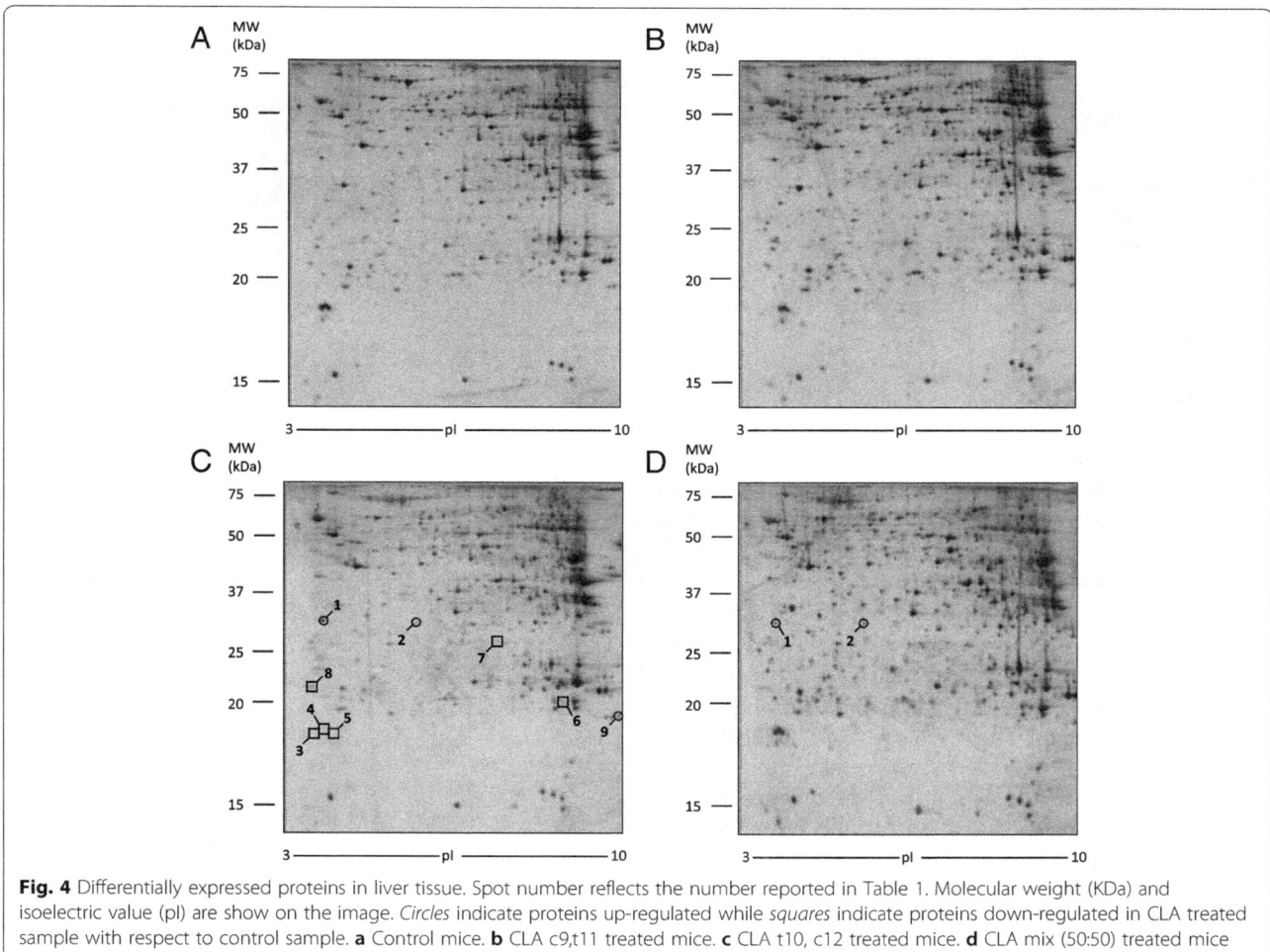

Fig. 4 Differentially expressed proteins in liver tissue. Spot number reflects the number reported in Table 1. Molecular weight (KDa) and isoelectric value (pI) are show on the image. *Circles* indicate proteins up-regulated while *squares* indicate proteins down-regulated in CLA treated sample with respect to control sample. **a** Control mice. **b** CLA c9,t11 treated mice. **c** CLA t10, c12 treated mice. **d** CLA mix (50:50) treated mice

Table 1 Proteins separated by 2-DE electrophoresis and identified by MS in liver tissue

Spot[a]	Identification (Swiss-Prot)[b]	Gene[c]	Sequence[c] coverage (%)	Spot[d] MW (KDa)	Spot[e] pI	Score[f]	Swiss[g] Prot access #
1	Annexin A5 (ANXA5)	Anxa5	72	35.8	4.8	631	P48036
2	Ketohexokinase (KHK)	Khk	61	32.8	5.8	475	P97328
3	Major urinary protein 6 (MUP6)	Mup6	52	20.7	4.7	284	P02762
4	Major urinary protein 2 (MUP2)	Mup2	73	20.7	4.9	227	P11589
5	Major urinary protein 2 (MUP2)	Mup2	51	20.7	4.9	96	P11589
6	Glutathione S-transferase P1 (GSTP1)	Gstp1	39	20.6	8.1	211	P19157
7	Bile salt sulfotransferase 2 (ST2A2)	Sult2a2	10	33.3	6.9	45	P50236
8	Alanine-TRNA ligase, cytoplasmic (SYAC)	Aars	1	106.9	5.4	34	Q8BGQ7
9	Peroxisomal acyl-coenzyme A oxidase 1 (ACOX1)	Acox1	15	74.7	8.6	177	Q9R0H0

[a]2-DE gel image spot number presented in Fig. 1
[b]Commonly used protein name
[c]Gene symbol
[d]Percentage of amino acid sequences for the identified protein
[e]MW and pI = molecular weight and isoelectric point of the protein
[f]Score = [−10 log (P)] and P is the absolute probability that the observed match between the experimental data and the database sequence is a random event, obtained with MASCOT for all proteins listed
[g]Swiss-Prot primary protein accession number

Results

Necroscopic analysis

After animal sacrifice, the necroscopic analysis showed that livers from CLA-fed mice were enlarged for fat accumulation (Fig. 1) and the degree of this phenomenon was different depending on the type of diet. Steatosis was mild in mice fed with CLA c9,t11 diet, moderate in mice fed with CLA mix diet, and severe in mice fed with CLA t10,c12 diet: this latter was also pale in comparison to all the other livers. This result was supported by the histological analysis (Fig. 2). Furthermore, in mice fed with CLA t10,c12, both white adipose tissue (WAT) and brown adipose tissue (BAT) completely disappeared as shown in Fig. 3.

Liver proteomic analysis

To evaluate whether the diet with different CLA isomers could modify proteins expression in liver tissue, we performed 2-DE analysis. Liver samples from mice treated with oleic acid were used as control, since no difference was found in proteomic profile between mice fed with oleic acid and mice fed with a standard chow. The analysis of control samples revealed a number of 900 spots on each gel, 450 of which were selected for PDQuest analysis (Fig. 4). Only the spots that were in accordance with the selection criterion (± twofold change) and statistically significant were excised and subjected to ESI-Q-TOF-MS/MS. All identified proteins are reported in Table 1. As shown in Fig. 4, in liver of mice treated with CLA t10,c12, a modification of nine spots was observed with respect to the control group. In particular, we found the down-regulation of six proteins: major urinary protein 6 (MUP6, spot # 3), major urinary protein 2 (MUP2, spot # 4 and 5), glutathione S-transferase

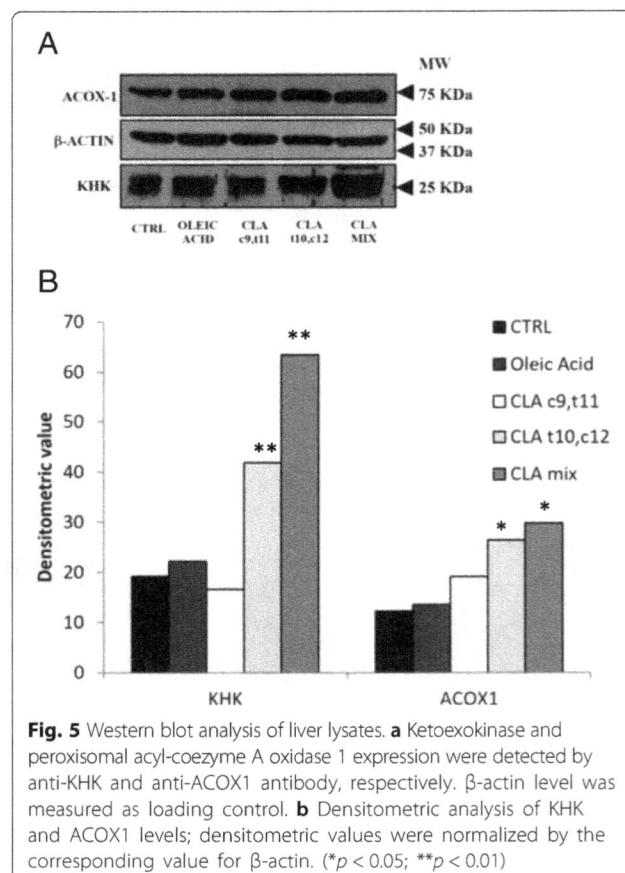

Fig. 5 Western blot analysis of liver lysates. **a** Ketoexokinase and peroxisomal acyl-coezyme A oxidase 1 expression were detected by anti-KHK and anti-ACOX1 antibody, respectively. β-actin level was measured as loading control. **b** Densitometric analysis of KHK and ACOX1 levels; densitometric values were normalized by the corresponding value for β-actin. (*$p < 0.05$; **$p < 0.01$)

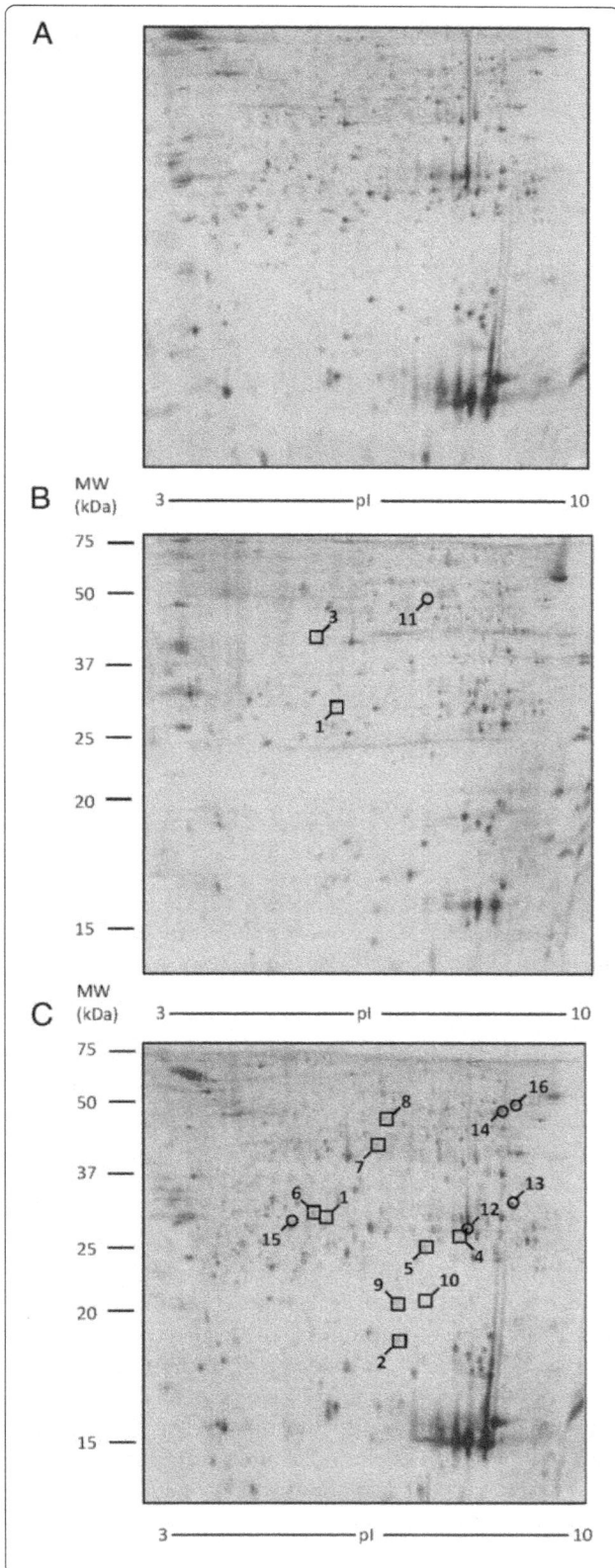

Fig. 6 2-DE images of proteins differentially expressed in white adipose tissue (WAT). Spot number reflects the number reported in Table 2. Molecular weight (KDa) and isoelectric value (pI) are show on the image. *Circles* indicate proteins up-regulated, while *squares* indicate proteins down-regulated in CLA treated sample with respect to control sample. **a** Control mice. **b** CLA c9,t11 treated mice. **c** CLA mix (50:50) treated mice

P1 (GSTP1, spot # 6), bile salt sulfotransferase 2 (ST2A2, spot # 7), alanine-TRNA ligase, and cytoplasmic (SYAC, spot # 8). Three proteins have been found up-regulated: annexin A5 (ANXA5, spot # 1), ketoexokinase (KHK, spot # 2), and peroxisomal acyl-coenzyme A oxidase 1 (ACOX1, spot # 9). Moreover, two of these proteins, ANXA5 and KHK, were also up-regulated in the liver of mice fed with CLA mix.

In order to confirm the result obtained by 2-DE analysis, we performed a western blot analysis using anti-ACOX1 and anti-KHK antibodies. As illustrated in Fig. 5, the expression of ACOX1 and KHK normalized by corresponding ß-actin was significantly increased in mice treated with CLA mix and CLA t10,c12.

Adipose tissue proteomic analysis

The study of proteomic profile of WAT extracts was performed using the same approach used for liver tissue (2-DE, spectrometry mass analysis and western blot confirmation). This analysis was not carried out in mice fed with CLA t10,c12, since no trace of adipose tissue was found in these mice. Also in this tissue, no differences were found between WAT proteomic profile from mice fed with oleic acid and mice fed with control diet: as a consequence, WAT samples from mice treated with oleic acid were used as control. The analysis of control samples revealed a number of 400 spots on each gel, 250 of which were selected for PDQuest analysis (Fig. 6). Only the spots that were in accordance with the selection criterion (± twofold change) and statistically significant were excised and subjected to ESI-Q-TOF-MS/MS (Table 2). Figure 6 shows that CLA mix treatment causes the down-regulation of nine proteins: indolethylamine *N*-methyltransferase (INMT, spot #1), destrin (DEST, spot # 2), glutathione S transferase theta-1 (GSTT1, spot # 4), mitochondrial peptide methionine sulfoxide reductase (MSRA, spot # 5), endoplasmic reticulum resistant protein 29 (ERP29, spot # 6), delta-amino levulinic acid dehydratase (HEM2, spot # 7), actin, alpha cardiac muscle 1 (ACTC, spot # 8), histone H2B type 1-B (H2B1B, spot # 9), and peptidyl prolyl cistrans isomerase C (PPIC, spot # 10). Five proteins were up-regulated: triosephosphate isomerase (TPIS, spot #12), galectin 3 (LEG-3 spot # 13), citrate synthase, mitochondrial (CISY, spot # 14), AP-5 complex subunit beta 1 (AP5B1, spot # 15), and elongation factor 1 alpha-1 (EF1A1, spot #16).

Table 2 Proteins separated by 2-DE electrophoresis and identified by MS in adipose tissue

Spot[a]	Identification (Swiss-Prot)[b]	Gene[c]	Sequence[c] coverage (%)	Spot[d] MW (KDa)	Spot[e] pI	Score[f]	Swiss[g] Prot access #
1	Indolethylamine N-methyltransferase (INMT)	iNMT	40	29.5	6.0	282	P40936
2	Destrin (DEST)	DSTN	41	18.4	8.2	126	Q9R0P5
3	Pyridoxal kinase (PDXK)	Pdxk	26	35.0	5.9	116	Q8K183
4	Glutathione S transferase theta-1 (GSTT1)	GSTT1	32	27.2	7.2	181	P30711
5	Mitochondrial peptide methionine sulfoxide reductase (MSRA)	Msra	19	23.8	6.7	27	Q9D6Y7
6	Endoplasmic reticulum resistant protein 29 (ERP29)	Erp29	29	25.7	5.7	185	P57759
7	Delta-amino levulinic acid dehydratase (HEM2)	Alad	20	36.0	6.3	263	P10518
8	Actin, alpha cardiac muscle 1 (ACTC)	Actc 1	38	41.8	5.2	606	P68033
9	Histone H2B type 1-B (H2B1B)	Hist1h2bb	27	13.8	10.3	67	Q64475
10	Peptidyl prolyl cistrans isomerase C (PPIC)	Ppic	14	22.8	7.0	172	P30412
11	2 Amino 3 ketobutyrate CoA ligase (KBL)	Goat	39	42.8	6.5	2133	O88986
12	Triosephosphate isomerase (TPIS)	Tip1	70	32.2	5.6	1581	P17751
13	Galectin 3 (LEG3)	Lgals3	29	27.6	8.5	500	P16110
14	Citrate synthase mitochondrial (CISY)	Cs	26	49.0	8.2	293	Q9CZU6
15	AP-5 complex subunit beta 1 (AP5B1)	Ap5b1	1	94.0	5.7	22	Q3TAP4
16	Elongation factor 1 alpha-1 (EF1A1)	Ef1a1	29	50.1	9.1	500	P10126

[a]2-DE gel image spot number presented in Fig. 1
[b]Commonly used protein name
[c]Gene symbol
[d]Percentage of amino acid sequences for the identified protein
[e]MW and pI = molecular weight and isoelectric point of the protein
[f]Score = [−10 log (P)] and P is the absolute probability that the observed match between the experimental data and the database sequence is a random event, obtained with MASCOT for all proteins listed
[g]Swiss-Prot primary protein accession number

Mice fed with a CLA c9,t11 isomer diet showed a down-regulation of indolethylamine N-methyltransferase (INMT, spot #1) and pyridoxal kinase (PDXK, spot #3) and an up-regulation of 2-amino-3-ketobutyrate coenzyme A ligase (KBL, spot # 11).

An anti-LEG-3 antibody was used for western blot analysis in order to confirm the 2-DE results. As shown in Fig. 7, the expression of LEG-3, normalized by corresponding β-actin, was significantly increased in mice treated with CLA mix.

Muscle tissue proteomic analysis

Extracts from muscle tissue were processed for proteomic analysis, mass spectrometry analysis, and finally for western blot analysis, to confirm the results. Since no differences were found between muscle proteomic profile from mice fed with oleic acid and mice fed with control diet, muscle samples from mice treated with oleic acid were used as control. In each gel, 700 spots were revealed and 420 of these selected for PDQuest analysis. Only the spots statistically different from control were excised and subjected to ESI-Q-TOF-MS/MS. Results from the MS analysis are reported in Table 3. CLA c9,t11 treatment modified the expression of two proteins, phosphoglucomutase-1 (PGM1, spot # 1) that

was down-regulated and galectin-1 (LEG1, spot # 4) that was up-regulated. Furthermore, the proteomic profile of mice fed with CLA t10,c12 shows the up-regulation of three proteins: two isoforms of fatty acid-binding protein, heart (FABPH, spots # 2 and 3) and fumarate hydratatase, mitochondrial (FUMH, spot # 5). The different protein expressions are also indicated in Fig. 8.

The western blot analysis, performed with an anti-LEG1 antibody, confirmed these results (Fig. 9).

Discussion

In the present study, we evaluated the proteomic profile of liver and WAT, in order to identify a proteomic pattern related to modifications that occurred after the administration of diet supplemented with different CLA isomers. We found differential effects using the separate isomers in comparison to the mixture of them: in this case, we have to take into account that in the mixture the amount of the individual isomers is the half, being the final concentration always 1 %. For interpretation of data obtained through proteomic analysis, we categorized all identified proteins into three groups: proteins disregulated in liver tissue, proteins disregulated in WAT, and proteins disregulated in muscle.

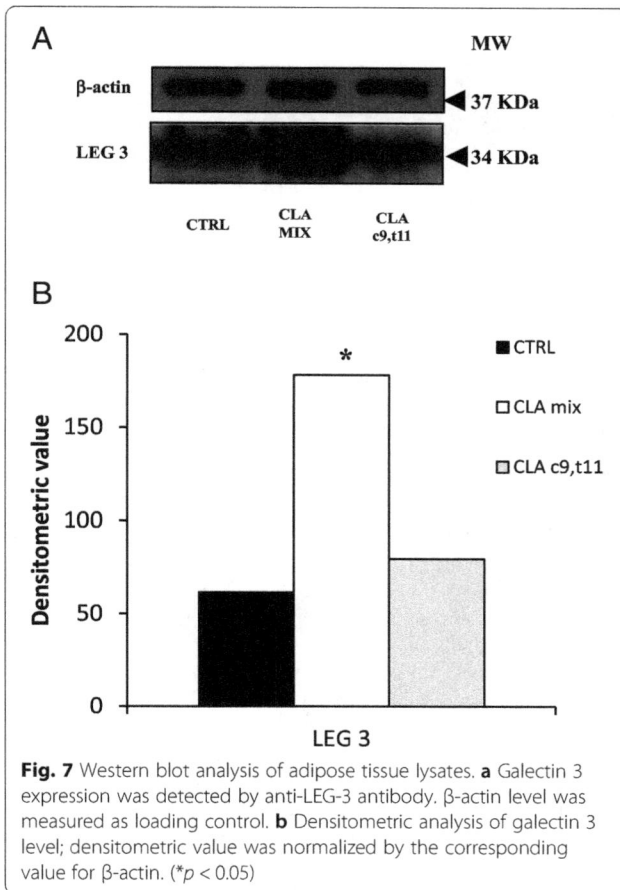

Fig. 7 Western blot analysis of adipose tissue lysates. **a** Galectin 3 expression was detected by anti-LEG-3 antibody. β-actin level was measured as loading control. **b** Densitometric analysis of galectin 3 level; densitometric value was normalized by the corresponding value for β-actin. (*$p < 0.05$)

Proteins disregulated in the liver tissue

We found an up-regulation of ketohexokinase (KHK) in mice fed with CLA t10,c12 isomer. Fructose is metabolized in the liver by fructokinase (KHK), which uses ATP to phosphorylate fructose to fructose-1-phosphate. Fructokinase exists in two isoforms: fructokinase C and fructokinase A, where fructokinase C is the principal isoform in liver and rapidly leads to an intracellular ATP depletion; fructokinase A, instead, metabolizes fructose slowly, without significant ATP consumption [15]. The metabolism of fructose results in nucleotide turnover and uric acid generation that may have a role in inducing mitochondrial oxidative stress and fat accumulation [20, 21]. The up-regulation of KHK was demonstrated in mice fed with a high-fat diet and correlates with steatosis and obesity: for this reason, it has been proposed as an early marker of obesity [25]. Another study shows that the metabolism of fructose by KHK results in intracellular production of ureic acid and that its blockade in intracellular compartment could inhibit the increase in fat accumulation due to fructose [22].

In animal cells, mitochondria, as well as peroxisomes, oxidizes long chain fatty acids via β-oxidation [28]. When cytosolic fatty acids accumulate as a consequence of an impairment of oxidative capacity in mitochondria, alternative pathways in the peroxisomes (β-oxidation) and in microsomes (ω-oxidation) are activated. In peroxisomal β-oxidation, ACOX-1 catalyzes the initial oxidation of very long fatty acids to acyl-CoA. In non-alcoholic fatty liver disease (NAFLD), where a triglyceride accumulation in hepatocytes (hepatic steatosis) is present, Kohjima et al. demonstrated that the expression of ACOX-1 was increased twofold compared with that in the normal liver [19]. The up-regulation of ACOX-1 with CLA t10,c12 isomer that we observed suggested an increase in fatty acid β-oxidation in peroxisomes.

The increase of ACOX-1 by dietary CLA has been previously described by Belury et al. [4] as a result of its activity on PPAR alpha [23], and in addition, it has been shown that it undergoes peroxisomal beta oxidation probably inducing PPAR alpha [1] and may interfere with other peroxisomal beta oxidation substrate [14].

Major urinary protein (MUP) family members are secreted proteins produced predominantly from the liver

Table 3 Proteins separated by 2-DE electrophoresis and identified by MS in muscle tissue

Spot[a]	Identification (Swiss-Prot)[b]	Gene[c]	Sequence[c] coverage (%)	Spot[d] MW (KDa)	Spot[e] pI	Score[f]	Swiss[g] Prot access #
1	Phosphoglucomutase-1 (PGM1)	Pgm1	45	61.7	6.1	816	Q9DOF7
2	Fatty acid-binding protein, heart (FABPH)	Fabp3	59	14.8	6.1	790	P11404
3	Fatty acid-binding protein, heart (FABPH)	Fabp3	66	14.8	6.1	533	P11404
4	Galectin-1 (LEG1)	Lgals1	31	15.2	5.3	135	P16045
5	Fumarate hydratase, mitochondrial (FUMH)	Fh	1	54.5	9.1	15	P97807

[a]2-DE gel image spot number presented in Fig. 1
[b]Commonly used protein name
[c]Gene symbol
[d]Percentage of amino acid sequences for the identified protein
[e]MW and pI = molecular weight and isoelectric point of the protein
[f]Score = [−10 log (P)] and P is the absolute probability that the observed match between the experimental data and the database sequence is a random event, obtained with MASCOT for all proteins listed
[g]Swiss-Prot primary protein accession number

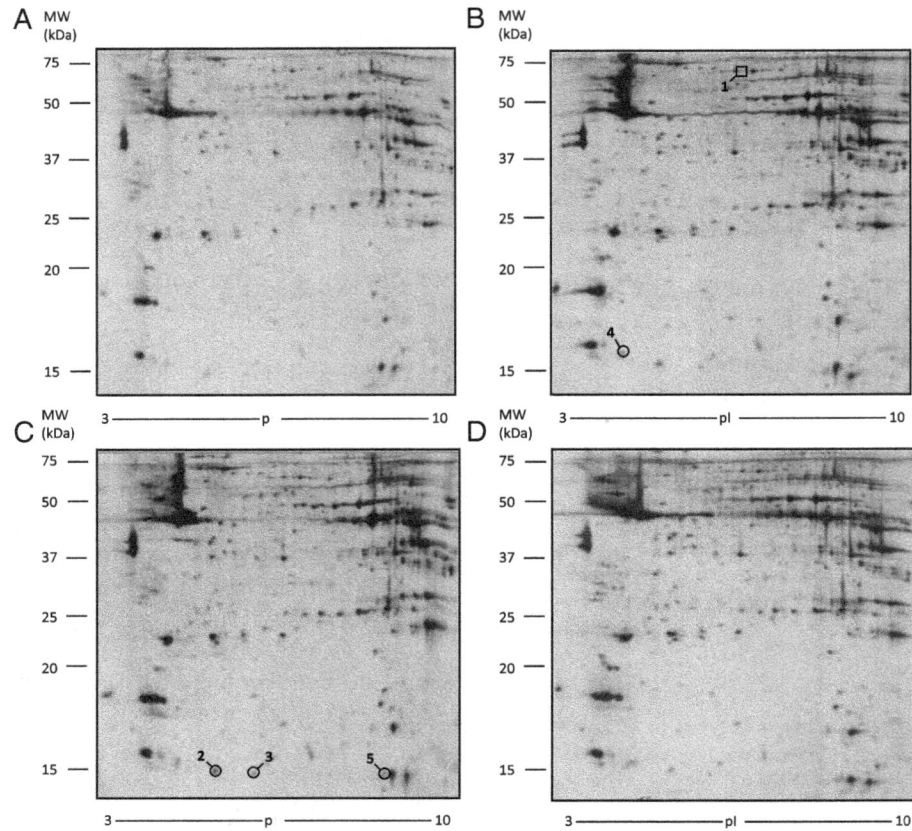

Fig. 8 Differentially expressed proteins in muscle tissue. Spot number reflects the number reported in Table 3. Molecular weight (KDa) and isoelectric value (pI) are show on the image. *Circles* indicate proteins up-regulated, while a square indicates proteins down-regulated in CLA treated sample with respect to control sample. **a** Control mice. **b** CLA c9,t11 treated mice. **c** CLA t10, c12 treated mice. **d** CLA mix (50:50) treated mice

and excreted into urine [9, 30]. Is well known that MUPs carry small hydrophobic ligands such as pheromones [13, 33], while their endocrine role is less clear. Scientists found that in addition to mediating chemical signaling, circulatory MUP1 regulates glucose and lipid metabolism in animals. Indeed, overexpression of MUP1 suppresses the expression of both glucogenic and lipogenic genes in liver [12, 35]. The role of the other MUPs member is not well documented and therefore requires further studies. In our experiments we found, in mice fed with CLA t10,c12, the down-regulation of other two members of MUP family, MUP2 and MUP6. None of the published reports highlights the effects of MUP2 and MUP6 on lipidic and glucidic metabolism; for this reason, we suggest that a down-regulation of MUP2 and MUP6 may have a role in the genesis of steatosis and they could be considered as markers of steatosis.

It has to be mentioned that liver steatosis by dietary CLA seems to be restricted to mice, since in models of obesity in rats, such as the Zucker, that develop fatty liver, CLA has actually an opposite effect [24], probably mediated by PPAR alpha-mediated activity [27].

Proteins disregulated in WAT

In WAT tissue, only the CLA mix treatment caused the up-regulation of three proteins related to lipid metabolisms: triosephosphate isomerase (TPIS), citrate synthase, mitochondrial (CISY), and galectin 3 (LEG-3). We suppose that the increased expression of these three proteins was determined by the effect of CLA t10,c12 isomer, since the CLA c9,t11 isomer did not modify the proteomic profile of WAT tissue.

The up-regulation of TPIS was demonstrated in rat fed with high-fat lipid diet by Saggerson [29]. In our experiments, we found the up-regulation of this protein in mice fed with CLA mix.

The acetyl-CoA, in order to be converted into fatty acids, must leave the mitochondria as citrate, and this reaction is operated by the CISY. Therefore, the citrate is cleaved into acetyl-CoA and oxaloacetate. Dietary supplementation with long-chain fatty monounsaturated

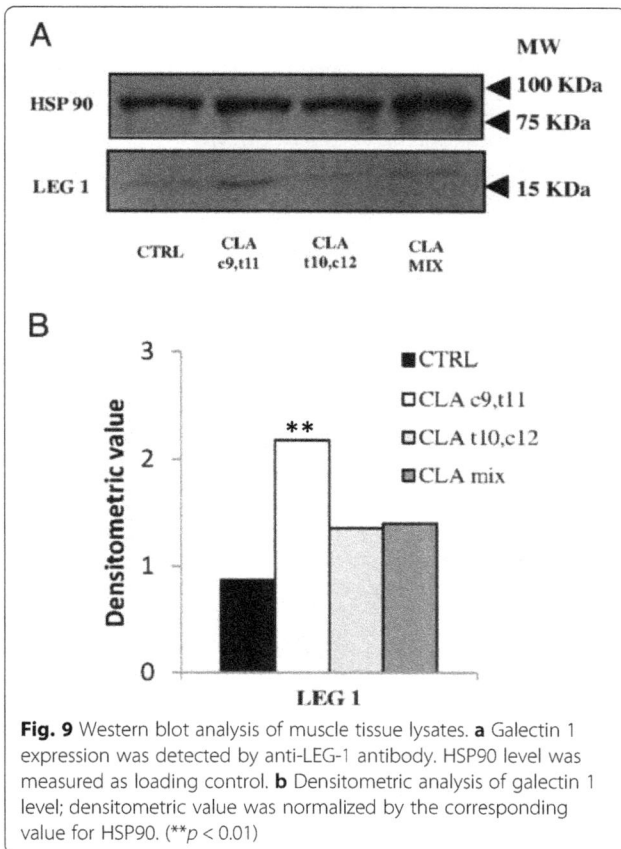

Fig. 9 Western blot analysis of muscle tissue lysates. **a** Galectin 1 expression was detected by anti-LEG-1 antibody. HSP90 level was measured as loading control. **b** Densitometric analysis of galectin 1 level; densitometric value was normalized by the corresponding value for HSP90. (**$p < 0.01$)

fatty acids significantly increases the CISY expression [34]. The up-regulation of CISY, in CLA mix treated mice, that we observed explains the increased acetyl-CoA bioavailability for fatty acids synthesis, and therefore, this protein can be considered as a possible marker of accumulation of fatty acids.

Galectin-3 is a 30-KDa lectin which has a C-terminal carbohydrate-recognition domain and an N-terminal domain comprising multiple repeat sequences. Kiwaki et al. demonstrated that adipose tissue synthesized galectin-3 and that the up-regulation of this protein might play a role in adipose tissue growth induced by high-fat diets [18]. In our experiments, we found the up-regulation of this protein in mice fed with CLA mix.

Proteins disregulated in muscle

In muscle tissues analyzed, we found a disregulation of three proteins: fatty acid-binding protein, heart (FABPH), fumarate hydratase mitochondrial (FUMH), and galectin-1 (LEG1).

More in detail, FABPH is a cytosolic protein belonging to the fatty acid-binding proteins family (FABPs), small ubiquitous proteins (~15 KDa) that have an high affinity with very long chain fatty acid. FABPH is expressed in cardiac and muscular tissue and it is involved in the

mitochondrial β-oxidation as very long chain fatty acids and acyl-CoA intracellular transporter. Tan et al. [32] demonstrated that FABPH may also interact with PPARα, nuclear receptors that induced mitochondrial and peroxisomal β-oxidation. The observed up-regulation of FABPH with CLA t10,c12 isomer suggests an increase in fatty acid β-oxidation in peroxisomes.

CLA t10,c12 induces also the up-regulation of FUMH, an enzyme involved in Krebs cycles that converts fumarate to malate: this could indicate an increase of lipid catabolism and a greater ATP availability in muscle tissues.

LEG1 belongs to a family of carbohydrates binding protein and it is primarily expressed in skeletal muscle [2]. Goldring et al. demonstrated that the addiction of LEG1 to cultures of dermal fibroblasts can induce their conversion into muscle cells [10, 11] and the presence of galectin-1 in cultured medium of mesenchymal human stem cells increases than 30 % the cells differentiation [31]. In our experiments, the up-regulation of LEG1 by CLA c9,t11 treatment could therefore indicate an enhancement in muscular cells differentiation, leading to an increase in lean body mass. Moreover, these data may have an important implication regarding muscle tissue repair after exercise [5]. It may also explain the effect of CLA on skeletal muscle metabolism as recently reviewed [17].

Conclusions

The mechanism of steatogenic action of CLA is clearly mediated by the increased expression of lipogenetic proteins: the up-regulation of ketohexokinase correlates with steatosis and obesity, while the up-regulation of the peroxisomal acyl-coenzyme A oxidase-1 suggests an increase in fatty acid β-oxidation in peroxisomes. The down-regulation of the major urinary proteins could be responsible for a PPAR-γ mediated lipogenesis. The two CLA isomers have different steatogenic effect, being the most evident effect due to the CLA t10, c12 isomer. Being both the tested isomers present in commercially available CLA mixture, we suggest caution in using it as a supplement in human diet. The effect on body lean mass seems to be exclusively due to the isomer CLA c9,t11.

Abbreviations
ACOX1: Peroxisomal acyl-coenzyme A oxidase 1; ACTC: Actin, alpha cardiac muscle; ANXA5: Annexin A5; AP5B1: AP-5 complex subunit beta 1; BAT: Brown adipose tissue; CISY: Citrate synthase, mitochondrial; CLA: Conjugated linoleic acid; DEST: Destrin; EF1A1: Elongation factor 1 alpha-1; ERP29: Endoplasmic reticulum resistant protein 29; FABPH: Fatty acid-binding protein, heart; FUMH: Fumarate hydratatase, mitochondrial; GSTP1: Glutathione S-transferase P1; GSTT1: Glutathione S transferase theta-1; H2B1B: Histone H2B type 1-B; HEM2: Delta-amino levulinic acid dehydratase; INMT: Indolethylamine N-methyltransferase; KBL: 2-Amino-3-ketobutyrate coenzyme A ligase; KHK: Ketoexokinase; LEG: Galectin; MSRA: Mitochondrial peptide methionine sulfoxide reductase; MUP: Major urinary protein; PDXK: Pyridoxal kinase; PGM1: Phosphoglucomutase-1; PPIC: Peptidyl prolyl

cistrans isomerase C; ST2A2: Bile salt sulfotransferase 2; SYAC: Alanine-TRNA ligase, cytoplasmic; TPIS: Triosephosphate isomerase; TFNA ligase: Cytoplasmic; WAT: White adipose tissue

Acknowledgements
The authors thank Dott. Luca Fabbiani for technical assistance in histological analysis.

Funding
This research was supported by institutional funds.

Authors' contributions
LDC and AI conceived the study and designed the experiments. ER, LDC, and CR conducted the animal studies and the proteomic analysis. LG analyzed the data. AI and ER wrote the paper. All authors read and approved the final manuscript.

Competing interests
The authors declare that they have no competing interests.

Author details
[1]"ProteoWork Lab", Dipartimento di Medicina Diagnostica, Clinica e di Sanità Pubblica, Università di Modena e Reggio Emilia, via Campi 287, 41125 Modena, Italy. [2]Dipartimento Chirurgico, Medico, Odontoiatrico e di Scienze Morfologiche con Interesse Trapiantologico, Oncologico e di Medicina Rigenerativa, Università di Modena e Reggio Emilia, via Campi 287, 41125 Modena, Italy.

References
1. Banni S, Petroni A, Blasevich M, Carta G, Angioni E, Murru E, Day BW, Melis MP, Spada S, Ip C. Detection of conjugated C16 PUFAs in rat tissues as possible partial beta-oxidation products of naturally occurring conjugated linoleic acid and its metabolites. Biochim Biophys Acta. 2004;1682:120–7.
2. Barondes SH, Cooper DN, Gitt MA, Leffler H. Galectins. Structure and function of a large family of animal lectins. J Biol Chem. 1994;269:20807–10.
3. Bellei E, Rossi E, Lucchi L, Uggeri S, Albertazzi A, Tomasi A, Iannone A. Proteomic analysis of early urinary biomarkers of renal changes in type 2 diabetic patients. Proteomics Clin. Appl. 2008;2(4):478–91.
4. Belury MA, Moya-Camarena SY, Liu K-L, Vanden Heuvel JP. Dietary conjugated linoleic acid induces peroxisome-specific enzyme accumulation and ornithine decarboxylase activity in mouse liver. J Nutr Biochem. 1997;8:579–84.
5. Cerri DG, Rodrigues LC, Stowell SR, Araujo DD, Coelho MC, Oliveira SR, Bizario JC, Cummings RD, Dias-Baruffi M, Costa MC. Degeneration of dystrophic or injured skeletal muscles induces high expression of galectin-1. Glycobiology. 2008;18:842–50.
6. Chadwick R. Nutrigenomics, individualism and public health. Proc Nutr Soc. 2004;63:161–6.
7. Chin SF, Liu W, Storkson JM, Ha YL, Pariza MW. Dietary sources of conjugated dienoic isomers of linoleic acids, a newly recognized class of anticarcinogens. J Fodd Compons Anal. 1992;5:185–97
8. Clement L, Poirier H, Niot I, Bocher V, Guerre-Millo M, Krief S, Staels B, Besnard P. Dietary trans-10, cis-12 conjugated linoleic acid induces hyperinsulinemia and fatty liver in the mouse. J Lipid Res. 2002;43:1400–9.
9. Finlayson JS, Asofsky R, Potter M, Runner CC. Major urinary protein complex of normal mice: origin. Science. 1965;149:981–2.
10. Goldring K, Jones GE, Thiagarajah R, Watt DJ. The effect of galectin-1 on the differentiation of fibroblasts and myoblasts in vitro. J Cell Sci. 2002;115:355–66.
11. Goldring K, Jones GE, Watt DJ. A factor implicated in the myogenic conversion of nonmuscle cells derived from the mouse dermis. Cell Transplant. 2000;9:519–29.
12. Hui X, Zhu W, Wang Y, Lam KS, Zhang J, Wu D, Kraegen EW, Li Y, Xu A. Major urinary protein-1 increases energy expenditure and improves glucose intolerance through enhancing mitochondrial function in skeletal muscle of diabetic mice. J Biol Chem. 2009;284:14050–7.
13. Hurst JL. Female recognition and assessment of males through scent. Behav Brain Res. 2009;200:295–303.
14. Iannone A, Petroni A, Murru E, Cordeddu L, Carta G, Melis MP, Bergamini S, Casa LD, Cappiello L, Carissimi R, et al. Impairment of 8-iso-PGF(2ALPHA) isoprostane metabolism by dietary conjugated linoleic acid (CLA). Prostaglandins Leukot Essent Fatty Acids. 2009;80:279–87.
15. Ishimoto T, Lanaspa MA, Le MT, Garcia GE, Diggle CP, Maclean PS, Jackman MR, Asipu A, Roncal-Jimenez CA, Kosugi T, et al. Opposing effects of fructokinase C and A isoforms on fructose-induced metabolic syndrome in mice. Proc Natl Acad Sci U S A. 2012;109:4320–5.
16. Kelley DS, Erickson KL. Modulation of body composition and immune cell functions by conjugated linoleic acid in humans and animal models: benefits vs. risks. Lipids. 2003;38:377–86.
17. Kim Y, Kim J, Whang KY, Park Y. Impact of conjugated linoleic acid (CLA) on skeletal muscle metabolism. Lipids. 2016;51:159–78.
18. Kiwaki K, Novak CM, Hsu DK, Liu FT, Levine JA. Galectin-3 stimulates preadipocyte proliferation and is up-regulated in growing adipose tissue. Obesity. 2007;15:32–9.
19. Kohjima M, Enjoji M, Higuchi N, Kato M, Kotoh K, Yoshimoto T, Fujino T, Yada M, Yada R, Harada N, et al. Re-evaluation of fatty acid metabolism-related gene expression in nonalcoholic fatty liver disease. Int J Mol Med. 2007;20:351–8.
20. Lanaspa MA, Cicerchi C, Garcia G, Li N, Roncal-Jimenez CA, Rivard CJ, Hunter B, Andres-Hernando A, Ishimoto T, Sanchez-Lozada LG, et al. Counteracting roles of AMP deaminase and AMP kinase in the development of fatty liver. PloS one. 2012a;7:e48801.
21. Lanaspa MA, Sanchez-Lozada LG, Choi YJ, Cicerchi C, Kanbay M, Roncal-Jimenez CA, Ishimoto T, Li N, Marek G, Duranay M, et al. Uric acid induces hepatic steatosis by generation of mitochondrial oxidative stress: potential role in fructose-dependent and -independent fatty liver. J Biol Chem. 2012b; 287:40732-40744.
22. Lanaspa MA, Sanchez-Lozada LG, Cicerchi C, Li N, Roncal-Jimenez CA, Ishimoto T, Le M, Garcia GE, Thomas JB, Rivard CJ, et al. Uric acid stimulates fructokinase and accelerates fructose metabolism in the development of fatty liver. PloS one. 2012c;7:e47948.
23. Moya-Camarena SY, Vanden Heuvel JP, Blanchard SG, Leesnitzer LA, Belury MA. Conjugated linoleic acid is a potent naturally occurring ligand and activator of PPARalpha. J Lipid Res. 1999;40:1426–33.
24. Nagao K, Inoue N, Wang YM, Shirouchi B, Yanagita T. Dietary conjugated linoleic acid alleviates nonalcoholic fatty liver disease in Zucker (fa/fa) rats. J Nutr. 2005;135:9–13.
25. Oh TS, Kwon EY, Choi JW, Choi MS, Yun JW. Time-dependent hepatic proteome analysis in lean and diet-induced obese mice. J Microbiol Biotechnol. 2011;21:1211–27.
26. Park Y, Storkson JM, Albright KJ, Liu W, Pariza MW. Evidence that the trans-10, cis-12 isomer of conjugated linoleic acid induces body composition changes in mice. Lipids. 1999;34:235–41.
27. Piras A, Carta G, Murru E, Lopes PA, Martins SV, Prates JA, Banni S. Effects of dietary CLA on n-3 HUFA score and N-acylethanolamides biosynthesis in the liver of obese Zucker rats. Prostaglandins Leukot Essent Fatty Acids. 2015;98:15–9.
28. Reddy JK, Hashimoto T. Peroxisomal beta-oxidation and peroxisome proliferator-activated receptor alpha: an adaptive metabolic system. Annu Rev Nutr. 2001;21:193–230.
29. Saggerson ED, Greenbaum AL. The effect of dietary and hormonal conditions on the activities of glycolytic enzymes in rat epididymal adipose tissue. Biochem J. 1969;115:405–17.
30. Shaw PH, Held WA, Hastie ND. The gene family for major urinary proteins: expression in several secretory tissues of the mouse. Cell. 1983;32:755–61.
31. Shoji H, Deltour L, Nakamura T, Tajbakhsh S, Poirier F. Expression pattern and role of galectin1 during early mouse myogenesis. Dev Growth Differ. 2009;51:607–15.
32. Tan NS, Shaw NS, Vinckenbosch N, Liu P, Yasmin R, Desvergne B, Wahli W, Noy N. Selective cooperation between fatty acid binding proteins and peroxisome proliferator-activated receptors in regulating transcription. Mol Cell Biol. 2002;22:5114–27.
33. Tirindelli R, Dibattista M, Pifferi S, Menini A. From pheromones to behavior. Physiol Rev. 2009;89:921–56.
34. Yang ZH, Miyahara H, Iwasaki Y, Takeo J, Katayama M. Dietary supplementation with long-chain monounsaturated fatty acids attenuates obesity-related metabolic dysfunction and increases expression of PPAR gamma in adipose tissue in type 2 diabetic KK-Ay mice. Nutr Metab. 2013;10:16.

5

Effect of different concentrations of omega-3 fatty acids on stimulated THP-1 macrophages

B. Allam-Ndoul[1], F. Guénard[1], O. Barbier[2] and M-C Vohl[1*]

Abstract

Background: Inflammation plays a central role in chronic diseases occurring in the contemporary society. The health benefits of omega-3 (n-3) fatty acids (FAs), mostly eicosapentaenoic acid (EPA) and docosahexaenoic acid (DHA), have been reported. However, their mechanisms of action are poorly understood. We explored dose and time effects of EPA, DHA, and a mixture of EPA + DHA on the expression of inflammatory genes in stimulated macrophages.

Methods: Lipopolysaccharide was used to stimulate human THP-1 macrophages. Cells were incubated in different conditions in the presence of n-3 FAs and LPS, and mRNA levels of inflammatory genes were measured by real-time PCR. Cytokine levels in culture media were measured.

Results: The mixture of EPA + DHA had a more effective inhibitory effect than either DHA or EPA alone, DHA being more potent than EPA. For both EPA and DHA, 75 μM of FAs had a more important anti-inflammatory effect than 10 or 50 μM. For gene expression, EPA had the greater action during the post-incubation (after LPS treatment) condition while DHA and EPA + DHA were more potent during the co-incubation (n-3 FAs and LPS). Cytokine concentrations decreased more markedly in the co-incubation condition.

Conclusions: These results suggest that in stimulated macrophages, expression levels of genes involved in inflammation are influenced by the dose, the type of n-3 FAs, and the time of incubation.

Keywords: EPA, DHA, LPS, Inflammation, mRNA

Background

Inflammation is a biological response to harmful chemical or physical stimuli. The purpose of an acute resolving inflammatory response is to protect the human body from damage and to re-establish homeostasis [24]. Several conditions such as inflammatory bowel disease, cardiovascular diseases (CVD), Alzheimer's disease, or cancers are caused by a persistent inflammation and their prevalence increase due to inappropriate responses arising in a chronic manner along with them [9, 20].

Fatty acids (FAs) are carboxylic acids with a variable number of carbon atoms, building a hydrocarbon chain, which finishes with carboxyl and methyl groups. Polyunsaturated FAs (PUFAs) contain more than one double bond in their backbone. Omega-6 (n-6) and omega-3 (n-3) are the two main families of FAs. Linoleic acid (LA) and alpha-linolenic acid (ALA) are, respectively, the precursors of n-6 and n-3 FAs. These FAs are called essential because they cannot be produced by the body and must be provided by the diet. The main FAs derived from n-6 FAs is arachidonic acid producing rather pro-inflammatory eicosanoids. FAs derived from ALA, namely eicosapentaenoic acid (EPA; 20:5n − 3) and docosahexaenoic acid (DHA; 22:6n − 3), produce eicosanoids with a less inflammatory profile [4]. Human being synthetizes EPA and DHA from their dietary precursor ALA at a very low rate. This makes dietary intake of EPA and DHA a more efficient source for their assimilation. In fact, their availability are increased when they

* Correspondence: marie-claude.vohl@fsaa.ulaval.ca
[1]Institute of Nutrition and Functional Foods (INAF), Laval University, Pavillon des Services, 2440 Hochelaga Blvd, Québec, Québec, Canada
Full list of author information is available at the end of the article

are found in the flesh of oily fish such as herring, mackerel, and salmon or in fish oil supplements [19].

n-3 FAs, particularly EPA and DHA, have been proven to exert beneficial effects on health. Over the past decades, mechanisms by which EPA and DHA impact inflammation have been investigated, demonstrating an improvement of cardiovascular health [10, 14], inflammation status [5], or cancer progression [3, 12] after their consumption.

Despite significant advances on health benefits associated with n-3 FAs, the dose needed to provide health benefits, the best window of time to consume them to fight efficiently against inflammation, and the mechanisms of action in preventing inflammation-related diseases are still unclear. Thus, the aim of the present study was to investigate the effect of 10, 50, and 75 μM EPA, DHA, and a mixture of EPA + DHA on the expression of inflammatory genes in stimulated THP-1 macrophages. The impact of the condition of incubation (preincubation, co-incubation, post-incubation) with n-3 FAs relative to macrophage stimulation was also evaluated.

Methods
Reagents and cell lines
Cell culture media, Roswell Park Memorial Institute (RPMI) 1640 medium, fetal bovine serum (FBS), penicillin and streptomycin media supplements, phorbol 12-myristate 13-acetate (PMA), and dimethyl sulfoxide (DMSO) were purchased from Thermo Scientific (Walthman, USA). Lipopolysaccharide (LPS) from *Escherichia coli* 0111:B4 (reference L2630) was purchased from Sigma (Saint Louis, USA). Phosphate-buffered saline (PBS) solution was obtained from Life Technologies (Burlington, Canada). EPA, DHA, and reagents for reverse transcription were obtained from Applied Biosystems (Oakville, Canada).

Cell culture and fatty acid treatment
The human THP-1 cell line, an acute monocytic leukemia cell line (American Type Culture Collection (ATCC), Rockville, MD, USA), was cultured in RPMI 1640 media supplemented with penicillin (100 U/ml) and streptomycin (100 μM/ml), 10% FBS at 37 °C in a 5% CO_2 incubator. Differentiation of monocytes into macrophages was induced with PMA. 9×10^5 cells per ml were seeded into six-well plates, with 200 nM of PMA for 72 h. Then, non-attached cells were removed by aspiration, adherent cells were washed three times with PBS, and then, cells were ready for experiments. The cells were incubated in different conditions: (1) in the post-incubation condition, the macrophages were stimulated during 18 h by LPS, before the addition of n-3 FAs for 24 h; (2) in the co-incubation condition, the cells were incubated during 24 h with LPS and n-3 FAs at the same time; (3) finally, in the pre-incubation

condition, the macrophages were incubated during 24 h into n-3 FAs and then stimulated during 18 h by an addition of LPS.

n-3 FAs and LPS preparation
All treatments were performed in triplicate, and the entire experiment was replicated independently three times. LPS was dissolved in PBS and diluted to a final concentration of 10 ng/ml prior to treatment. Stock solutions of FAs (EPA-DMSO 33×10^4 μM and DHA-DMSO 76×10^4 μM) prepared in serum-free RPMI 1640 medium were diluted in culture medium to obtain 10, 50, and 75 μM concentrations. Fresh FAs and LPS were prepared before every experiment from the frozen stock solution. The cells were thereafter incubated with LPS and EPA, DHA, or EPA + DHA (ratio 1:1) for 24 h. Controls in this experiment were THP-1 cells incubated with the vehicle, DMSO, and LPS.

Cell proliferation and cytotoxicity assay
A viability test was performed to exclude cytotoxicity of EPA, DHA, and EPA + DHA concentrations used. Briefly, cell cytotoxicity was assessed by measuring the activity of mitochondrial dehydrogenase. 3-(4,5-Dimethyl-2-thiazol)-2,5-diphenyl-2h-tetrazolium bromide (MTT) reagent was used. After incubation at 37 °C for 1 h, the absorbance at 490 nm was assayed using an ELISA plate reader (Biotech).

RNA isolation and quantitative real-time PCR
After 24 h, following the protocol provided, total RNA was extracted using RNeasy Mini Kit (Qiagen). RNA quality and integrity were tested on 1.5% agarose gel electrophoresis with ethidium bromide staining. Absorption spectroscopy at 260/280 was used to determine RNA concentrations. Then, complementary DNA (cDNA) was produced from RNA using High Capacity Transcription Kit (Applied Biosystems). The expression of several inflammatory genes (*SOCS1*, *TNFAIP3*, *TNFA*, *IL1B*, *IL6*, *MCP1*, *PTGS2*) was assessed using real-time PCR. PCR samples were normalized against 18S gene expression. Applied Biosystems provided primers and TaqMan® probes (Table 1).

Cytokine measurements
Cytokines, TNFA, IL1B, IL6, and MCP1, were assessed in collected media, using the Bio-Plex Pro Human Chemokine kit (Bio-Rad Laboratories Canada Ltd., Mississauga, ON, Canada) according to the manufacturer's instructions.

Statistical analyses
Statistical analyses were done using SAS software (version 9.2). Experimental results were reported as mean ± SE.

Table 1 Probe sets for real-time PCR

	5′ Forward primer 3′ Reverse primer
SOCS1	TCCTGAGGAGCGGGAGGAGTGGAC
	GTCCACTCCTCCCGCTCCTCAGGA
TNFAIP3	GAAAACGACGGTGACGGCATTGC
	GCAATGCCGTCCGTCGTCGTTTTC
TNFA	CCATGTTGTAGCAAACCCTCAAGCT
	AGCTTGAGGGTTTGCTACAACATGG
IL1B	CAGATGAAGTGCTCCTTCCAGGACC
	GGTCCTGGAAGGAGCACTTCATCTG
MCP1	CGCTCAGCCAGATGCAATCAATGCC
	GGCATTGATTGCATCTGGCTGAGCG
PTGS2	CTGGGCCATGGGGTGGACTTAAATC
	GATTTAAGTCCACCCCATGGCCCAG
IL6	TCAGCCCTGAGAAAGGAGACATGTA
	TACATGTCTCCTTTCTCAGGGCGA
18S	CCATTGGAGGGCAAGTCTGGTGCCA
	TGGCACCAGACTTGCCCTCCAATGG

Analysis of variance was used to compare between group means. A significant overall F test was followed by post hoc comparisons using the LS means procedure. The level of significance was defined at $P < 0.05$ for all.

Results

Cytotoxicity assay

The effect of EPA, DHA, and EPA + DHA on THP-1 macrophage viability was performed using the MTT assay. After 24-h incubation of the cells with 10, 50, and 75 μM EPA, DHA, and EPA + DHA, the test was done. All concentrations of each n-3 FA investigated did not have any effect on cell viability (data not shown).

Influence of EPA, DHA, and EPA + DHA on inflammatory gene expression

The cells were cultivated in three conditions. First, the macrophages were incubated in FAs before being stimulated (pre-incubation). In the second condition, inflammation and treatment with n-3 FAs were done at the same time (co-incubation). Finally, in the last condition, inflammation was triggered before adding the FAs (post-incubation). In the presence of LPS stimulation, there was a global increase of gene expression levels of inflammatory genes compared with the control (dotted line, Fig. 1). After the addition of n-3 FAs in the culture medium, a global suppression of *IL6*, *TNFA*, *IL1B*, *MCP1*, *TNFAIP3*, and *PTGS2* expression was seen. The effect was more pronounced with the mixture EPA + DHA than with either EPA or DHA alone. The

incubation of cells with n-3 FAs had different effects depending on the FAs. Except for *MCP1* for which the post-incubation and co-incubation conditions had the same effect, the post-incubation with EPA was more efficient on reducing *IL6*, *TNFA*, *IL1B*, and *TNFAIP3* gene expression than the co-incubation and the pre-incubation. For treatment with either DHA or the mixture EPA + DHA, the co-incubation of THP-1 cells in these FAs was more potent than the pre- and post-incubation for all the studied genes. A dose effect was observed on gene expression levels; incubation of cells in 75 μM of any FAs decreased their expression more efficiently than incubation in 10 and 50 μM. LPS stimulation increased *SOCS1* expression. A regulation of this gene was seen only with 75 μM of each n-3 FA, which further increased *SOCS1* expression. No condition-dependant modulation of *SOCS1* was seen.

Influence of EPA, DHA, and EPA + DHA on cytokine secretion

Since the results obtained in the co-incubation and the post-incubation conditions were the most interesting, cytokine measurements were done for these two conditions.

In the LPS-stimulated condition, compared to the control condition (LPS−), there was an increased production of cytokines (Fig. 2). When EPA, DHA, or the mixture EPA + DHA was added to the cultured medium, for each cytokine, a decreased secretion was observed. This diminution was more important in the co-incubation than in the post-incubation condition. A dose effect was also noted; 75 μM of each n-3 FA decreased cytokine concentrations more effectively than 10- and 50-μM doses. FA-specific effects were also seen. DHA and EPA + DHA downregulated cytokine secretion more efficiently than EPA. For IL1B and IL6, the co-incubation with DHA and EPA + DHA restored secretion back to the basal level. This phenomenon was not observed in cells incubated with EPA.

Discussion

Because of the health benefits associated with DHA and EPA, several international agencies and organizations have put together recommendations for EPA and DHA supplementation and for fish consumption [10]. This initiative enabled not only health promotion but also the reduction of the risk of several chronic inflammatory diseases [3, 23]. Although much has been learn about n-3 FAs, many questions remain, including the dose-response effect on clinical outcomes as well as the differential effects on health of EPA and DHA.

The objective of the present study was to investigate the effect of different concentrations of EPA, DHA, and EPA + DHA on inflammatory markers, in stimulated

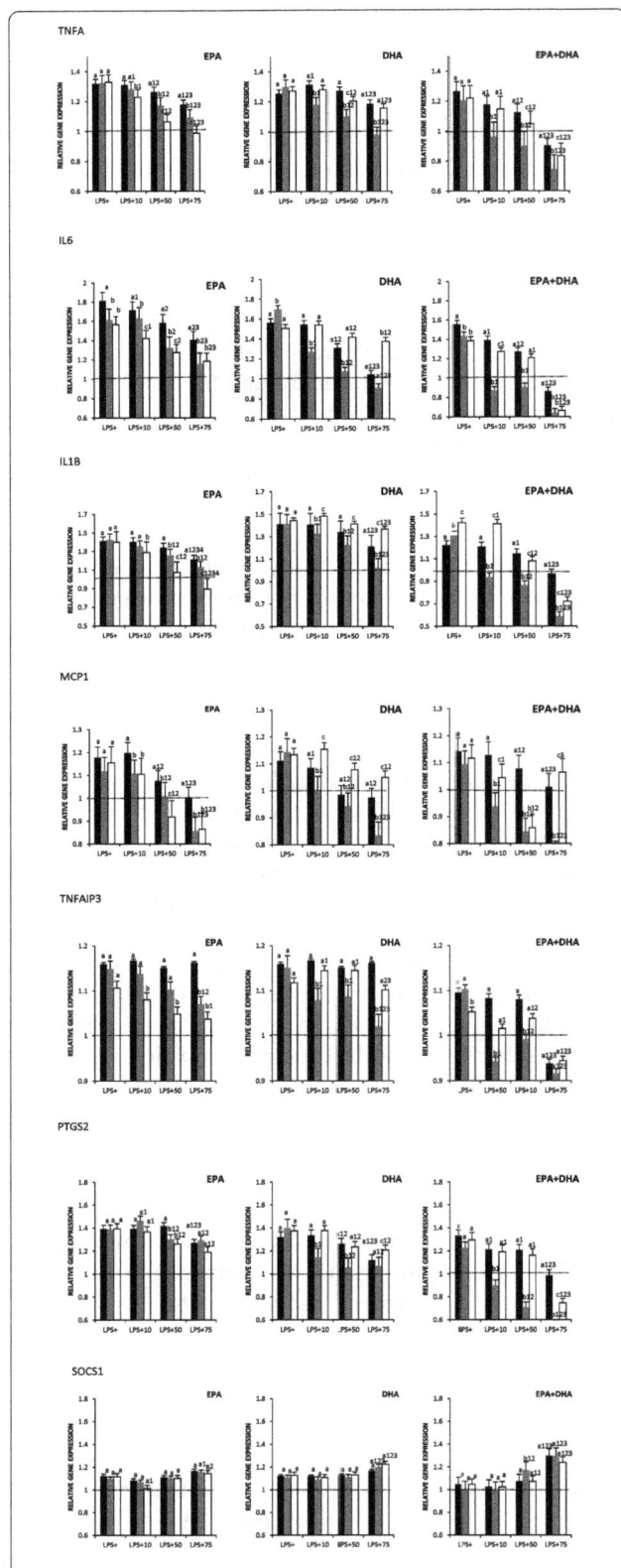

Fig. 1 Influence of n-3 FAs on gene expression. The total RNA was extracted using RNeasy Mini, then cDNA was produced from the RNA. The expression of *SOCS1*, *TNFAIP3*, *TNFA*, *IL1B*, *IL6*, *MCP1*, and *PTGS2* was assessed using real-time PCR. PCR samples were normalized against 18S gene expression. Gene expression was measured under three conditions. [a, b, c]Represents the differences ($P \leq 0.05$) between each of these conditions (pre-incubation [*black bars*], co-incubation [*gray bars*], and post-incubation [*white bars*]). [1]$P \leq 0.05$ represents the difference between different concentrations relative to LPS+ within the same condition; [2]$P \leq 0.05$ represents the difference between different concentrations relative to 10 µM within the same condition; and [3]$P \leq 0.05$ represents the difference between different concentrations relative to 50 µM within the same condition

THP-1 macrophages. It is well accepted that EPA and DHA are associated with a lower risk of inflammatory diseases [7]. Their health effects are usually studied as a sum or combination. Thus, little is known about the potential health effect of EPA compared to DHA. Nevertheless, few studies have shown EPA- or DHA-specific effects on inflammation. Gorjao and collaborators reported different effects of EPA and DHA on endothelial cells, insulin-secreting cells, and leukocyte function [8]. In a study on RAW 264.7 macrophages, Honda et al. demonstrated that EPA and DHA attenuated cell inflammatory activities and more importantly that their respective effect changed in potency depending on the investigated cytokines (IL6 and TNFA) [11]. Finally, an investigation of the effect of EPA and DHA on THP-1 macrophages showed that EPA and DHA had a differential effect on cytokine transcription [17]. It is important to further understand the specific effect of n-3 FAs on inflammatory mechanisms and to know whether they have complementary, shared, or divergent effects. A previous study by our research group [2] investigated the effect of 50 and 10 µM EPA, DHA, and EPA + DHA on non-stimulated macrophages. This study firstly showed that in non-inflammatory conditions, EPA and DHA had a varying effect on the expression of inflammatory genes and that the anti-inflammatory effect was dose-dependent [2].

In the present study, our ultimate goal was to investigate the anti-inflammatory effects of n-3 FAs in inflamed cells. In this perspective, the current study investigated the effect of EPA, DHA, and EPA + DHA on stimulated THP-1 macrophages. n-3 FA effects were tested on seven genes involved in inflammation. An incubation of these macrophages into 100 ng/ml LPS for 18 h allowed mimicking an inflammatory state. Stimulation with LPS increased expression levels of inflammatory genes.

The combination of EPA + DHA (1:1) had a more potent anti-inflammatory action than DHA and EPA alone, DHA being a better inhibitor of the studied gene expression than EPA. This implies that giving a mixture of EPA + DHA (1:1) seems to have the best anti-inflammatory effect.

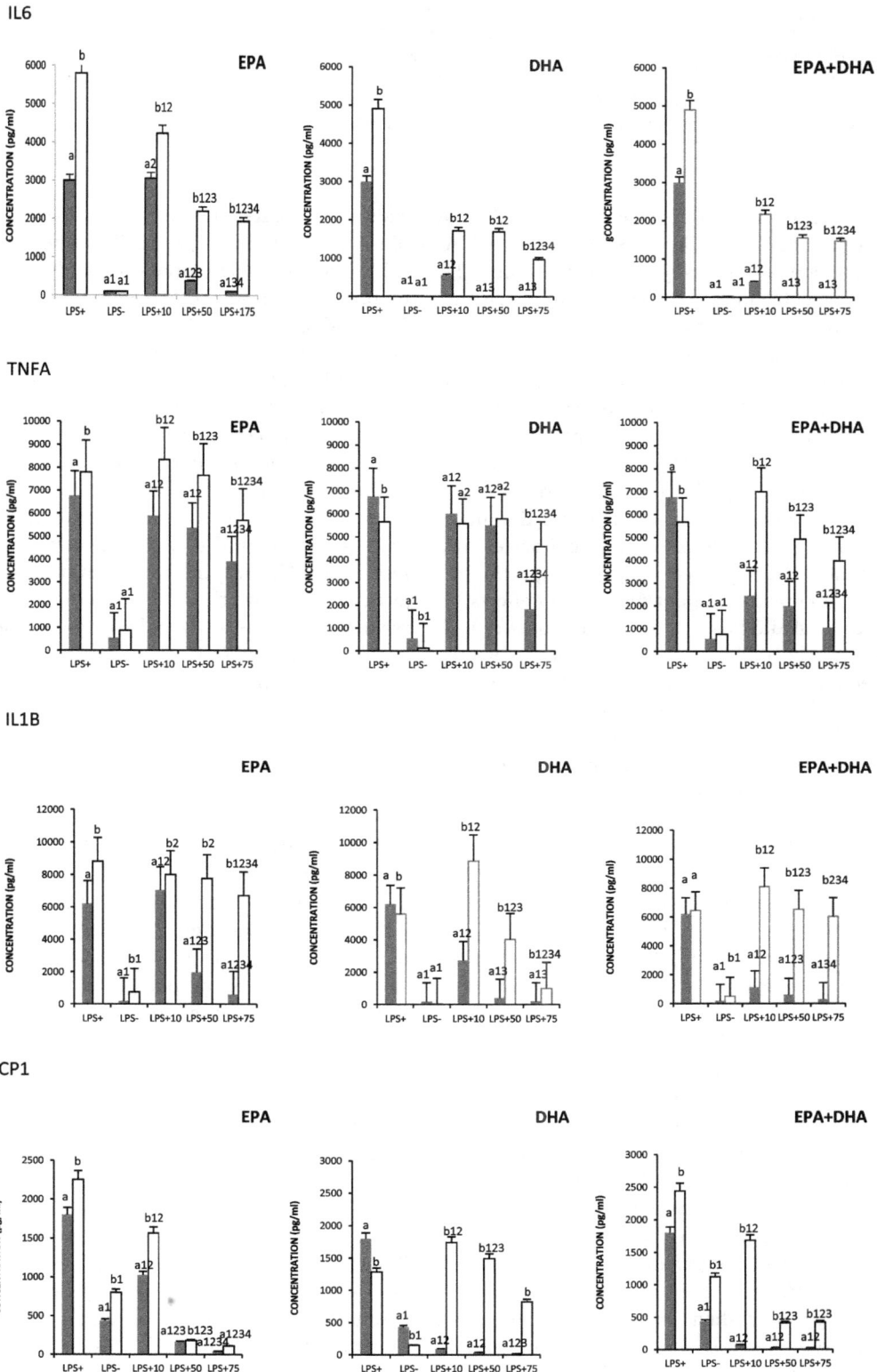

Fig. 2 (See legend on next page.)

(See figure on previous page.)

Fig. 2 Influence of n-3 FAs on cytokine secretion. TNFA, IL1B, IL6, and MCP1 were assessed in collected media of cell cultures. [a, b]Represents the differences ($P \leq 0.05$) between each condition (co-incubation [*gray bars*] and post-incubation [*white bars*]). [1]$P \leq 0.05$ represents the difference between different concentrations relative to LPS+ within the same condition; [2]$P \leq 0.05$ represents the difference between different concentrations relative to LPS− within the same condition; [3]$P \leq 0.05$ represents the difference between different concentrations relative to 10 µM within the same condition; and [4]$P \leq 0.05$ represents the difference between different concentrations relative to 50 µM within the same condition

The dose of 75 µM was more powerful than 10 and 50 µM. A treatment of T cells with 12.5 µM EPA or DHA during 24 h was done by Verlengia and collaborators [22]. Using the microarray technique, the expression of specific selected genes involved in cytokine production, cell production, signal transduction, and apoptosis was changed. DHA increased the expression of 62% of the studied genes against 33% for EPA. In Raji cells which were treated in the same conditions, 25.9% of the studied genes were regulated by EPA against 8.4% by DHA. Only 3% of the genes were regulated by the two n-3 FAs [22]. These results suggest that molecular mechanisms responsible for the modulatory effect of EPA and DHA on T lymphocytes are different and that DHA regulated a bigger proportion of studied genes. In line with different modulatory effects of EPA and DHA revealed by us and others, an effect of n-3 FAs on heart rate mediated by DHA rather than EPA was previously demonstrated in a supplementation study among humans [15]. High heart rate (HR) has long been associated with CVD morbidity in epidemiological studies. It has been proven that fish oil intake reduced HR mostly in individuals with a high baseline HR and when taken for a long intervention period. In fact, DHA alone (2.8 g/day) diminished HR by 7% in post-menopausal women and DHA but not EPA reduced HR by 3.5 beats per minute and 2.2 beats per minute, respectively, in hyperlipidemic and healthy males [15].

Regarding cytokine production, it was mostly inhibited with the mixture of EPA + DHA. This inhibition was more pronounced than the one observed with either DHA or EPA alone, DHA being more efficient than EPA. Weldon et al. investigated the action of n-3 FAs on cytokine expression in THP-1 macrophages [17]. Pre-treatment with 100 µM EPA and DHA decreased LPS-stimulated THP-1 cell secretion of TNFA, IL1B, and IL6 compared to control. Even though the effect of the mixture of EPA + DHA was not investigated, the effect of DHA was more important than the one observed with EPA. Similar results were obtained when a lower dose was used, 25 µM DHA decreased the production of IL6 and IL1B more potently than EPA in LPS-stimulated THP-1 macrophages. A similar observation has been reported after addition of EPA and DHA to the culture media of RAW 264.7 macrophages [11]. It must also be noted that in the present study, n-3 FAs decreased IL6 secretion to a greater extent than other cytokines.

This corroborates the fact that anti-inflammatory effects of n-3 FAs were cytokine specific rather than global.

To our knowledge, only one study has been designed to provide a head-to-head comparison of the effect of EPA and DHA on inflammation markers as a primary outcome. Allaire and collaborators provided 2.7 g/day of EPA and DHA for 10 weeks to healthy people with abdominal obesity. The group which had DHA supplement had a greater reduction of plasma IL8 levels and greater increase of adiponectin concentration [1].

The present study showed that in inflammatory conditions, DHA has a better anti-inflammatory effect than EPA. It also showed that the mixture EPA/DHA at a 1:1 ratio more efficiently inhibits inflammation. In human subjects, n-3 FAs have been shown to modulate inflammation-related conditions such as hypertension, dyslipidemia, or insulin resistance [4]. However, it should be noted that, up to now, most trials have not considered that the relative proportion of EPA and DHA may influence the results. This phenomenon might, at least in part, explain the relative controversy on the beneficial effect of n-3 FAs on several conditions. Luis and collaborators [13] have investigated on Wistar Kyoto rats the effect of a supplementation with different ratios of EPA + DHA on markers of CVD and oxidative stress. EPA + DHA at a 1:1 ratio triggered the most important improvement of the risk factor for type 2 diabetes and reduction of oxidative stress. It is important to point out the fact that in most studies, supplements used have a greater proportion of EPA than DHA. Since DHA appears to have a more important anti-inflammatory action, it might be interesting to reconsider their ratio in supplements, at least for inflammatory diseases.

At the present time, there is no consensus on the ideal n-3 FA intake. Nutritional guidelines have been set by several governments (France, Belgium, Canada) and health organizations (Food and Agriculture Organization, American Dietetic Association) [21]. For instance, the American Heart Association (AHA) recommends that all adults eat fish at least twice a week, which provides 500 mg n-3 FAs/day. It is also recommended for people with documented coronary heart diseases to consume 1 g EPA and DHA/day for secondary prevention [6]. Mozaffarian and collaborators recently reviewed facts concerning EPA and DHA possible shared or complementary effects [16]. In human and animal studies, EPA and DHA reduced platelet aggregation, modulate inflammation, and lower plasma triglyceride

(TG) levels. Clinical and observational studies show that DHA increases high-density lipoprotein particles, favors the proportion of large low-density lipoprotein, and causes stronger TG-lowering effects. Mozaffarian et al. concluded that EPA and DHA have complementary and shared benefits. In a study led by Robinson et al., 3T3-L1 adipocytes were incubated in 125 µM of several fatty acids among which are EPA and DHA. Results have shown that DHA increased cellular adiponectin mRNA and secreted adiponectin protein to a greater extent (40% more, $P < 0.05$) than EPA [18].

Unfortunately, scientific evidences are still lacking to make quantitative recommendation about the ratio and the dose of EPA and DHA that should be taken to prevent inflammatory diseases. However, it is known that n-3 FAs have anti-inflammatory effects and thus their consumption should be favored. Additional experimental, clinical, and observational investigations are necessary to better understand the complementary and shared effects of EPA and DHA on various clinical outcomes.

A dose effect was obvious for the studied genes; 75 µM of each FA had a stronger anti-inflammatory effect than 10 and 50 µM. It must be noted that a decrease of the expression of all genes except for *SOCS1* was seen after the addition of 75 µM n-3 FAs. *SOCS1* gene expression was increased. This gene encodes for a suppressor of cytokine signaling. This result suggests that 75 µM but not 10 or 50 µM of EPA, DHA, or EPA + DHA was able to increase *SOCS1* expression. *SOCS1* being an anti-inflammatory gene, here again, a protective effect of n-3 FAs is showed.

We tested the effect of three different concentrations of each n-3 FA in three different cell culture conditions. In the first condition, the macrophages were incubated in FAs before being stimulated (pre-incubation); in the second, the inflammation and the treatment with n-3 FAs were done at the same time (co-incubation); and in the last condition, inflammation was triggered before adding the FAs (post-incubation). In the post-incubation condition, the anti-inflammatory effect of EPA was greater for *IL6*, *IL1B*, *TNFA*, and *TNFAIP3*. As far as *MCP1* was concerned, the post- and co-incubation had the same effect. EPA + DHA had the best anti-inflammatory effect during the co-incubation for all genes except for *SOCS1* where no differences were observed between each condition. Concerning cytokine secretion, the co-incubation seems to be the better condition for EPA, DHA, and EPA + DHA. Globally, findings from gene expression and cytokine production suggest that according to the inflammatory environment, the action of each n-3 FA could be different. Thus, EPA seems to have a greater anti-inflammatory effect on a situation where an inflammatory state is already present; this can be associated to a resolution of inflammation. DHA and the mixture EPA + DHA

have a more potent action when they were added at the same time with LPS. This suggests that starting to take EPA and DHA at the same moment with the installation of inflammation might bring out their best anti-inflammatory effects. Even if the anti-inflammatory effect of n-3 FAs on the pre-incubation condition is the less important, a dose effect does exist. It suggests that the protective effect of n-3 FAs among healthy subjects might be visible but less obvious than the one observed among people with pre-existing inflammatory conditions. Current recommendations concerning the consumption of n-3 FAs are available not only as primary prevention of healthy people but also as secondary prevention for people suffering of coronary heart disease or having high TG levels. Human studies investigating the impact of n-3 FA intake against non-CVD were unfortunately not consistent with the data collected in preclinical studies. This is why consensus recommendation has not yet been made regarding the possible curative effects of these FAs or their ability to prevent inflammatory disorders. Further investigations are needed to build more precise recommendations which would take into account the body inflammatory state, the best n-3 FAs, and the dose to provide in different inflammatory states.

Conclusions

The n-3 FAs do not have the same anti-inflammatory effect, and depending on the inflammatory state, their action can be different. This observation adds to the complexity concerning the dose and ratio of n-3 FAs for optimal health benefits. In fact, their action seems to depend on their respective dose when used alone, the ratio of each of them when used in combination, and also the inflammatory environment at the time of their consumption.

Abbreviations
ALA: Alpha-linolenic acid; DHA: Docosahexaenoic acid; DMSO: Dimethyl sulfoxide; EPA: Eicosapentaenoic acid; FAs: Fatty acids; FBS: Fetal bovine serum; LA: Linoleic acid; LPS: Lipopolysaccharide; n-3: Omega-3; n-6: Omega-6; PMA: Phorbol 12-myristate 13-acetate; PUFAs: Polyunsaturated FAs; RNA: Ribonucleic acid; RPMI: Roswell Park Memorial Institute

Acknowledgements
The authors would like to acknowledge the contribution of Alain Houde for the technical assistance.

Funding
This work was supported by a grant from the Natural Sciences and Engineering Research Council of Canada (grant number: 48031–2012).

Authors' contributions
BA-N and M-CV conceived and designed the experiments. BA-N and FG analyzed the data. BA-N, M-CV, and OB interpreted the data. BA-N wrote the paper. All authors read and approved the final manuscript.

Competing interests
The authors declare that they have no competing interests.

Author details

[1]Institute of Nutrition and Functional Foods (INAF), Laval University, Pavillon des Services, 2440 Hochelaga Blvd, Québec, Québec, Canada. [2]Laboratory of Molecular Pharmacology, CHU de Québec Research Center, 2705 Laurier Blvd, Québec, Québec G1V 4G2, Canada.

References

1. Allaire J, Couture P, Leclerc M, Charest A, Marin J, Lepine MC, Talbot D, Tchernof A, Lamarche B. A randomized, crossover, head-to-head comparison of eicosapentaenoic acid and docosahexaenoic acid supplementation to reduce inflammation markers in men and women: the Comparing EPA to DHA (ComparED) Study. Am J Clin Nutr. 2016;104:280–7.
2. Allam-Ndoul B, Guenard F, Barbier O, Vohl MC. Effect of n-3 fatty acids on the expression of inflammatory genes in THP-1 macrophages. Lipids Health Dis. 2016;15:69.
3. Astorg P. Dietary N-6 and N-3 polyunsaturated fatty acids and prostate cancer risk: a review of epidemiological and experimental evidence. Cancer Causes Control. 2004;15:367–86.
4. Calder PC. Mechanisms of action of (n-3) fatty acids. J Nutr. 2012;142:592S–9S.
5. Calder PC. n-3 fatty acids, inflammation and immunity: new mechanisms to explain old actions. Proc Nutr Soc. 2013;72:326–36.
6. Flock MR, Harris WS, Kris-Etherton PM. Long-chain omega-3 fatty acids: time to establish a dietary reference intake. Nutr Rev. 2013 71:692–707.
7. Gopinath B, Buyken AE, Flood VM, Empson M, Rochtchina E, Mitchell P. Consumption of polyunsaturated fatty acids, fish, and nuts and risk of inflammatory disease mortality. Am J Clin Nutr. 2011;93:1073–9.
8. Gorjao R, Azevedo-Martins AK, Rodrigues HG, Abdulkader F, Arcisio-Miranda M, Procopio J, Curi R. Comparative effects of DHA and EPA on cell function. Pharmacol Ther. 2009;122:56–64.
9. Guerra I, Bermejo F. Biosimilars in inflammatory bowel disease: management and care. Rev Esp Enferm Dig. 2015;107:389.
10. Harris WS. Omega-3 fatty acids and cardiovascular disease: a case for omega-3 index as a new risk factor. Pharmacol Res. 2007;55:217–23.
11. Honda KL, Lamon-Fava S, Matthan NR, Wu D, Lichtenstein AH. EPA and DHA exposure alters the inflammatory response but not the surface expression of Toll-like receptor 4 in macrophages. Lipids. 2015;50:121–9.
12. Leitzmann MF, Stampfer MJ, Michaud DS, Augustsson K, Colditz GC, Willett WC, Giovannucci EL. Dietary intake of n-3 and n-6 fatty acids and the risk of prostate cancer. Am J Clin Nutr. 2004;80:204–16.
13. Lluis L, Taltavull N, Munoz-Cortes M, Sanchez-Martos V, Romeu M, Giralt M, Molinar-Toribio E, Torres JL, Perez-Jimenez J, Pazos M, Mendez L, Gallardo JM, Medina I, Nogues MR. Protective effect of the omega-3 polyunsaturated fatty acids: eicosapentaenoic acid/docosahexaenoic acid 1:1 ratio on cardiovascular disease risk markers in rats. Lipids Health Dis. 2013;12:140.
14. Lu J, Borthwick F, Hassanali Z, Wang Y, Mangat R, Ruth M, Shi D, Jaeschke A, Russell JC, Field CJ, Proctor SD, Vine DF. Chronic dietary n-3 PUFA intervention improves dyslipidaemia and subsequent cardiovascular complications in the JCR:LA-cp rat model of the metabolic syndrome. Br J Nutr. 2011;105:1572–82.
15. Mori TA, Bao DQ, Burke V, Puddey IB, Beilin LJ. Docosahexaenoic acid but not eicosapentaenoic acid lowers ambulatory blood pressure and heart rate in humans. Hypertension. 1999;34:253–60.
16. Mozaffarian D, Geelen A, Brouwer IA, Geleijnse JM, Zock PL, Katan MB. Effect of fish oil on heart rate in humans: a meta-analysis of randomized controlled trials. Circulation. 2005;112:1945–52.
17. Mullen A, Loscher CE, Roche HM. Anti-inflammatory effects of EPA and DHA are dependent upon time and dose-response elements associated with LPS stimulation in THP-1-derived macrophages. J Nutr Biochem. 2010;21:444–50.
18. Oster RT, Tishinsky JM, Yuan Z, Robinson LE. Docosahexaenoic acid increases cellular adiponectin mRNA and secreted adiponectin protein, as well as PPARgamma mRNA, in 3T3-L1 adipocytes. Appl Physiol Nutr Metab. 2010;35:783–9.
19. Siriwardhana N, Kalupahana NS, Moustaid-Moussa N. Health benefits of n-3 polyunsaturated fatty acids: eicosapentaenoic acid and docosahexaenoic acid. Adv Food Nutr Res. 2012;65:211–22.
20. Stark AK, Sriskantharajah S, Hessel EM, Okkenhaug K. PI3K inhibitors in inflammation, autoimmunity and cancer. Curr Opin Pharmacol. 2015;23:82–91.
21. Tvrzicka E, Kremmyda LS, Stankova B, Zak A. Fatty acids as biocompounds: their role in human metabolism, health and disease—a review. Part 1: classification, dietary sources and biological functions. BiomedPapMedFacUniv PalackyOlomoucCzechRepub. 2011;155:117–30.
22. Verlengia R, Gorjao R, Kanunfre CC, Bordin S, Martins De LT, Martins EF, Curi R. Comparative effects of eicosapentaenoic acid and docosahexaenoic acid on proliferation, cytokine production, and pleiotropic gene expression in Jurkat cells. J Nutr Biochem. 2004;15:657–65.
23. Weylandt KH, Serini S, Chen YQ, Su HM, Lim K, Cittadini A, Calviello G. Omega-3 polyunsaturated fatty acids: the way forward in times of mixed evidence. Biomed Res Int. 2015;2015:143109.
24. Yaqoob P, Calder P. Effects of dietary lipid manipulation upon inflammatory mediator production by murine macrophages. Cell Immunol. 1995;163:120–8.

6

The PBMC transcriptome profile after intake of oxidized versus high-quality fish oil

Mari C. W. Myhrstad[1*], Inger Ottestad[2,1], Clara-Cecilie Günther[3], Einar Ryeng[4], Marit Holden[3], Astrid Nilsson[5], Kirsti W. Brønner[6], Achim Kohler[5,7], Grethe I. A. Borge[5], Kirsten B. Holven[2,8] and Stine M. Ulven[1,2]

Abstract

Background: Marine long-chain polyunsaturated fatty acids are susceptible to oxidation, generating a range of different oxidation products with suggested negative health effects. The aim of the present study was to utilize sensitive high-throughput transcriptome analyses to investigate potential unfavorable effects of oxidized fish oil (PV: 18 meq/kg; AV: 9) compared to high-quality fish oil (PV: 4 meq/kg; AV: 3).

Methods: In a double-blinded randomized controlled study for seven weeks, 35 healthy subjects were assigned to 8 g of either oxidized fish oil or high quality fish oil. The daily dose of EPA+DHA was 1.6 g. Peripheral blood mononuclear cells were isolated at baseline and after 7 weeks and transcriptome analyses were performed with the illuminaHT-12 v4 Expression BeadChip.

Results: No gene transcripts, biological processes, pathway or network were significantly changed in the oxidized fish oil group compared to the fish oil group. Furthermore, gene sets related to oxidative stress and cardiovascular disease were not differently regulated between the groups. Within group analyses revealed a more prominent effect after intake of high quality fish oil as 11 gene transcripts were significantly (FDR < 0.1) changed from baseline versus three within the oxidized fish oil group.

Conclusion: The suggested concern linking lipid oxidation products to short-term unfavorable health effects may therefore not be evident at a molecular level in this explorative study.

Keywords: Oxidized fish oil, n-3 fatty acids, PBMCs, Transcriptome, Human intervention

Background

Fish oil (FO) is associated with reduced risk of coronary heart disease (CHD) and CHD deaths [1, 2]; thus, the use of supplements containing n-3 fatty acids are recommended for CHD prevention among those who do not eat fish in accordance with the food recommendations [3–5]. Long-chain polyunsaturated fatty acids (LCPU-FAs), including n-3 fatty acids in marine oils, are susceptible to oxidation, and consequently, lipid oxidation products are generated [6–8]. For several years, the

voluntary monographs by the Global Organization for eicosapentaenoic acid (EPA) and docosahexaenoic acid (DHA) Omega-3s (GOED) have served as the quality standard of the industry, giving recommendations for the content of lipid oxidation products, such as a maximum peroxide value (PV) of 5 meq/kg (milliequivalents per kilogram) and a maximum anisidine value (AV) of 20 [9]. Other monographs exists, such as the European pharmacopeia recommending a PV at 5 or 10 meq/kg and an AV at 30 or 15, depending on the content of marine n-3s. The quality of the FO, in terms of the oxidative status, can be camouflaged by encapsulation, additives, and flavorings [10], and a variation in the oxidative status of n-3 supplements and vegetable oils has been reported [11–13].

* Correspondence: mari.myhrstad@hioa.no
[1]Department of Health, Nutrition and Management, Faculty of Health Sciences, Oslo and Akershus University College of Applied Sciences, P.O. Box 4St. Olavs plass, 0130 Oslo, Norway
Full list of author information is available at the end of the article

Concerns related to a regular consumption of oxidized marine oils and negative health effects have been raised [10, 14, 15]. If lipid oxidation products from the diet are absorbed in humans, these highly reactive compounds may cause oxidative damage to macromolecules such as proteins, carbohydrate, DNA, and lipids thereby altering their function [16]. Highly reactive lipid compounds may also act as signaling molecules that alter gene functions and thereby influence health via cellular sensing mechanisms [16].

Cell studies have indicated that lipid oxidation products are involved in pathophysiological processes due to their reactivity [7, 17–19], and oxidized n-3 fatty acids have been shown to increase the antioxidant defense system and to enhance endoplasmic reticulum (ER) stress in human intestinal Caco-2/TC7 cells [20]. Some animal studies show serious biological effects from the intake of oxidized lipids [21], but there are few studies investigating the intake of oxidized lipids in concentrations more similar to daily life. However, mice fed on a high-fat diet containing weakly oxidized n-3 fatty acids for 8 weeks increased the plasma level of n-3 oxidation products and inflammatory markers [20]. The intake of oxidized vegetable oils has been shown to increase the postprandial level of plasma lipid oxidation products and markers related to coronary vascular disease in humans [22–26]. Discrepancies exist, and we have previously reported that the intake of oxidized fish oil for 7 weeks did not change the plasma levels of peroxidation products of LCPUFAs, serum level of oxidized LDL-cholesterol, or selected markers of oxidative stress and inflammation [27, 28]. However, lipid oxidation generates a variety of reactive compounds [6–8], and no single biomarker reflects the total in vivo lipid oxidation and oxidative stress status. In addition, the circulating oxidative stress markers may not be sensitive enough to reflect a local change in the cellular oxidative stress status. Other approaches including more sensitive techniques to accurately measure the influence of lipid oxidation products at a molecular level are therefore required.

Transcriptome analyses examine the mRNA transcript level in a given cell population and reflect the genes that are actively expressed at a given time. Changes in the transcriptome profile occur prior to changes in protein levels. Transcriptomics has therefore shown to be a valuable and sensitive technique measuring early changes related to a dietary challenge [29, 30]. The peripheral blood mononuclear cells (PBMCs) include monocytes and lymphocytes. In the circulation, PBMCs are exposed to environmental factors and metabolic tissues and may therefore reflect systemic health. It is well known that dietary factors modulate the gene expression in PBMCs [31–35]. In the same intervention trials as presented here, we have previously shown that the intake of high-

quality FO modulated the transcriptional profile in human PBMCs and changes in the gene transcripts related to cell cycle, apoptosis, and ER stress were observed [36]. The potential of transcriptome analyses to detect early changes caused by a nutritional challenge encourages us to further investigate whether the intake of oxidized fish oil (oxFO) could alter the gene expression profile in PBMCs compared to high-quality FO in healthy subjects.

Methods

Subjects

The intervention study took place at Akershus University College, Norway, between September and December 2009. Thirty-five young healthy subjects (10 men and 25 women, aged 28.0 ± 8.1 years) with body mass index (BMI) and serum lipids within the normal range were included. Subjects enrolled in the present study are shown in Fig. 1. The detailed description of the protocol, participant recruitment and enrolment, inclusion and exclusion criteria, and compliance are published in detail elsewhere [28].

Study design

This study was a part of a randomized controlled double-blinded three-arm parallel group study, designed to investigate the health effects from the intake of fish oil with different oxidative quality [28]. In the present study, data from two of the intervention arms are included, as shown in Fig. 1. All subjects received 16 capsules each day, containing 8 g FO per day, of which 1.6 g was n-3 fatty acids (0.7 g/d EPA + 0.9 g/d DHA). Both FOs were originating from the same batch of cod liver oil (Gadidae sp., TINE EPA/DHA Oil 1200) provided by TINE SA (Oslo, Norway), and they were identical except for the oxidative status level. The intervention group received either oxidized oxFO (PV, 18 meq/kg; AV, 9; n, 18) or FO (PV, 4 meq/kg; AV, 3; n, 17) (Table 1). Further characterization of the encapsulated oils have previously been published [28]. The subjects were instructed to take the capsules with food (minimum two meals). Blood samples were collected at baseline and after 3 and 7 weeks of intervention. The blood samples after 7 weeks are utilized in the current study. Prior to the baseline visit, the subjects underwent a 4-week marine n-3 fatty acid washout period. During the first 3 weeks of the intervention period, the subjects conducted a fully controlled isoenergetic diet. The food items given did not contain any marine n-3 fatty acids, and the food provided has previously been described in detail elsewhere [28]. The intake of dietary supplements and marine n-3 fatty acids was not allowed during the intervention period.

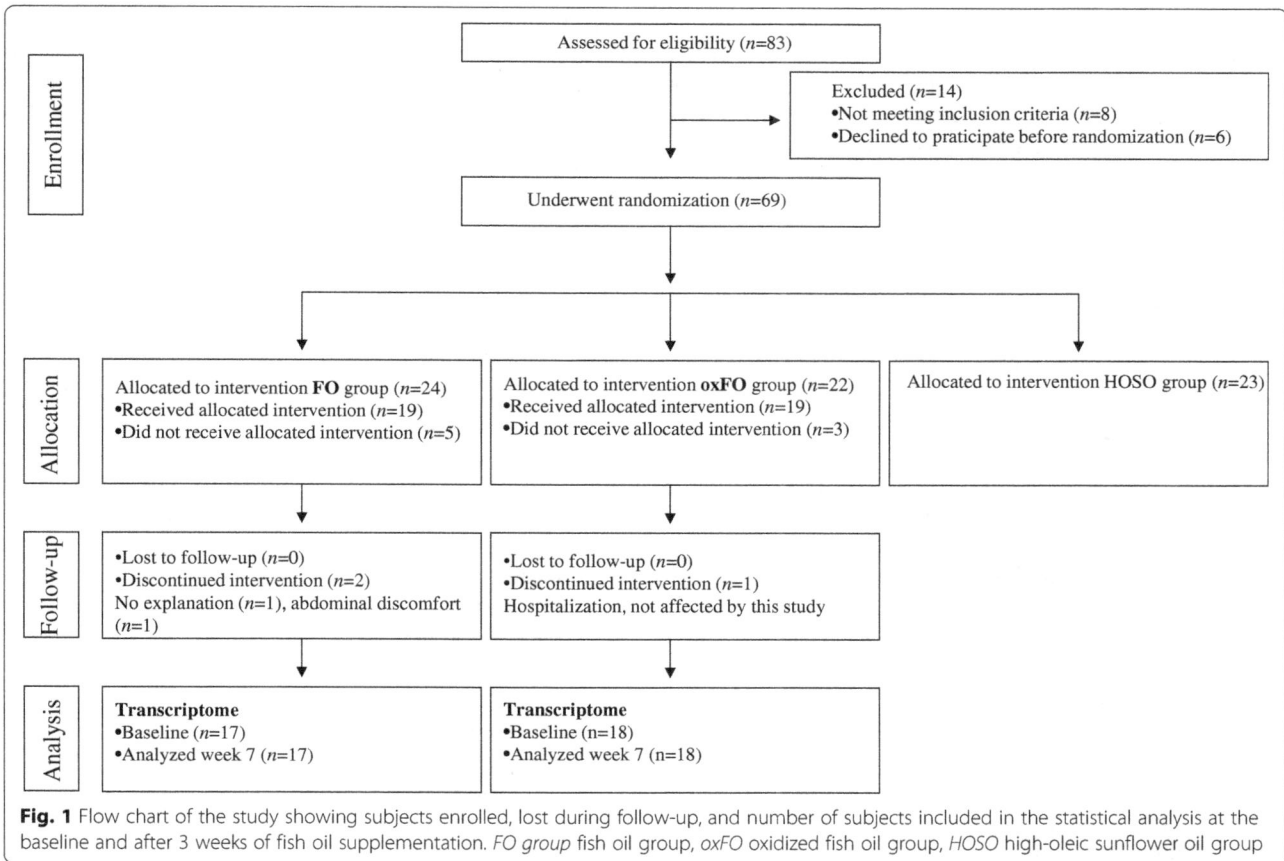

Fig. 1 Flow chart of the study showing subjects enrolled, lost during follow-up, and number of subjects included in the statistical analysis at the baseline and after 3 weeks of fish oil supplementation. *FO group* fish oil group, *oxFO* oxidized fish oil group, *HOSO* high-oleic sunflower oil group

PBMCs and RNA isolation

After blood collection, the PBMCs were isolated by using the BD Vacutainer Cell Preparation tubes according to the manufacturer's instructions (Becton, Dickinson and Company, NJ 07417, USA). Pellets were frozen and stored at −80 °C for further RNA isolation.

Table 1 Characterization of the encapsulated oil

	oxFO	FO
Omega-3 fatty acids		
EPA (20: 5n-3) (g/100 g)	9.1	9.0
DHA (22: 6n-3) (g/100 g)	11.2	11.1
DPA (22 : 5n-3) (g/100 g)	1.1	1.1
Oxidation level		
PV (meq/kg)	18	4
AV	9	3
TOTOX (2 × PV + AV)	45	11
Volatile oxidation products of omega-3 FA		
Pentanal (µg/100 g)	137.8	6.2
1-penten-3-ol (µg/100 g)	132.4	12.8

oxFO oxidized fish oil, *FO* fish oil, *EPA* eicosapentaenoic acid, *DHA* docosahexaenoic acid, *DPA* docosapentaenoic acid, *PV* peroxide value, *AV* anisidine value, *TOTOX* total oxidation

Total RNA was isolated from all PBMC samples using the RNeasy Mini Kit (Qiagen) with lysis buffer-added β-mercaptoethanol according to the manufacturer's instructions and stored at −80 °C. RNA quantity and quality measurements were performed using the ND 1000 Spectrophotometer (Saveen & Werner AB, Limhamn, Sweden) and Agilent Bioanalyser (Agilent Technologies Inc., CA 95051, USA), respectively. One sample had a RNA integrity number (RIN) score of 3.3, and all other samples were above 8 (mean = 9.6). Nanodrop analysis did not indicate any contamination in the RNA samples. The total numbers of monocytes and lymphocytes were measured in EDTA plasma at a routine laboratory (Fürst Medical Laboratory, Oslo, Norway).

Microarray hybridization

Labeled extracts were prepared using the Illumina Total-Prep RNA Amplification Kit (Illumina Inc., CA 92122, USA) according to manufacturer's instructions. The labeled extracts were hybridized on an Illumina HumanHT-12 v4 Expression BeadChip and scanned on an Illumina HiScan microarray scanner (Illumina Inc., CA 92122, USA). Illumina GenomeStudio was used to transform bead-level data to probe-level intensity values and statistics, which were exported raw (unfiltered, non-normalized) for bioinformatic analysis. After hybridization and scanning, a manual quality control step was performed, looking at density plots and hierarchical clustering of raw probe densities. All samples, including the one with RIN < 8 were displaying good characteristics and included in further analysis.

Microarray data analyses

The Illumina intensities were quantile-normalized. To improve statistical power, probes without a detectable expression (detection p value > 0.01) in at least 10 % of the samples were discarded from further analysis. From the 48,000 probes presented on the HumanHT-12 v4 microarray, 21,236 were defined as expressed in the PBMCs and included in the analyses. Changes in gene expression were obtained by calculating $\log_2$ ratios between the baseline and after 7-week intensities, and the two intervention groups were compared with regard to this ratio. Differentially expressed genes between groups were identified using the Linear Models for Microarray (Limma) data [37] package from Bioconductor (http://www.bioconductor.org) performed with the R software. For the within-group analyses, the $\log_2$ intensities at 7 weeks and baseline were compared and differentially expressed genes within each group were identified using Limma.

Genes with a nominal p value < 0.05 were defined as differentially regulated and subjected to further gene ontology, pathway, and network analyses using the Database for Annotation, Visualization and Integrated Discovery (DAVID) software tool version 6.7 (http://david.abcc.ncifcrf.gov) and MetaCore (GeneGo, division of Thomson Reuters, St. Joseph, MI, USA). For the DA-VID analyses, the list of differential regulated genes was compared to a reference list of Homo sapiens and biological processes containing more than 10 genes and a false discovery rate (FDR) q value < 0.05 were considered significantly modulated. Pathways and networks identified in MetaCore with a FDR q value < 0.05 were considered significantly modulated.

Gene Set Enrichment Analyses (GSEA) (http://www.broad.mit.edu/gsea/) were applied on the genes defined as expressed in PBMCs (21,236) for comparison of the transcriptome profile between the two groups. The gene sets in the collection of C2 canonical pathways (cps) and C5 biological process (bp) from Molecular Signatures Database (MSigDB v5.0) were used separately. In addition, six gene set collections associated with oxidative stress and cardiovascular disease were created using a gene set browser (MSigDB v5.0) on the Broad Institute website (http://software.broadinstitute.org/gsea/msigdb/search.jsp) using the keywords stepwise: "oxidative AND stress," "oxidative AND damage," "hypoxi*," "cardiovascular*," "immune AND response," and "inflammation".

Permutation (1000) was performed on phenotypes, and gene sets were defined as significantly changed when FDR q value < 0.25 as recommended for explorative analyses by the Broad Institute (http://www.broad.mit.edu/gsea/). The minimum information about a microarray experiment (MIAME) standards [38] were followed in the analysis and storage of data.

Results

The subjects included in the study were young and middle-aged adults (28.0 ± 8.1 years), and the characteristics of the subjects have previously been described [28]. In short, no differences in age, BMI, or serum lipids were observed between the oxFO ($n = 18$) and the FO groups ($n = 17$) at baseline or after 7 weeks of intervention (Table 2). Additionally, no differences in plasma fatty acids, including the level of long-chained n-3 fatty acids, were observed between the two groups after the intervention period as previously described [28]. The number of monocytes and lymphocytes were the same between the two groups at baseline and after 7 weeks of intervention (data not shown).

Gene expression profiling in PBMCs

Microarray hybridization was performed on RNA from PBMCs collected at baseline and after 7 weeks of supplementation with oxFO ($n = 18$) or FO ($n = 17$).

The differences in gene expression between the two groups were determined by a moderated t test (Limma), by comparing the relative change from baseline to 7 weeks of intervention among the 21,236 expressed genes. In total, 402 gene transcripts were found to be differentially expressed between the two intervention groups ($p < 0.05$) (Additional file 1: Table S1). However, no gene transcripts were significantly differentially expressed (FDR q value <0.1) between the two groups when adjusting for multiple testing (Additional file 1: Table S1). To identify differences across the two intervention groups related to biological processes, pathways, and networks, we analyzed functional relationships among the 402 differentially expressed gene transcripts obtained with Limma ($p < 0.05$). There was no significantly regulated biological processes, pathways, or networks between the two groups after 7 weeks using the software tools DAVID or MetaCore (FDR q value < 0.05, data not shown).

GSEA was used to test whether groups of genes involved in the same biological process or pathway were changed after intake of oxFO compared to FO among all the 21,236 defined expressed genes. We could not detect any differences between the two groups when using the C2 cp or the C5 bp gene set collection (MSigDB v5.0) (FDR q value < 0.25) (Additional files 2 and 3: Table S2 and S3). In addition, GSEA was used to test whether gene sets associated with oxidative stress, inflammation,

Table 2 Baseline characteristic and serum blood values at baseline

	FO (n 17)		oxFO (n 18)		
	Baseline		Baseline		
	Mean/median	SD/25–75 pers	Mean/median	SD/25–75 pers	p
Male/female (n)	5/12		5/13		
Age (year)	25	23–32	22	21–28	0.202
BMI (kg/m²)	22.1	2.5	22.2	1.7	0.849
Total-C (mmo/l)	4.6	0.8	4.7	0.9	0.646
LDL-C (mmol/l)	2.5	0.8	2.7	0.8	0.431
HDL-C (mmol/l)	1.5	0.3	1.4	0.4	0.598
TG (mmol/l)	0.8	0.7–0.9	0.9	0.5–1.5	0.921

Data are presented as mean and standard deviation (SD) or median (25–75 percentile), and differences between the groups were calculated using independent-samples t test or Mann-Whitney U test. p values <0.05 were considered significant

oxFO oxidized fish oil, FO fish oil, Total-C total cholesterol, LDL-C low-density lipoprotein cholesterol, HDL-C high-density lipoprotein cholesterol, TG triglycerides

and cardiovascular disease were differently changed during the intervention in the oxFO group compared to the FO group. However, these gene sets were not significantly changed in the two FO groups (Table 3).

A moderated t test (Limma) was used to identify regulated gene transcripts within the two intervention groups separately, by comparing the transcript level at 7 weeks to the level at baseline. In total, 345 and 667 gene transcripts ($p < 0.01$) among the defined expressed genes were regulated within the oxFO or FO group after 7 weeks, respectively. Of these, 3 (oxFO) and 11 (FO) gene transcripts were significantly regulated when adjusting for multiple testing (FDR q value <0.1) (Table 4). Two of the gene transcripts (CD55 and SNORD13) were overlapping and significantly downregulated in both groups. BAK1 mRNA

Table 3 GSEA analyses. Gene sets associated with oxidative stress and cardiovascular diseases created using a gene set browser (Molecular Signatures Database v5.0)

GSEA gene set collection[a]	# gene sets in collection[b]	Regulated gene sets oxFO vs FO (FDR q value < 0.25)
oxidative AND stress	46	0
oxidative AND damage	5	0
hypoxi*	65	0
cardiovascular*	13	0
immune AND response	147	0
inflammation	29	0

number of gene sets, FDR false discovery rate
* indicates truncated search words
[a]Collections of gene sets were obtained using a gene set browser from the Broad Institute website http://software.broadinstitute.org/gsea/msigdb/search.jsp by the listed keywords
[b]Number of gene sets passing the gene set size filter (min 10 genes, max 500 genes)

was significantly increased from the baseline within the oxFO group only. In addition, the gene transcripts shown in Table 2 were regulated in the same direction within the two groups after 7 weeks. To explore the biological processes modulated within each intervention group, the lists of 345 and 667 changed gene transcripts were subjected to functional analyses separately. Several biological processes were significantly modulated within each intervention group (Table 5). Modulated biological processes after 7 weeks within the oxFO group and FO group were related to translation elongation, translation, and apoptosis, whereas only cell cycle was modulated after intake of oxFO (Table 5).

Discussion

In the present study, the consumption of oxFO for 7 weeks did not alter the transcriptome profile in PBMCs in healthy subjects when compared to the intake of high-quality FO in a randomized controlled intervention study. Within-group analyses revealed a more prominent effect after intake of high-quality FO as more gene transcripts were changed from the baseline than within the oxFO group. The current study is to our knowledge the first to investigate effects at a molecular level after the intake of oxFO using high-throughput sensitive transcriptome analyses.

The intake of lipid oxidation products may disturb the normal redox state of the cell, alter normal cell function and signaling [7, 16], and ultimately lead to modulation of gene expression [39]. In a previous study with mice, the intake of moderately oxidized n-3 PUFA for 8 weeks induced oxidative stress in the intestine and enhanced

Table 4 Significantly changed gene transcripts identified with Limma (FDR q value < 0.1) within the oxFO or FO group after 7 weeks of intervention

	FC within groups from baseline		FDR q value	
Gene	oxFO	FO	oxFO	FO
CD55	0.83	0.85	0.00	0.01
SNORD13	0.63	0.60	0.04	0.01
VNN2	0.90	0.80	0.59	0.01
SNORA12	0.82	0.70	0.59	0.03
RSBN1L	0.92	0.88	0.59	0.03
VNN2	0.87	0.77	0.62	0.04
LOC80054	1.05	1.09	0.62	0.09
POLR1D	0.96	0.90	0.66	0.09
SERPINB9	0.98	0.85	0.92	0.09
RAB11FIP2	0.99	0.90	0.92	0.09
SNORD12C	0.91	0.88	0.59	0.10
BAK1	1.13	1.08	0.04	0.24

oxFO oxidized fish oil, FO fish oil, FC fold change from baseline, FDR false discovery rate

Table 5 Enriched biological processes within the oxFO and FO groups after 7 weeks of intervention among the regulated genes obtained with Limma analysis ($p < 0.05$)

Enriched BP oxFO	Fold enrichment	FDR %
GO:0006414~translational elongation	9.52	0.00
GO:0007049~cell cycle	2.48	0.02
GO:0006412~translation	3.49	0.03
GO:0000280~nuclear division	4.08	0.07
GO:0007067~mitosis	4.08	0.07
GO:0000087~M phase of mitotic cell cycle	4.01	0.08
GO:0048285~organelle fission	3.92	0.10
GO:0000278~mitotic cell cycle	3.12	0.11
GO:0022402~cell cycle process	2.38	0.85
GO:0051301~cell division	3.04	1.19
GO:0022403~cell cycle phase	2.63	1.23
GO:0042981~regulation of apoptosis	1.99	2.62
GO:0043067~regulation of programmed cell death	1.97	2.98
GO:0010941~regulation of cell death	1.97	3.13
GO:0000279~M phase	2.73	3.15
GO:0051726~regulation of cell cycle	2.71	3.34
GO:0051338~regulation of transferase activity	2.59	3.37
Enriched BP FO		
GO:0006414~translational elongation	9.22	0.00
GO:0006412~translation	3.83	0.00
GO:0006916~anti-apoptosis	3.80	0.00
GO:0043066~negative regulation of apoptosis	2.53	0.14
GO:0043069~negative regulation of programmed cell death	2.49	0.18
GO:0060548~negative regulation of cell death	2.48	0.18
GO:0043067~regulation of programmed cell death	1.88	0.23
GO:0010941~regulation of cell death	1.87	0.25
GO:0042981~regulation of apoptosis	1.85	0.39
GO:0042254~ribosome biogenesis	3.36	2.73
GO:0006917~induction of apoptosis	2.21	4.20
GO:0012502~induction of programmed cell death	2.21	4.32

oxFO oxidized fish oil, FO fish oil, BP biological processes, FDR false discovery rate

plasma inflammatory markers and gene expression analyses showed an increase in the glucose-regulated protein 78 (GRP78) and glutathione peroxidase 2 (GPx2) mRNA [20]. We have previously not been able to detect changes in markers of oxidative stress such as urinary 8-iso-PGF2a, plasma a-tocopherol, plasma 4-hydroxy-2-

hexenal and plasma 4-hydroxy-2-nonenal or glutathione, CAT activity, and GPx activity in erythrocytes or inflammatory markers in the same study after intake of oxFO compared to high-quality FO [27, 28]. Furthermore, the intake of oxFO, containing lipid oxidation products, did not alter biological processes or gene sets related to oxidative stress when compared to fish oil in the current study.

When the groups were analyzed separately, the mRNA level of BAK1 was significantly increased from baseline within the oxFO group. The BAK1 protein is localized to the mitochondria and functions to induce apoptosis. This protein also interacts with the tumor suppressor p53 after exposure to cellular stress [40], and the increased BAK1 mRNA level could be caused by the intake of lipid oxidation products in the oxFO group. BAK and BAX were recently shown to be involved in eicosanoid metabolism independent of apoptotic functions [41]. The increase in BAK1 mRNA may therefore be related to the eicosanoid precursor EPA and DHA, presented in equal amounts in the two fish oils. BAK1 mRNA was also increased from the baseline within the FO group, although not significantly (Table 4), and biological processes related to apoptosis were regulated within both fish oil groups.

Biological processes related to translation elongation, translation, and apoptosis were enriched within both groups, while biological processes related to cell cycle was only enriched within the oxFO group. However, we have previously shown that the intake of high-quality FO regulated gene transcripts related to apoptosis, cell cycle, and ER stress when compared to the intake of high-oleic sunflower oil [36]. Our data is in accordance with Bouwens et al.'s, who also demonstrated that the expression of genes involved in pathways related to processes such as transcription, translation, and cell cycle were regulated in PBMCs after the intake of FO (1.8 g/day EPA+DHA) for 26 weeks in elderly subjects [31]. Thus, processes related to the translation, apoptosis, and cell cycle may be modulated after the intake of fish oil independent of oxidative status. These processes and pathways are involved in normal cellular functions and may ultimately influence whole body health. We did not detect any regulated pathways or processes related to lipid metabolism, antioxidant defense, and inflammation as previously reported after n-3 supplementation [31, 42–44]. This could be explained by the inclusion of healthy subjects in the current study, and the results may be different in subjects with elevated levels of inflammation, oxidative stress, or serum lipids.

CD55 was downregulated from the baseline within both groups and independent of the oxidative status of the fish oils. CD55 is part of the complement system and has been suggested to play a role in the pathogenesis of atherosclerosis [45]. CD55 deficiency has also been shown to protect apoE$^{-/-}$ mice from atherosclerosis [46]. The downregulation of CD55 mRNA by fish oil may thus be one of the mechanisms by which fish oil can exert its beneficial effect.

The changes in the oxidative status of the oil as measured by increased PV and AV occur prior to a measurable reduction in the concentration of fatty acids. Thus, the oxidized and the non-oxidized FO contained an equal amount of fatty acids, including n-3 fatty acids (Table 1). The similar transcriptome profile may therefore be explained by the similar fatty acid profile of the FOs [28] as they originated from the same batch.

Conflicting results related to the prevention of cardiovascular diseases by marine LCPUFAs have recently been published [47]. It has been suggested that the oxidation of the marine oils may be responsible for the lack of effect [15]. A recent study investigating the effect of omega-3 supplements with different oxidation level on circulating lipid parameters showed a reduction in plasma triglycerides independent of the oxidative status of the fish oil. However, a beneficial effect on plasma total cholesterol was only evident in the group consuming less oxidized fish oil [48]. In the current study, a more prominent effect was evident after the intake of FO as 11 gene transcripts were significantly (FDR < 0.1) changed from baseline whereas 3 within the oxFO group (Table 4). Whether this is related to the oxidative status of the fish oils is currently not known and needs further investigations.

The present study was originally designed to investigate the effect of oxFO on the circulating markers of oxidative stress, inflammation, and plasma lipids compared to high-quality FO, and the power of the study was calculated based on the relative change in plasma n-3 compared to the high-oleic sunflower oil [28]. We cannot rule out the possibility that the current study lacks the power to detect differences between the two FO groups when it comes to the transcriptome profile. However, transcriptome analyses in PBMCs represent a sensitive high-throughput method to detect changes caused by diet [30]. To increase the power in the current study, we included analyses where genes were grouped based on involvement in the same biological process, pathway, or network.

The strengths of the present study are that the study design was performed as a blinded randomized controlled trial with high compliance, as described in more detail elsewhere [28]. The transcriptome analyses have been performed with an exploratory approach where the identification of regulated gene transcripts, biological processes, and networks was done with several data analysis strategies. The major limitation is the relatively low daily dose of oxidized lipids (PV/AV) administered and the relatively short intervention period. The study group included healthy subjects, and we cannot rule out that by using another study group more susceptible to the intake of oxFO, this would have led to different results. There is also a chance that other cellular compartments

or tissues such as the intestine may have been affected by the intake of oxFO in the present study.

Conclusion

By using a transcriptome approach, we aimed to investigate the effects at the molecular level prior to changes in circulating markers. The results demonstrate that the short-term consumption of oxidized fish oil in healthy subjects did not alter the transcriptome profile in PBMCs compared to the intake of high-quality FO. Whether these results are applicable for other oxidized marine oils, longer interventions, or valid in subjects with elevated levels of inflammation and oxidative stress needs to be addressed.

Abbreviations
AV: anisidine value; CHD: coronary heart disease; FC: fold change; FDR: false discovery rate; FO: fish oil; LCPUFAs: long-chain polyunsaturated fatty acids; meq/kg: milliequivalents per kilogram; oxFO: oxidized fish oil; PBMCs: peripheral blood mononuclear cells; PV: peroxide value.

Acknowledgements
The microarray analyses were performed by the Genomics Core Facility, Norwegian University of Science and Technology, and NMC—a national technology platform supported by the Functional Genomics (FUGE) program of the Research Council of Norway.

Funding
This study was supported by the Research Council of Norway (project no. 184813/110), Oslo, the Akershus University College of Applied Sciences, Norway; the University of Oslo, Norway; and the Throne Holst Foundation for Nutrition Research.

Authors' contributions
MCWM designed research and developed the research plan, carried out the microarray and statistical analyses, interpretation of data and drafted the manuscript. IO designed research and developed the research plan, performed statistical analyses and drafted the manuscript. C-CG carried out microarray analyses. ER carried out microarray analyses. MH carried out microarray analyses. AN designed research and developed research plan. KWB designed research and developed the research plan. AK carried out statistical analyses and interpretation of data. GIAB designed research and developed the research plan, interpretation of data. KBH designed research and developed the research plan, interpretation of data and drafted the manuscript. SMU designed research and developed the research plan, interpretation of data and draftet the manuscript. All authors read and approved the final manuscript.

Competing interests
Kirsti W. Brønner is a clinical nutritionist/project manager at the TINE SA R&D Center, Norway, with no financial interest. Kirsten B. Holven and Stine M. Ulven have received research funding from TINE SA but declare no conflict of interest. Mari C. W. Myhrstad, Inger Ottestad, Clara-Cecilie Günther, Einar Ryeng, Marit Holden, Astrid Nilsson, Achim Kohler, and Grethe I. A. Borge declare no conflict of interest.

Author details
[1]Department of Health, Nutrition and Management, Faculty of Health Sciences, Oslo and Akershus University College of Applied Sciences, P.O. Box 4St. Olavs plass, 0130 Oslo, Norway. [2]Department of Nutrition, Institute for Basic Medical Sciences, University of Oslo, P.O. Box 1046Blindern, 0317 Oslo, Norway. [3]Norwegian Computing Center, 0314 Oslo, Norway. [4]Department of Cancer Research and Molecular Medicine, Norwegian University of Science

and Technology, 7489 Trondheim, Norway. ⁵Nofima AS Norwegian Institute of Food, Fisheries and Aquaculture Research, PB 210, Aas N-1431, Norway. ⁶TINE SA, Centre for Research and Development, P.O. Box 7Kalbakken, 0902 Oslo, Norway. ⁷Department of Mathematical Sciences and Technology (IMT), Norwegian University of Life Sciences, 1432 Ås, Norway ⁸Norwegian National Advisory Unit on Familial Hypercholesterolemia, Department of Endocrinology, Morbid Obesity and Preventive Medicine, Oslo University Hospital Rikshospitalet, P.O Box 4950Nydalen, Oslo, Norway.

References

1. Dietary supplementation with n-3 polyunsaturated fatty acids and vitamin E after myocardial infarction: results of the GISSI-Prevenzione trial. Gruppo Italiano per lo Studio della Sopravvivenza nell'Infarto miocardico. 1999 Lancet 354:447-55.
2. Yokoyama M et al. Effects of eicosapentaenoic acid on major coronary events in hypercholesterolaemic patients (JELIS): a randomised open-label, blinded endpoint analysis. Lancet. 2007;369:1090-8. doi:10.1016/S0140-6736(07)60527-3.
3. Gebauer SK, Psota TL, Harris WS, Kris-Etherton PM. n-3 fatty acid dietary recommendations and food sources to achieve essentiality and cardiovascular benefits. Am J Clin Nutr. 2006;83:1526S-35.
4. Lichtenstein AH et al. Summary of American Heart Association Diet and Lifestyle Recommendations revision 2006. Arterioscler Thromb Vasc Biol. 2006;26:2186-91. doi:10.1161/01.ATV.0000238352.25222.5e.
5. Mozaffarian D. Fish and n-3 fatty acids for the prevention of fatal coronary heart disease and sudden cardiac death. Am J Clin Nutr. 2008;87:1991S-6.
6. Catala A. Lipid peroxidation of membrane phospholipids generates hydroxy-alkenals and oxidized phospholipids active in physiological and/or pathological conditions. Chem Phys Lipids. 2009;157:1-11. doi:10.1016/j.chemphyslip.2008.09.004.
7. Esterbauer H, Schaur RJ, Zollner H. Chemistry and biochemistry of 4-hydroxynonenal, malonaldehyde and related aldehydes. Free Radic Biol Med. 1991;11:81-128.
8. Siddiqui RA, Harvey K, Stillwell W. Ant cancer properties of oxidation products of docosahexaenoic acid. Chem Phys Lipids. 2008;153:47-56. doi:10.1016/j.chemphyslip.2008.02.009.
9. (GOED) GOfEaDo-s (2006) Global Organization for EPA and DHA omega-3s (GOED) GOED
10. (VKM) NSCfFS (2012) Description of the processes in the value chain and risk assessment of decomposition substances and oxidation products in fish oils (08-504-4-final). vol 08-504-4-final.
11. Albert BB et al. Fish oil supplements in New Zealand are highly oxidised and do not meet label content of n-3 PUFA. Sci Rep. 2015;5:7928. doi:10.1038/srep07928.
12. Halvorsen BL, Blomhoff R. Determination of lipid oxidation products in vegetable oils and marine omega-3 supplements. Food Nutr Res. 2011; 55 doi:10.3402/fnr.v55i0.5792
13. Kolanowski W. Omega-3 LC PUFA contents and oxidative stability of encapsulated fish oil dietary supplements. Int J Food Prop. 2010;13:498-511. doi:10.1080/10942910802652222.
14. (BIOHAZ) EPoBH. Scientific opinion on fish oil for human consumption. Food hygiene, including rancidity. EFSA J. 2010;8:48. doi:10.2903/j.efsa.2010.1874.
15. Albert BB, Cameron-Smith D, Hofman PL, Cutfield WS. Oxidation of marine omega-3 supplements and human health. Biomed Res Int. 2013;2013: 464921. doi:10.1155/2013/464921.
16. Halliwell B, Chirico S. Lipid peroxidation: its mechanism, measurement, and significance. Am J Clin Nutr. 1993;57:715S-24. discussion 724S-725S.
17. Niki E. Lipid peroxidation: physiological levels and dual biological effects. Free Radic Biol Med. 2009;47:469-84. doi:10.1016/j.freeradbiomed.2009.05.032.
18. Riahi Y, Cohen G, Shamni O, Sasson S. Signaling and cytotoxic functions of 4-hydroxyalkenals. Am J Physiol Endocrinol Metab. 2010;299:E879-86. doi:10.1152/ajpendo.00508.2010.
19. Sayre LM, Lin D, Yuan Q, Zhu X, Tang X. Protein adducts generated from products of lipid oxidation: focus on HNE and one. Drug Metab Rev. 2006; 38:651-75. doi:10.1080/03602530600959508.
20. Awada M et al. Dietary oxidized n-3 PUFA induce oxidative stress and inflammation: role of intestinal absorption of 4-HHE and reactivity in intestinal cells. J Lipid Res. 2012;53:2069-80. doi:10.1194/jlr.M026179.
21. Esterbauer H. Cytotoxicity and genotoxicity of lipid-oxidation products. Am J Clin Nutr. 1993;57:779S-85. discussion 785S-786S.
22. Staprans I, Hardman DA, Pan XM, Feingold KR. Effect of oxidized lipids in the diet on oxidized lipid levels in postprandial serum chylomicrons of diabetic patients. Diabetes Care. 1999;22:300-6.
23. Staprans I, Rapp JH, Pan XM, Kim KY, Feingold KR. Oxidized lipids in the diet are a source of oxidized lipid in chylomicrons of human serum. Arterioscler Thromb. 1994;14:1900-5.
24. Sutherland WH, de Jong SA, Hessian PA, Williams MJ. Ingestion of native and thermally oxidized polyunsaturated fats acutely increases circulating numbers of endothelial microparticles. Metabolism. 2010;59:446-53. doi:10.1016/j.metabol.2009.07.033.
25. Sutherland WH, de Jong SA, Walker RJ, Williams MJ, Murray Skeaff C, Duncan A, Harper M. Effect of meals rich in heated olive and safflower oils on oxidation of postprandial serum in healthy men. Atherosclerosis. 2002;160:195-203.
26. Wallace AJ, Sutherland WH, Mann JI, Williams SM. The effect of meals rich in thermally stressed olive and safflower oils on postprandial serum paraoxonase activity in patients with diabetes. Eur J Clin Nutr. 2001;55:951-8. doi:10.1038/sj.ejcn.1601250.
27. Ottestad I et al. Intake of oxidised fish oil does not affect circulating levels of oxidised LDL or inflammatory markers in healthy subjects. Nutr Metab Cardiovasc Dis. 2013;23:e3-4. doi:10.1016/j.numecd.2012.08.009.
28. Ottestad I et al. Oxidised fish oil does not influence established markers of oxidative stress in healthy human subjects: a randomised controlled trial Br J Nutr. 2011:1-12 doi:10.1017/S0007114511005484
29. Afman L, Milenkovic D, Roche HM. Nutritional aspects of metabolic inflammation in relation to health-insights from transcriptomic biomarkers in PBMC of fatty acids and polyphenols. Mol Nutr Food Res. 2014. doi:10.1002/mnfr.201300559.
30. de Mello VD, Kolehmanien M, Schwab U, Pulkkinen L, Uusitupa M. Gene expression of peripheral blood mononuclear cells as a tool in dietary intervention studies: what do we know so far? Mol Nutr Food Res. 2012;56: 1160-72. doi:10.1002/mnfr.201100685.
31. Bouwens M et al. Fish-oil supplementation induces antiinflammatory gene expression profiles in human blood mononuclear cells. Am J Clin Nutr. 2009;90:415-24. doi:10.3945/ajcn.2009.27680.
32. de Mello VD et al. The effect of fatty or lean fish intake on inflammatory gene expression in peripheral blood mononuclear cells of patients with coronary heart disease. Eur J Nutr. 2009;48:447-55. doi:10.1007/s00394-009-0033-y.
33. Kolehmainen M et al. Bilberries reduce low-grade inflammation in individuals with features of metabolic syndrome. Mol Nutr Food Res. 2012;56:1501-10. doi:10.1002/mnfr.201200195.
34. Radler U et al. A combination of (omega-3) polyunsaturated fatty acids, polyphenols and L-carnitine reduces the plasma lipid levels and increases the expression of genes involved in fatty acid oxidation in human peripheral blood mononuclear cells and HepG2 cells. Ann Nutr Metab. 2011; 58:133-40. doi:10.1159/000327150.
35. van Dijk SJ, Feskens EJ, Bos MB, de Groot LC, de Vries JH, Muller M, Afman LA. Consumption of a high monounsaturated fat diet reduces oxidative phosphorylation gene expression in peripheral blood mononuclear cells of abdominally overweight men and women. J Nutr. 2012;142:1219-25. doi:10.3945/jn.111.155283.
36. Myhrstad MC et al. Fish oil supplementation induces expression of genes related to cell cycle, endoplasmic reticulum stress and apoptosis in peripheral blood mononuclear cells: a transcriptomic approach. J Intern Med. 2014;276:498-511. doi:10.1111/joim.12217.
37. Smyth GK. Linear models and empirical Bayes methods for assessing differential expression in microarray experiments. Stat Appl Genet Mol Biol. 2004;3:Article3. doi:10.2202/1544-6115.1027.
38. Brazma A et al. Minimum information about a microarray experiment (MIAME)-toward standards for microarray data. Nat Genet. 2001;29:365-71. doi:10.1038/ng1201-365.
39. Allen RG, Tresini M. Oxidative stress and gene regulation. Free Radic Biol Med. 2000;28:463-99.
40. Mathai JP, Germain M, Shore GC. BH3-only BIK regulates BAX, BAK-dependent release of Ca2+ from endoplasmic reticulum stores and mitochondrial apoptosis during stress-induced cell death. J Biol Chem. 2005;280:23829-36. doi:10.1074/jbc.M500800200.
41. Zhang T, Walensky LD, Saghatelian A. A nonapoptotic role for BAX and BAK in eicosanoid metabolism. ACS Chem Biol. 2015;10:1398-403. doi:10.1021/acschembio.5b00168.

42. Schmidt S, Stahl F, Mutz KO, Scheper T, Hahn A, Schuchardt JP. Different gene expression profiles in normo- and dyslipidemic men after fish oil supplementation: results from a randomized controlled trial. Lipids Health Dis. 2012a 11:105 doi:10.1186/1476-511X-11-105

43. Schmidt S, Stahl F, Mutz KO, Scheper T, Hahn A, Schuchardt JP. Transcriptome-based identification of antioxidative gene expression after fish oil supplementation in normo- and dyslipidemic men. Nutr Metab 2012b 9:45 doi:10.1186/1743-7075-9-45

44. Vedin I et al. Effects of DHA-rich n-3 fatty acid supplementation on gene expression in blood mononuclear leukocytes: the OmegAD study. PLoS One. 2012;7:e35425. doi:10.1371/journal.pone.0035425.

45. Kostner KM. Activation of the complement system: a crucial link between inflammation and atherosclerosis? Eur J Clin Invest. 2004;34:800–2. doi:10.1111/j.1365-2362.2004.01431.x.

46. Lewis RD, Perry MJ, Guschina IA, Jackson CL, Morgan BP, Hughes TR. CD55 deficiency protects against atherosclerosis in ApoE-deficient mice via C3a modulation of lipid metabolism. Am J Pathol. 2011;179:1601–7. doi:10.1016/j.ajpath.2011.06.015.

47. Rizos EC, Ntzani EE, Bika E, Kostapanos MS, Elisaf MS. Association between omega-3 fatty acid supplementation and risk of major cardiovascular disease events: a systematic review and meta-analysis. JAMA. 2012;308: 1024–33. doi:10.1001/2012.jama.11374.

48. Garcia-Hernandez VM, Gallar M, Sanchez-Soriano J, Micol V, Roche E, Garcia-Garcia E. Effect of omega-3 dietary supplements with different oxidation levels in the lipidic profile of women: a randomized controlled trial. Int J Food Sci Nutr. 2013;64:993–1000. doi:10.3109/09637486.2013.812619.

7

Bioavailability of transgenic microRNAs in genetically modified plants

Jian Yang[1], Cecilia Primo[1], Ismail Elbaz-Younes[1] and Kendal D. Hirschi[1,2*] (iD)

Abstract

Background: Transgenic expression of small RNAs is a prevalent approach in agrobiotechnology for the global enhancement of plant foods. Meanwhile, emerging studies have, on the one hand, emphasized the potential of transgenic microRNAs (miRNAs) as novel dietary therapeutics and, on the other, suggested potential food safety issues if harmful miRNAs are absorbed and bioactive. For these reasons, it is necessary to evaluate the bioavailability of transgenic miRNAs in genetically modified crops.

Results: As a pilot study, two transgenic Arabidopsis lines ectopically expressing unique miRNAs were compared and contrasted with the plant bioavailable small RNA MIR2911 for digestive stability and serum bioavailability. The expression levels of these transgenic miRNAs in Arabidopsis were found to be comparable to that of MIR2911 in fresh tissues. Assays of digestive stability in vitro and in vivo suggested the transgenic miRNAs and MIR2911 had comparable resistance to degradation. Healthy mice consuming diets rich in Arabidopsis lines expressing these miRNAs displayed MIR2911 in the bloodstream but no detectable levels of the transgenic miRNAs.

Conclusions: These preliminary results imply digestive stability and high expression levels of miRNAs in plants do not readily equate to bioavailability. This initial work suggests novel engineering strategies be employed to enhance miRNA bioavailability when attempting to use transgenic foods as a delivery platform.

Keywords: Dietary microRNAs, Genetically modified organisms, Bioavailability, Digestive stability, MIR2911, Mice

Background

Since 1996, genetically modified (GM) crops have been commonly consumed by the general public [1]. Excitement has also been generated that some of these GM plants can help alleviate diseases and malnutrition [2, 3]. The current safety assessments for these commercial crops predominately focus on the transgenic protein(s) [4, 5]. However, agrobiotechnology often expresses novel RNA molecules in crops. Both the safety and therapeutic potential of transgenic RNAs in GM crops should be thoughtfully addressed [6].

Both microRNAs (miRNAs) and small interfering RNAs (siRNAs) are classes of small RNAs (sRNAs) that regulate gene expression [7]. RNA interference (RNAi) is an umbrella term that defines conditions where a sRNA directs sequence-specific gene repression. The prevailing view is that dietary sRNAs are not absorbed by consumers [8–13]; however, recent studies suggest that consumers may absorb and circulate dietary RNAs [14–19]. The uptake of GM diet-derived RNAs in controlled animal feeding studies should be carefully examined in order to establish guidelines for risk assessment and therapeutic applications.

Bioavailability is defined as the portion of a substance that reaches systemic circulation, and the bioavailability of dietary sRNAs appears to be low [13, 20, 21]. However, sRNAs ingested from plant-based foods may act as potent bioactives and have been implicated in reversing specific diseases in several cases [15–18, 20, 22, 23]. Meanwhile, numerous groups have found that dietary sRNAs are not bioavailable in animals [8, 9, 13]. The ability/inability to detect these dietary sRNAs in consumers has been attributed to a variety of potential differences among research groups, including methodology inconsistencies, contamination, and detection sensitivity issues [20, 24–26]. To date, research labs that have successfully demonstrated serum uptake of plant-based

* Correspondence: kendalh@bcm.edu
[1]USDA/ARS Children's Nutrition Research Center, Baylor College of Medicine, 1100 Bates Street, Houston, TX 77030, USA
[2]Vegetable and Fruit Improvement Center, Texas A&M University, College Station, TX 77845, USA

sRNAs have not addressed bioavailability of transgenic miRNAs in plant-based diets. One of the concerns of GM crops is the introduction of foreign genes into crops and its unpredictable consequences. For example, it is theoretically possible that transgenic miRNAs possess unique chemical modifications which allow them to be more bioavailable than a native miRNA. As a result, the characterization of the bioavailability of transgenic foreign miRNAs is warranted.

Our group has successfully demonstrated that the plant-based sRNA MIR2911, found in a melody of vegetables, is more stable during digestion and is bioavailable to mice fed vegetable-based diets [14, 21, 27, 28]. Here we report the characterization of the digestive stability and dietary uptake of two miRNAs that are expressed in transgenic plants at levels comparable to the MIR2911 in fresh tissues. This small sampling of Arabidopsis lines suggests that transgenic miRNAs may not be readily bioavailable.

Methods
Generation of transgenic plant lines
The transgenic Arabidopsis line expressing the artificial miRNA termed amiR-RICE sequence (5′-UUU GGA AGC AAA GAA GCG GUG -3′) was obtained from Dr. Xiuren Zhang (Zhang et al.; personal communication 2015). The binary construct for overexpression of a murine miRNA mmu-miR146a (5′-UGA GAA CUG AAU UCC AUG GGU U -3′) in Arabidopsis was made using the Gateway system (Invitrogen, Carlsbad, CA). The destination vector pBA-DC [29] and template entry vector pENTR-amiR-CPC3-159a [29] were provided by Dr. Xiuren Zhang, and mmu-miR146a was cloned into the entry vector as previously described [29]. The sequences of the cloning primers which contained the incorporated mmu-miR146a sequences were as follows: forward-5′-AAG ATA GAT CTT GAT CTG ACG ATG GAA GAA CCT GTG AAA TTC AGT TCT TGC ATG AGT TGA GCA GGG TA -3′; reverse-5′-AAG ACC CGG GAT GAA CCC ATG GAA TTC AGT TCT CAG AAG AGT AAA AGC CAT TA -3′ (mmu-miR146a business and passenger strand sequences are underlined). The growth conditions of Arabidopsis line were as described [30]. Transgenic lines were distinguished from untransformed by BASTA selection. Homozygous lines harboring the transgenic mmu-miR146a constructs were selected by segregation analysis in the T3 generation. The lines were analyzed by qRT-PCR for mmu-miR146a expression, and the lines displaying the most robust shoot expression in adult plants grown on soil for 45 days (stage 6.50, https://www.arabidopsis.org/portals/education/growth.jsp) were used for diet preparation. From here on, the transgenic Arabidopsis lines used for mouse feeding

studies and overexpressing amiR-RICE and mmu-miR146a are referred to as tg-RICE and tg-146, respectively.

Plant diet preparation
The shoot tissues from approximately 45-day-old tg-RICE or tg-146 plants were harvested and freeze dried to 30% of fresh weight, and the dried tissues was then finely ground and mixed with finely ground chow (Teklad 2914, Envigo, UK) and water at 1:2:2 weight ratios, according to procedures described previously [14] and stored at −20 °C until use.

Degradation of miRNAs in transgenic plant diets
After preparation, the diets were incubated at room temperature. A 10–20-mg fraction of diet was removed at 1, 4, and 24 h to assay the stability of miRNAs within the diet [31]. To isolate total RNA from the plant diet, the miRNEASY RNA isolation kit (Qiagen, Valencia, CA) was used according to the manufacturer's instructions. Fifty femtomoles of an artificial miRNA termed C7 was used as an exogenous spike-in control.

Animal feeding studies
The experimental protocol involving mice was approved by the Institutional Animal Care and Use Committee of Baylor College of Medicine. Specifically, the institutional animal protocols AN-2624, AN-6438, and AN-6454 cover the experiments performed in this study. All mice were obtained from the Center for Comparative Medicine at Baylor College of Medicine. Male ICR mice at 8 to 10 weeks old were used in all feeding studies, which were replicated at least three times; the results shown are representative of the biological replicates. Mice were fed with the plant diets for 3 days before they were sacrificed. Each day, 5 g of the plant diet that contained 1 g of dried plant material was fed to each mouse. The daily intake of plant material per mouse is equivalent to 3.3 g of fresh plant tissue.

Serum collection and RNA extraction
Blood was collected via cardiac puncture as previously described [14]. Sera were separated at room temperature followed by centrifugation to remove all blood cells and debris. Total RNA was extracted from 100 μL of sera using the miRNEASY Kit following the manufacturer's recommendations.

Analysis of miRNA levels by qRT-PCR
TaqMan miRNA Assays for let-7dgi [32], C7, amiR-RICE, mmu-miR146a, MIR2911, and MIR168a were obtained from Life Technologies (Carlsbad, CA). Total RNA isolated was used in each reverse transcription (RT) reaction, as previously described [14]. To quantify miRNA levels in Arabidopsis, plant shoot material was

ground to a fine powder in liquid nitrogen and then 10–20 mg was subjected to RNA isolation using the miRNeasy kit; 50 fmol of synthetic C7 was spiked into the plant Qiazol lysate as an exogenous RNA control. qRT-PCR was performed using a Biorad CFX96 Real-Time PCR Detection System, and data were analyzed using Biorad CFX software. Delta-Delta-Ct method was used to calculate the relative levels of miRNAs. Absolute concentrations of miRNAs were calculated based on standard curves obtained from serial dilutions of synthetic miRNAs [14] (Additional file 1: Figure S1).

Preparation of synthetic miRNAs

Synthetic miRNAs were obtained from Integrated DNA Technologies (Coralville, IA) with 5′-phosphorylation and 2-O-methylation at the 3′ end nucleotide, to mimic the chemistry of plant-derived miRNAs. The sequence of the miRNAs were as follows: MIR-2911 5′-GGC CGG GGG ACG GGC UGG GA -3′; MIR-168a 5′-UCG CUU GGU GCA GAU CGG GAC -3′; amiR-RICE 5′-UUU GGA AGC AAA GAA GCG GUG -3′; mmu-miR146a 5′-UGA GAA CUG AAU UCC AUG GGU U -3′; C7 5′-GGA UCA UCU CAA GUC UUA CGU -3′; and MIR161 5′- UCA AUG CAU UGA AAG UGA CUA -3′. For gavage feeding, miRNAs were diluted in RNase-free phosphate-buffered saline (PBS), and each animal was fed 400 pmol of each miRNA in 300-µL volume [14].

In vitro digestion of miRNAs with porcine enzymes

In vitro digestion conditions were as previously described [33, 34]. Briefly, the gastric phase was composed of a gastric electrolyte solution (7.8 mM K^+, 72.2 mM Na^+, 70.2 mM Cl^-, 0.9 $H_2PO_4^-$, 25.5 mM HCO_3^-, 0.1 mM Mg^{2+}, 1.0 mM NH_4^+, 0.15 mM Ca^{2+}) with pH adjusted by 1 N HCl to 2.0 and porcine pepsin (80 mg/mL) (Sigma, St. Louis, MO); the intestinal phase was formed by adding to the gastric phase an intestinal electrolyte solution (7.8 mM K^+, 72.2 mM Na^+, 124.4 mM Cl^-, 55.5 $H_2PO_4^-$, 85 mM HCO_3^-, 0.33 mM Mg^{2+}, 0.6 mM Ca^{2+}), 24 mg/mL of bile extract (Sigma, St. Louis, MO), and 40 mg/mL of porcine pancreatin (Sigma, St. Louis, MO) and 1 N NaOH to adjust the pH to 7.0. One-milliliter PBS solution containing 10 pmol each of MIR2911, C7, amiR-RICE, and mmu-miR146a synthetic miRNAs was first mixed with 1-mL gastric phase and digested with slow rotation at 37 °C for 60 min. The digestion mixture was then mixed with intestinal phase and digested with slow rotation at 37 °C for an additional 75 min. One hundred microliters of samples were removed at 30 min, 60 min of the gastric phase, and 5, 30, and 75 min of the intestinal phase for analysis of the levels of surviving miRNAs. One hundred microliters of pre-digestion samples were used as controls for calculating

the percentage of surviving miRNAs. MIR161 was used as an exogenous spike-in control.

In vivo digestion of gavaged miRNAs

ICR mice were fed purified diet (AIN-76a) for 7 days and then gavage-fed 400 pmol of MIR2911, C7, amiR-RICE, and mmu-miR146a. miRNA levels from the intestine were assessed 1 h post-gavage from the intestinal contents by flushing the excised intestines with 1 mL of PBS. One hundred microliters of the homogenized intestinal content was subject to RNA isolation and qRT-PCR analysis. MIR161 was used as an exogenous spike-in control.

Assaying miRNA levels from diets in the small intestines

Mice fed transgenic diets and chow were used for this assay. The levels of miRNAs from the small intestine were determined using the intestinal contents collected by flushing the excised small intestines with 1 mL of PBS solution. One hundred microliters of the homogenized intestinal contents were analyzed by qRT-PCR for the levels of miRNAs.

Statistical analysis

Statistical analyses were performed with the Student t test formula in Microsoft Excel. Significance was set at $p < 0.05$. Data were presented as means ± SEMs.

Results

Levels of transgenic miRNAs in plants

Arabidopsis was used for creating transgenic foods as it is a well-characterized model system [35]. Arabidopsis lines were engineered that express two miRNAs, amiR-RICE and mmu-miR146a. amiR-RICE is an artificial miRNA whose sequence has no homology to either plant or animal endogenous miRNAs, while mmu-miR146a's sequence is identical to the endogenous murine miRNA [36]. The expression level of amiR-RICE lines has been characterized (Xiuren Zhang; personal communication 2015). For mmu-miR146a, plant lines that showed the most robust expression were used for further studies (Additional file 2: Figure S2). qRT-PCR quantification results demonstrated that the expression levels of amiR-RICE and mmu-miR146a reached levels of 22.9 and 26.3 fmol/g of fresh weight, respectively, which is similar to the levels of MIR2911 in fresh shoot tissues (approximately 18–19 fmol/g) (Fig. 1).

Levels of transgenic miRNAs in diets

Our previous studies demonstrate that dietary abundance of miRNAs can change during diet degradation and impact uptake in consumers [31]. Levels of amiR-RICE and mmu-miR146a were assayed to determine their stability relative to that of MIR2911, in the diets

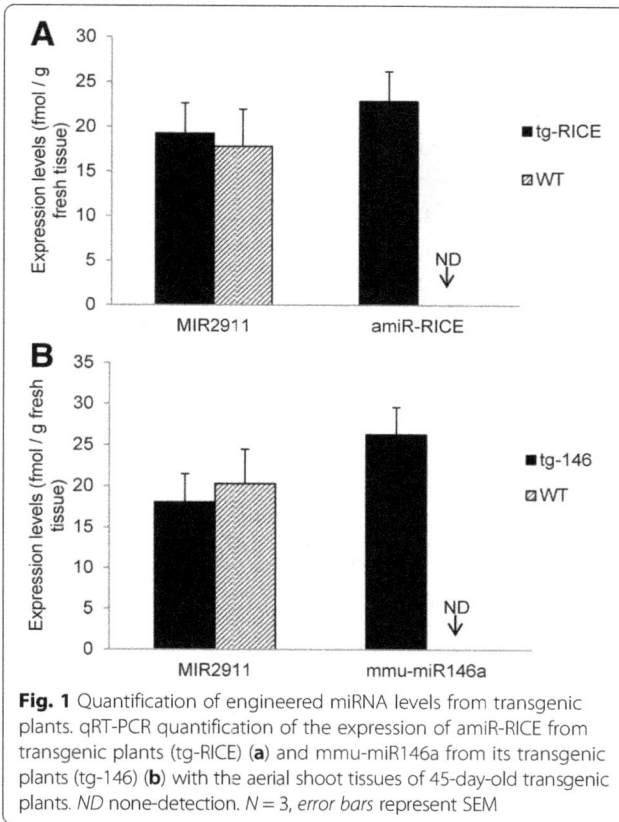

Fig. 1 Quantification of engineered miRNA levels from transgenic plants. qRT-PCR quantification of the expression of amiR-RICE from transgenic plants (tg-RICE) (**a**) and mmu-miR146a from its transgenic plants (tg-146) (**b**) with the aerial shoot tissues of 45-day-old transgenic plants. *ND* none-detection. *N* = 3, *error bars* represent SEM

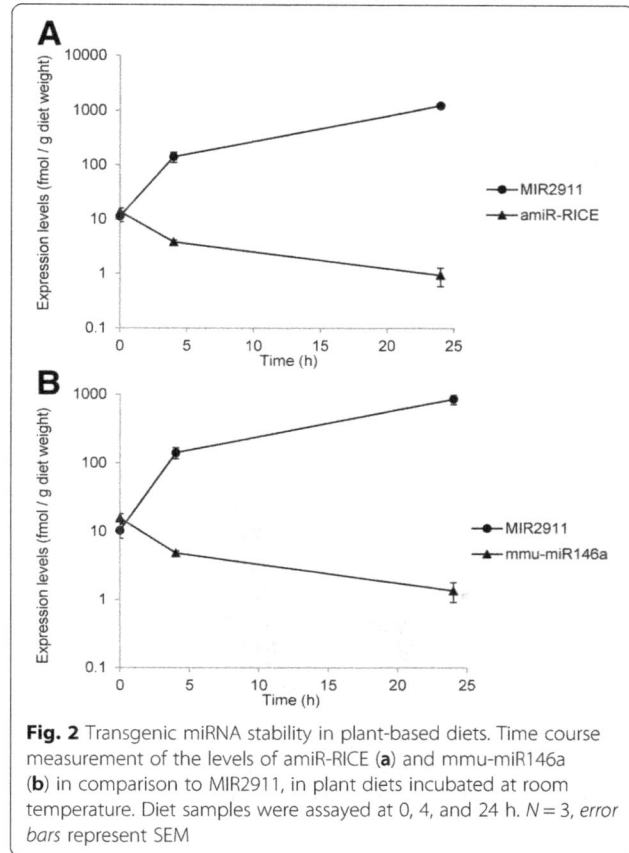

Fig. 2 Transgenic miRNA stability in plant-based diets. Time course measurement of the levels of amiR-RICE (**a**) and mmu-miR146a (**b**) in comparison to MIR2911, in plant diets incubated at room temperature. Diet samples were assayed at 0, 4, and 24 h. *N* = 3, *error bars* represent SEM

that were incubated at room temperature. The abundance of amiR-RICE and mmu-miR146a decreased gradually over time by approximately 10-fold, to approximately 1 fmol/g of diet, while MIR2911's abundance, as we have demonstrated previously [31], was amplified by more than 85-fold after 24 h in the chow (Fig. 2).

Digestive stability of transgenic miRNAs

One of the main factors affecting bioavailability is the digestive stability of the nutrients [33]. Synthetic forms of the plant-based transgenic miRNAs, amiR-RICE and mmu-miR146a, were tested for their digestive stability using both an in vitro and in vivo assay. This was performed in comparison to MIR2911 and C7, which have been shown to have vastly different digestive stability in an in vitro assay, with MIR2911 being 10-fold more stable than C7 [27]. The in vitro digestion assay contained porcine digestion enzymes and demonstrated that amiR-RICE had similar digestive stability compared to MIR2911, while mmu-miR146a was significantly less stable than MIR2911, with surviving percentage in the intestinal phase after 75 min for mmu-miR146a being 0.39% comparing to 1.11% for MIR2911 (Fig. 3a). In the in vivo assay, gavage-fed synthetic miRNAs demonstrated much higher sensitivity to the murine digestive enzymes in vivo compared to the in vitro porcine system. After an

hour, amiR-RICE had an approximately threefold higher survival percentage after gavage feeding compared to MIR2911 in the small intestines (0.0014% for amiR-RICE compared to 0.00045% for MIR2911) (Fig. 3b). Due to high background detection of endogenous mmu-miR146a in the murine intestines, the in vivo stability of mmu-miR146a was not analyzed (data not shown).

Bioavailability of transgenic miRNAs

When testing the bioavailability of the transgenic miRNAs using mice fed the plant diets, we concurrently analyzed the uptake of dietary miRNAs in circulation and the miRNA levels in the gut. The analysis of the gut content of the mice fed the transgenic plant diets revealed a difference in the surviving levels in the small intestines between MIR2911 and amiR-RICE or mmu-miR146a. On average, MIR2911 had a total abundance of about 238 fmol per mouse, while amiR-RICE only had about 2.7 fmol per mouse. mmu-miR146a was at a much higher level at around 38 fmol per mouse than amiR-RICE. However, a similar level was also detected in the chow-fed mice when they did not consume the transgenic plant material, suggesting that this mmu-miR146a was not derived from the diet (Fig. 4).

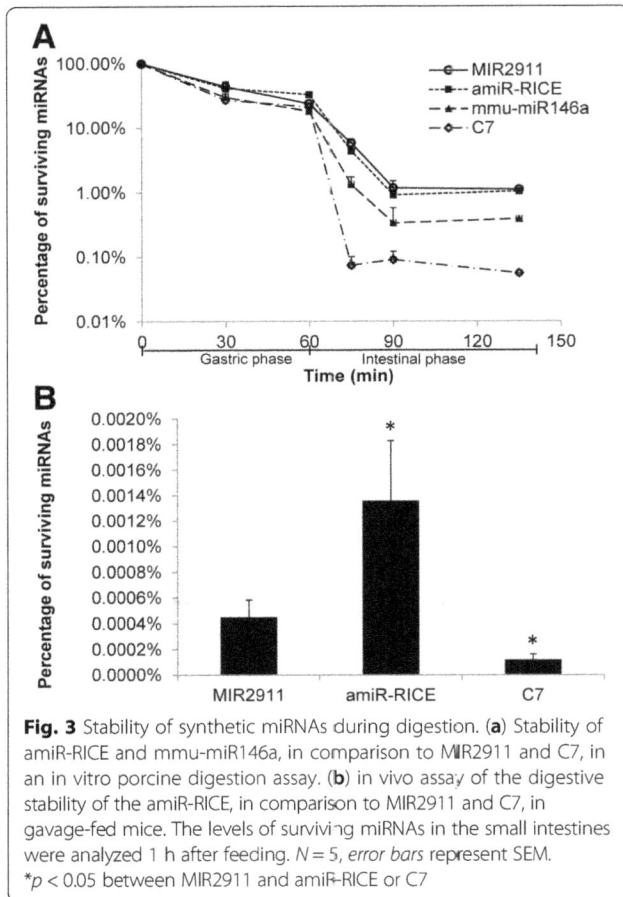

Fig. 3 Stability of synthetic miRNAs during digestion. (**a**) Stability of amiR-RICE and mmu-miR146a, in comparison to MIR2911 and C7, in an in vitro porcine digestion assay. (**b**) in vivo assay of the digestive stability of the amiR-RICE, in comparison to MIR2911 and C7, in gavage-fed mice. The levels of surviving miRNAs in the small intestines were analyzed 1 h after feeding. $N = 5$, *error bars* represent SEM. *$p < 0.05$ between MIR2911 and amiR-RICE or C7

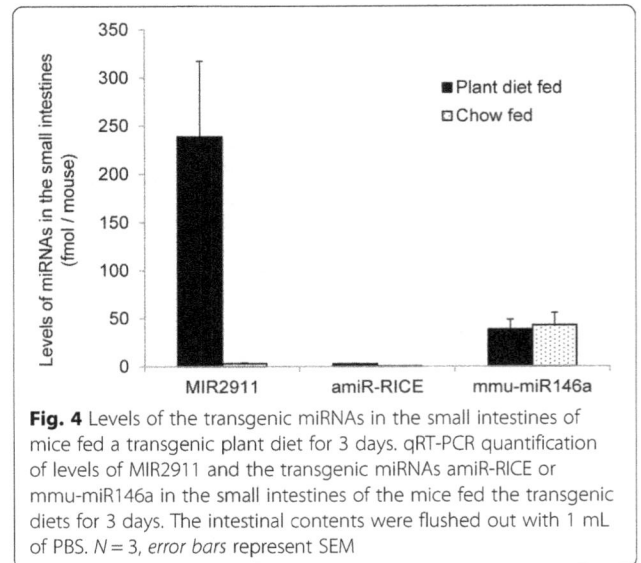

Fig. 4 Levels of the transgenic miRNAs in the small intestines of mice fed a transgenic plant diet for 3 days. qRT-PCR quantification of levels of MIR2911 and the transgenic miRNAs amiR-RICE or mmu-miR146a in the small intestines of the mice fed the transgenic diets for 3 days. The intestinal contents were flushed out with 1 mL of PBS. $N = 3$, *error bars* represent SEM

In vitro and in vivo digestion assays demonstrated that amiR-RICE is at least as stable as MIR2911 (Fig. 3). However, when we analyzed sera from mice gavage fed 400 pmol of synthetic amiR-RICE, these miRNAs were not readily bioavailable (Fig. 5a). Mice fed diets supplemented with transgenic plant materials for 3 days also had negligible serum levels of the transgenic miRNAs. Furthermore, attempts to detect other plant miRNAs that have been reported by others to be bioavailable, albeit from other plant-based diets, were not successful (Additional file 3: Figure S3), However, the levels of MIR2911 in mice fed the plant diets (28.5 fM, or 1.3×10^7 copies per mouse) were more than fivefold higher than animals receiving the chow-based diet (5.2 fM, or 2.3×10^6 copies per mouse) (Fig. 5b). The enhanced levels of MIR2911 in the transgenic diet-fed mice served as a positive control for consumption of the diets and detection of plant-based RNAs in the mouse sera.

Discussion

Disagreements are common but crucial in science; the nascent field of dietary sRNAs is certainly no stranger

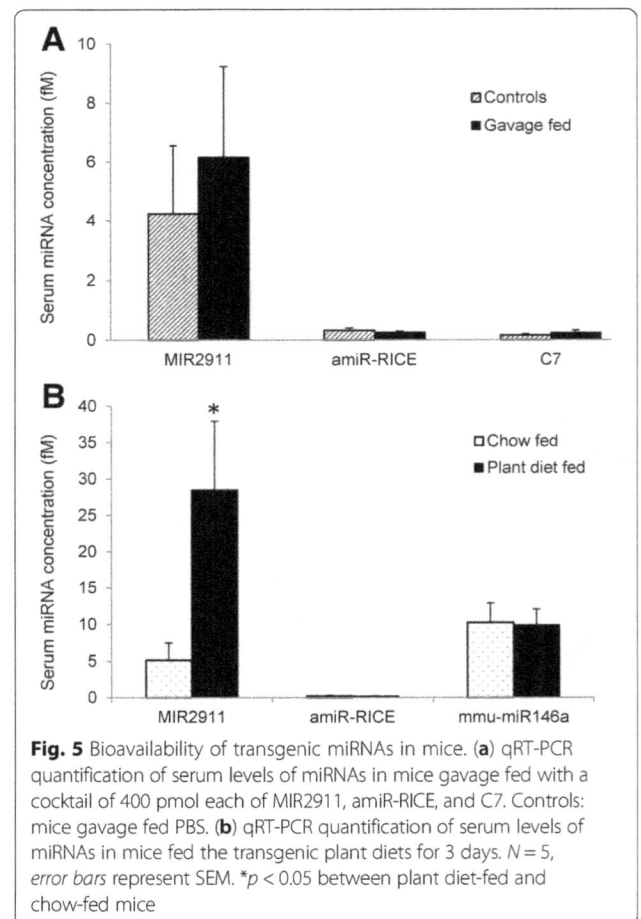

Fig. 5 Bioavailability of transgenic miRNAs in mice. (**a**) qRT-PCR quantification of serum levels of miRNAs in mice gavage fed with a cocktail of 400 pmol each of MIR2911, amiR-RICE, and C7. Controls: mice gavage fed PBS. (**b**) qRT-PCR quantification of serum levels of miRNAs in mice fed the transgenic plant diets for 3 days. $N = 5$, *error bars* represent SEM. *$p < 0.05$ between plant diet-fed and chow-fed mice

to these controversies [20]. Transgenic crops can express populations of miRNAs not found in nature, and in view of the conflicting reports inferring bioavailability of diet-derived miRNAs, the disagreements among scientists are profound because they impact the way agencies and agrobiotechnology regulate and use this technology.

The two plant-derived transgenic miRNAs tested here demonstrated modest digestive stability (Fig. 3) and were abundant in the transgenic plants (Fig. 1); however, they were not readily bioavailable when fed to healthy mice (Fig. 5). Our group has also been unable to reliably detect (<32 Ct) canonical plant-based miRNAs in the sera of mice consuming plant-based diets (Additional file 3: Figure S3; (28)). Future analysis should be performed with mice fed with the transgenic plants for longer intervals and detection measured in the intestine as well as in organs outside the gastro-intestinal tract.

A variety of plant-based miRNAs can be found within the plant cellular matrix and may be coupled with other plant molecules such as proteins and polysaccharides [33]. These alterations may provide a conduit for dietary plant-derived miRNA uptake [33]. Using in vitro experiments, miR168a in soybean and mir166 in rice demonstrate more resistance to degradation than miR168a from rice and mir166 from soybean [33]. There are no sequence differences between these miRNAs; thus, it has been proposed that plant-specific mechanisms afford varying levels of protection from degradation. If this is true, bioavailability tests in transgenic Arabidopsis lines may not equate to bioavailability in other transgenic plants. Plant-specific exosome-like nanoparticles (EPDENs) may also mediate interspecies communication [37], but it remains an open question if these effects are mediated by miRNAs. In milk, specific miRNAs appear to be encapsulated in exosomes conferring protection against degradation and facilitating uptake [18, 19]. These mechanisms may facilitate bioavailability of selected plant-based miRNAs, but with the two miRNAs tested here, they did not provide a conduit for absorption of the specific transgenic miRNAs tested here.

While these two transgenic miRNAs do not appear to be bioavailable in healthy mice, disease and nutritional status are important influences controlling consumer nutrient absorption [38]. A confluence of diet and health issues converges to influence uptake of plant-based genetic material [14, 21, 28]. Pharmacological regimes also facilitate the detection of gavage-fed miRNAs. Future work will focus on assaying bioavailability of GM-derived miRNAs under these more permissive conditions.

Preparation methods could enhance the bioavailability of sRNAs in plant-based diets [16, 23]. For traditional

nutrients, various strategies, including thermal processing, soaking, and fermentation, aim to increase the physicochemical accessibility of the nutrients while decreasing the content of antinutrients [39]. Future work will need to be directed at how food processing and preparation practices impact the dietary sRNA quality of plant-based foods.

MIR2911 has several features that facilitate its bioavailability that do not appear to be characteristics of the miRNAs tested here: first, the GC-rich MIR2911 has a high digestive stability [16, 27]; secondly, a protein complex protects MIR2911 [27]; third, synthesis via rRNA degradation dramatically increases MIR2911 abundance post-harvest [31]. The difference in intestinal levels of MIR2911 and the transgenic miRNAs could be explained by the degradation of the ribosomal RNAs that generate increased levels of MIR2911 [31]. In order for transgenic miRNAs to become more bioavailable, strategies need to be deployed that co-opt some or all of these tactics. It is interesting that one of the two transgenic miRNAs tested, amiR-RICE, was found to have similar digestive stability to MIR2911 in the in vitro system, or when gavage fed to the mice, but was not bioavailable. We posit this could be caused by either selective transport by the gut or differential stability or metabolism within the cells or in circulation.

Low bioavailability of the plant-based miRNAs does not negate potential bioactivity. Curcumin, a plant-based product, exhibits poor systemic bioavailability but still has potent pharmacological effects [40]. Like curcumin, emerging studies demonstrate that femtomolar amounts of a specific miRNA altered the fate of a targeted cell [41]. The miRNAs released by cancer cells can act as hormones [42, 43]. Additionally, evidence suggests that plant sRNAs have therapeutic effects that are sequence independent [44], allowing speculation that it is the additive abundance of trace amounts of a variety of different plant-based sRNAs that confer biological activity. Low amounts of miRNAs may have biological functions that could revolutionize our concepts of plant-based bioactives.

Conclusions

Studies continue to suggest cross-kingdom gene regulation by dietary miRNAs; meanwhile, the majority of work has questioned the validity of these reports [20, 24, 45, 46]. This pilot study suggests that the two transgenic miRNAs tested are not readily bioavailable to healthy consumers and therapeutic plant-based dietary miRNAs may need to focus on establishing conditions that allow miRNAs to overcome the obstacles hindering bioavailability.

Acknowledgements
We thank Dr. Xiuren Zhang for providing reagents and consultation in generating transgenic Arabidopsis lines overexpressing microRNAs.

Funding
This research was supported by the United States Department of Agriculture (USDA) 3092-51000-056-00D.

Authors' contributions
JY and KDH designed all the studies. CP and IE-Y carried out the in vivo digestion experiments. JY carried out all other experiments. JY and KDH wrote the paper. All authors read and approved the final manuscript.

Competing interests
The authors declare that they have no competing interests.

References
1. James C. A global overview of biotech (GM) crops: adoption, impact and future prospects. GM Crops. 2010;1:8–12.
2. Sakakibara K, Saito K. Review: genetically modified plants for the promotion of human health. Biotechnol Lett. 2006;28:1983–91.
3. Gartland KMA, Bruschi F, Duncan M, Gahan PB, et al. Progress towards the 'Golden Age' of biotechnology. Curr Opin Biotechnol. 2013;24 Suppl 1:S6–13.
4. Kuiper HA, Kleter GA, Noteborn HP, Kok EJ. Assessment of the food safety issues related to genetically modified foods. Plant J. 2001;27:503–28.
5. Varzakas TH, Chryssochoidis G, Argyropoulos D. Approaches in the risk assessment of genetically modified foods by the Hellenic Food Safety Authority. Food Chem Toxicol. 2007;45:530–42.
6. Ramon M, Devos Y, Lanzoni A, Liu Y, et al. RNAi-based GM plants: food for thought for risk assessors. Plant Biotechnol J. 2014;12:1271–3.
7. Levine E, Zhang Z, Kuhlman T, Hwa T. Quantitative characteristics of gene regulation by small RNA. PLoS Biol. 2007;5:e229.
8. Dickinson B, Zhang Y, Petrick JS, Heck G, et al. Lack of detectable oral bioavailability of plant microRNAs after feeding in mice. Nat Biotechnol. 2013;31:965–7.
9. Witwer KW, McAlexander MA, Queen SE, Adams RJ. Real-time quantitative PCR and droplet digital PCR for plant miRNAs in mammalian blood provide little evidence for general uptake of dietary miRNAs: limited evidence for general uptake of dietary plant xenomiRs. RNA Biol. 2013;10:1080–6.
10. Petrick JS, Brower-Toland B, Jackson AL, Kier LD. Safety assessment of food and feed from biotechnology-derived crops employing RNA-mediated gene regulation to achieve desired traits: a scientific review. Regul Toxicol Pharmacol. 2013;66:167–76.
11. Petrick JS, Moore WM, Heydens WF, Koch MS, Sherman JH. A 28-day oral toxicity evaluation of small interfering RNAs and a long double-stranded RNA targeting vacuolar ATPase in mice. Regul Toxicol Pharmacol. 2015;71:8–23.
12. Knudsen I, Poulsen M. Comparative safety testing of genetically modified foods in a 90-day rat feeding study design allowing the distinction between primary and secondary effects of the new genetic event. Regul Toxicol Pharmacol. 2007;49:53–62.
13. Snow JW, Hale AE, Isaacs SK, Baggish AL, Chan SY. Ineffective delivery of diet-derived microRNAs to recipient animal organisms. RNA Biol. 2013;10:1107–16.
14. Yang J, Farmer LM, Agyekum AAA, Elbaz-Younes I, Hirschi KD. Detection of an abundant plant-based small RNA in healthy consumers. PLoS One. 2015;10:e0137516. p. 0137511–0137514.
15. Chin AR, Fong MY, Somlo G, Wu J, et al. Cross-kingdom inhibition of breast cancer growth by plant miR159. Cell Res. 2016;20(2):217–28.
16. Zhou Z, Li X, Liu J, Dong L, et al. Honeysuckle-encoded atypical microRNA2911 directly targets influenza A viruses. Cell Res. 2015;25:39–49.
17. Zhang L, Hou D, Chen X, Li D, et al. Exogenous plant MIR168a specifically targets mammalian LDLRAP1: evidence of cross-kingdom regulation by microRNA. Cell Res. 2012;22:107–26.
18. Zempleni J, Baier SR, Hirschi KD. Diet-responsive MicroRNAs are likely exogenous. J Biol Chem. 2015;290:25197.
19. Baier SR, Nguyen C, Xie F, Wood JR, Zempleni J. MicroRNAs are absorbed in biologically meaningful amounts from nutritionally relevant doses of cow milk and affect gene expression in peripheral blood mononuclear cells, HEK-293 kidney cell cultures, and mouse livers. J Nutr. 2014;144:1495–500.
20. Witwer KW, Hirschi KD. Transfer and functional consequences of dietary microRNAs in vertebrates: concepts in search of corroboration: negative results challenge the hypothesis that dietary xenomiRs cross the gut and regulate genes in ingesting vertebrates, but important questions persist. Bioessays. 2014;36:394–406.
21. Yang J, Hirschi KD, Farmer LM. Dietary RNAs: new stories regarding oral delivery. Nutrients. 2015;7:3184–99.
22. Mlotshwa S, Pruss GJ, MacArthur JL, Endres MW, et al. A novel chemopreventive strategy based on therapeutic microRNAs produced in plants. Cell Res. 2015;25:521–4.
23. Pastrello C, Tsay M, McQuaid R, Abovsky M, et al. Circulating plant miRNAs can regulate human gene expression in vitro. Sci Rep. 2016;6:32773.
24. Witwer KW. Diet-responsive mammalian miRNAs are likely endogenous. J Nutr. 2014;144:1880–1.
25. Bagci C, Allmer J. One step forward, two steps back; xeno-microRNAs reported in breast milk are artifacts. PLoS One. 2016;11:e0145065.
26. Auerbach A, Vyas G, Li A, Halushka M, Witwer K. Uptake of dietary milk miRNAs by adult humans: a validation study. F1000Res. 2016;5:721.
27. Yang J, Hotz T, Broadnax L, Yarmarkovich M, et al. Anomalous uptake and circulatory characteristics of the plant-based small RNA MIR2911. Sci Rep. 2016;6:1–9.
28. Yang J, Farmer LM, Agyekum AAA, Hirschi KD. Detection of dietary plant-based small RNAs in animals. Cell Res. 2015;25:517–20.
29. Zhang X, Yuan YR, Pei Y, Lin SS, et al. Cucumber mosaic virus-encoded 2b suppressor inhibits Arabidopsis Argonaute1 cleavage activity to counter plant defense. Genes Dev. 2006;20:3255–68.
30. Tsuzuki M, Takeda A, Watanabe Y. Recovery of dicer-like 1-late flowering phenotype by miR172 expressed by the noncanonical DCL4-dependent biogenesis pathway. RNA. 2014;20:1320–7.
31. Yang et al. Mol Nutr Food Res. http://onlinelibrary.wiley.com/doi/10.1002/mnfr.201600974/abstract;jsessionid=123206D8B1EA5E15E9516E804C2927AC.f04t04.
32. Chen X, Liang H, Guan D, Wang C, et al. A combination of Let-7d, Let-7g and Let-7i serves as a stable reference for normalization of serum microRNAs. PLoS One. 2013;8:e79652.
33. Philip A, Ferro VA, Tate RJ. Determination of the potential bioavailability of plant microRNAs using a simulated human digestion process. Mol Nutr Food Res. 2015;59:1962–72.
34. Minekus M, Alminger M, Alvito P, Ballance S, et al. A standardised static in vitro digestion method suitable for food—an international consensus. Food Funct. 2014;5:1113–24.
35. Huala E, Dickerman AW, Garcia-Hernandez M, Weems D, et al. The Arabidopsis Information Resource (TAIR): a comprehensive database and web-based information retrieval, analysis, and visualization system for a model plant. Nucleic Acids Res. 2001;29:102–5.
36. Dai Y, Jia P, Fang Y, Liu H, et al. miR-146a is essential for lipopolysaccharide (LPS)-induced cross-tolerance against kidney ischemia/reperfusion injury in mice. Sci Rep. 2016;6:1–11.
37. Mu J, Zhuang X, Wang Q, Jiang H, et al. Interspecies communication between plant and mouse gut host cells through edible plant derived exosome-like nanoparticles. Mol Nutr Food Res. 2014;58:1561–73.
38. Krehl WA. Factors affecting utilization and requirements. Vitamins and minerals. Am J Clin Nutr. 1962;11:389–99.
39. Hotz C, Gibson RS. Traditional food-processing and preparation practices to enhance the bioavailability of micronutrients in plant-based diets. J Nutr. 2007;137:1097–100.
40. Schiborr C, Kocher A, Behnam D, Jandasek J, et al. The oral bioavailability of curcumin from micronized powder and liquid micelles is significantly increased in healthy humans and differs between sexes. Mol Nutr Food Res. 2014;58:516–27.
41. Bryniarski K, Ptak W, Martin E, Nazimek K, et al. Free extracellular miRNA functionally targets cells by transfecting exosomes from their companion cells. PLoS One. 2015;10:1–22.
42. Fabbri M, Paone A, Calore F, Galli R, et al. MicroRNAs bind to Toll-like receptors to induce prometastatic inflammatory response. Proc Natl Acad Sci U S A. 2012;109:E2110–6.
43. Galli R, Paone A, Fabbri M, Zanesi N, et al. Toll-like receptor 3 (TLR3) activation induces microRNA-dependent reexpression of functional RARβ and tumor regression. Proc Natl Acad Sci U S A. 2013;110:9812–7.

8

Hepatic transcriptome implications for palm fruit juice deterrence of type 2 diabetes mellitus in young male Nile rats

Soon-Sen Leow[1]*(iD), Julia Bolsinger[2], Andrzej Pronczuk[2], K. C. Hayes[2] and Ravigadevi Sambanthamurthi[1]*

Abstract

Background: The Nile rat (NR, *Arvicanthis niloticus*) is a model of carbohydrate-induced type 2 diabetes mellitus (T2DM) and the metabolic syndrome. A previous study found that palm fruit juice (PFJ) delayed or prevented diabetes and in some cases even reversed its early stages in young NRs. However, the molecular mechanisms by which PFJ exerts these anti-diabetic effects are unknown. In this study, the transcriptomic effects of PFJ were studied in young male NRs, using microarray gene expression analysis.

Methods: Three-week-old weanling NRs were fed either a high-carbohydrate diet (%En from carbohydrate/fat/protein = 70:10:20, 16.7 kJ/g; $n = 8$) or the same high-carbohydrate diet supplemented with PFJ (415 ml of 13,000-ppm gallic acid equivalent (GAE) for a final concentration of 5.4 g GAE per kg diet or 2.7 g per 2000 kcal; $n = 8$). Livers were obtained from these NRs for microarray gene expression analysis using Illumina MouseRef-8 Version 2 Expression BeadChips. Microarray data were analysed along with the physiological parameters of diabetes.

Results: Compared to the control group, 71 genes were up-regulated while 108 were down-regulated in the group supplemented with PFJ. Among hepatic genes up-regulated were apolipoproteins related to high-density lipoproteins (HDL) and genes involved in hepatic detoxification, while those down-regulated were related to insulin signalling and fibrosis.

Conclusion: The results obtained suggest that the anti-diabetic effects of PFJ may be due to mechanisms other than an increase in insulin secretion.

Keywords: Palm fruit juice, Oil palm phenolics, Antioxidants, Diabetes, Metabolic syndrome, Gene expression, Nile rat

Background

Nutritional overload and sedentary lifestyle give rise to the prevalence of type 2 diabetes mellitus (T2DM) in modern societies, and this chronic disease is estimated to reach 439 million cases by 2030 [87]. Although T2DM is a disease of adults, it is an increasingly common diagnosis among adolescents in high-risk countries such as Asia, the Middle East, and the USA [46]. T2DM is characterised by insulin resistance, declining insulin production and eventual pancreatic β cell failure [71]. This leads to a decrease in glucose transport into liver, muscle and fat cells and an increase in circulating glucose. T2DM is often associated with increasing obesity, via a combination of clinical abnormalities known as the metabolic syndrome, which comprises insulin resistance, visceral adiposity, hypertension, atherogenic dyslipaemia and endothelial dysfunction [32]. These conditions are interrelated and share common mediators, pathways and pathophysiological mechanisms [50]. The metabolic syndrome is a state of chronic low-grade inflammation linked to aberrant energy metabolism as a consequence of complex interplay between genetic and environmental factors [57].

Due to the growing concern over T2DM and the metabolic syndrome, animal models that mimic these human diseases are needed to assess possible anti-diabetic preventative or therapeutic measures [128]. The Nile rat (NR), also known as the African grass rat

* Correspondence: ssleow@mpob.gov.my; raviga@mpob.gov.my
[1]Malaysian Palm Oil Board, No. 6, Persiaran Institusi, Bandar Baru Bangi, 43000 Kajang, Selangor, Malaysia
Full list of author information is available at the end of the article

(*Arvicanthis niloticus*), has been described as a relevant model of T2DM and the metabolic syndrome, as it allows for detailed nutritional modelling of diet-induced T2DM similar to that in humans. The NR spontaneously develops hyperinsulinaemia, hyperglycaemia with dyslipaemia and hypertension in the early phase of the disease [14, 16, 21, 85]. Further characterisation revealed that NRs develop liver steatosis, abdominal fat accumulation, nephropathy, atrophy of pancreatic islets of Langerhans and fatty streaks in the aorta, as well as hypertension [14, 16, 21, 85]. Males are more prone than females, with rapid progression to T2DM depending on the glycaemic load of the challenge diet and cumulative glycaemic load [15]. Although diet challenge appears as the primary factor and dietary intervention can modulate the development of T2DM and metabolic syndrome in NRs, genetic susceptibility also plays a pivotal role, similar to humans. This rodent model thus represents a novel system of gene-diet interactions affecting energy utilisation that can provide insights into the prevention and treatment of diabetes, as well as the metabolic syndrome [14, 21]. As in humans, the NR is sensitive to the daily glycaemic load and as such reliably mirrors the course of T2DM and the metabolic syndrome observed in humans [14].

At present, no cure has been found for T2DM and the metabolic syndrome. Treatment methods normally suggested include lifestyle modifications, treatment of obesity that induces weight reduction, oral anti-diabetic medication that reduces intestinal glucose absorption, increases insulin sensitivity or exerts insulin-sensitising effects or lastly insulin injections [87]. All the above measures have been shown to prevent T2DM in the NR. However, current research strongly supports the concept that the consumption of certain fruits and plant-derived foods is inversely correlated with prevalence of T2DM and the metabolic syndrome [8, 35, 80]. A great array of phenolic compounds may exert anti-diabetic effects either directly or indirectly [1]. Phenolic compounds may influence glucose metabolism by several mechanisms, such as inhibition of carbohydrate digestion and glucose absorption in the small intestine, stimulation of insulin secretion from pancreatic β cells, modulation of hepatic gluconeogenesis, activation of insulin receptors and glucose uptake in insulin-sensitive tissues (thus enhancing insulin sensitivity) and modulation of gut flora activity, as well as modulation of intracellular signalling pathways and gene expression influencing glucose utilisation [26, 47, 79]. Some examples of plant phenolic compounds which were found to display anti-diabetic effects in humans include resveratrol [82, 110], olive leaf extracts [28, 125], pomegranate juice [88] and green tea extracts [61, 69].

The oil palm (*Elaeis guineensis*) fruit contains phenolic compounds [99], which are extracted from the aqueous vegetation liquor produced during oil palm milling. Palm fruit juice (PFJ) consists mainly of phenolic acids, including three caffeoylshikimic acid isomers and *p*-hydroxybenzoic acid [99]. PFJ has been shown to display antioxidant properties and confer positive outcomes on degenerative diseases in various animal models without evidence of toxicity [16, 22, 65–68, 99, 100, 103]. In relation to T2DM, we have previously shown that PFJ blocked T2DM progression in 12-week-old male NRs, with a substantial decrease in blood glucose after 17 weeks of treatment [100]. In addition, PFJ delayed T2DM onset or completely prevented it during the intervention period and even reversed advancing T2DM in young NRs [16]. PFJ has also been shown to deter T2DM complications, including retinopathy and nephropathy in NRs [14, 21, 85], not unlike other plant polyphenols [5]. PFJ thus has demonstrated anti-diabetic effects. However, the detailed molecular mechanisms by which PFJ effects these changes in NRs have yet to be explored, prompting the microarray gene expression analysis in the present study.

Methods

Animal feeding and sample collection

Three-week-old male NRs ($n = 16$) were divided into two groups, controls without PFJ ($n = 8$) and PFJ ($n = 8$). We chose to study 3-week-old Nile rats for 4 weeks in this study as this window of development is the most sensitive to the development of nutritionally induced T2DM in the NR and thus provides the highest chances of altering this development through the application of PFJ. This would help pinpoint the gene expression changes caused by PFJ in deterring the occurrence of diabetes more efficiently [16, 21]. Early diabetes (7 weeks of age) in Nile rats is detected by random blood glucose levels, whereas diabetic fasting blood glucose does not always manifest until 12 weeks of age [85]. In addition, only males were used in this experiment as they develop T2DM more readily than females, presumably based on sex hormone differences [21]. NRs in the control group were fed a semi-purified high-carbohydrate diet ad libitum (% En from carbohydrate/fat/protein = 70:10:20, 16.7 kJ/g), while those in the PFJ group were given liquid PFJ incorporated directly into the same diet (415 ml of 13,000 ppm gallic acid equivalent (GAE) for a final concentration of 5.4 g GAE per kg diet or 2.7 g per 2000 kcal (daily human equivalent)) (Table 1). The composition of PFJ was as described previously [99], with major phenolic components being three caffeoylshikimic acid isomers and *p*-hydroxybenzoic acid. Body weight was assessed throughout the feeding period, as were food (in g/d and kJ/d) and fluid intakes. After 4 weeks, random and fasting blood glucose levels were assessed, along with terminal organ weights, plasma lipids and insulin. All experiments and procedures were approved by the Brandeis University Institutional Animal Care and Use Committee.

Food efficiency

Food efficiency was calculated by dividing body weight gain (in g/d) by caloric intake (in kJ/d) and multiplying the result by 1000. Results represent the body weight gained (g) per 1000 kJ consumed.

Random and fasting blood glucose

Blood glucose was measured in O_2/CO_2-anaesthetised NRs from a drop of tail blood, obtained by lancet puncture of the lateral tail vein using an Elite XL glucometer (Bayer Co., Elhart, IN). Random blood glucose (RBG) was assessed in non-fasted NRs between 9 and 10 am on non-feeding days (semi-purified diets were replenished three times per week). Fasting blood glucose (FBG) was measured at about 9 to 10 am after 16 h of overnight food deprivation.

Terminal organ weights

Organs (livers, kidneys, caecum and adipose) were weighed after excision, and their weights (in g) were divided by the terminal body weight (in g) to obtain a percentage. The livers were snap-frozen in liquid nitrogen and stored at −80 °C until the total RNA extraction process for gene expression analysis. The relative carcass weight (as percentage body mass) was determined by weighing lean body mass (after exsanguination and excision of all organs) and dividing it by the terminal body weight (in g). Carcass weight was included as an indicator of muscle growth. Body length (nose to base of tail, in cm) was also included as a parameter of growth.

Plasma biochemical measurements

Plasma triacylglycerol (TG) and total cholesterol (TC) were determined spectrophotometrically using Infinity™ kits (Thermo Fisher Scientific Inc., Middletown, VA, TG ref # TR22421, TC ref # TR13421). Plasma insulin was determined with an ELISA kit for rat/mouse insulin (Linco Research, EMD Millipore, Billerica, MA, ref # EZRMI-13K), according to the manufacturer's protocol.

Statistical analyses

Statistical analyses on physiological and biochemical parameters were performed using the Super ANOVA statistical software (Abacus Concepts, Inc., Berkeley, CA). Two-tailed unpaired Student's t test was performed, and differences with p values of less than 0.05 were considered statistically significant.

Microarray gene expression analysis

Total RNA isolation from frozen NR livers was conducted using the RNeasy Plus Mini Kit (Qiagen, Inc., Valencia, CA) and QIAshredder homogenisers (Qiagen, Inc., Valencia, CA), preceded by grinding in liquid nitrogen using mortars and pestles. The total RNA samples obtained were subjected to NanoDrop 1000A Spectrophotometer (Thermo Fisher

Table 1 Composition of high-carbohydrate diet

Component	Amount (g/kg)
% En	
Carbohydrate	70
Fat	10
Protein	20
En (kJ/g)	16.7
Ingredients (g/kg)	
Casein	100
Lactalbumin	100
Dextrose	350
Corn starch	288 (+60 with gel)[a]
Fat	44
Butter (g of fat)	8
Tallow	15
Soybean oil	23
Mineral mix[b]	44
Vitamin mix[c]	11
Choline chloride	3
Cholesterol	0.6

[a]60 g corn starch was added to 800 ml water to form a gel or added to 375 ml water + 415 ml PFJ (13,000 ppm GAE for a final concentration of 5.4 g GAE per kg diet or 2.7 g per 2000 kcal)
[b]Ausman-Hayes salt mix. Mineral mix contained the following (g/kg mix): magnesium oxide, 320; calcium carbonate, 290.5; potassium phosphate dibasic, 312.2; calcium phosphate dibasic, 72.6; magnesium sulphate, 98.7; sodium chloride, 162.4; ferric citrate, 26.6; potassium iodide, 0.77; manganese sulphate, 3.66; zinc chloride, 0.24; cupric sulphate, 0.29; chromium acetate, 0.044; sodium selenite, 0.004
[c]Hayes-Cathcart vitamin mix. Vitamin mix contained the following (g/kg mix): D-α-tocopheryl acetate (500 IU/g), 15; inositol, 5; niacin, 3; calcium pantothenate, 1.6; retinyl palmitate (500,000 IU/g), 1.5; cholecalciferol (400,000 IU/g), 0.1; menadione, 0.2; biotin, 0.02; folic acid, 0.2; riboflavin, 0.7; thiamin, 0.6; pyridoxine HCl, 0.7; cyanocobalamin, 0.001; dextrin, 972

Scientific, Waltham, MA) measurement for yield and purity assessment. Integrity of the total RNA samples was then assessed using the Agilent 2100 Bioanalyzer (Agilent Technologies, Santa Clara, CA) and Agilent RNA 6000 Nano Chip Assay Kit (Agilent Technologies, Santa Clara, CA).

Amplification of total RNA samples which were of high yield, purity and integrity was performed using the Illumina TotalPrep RNA Amplification Kit (Ambion, Inc., Austin, TX). The complementary ribonucleic acid (cRNA) produced was then hybridised to the Illumina MouseRef-8 Version 2 Expression BeadChip (Illumina, Inc., San Diego, CA), using the Direct Hybridization Kit (Illumina, Inc., San Diego, CA). As each MouseRef-8 BeadChip enables the interrogation of eight samples in parallel, a total of eight cRNA samples were used in the microarray experiment, by selecting four total RNA samples with the highest RNA integrity numbers and 28S/18S ribosomal RNA (rRNA) ratios within each condition. Microarray hybridisation, washing and scanning were conducted according to the manufacturer's instructions. The raw gene expression data obtained are available at Gene Expression Omnibus [33] (accession number: GSE64901).

Quality control of the hybridisation, microarray raw data extraction and initial analysis were performed using the Illumina BeadStudio software (Illumina, San Diego, CA). Outlier samples were also removed via hierarchical clustering analysis provided by the Illumina GenomeStudio software, via different distance metrics including correlation, absolute correlation, Manhattan and Euclidean distance metrics. Gene expression values were normalised using the rank invariant method, and genes which had a detection level of more than 0.99 in either the control or treatment samples were considered significantly detected.

To filter the data for genes which changed significantly in terms of statistics, the Illumina Custom error model was used and genes were considered significantly changed at a differential score of more than 13, which was equivalent to a p value <0.05. Two-way (gene and sample) hierarchical clustering of the significant genes was then performed using the TIGR MeV software to ensure that the replicates of each condition were clustered to each other. The Euclidean distance metric and average linkage method were used to carry out the hierarchical clustering analysis. The genes and their corresponding data were then exported into the Microsoft Excel software for further analysis. To calculate fold changes, an arbitrary value of 10 was given to expression values which were less than 10. Fold changes were then calculated by dividing the mean values of signal Y (treatment) with those of signal X (control) if the genes were up-regulated and vice versa if the genes were down-regulated.

Changes in biological pathways and gene ontologies (biological processes) were then assessed via functional enrichment analysis, using the GO-Elite software. The GO-Elite software ranks WikiPathways [58, 92] and gene ontologies based on the hypergeometric distribution. WikiPathways and gene ontologies which had permuted p values of less than 0.05, numbers of genes changed of more than or equal to 2 and Z scores of more than 2 were considered significantly changed. In this study, up-regulated and down-regulated genes were analysed separately in the functional enrichment analysis but were viewed together in each WikiPathway, using the PathVisio software [122]. For each of these WikiPathways, boxes coloured yellow indicate genes which were up-regulated while those coloured blue indicate genes which were down-regulated. The fold changes of the genes were indicated next to their boxes.

Changes in regulatory networks were also analysed through the use of the Ingenuity Pathways Analysis software (Ingenuity® Systems, Redwood City, CA). A network is a graphical representation of the molecular relationships between genes or gene products. Genes or gene products were represented as nodes, and the biological relationship between two nodes was represented as an edge (line). The intensity of the node colour indicates the degree of up-regulation (red) or down-regulation (green). Nodes were displayed using various shapes that represented the functional class of the gene product. Edges were displayed with various labels that described the nature of the relationship between the nodes.

Real-time qRT-PCR validation

Two-step real-time quantitative reverse transcription-polymerase chain reaction (qRT-PCR) was conducted using TaqMan Gene Expression Assays (Applied Biosystems, Foster City, CA) to validate the microarray data obtained. This was performed on six differentially expressed target genes of interest (Table 2), which were selected based on the microarray data analysis performed. The same aliquots of total RNA samples used in the microarray experiments were utilised for this analysis. Primer and probe sets for the selected genes were obtained from the ABI Inventoried Assays-On-Demand (Applied Biosystems, Foster City, CA).

Briefly, reverse transcription to generate first-strand complementary deoxyribonucleic acid (cDNA) from total RNA was conducted using the High-Capacity cDNA Reverse Transcription Kit (Applied Biosystems, Foster City, CA). Real-time PCR was then performed on the first-strand cDNA generated using a 25 μL reaction volume in an Applied Biosystems 7000 Real-Time PCR System (Applied Biosystems, Foster City, CA) using the following conditions: 50 °C, 2 min, 1 cycle; 95 °C, 10 min, 1 cycle; 95 °C, 15 s and 60 °C, 1 min, 40 cycles. For gene expression measurements, reactions for each biological replicate and non-template control (NTC) were performed in duplicates. For amplification efficiency determination, reactions were performed in triplicates.

Quality control of the replicates used, real-time qRT-PCR data extraction and initial analysis were conducted using the 7000 Sequence Detection System software (Applied Biosystems, Foster City, CA). A manual threshold of 0.6000 and an auto baseline were applied in order to obtain the threshold cycle (Ct) for each measurement taken. The threshold was chosen as it intersected the exponential phase of the amplification plots [19]. The criteria for quality control of the data obtained include ΔCt less than 0.5 between technical replicates and ΔCt more than 5.0 between samples and NTCs [86].

Relative quantification of the target genes of interest was performed using the qBase 1.3.5 software (Center for Medical Genetics, Ghent University Hospital, Ghent,

Table 2 Genes selected for the real-time qRT-PCR validation experiment

Symbol	Definition	Accession	Assay ID
Target genes			
Apoc1	Apolipoprotein C-I	NM_007469	Mm00431816_m1
Apoc3	Apolipoprotein C-III	NM_023114	Mm00445670_m1
Map3k11	Mitogen-activated protein kinase kinase kinase 11	NM_022012	Mm00491529_m1
Map3k2	Mitogen-activated protein kinase kinase kinase 2	NM_011946	Mm00442451_m1
Pik3r3	Phosphatidylinositol 3-kinase, regulatory subunit, polypeptide 3 (p55)	NM_181585	Mm00725026_m1
Stxbp2	Syntaxin binding protein 2	NM_011503	Mm00441589_m1
Reference genes			
Cct6a	Chaperonin containing Tcp1, subunit 6a (zeta)	NM_009838	Mm00486818_m1
Hpd	4-hydroxyphenylpyruvic acid dioxygenase	NM_008277	Mm00801734_m1
Nipbl	Nipped-B homologue (Drosophila)	NM_027707	Mm01297452_m1
Trim39	Tripartite motif-containing 39	NM_178281	Mm01273530_m1

The six target genes were selected based on their functional significance, their statistical significance, their presence as single splice transcripts in microarrays and their availability as Taqman assays designed across splice junctions. From the microarray data obtained, four candidate reference genes were also chosen to be tested for expression stability across the groups, with the three most stable ones being finally selected for relative quantification of the target genes

Belgium) [48], which takes into account the calculations of amplification efficiencies and multiple housekeeping genes. Expression levels of target genes were normalised to the geometric mean of the three most stable reference genes, selected out of the four tested (Table 2). Stability of these reference genes was assessed using the geNorm 3.5 software (Center for Medical Genetics, Ghent University Hospital, Ghent, Belgium) [123].

Results

Physiological and biochemical parameters

NRs fed the PFJ-supplemented diet consumed about 15 % fewer calories ($p < 0.05$) than control rats and were associated with significantly lower body weights ($p < 0.05$) (Table 3). Fluid intake did not significantly differ between the two groups. NRs in the PFJ group had less adipose tissue ($p < 0.05$) and a tendency for greater carcass weight (an indicator of lean body mass) and food efficiency. Their caeca were heavier too ($p < 0.05$) compared to the control group. NRs in the PFJ group had significantly lower levels of RBG ($p < 0.05$) and plasma TG ($p < 0.05$) compared to the control group, whereas no significant differences in overnight FBG were observed. Although TC in the PFJ group was slightly greater than that in the control group, it was not significant ($p > 0.05$). Insulin levels also did not differ between the two groups. Liver and kidney weights as percentages of body weights were similar between groups.

Microarray gene expression

Analysis of microarray gene expression of the NR livers revealed that 71 genes were up-regulated, while 108 genes were down-regulated in the PFJ group compared to the control group (Table 4). A few apolipoprotein genes, including *Apoa1*, *Apoa2*, *Apoc1* and *Apoc3*, were up-regulated in the PFJ group. Several cytochrome P450 genes involved in phase I detoxification, such as *Cyp1a2*, *Cyp2c67*, *Cyp2e1* and *Cyp4f14*, were also up-regulated. Three phase II detoxification genes, i.e. *Ugt2b36*, *Cat* and *Gsto2*, were up-regulated as well. On the other hand, genes down-regulated in the PFJ group include those involved in the insulin-signalling pathway, such as phosphatidylinositol kinases, *Pik3r3* and *Pi4ka*, as well as mitogen-activated protein triple kinases, *Map3k2* and *Map3k11*. Two genes related to fibrosis induction, *Pcolce* and *Plod2*, were also down-regulated in the PFJ group.

Functional enrichment analysis showed that various biological pathways (Table 5) and gene ontologies (biological processes) (Table 6) were differentially regulated in NRs given PFJ compared to controls. Among Wiki-Pathways up-regulated by PFJ were those of tryptophan metabolism, methylation, fatty acid omega oxidation, nuclear receptors in lipid metabolism and toxicity, complement and coagulation cascades, urea cycle and metabolism of amino groups, retinol metabolism, metapathway biotransformation, one-carbon metabolism and nuclear receptors, as well as cytochrome P450s. Down-regulated WikiPathways include regulation of actin cytoskeleton, insulin signalling and TNF-alpha NF-κβ signalling. In relation to T2DM, a significant observation was that the insulin-signalling pathway was down-regulated in the PFJ group (Fig. 1).

Up-regulated gene ontologies (biological processes) of interest include negative feedback of very-low-density lipoprotein particle remodelling, negative feedback of receptor-mediated endocytosis, negative feedback of very-low-density lipoprotein particle clearance, negative feedback of lipid catabolic process, macromolecular

Table 3 Diabetes assessment parameters of 3-week-old male NRs fed either a high-carbohydrate diet only or a high-carbohydrate diet supplemented with PFJ for 4 weeks

Group	Control (n = 8)		PFJ (n = 8)	
	Mean	SD	Mean	SD
Body weight (g)				
Initial (3 weeks old)	37	7	35	8
After 4 weeks	77[a]	8	70[a]	10
Food intake				
g/d	8[a]	1	7[a]	1
kJ/d	134[a]	25	117[a]	13
kcal/d	32[a]	6	28[a]	3
Food efficiency (g body weight gained/ 1000 kJ)	10.7	1.3	11.1	0.9
Fluid intake (ml/d)	18	7	21	7
Random blood glucose (RBG) (mg/dl)				
After four weeks	241[a]	133	128[a]	121
Fasting blood glucose (FBG) (mg/dl)				
After four weeks	77	38	70	22
Terminal organ weight (% body weight)				
Liver	3.6	0.6	3.6	0.5
Kidneys	0.8	0.2	0.9	0.2
Caecum	1.4[a]	0.4	1.9[a]	0.6
Adipose				
Epididymal	2.9[a]	0.5	2.4[a]	0.8
Perirenal	1.4[a]	0.4	1.1[a]	0.4
Brown fat	1.7[a]	0.2	1.5[a]	0.3
Total fat	6.0[a]	0.8	5.1[a]	1.1
Carcass	73	2	75	5
Body length (cm)	12.9[a]	0.4	12.4[a]	0.7
Plasma lipids (mmol/l)				
Total cholesterol (TC)	3.9	1.3	4.7	2.8
Triacylglycerol (TG)	2.8[a]	1.3	1.9[a]	0.5
Insulin (pmol/l)	0.6	0.3	0.6	0.4

Values sharing a common superscript are significantly different from each other ($p < 0.05$) by two-tailed unpaired Student's t test

complex remodelling, positive feedback of cholesterol esterification, negative feedback of lipid biosynthetic process, cellular response to lipid, cellular response to steroid hormone stimulus, negative feedback of cellular catabolic process, oxidation-reduction process, cellular response to peptide hormone stimulus and cellular carbohydrate metabolic process, as well as positive feedback of signal transduction. On the other hand, downregulated gene ontologies (biological processes) of interest include mammalian target of rapamycin (mTOR) signalling cascade, microtubule polymerisation, cell-cell junction organisation, cell activation involved in immune response, methylation, cell adhesion and catalytic activity, as well as negative feedback of protein phosphorylation.

Network analysis using the Ingenuity Pathways Analysis software showed that several apolipoproteins including apolipoproteins A1, A2 and C3 were upregulated by PFJ (Fig. 2). In addition, apolipoprotein C1 was up-regulated as well (Table 4).

Real-time qRT-PCR validation

To confirm the microarray results, the expression levels of six selected target genes were measured using real-time quantitative reverse transcription-polymerase chain reaction (qRT-PCR). From the four selected candidate reference genes tested, analysis using the geNorm 3.5 software [123] showed that *Hpd*, *Nipbl* and *Trim39* were more stable than *Cct6a*. Hence, the former three were selected as the reference genes to normalise the expression values of the target genes. The directions of fold changes of the target genes obtained from the real-time qRT-PCR technique as quantified by the qBase software [48] were comparable to those obtained from the microarray technique (Fig. 3). However, the magnitudes of fold changes obtained using real-time qRT-PCR were consistently lower than those obtained using microarrays.

Discussion

Rapid economic progress has resulted in lifestyle changes, especially in diet and physical activity. In combination with aging populations, this has resulted in a worldwide epidemic of obesity, T2DM and metabolic syndrome [105]. In the USA, the prevalence of obesity which leads to T2DM and the metabolic syndrome has risen, even as the intake of fat is reduced. This has been referred to as the American Paradox [17], and high-carbohydrate intake has been suggested to be the cause of the problem [9].

Many phenolic-rich extracts have been suggested to be beneficial in preventing or treating T2DM and its related complications. In line with this, we have previously shown that providing PFJ at 1800 mg/L GAE ad libitum as the sole drinking fluid for 17 weeks blocked T2DM and metabolic syndrome progression in 12-week-old male NRs, as evidenced by normalisation of initially elevated blood glucose and plasma lipids [15, 16, 100]. The anti-diabetic effects of PFJ appeared relatively independent of starting age, and no impairment of energy intake or body weight dynamics have been observed in mature NRs, nor were any other toxic effects attributed to it [16]. In addition, PFJ protection against blood glucose elevation has also previously been shown to occur independently of diet (chow or semi-purified, moderate or high carbohydrate), study duration, initial blood glucose or application method [16]. PFJ may thus represent a

Table 4 List of genes significantly regulated by PFJ

Symbol	Definition	Differential score	Fold change
Up-regulated genes			
Sds	Serine dehydratase	51.92	4.95
Plekhb1	Pleckstrin homology domain containing, family B (evectins) member 1	45.01	3.66
Npc1l1	Niemann-Pick C1-like 1	30.36	7.41
EG240549	Predicted gene, EG240549	25.98	3.13
F7	Coagulation factor VII	23.44	3.08
Ecm1	Extracellular matrix protein 1	23.18	2.32
Enpp2	Ectonucleotide pyrophosphatase/phosphodiesterase 2	21.76	2.50
Ugt2b36	UDP glucuronosyltransferase 2 family, polypeptide B36	21.09	2.98
Hdac3	Histone deacetylase 3	20.37	2.93
Cspg5	Chondroitin sulphate proteoglycan 5	20.27	2.05
Cyp2c67	Cytochrome P450, family 2, subfamily c, polypeptide 67	20.06	14.08
Specc1l	SPECC1-like	20.05	1.83
Cps1	Carbamoyl-phosphate synthetase 1, nuclear gene encoding mitochondrial protein XM_993466	19.42	2.78
Hbb-b1	Haemoglobin, beta adult major chain	19.19	2.14
Tnrc6a	Trinucleotide repeat containing 6a	19.03	1.58
Rps7	Ribosomal protein S7	18.21	1.76
Apoc1	Apolipoprotein C-I	17.47	13.49
Cyp2e1	Cytochrome P450, family 2, subfamily e, polypeptide 1	16.93	2.33
Ifrd1	Interferon-related developmental regulator 1	16.84	1.94
Mup2	Major urinary protein 2, transcript variant 1	16.51	197.62
Rpn2	Ribophorin II	16.41	2.07
Asl	Argininosuccinate lyase	16.33	1.85
Ptprt	Protein tyrosine phosphatase, receptor type, T	16.06	2.78
Bcdo2	Beta-carotene 9', 10'-dioxygenase 2	16.00	2.43
Zfhx2	Zinc finger homeobox 2	15.95	1.77
Mthfd1	Methylenetetrahydrofolate dehydrogenase (NADP+ dependent), methenyltetrahydrofolate cyclohydrolase, formyltetrahydrofolate synthase	15.95	1.54
Rnf215	Ring finger protein 215	15.91	1.63
Gne	Glucosamine	15.82	2.54
Cyp4f14	Cytochrome P450, family 4, subfamily f, polypeptide 14	15.60	2.55
Zxda	Zinc finger, X-linked, duplicated A	15.35	1.51
Nat1	N-acetyltransferase 1 (arylamine N-acetyltransferase)	15.26	2.05
Cat	Catalase	15.23	2.84
Tyms-ps	Thymidylate synthase, pseudogene	15.16	1.69
F5	Coagulation factor V	15.12	2.38
Fbxo7	F-box only protein 7	14.96	1.71
Apoa2	Apolipoprotein A-II	14.91	2.67
Hagh	Hydroxyacyl glutathione hydrolase	14.87	1.64
Alas1	Aminolevulinic acid synthase 1	14.80	10.33
Inmt	Indolethylamine N-methyltransferase	14.79	2.62
620807.00	Predicted gene, 620807	14.78	106.29

Table 4 List of genes significantly regulated by PFJ *(Continued)*

Hsd17b10	Hydroxysteroid (17-beta) dehydrogenase 10, nuclear gene encoding mitochondrial protein	14.75	2.30
Nr1i3	Nuclear receptor subfamily 1, group I, member 3	14.63	2.02
Nit2	Nitrilase family, member 2	14.58	1.99
Tbc1d15	TBC1 domain family, member 15	14.57	1.71
Apoc3	Apolipoprotein C-III	14.56	2.77
ORF61	Open reading frame 61	14.51	1.54
Ephx1	Epoxide hydrolase 1, microsomal	14.36	2.98
Serpina1d	Serine (or cysteine) peptidase inhibitor, clade A, member 1d	14.26	13.47
Stab1	Stabilin 1	14.19	2.00
Ifitm2	Interferon induced transmembrane protein 2	14.05	1.55
Hmgcs2	3-hydroxy-3-methylglutaryl-Coenzyme A synthase 2, nuclear gene encoding mitochondrial protein	14.03	5.41
Serpina1b	Serine (or cysteine) preptidase inhibitor, clade A, member 1b	14.03	13.48
Tmem132e	Transmembrane protein 132E	13.98	1.99
Syvn1	Synovial apoptosis inhibitor 1, synoviolin	13.97	1.78
Cyp1a2	Cytochrome P450, family 1, subfamily a, polypeptide 2	13.92	2.38
Reln	Reelin	13.90	2.44
Fzd7	Frizzled homologue 7 (Drosophila)	13.87	1.96
F13b	Coagulation factor XIII, beta subunit	13.83	2.30
Rpl36al	Ribosomal protein l36a-like	13.73	1.79
Klkb1	Kallikrein B, plasma 1	13.72	2.29
Sdf2	Stromal cell derived factor 2	13.53	1.44
3110049J23Rik	RIKEN cDNA 3110049 J23 gene	13.44	1.70
2810004N20Rik	RIKEN cDNA 2810004 N20 gene	13.40	1.74
Rxrg	Retinoid X receptor gamma	13.36	2.29
Ces3	Carboxylesterase 3	13.20	4.77
Sec16b	SEC16 homologue B (Saccharomyces cerevisiae)	13.20	2.31
Gsto2	Glutathione S-transferase omega 2	13.17	2.33
5830404H04Rik	RIKEN cDNA 5830404H04 gene	13.14	1.90
Creld1	Cysteine-rich with EGF-like domains 1	13.13	1.46
Mat1a	Methionine adenosyltransferase I, alpha	13.04	14.39
Apoa1	Apolipoprotein A-I	13.02	25.82
Down-regulated genes			
St3gal6	ST3 beta-galactoside alpha-2,3-sialyltransferase 6	−13.09	−21.14
Btbd3	BTB (POZ) domain containing 3	−13.12	−2.51
Wbp2	WW domain binding protein 2	−13.12	−1.47
LOC100045542	Predicted: similar to FERMRhoGEF (Arhgef) and pleckstrin domain protein 1	−13.14	−3.04
Shmt2	Serine hydroxymethyltransferase 2 (mitochondrial), nuclear gene encoding mitochondrial protein	−13.19	−1.69
Clptm1l	CLPTM1-like	−13.24	−1.48
Cox10	COX10 homologue, cytochrome c oxidase assembly protein, heme A: farnesyltransferase (yeast), nuclear gene encoding mitochondrial protein	−13.26	−1.54
Gpr107	G protein-coupled receptor 107	−13.27	−1.82

Table 4 List of genes significantly regulated by PFJ *(Continued)*

Dnajc10	Dnaj (Hsp40) homologue, subfamily C, member 10	−13.29	−1.55
Plod2	Procollagen-lysine, 2-oxoglutarate 5-dioxygenase 2	−13.29	−2.74
Magee1	Melanoma antigen, family E, 1	−13.31	−4.06
Ppp1r16a	Protein phosphatase 1, regulatory (inhibitor) subunit 16A	−13.35	−2.19
Prkcbp1	Protein kinase C binding protein 1	−13.36	−2.04
Map3k11	Mitogen-activated protein kinase kinase kinase 11	−13.37	−1.48
Marcks	Myristoylated alanine rich protein kinase C substrate	−13.38	−1.47
Tex9	Testis expressed gene 9	−13.39	−2.46
Cog1	Component of oligomeric golgi complex 1	−13.40	−1.51
Slc39a13	Solute carrier family 39 (metal ion transporter), member 13	−13.40	−2.66
Fam110b	Family with sequence similarity 110, member B	−13.43	−3.23
Cox6b1	Cytochrome c oxidase, subunit VIb polypeptide 1	−13.44	−1.45
Stxbp2	Syntaxin binding protein 2	−13.45	−1.68
Ino80b	INO80 complex subunit B	−13.45	−2.52
Nap1l4	Nucleosome assembly protein 1-like 4	−13.45	−1.55
Flii	Flightless I homologue (*Drosophila*)	−13.47	−1.63
Ahdc1	AT hook, DNA binding motif, containing 1	−13.55	−1.63
Nol5a	Nucleolar protein 5A	−13.69	−1.52
2400001E08Rik	RIKEN cDNA 2400001E08 gene	−13.75	−1.77
Prmt5	Protein arginine N-methyltransferase 5	−13.77	−1.79
Tinagl	Tubulointerstitial nephritis antigen-like	−13.78	−3.14
Parl	Presenilin associated, rhomboid-like	−13.84	−1.51
Zmat5	Zinc finger, matrin type 5	−13.85	−1.86
Calm3	Calmodulin 3	−13.86	−2.15
Ak3l1	Adenylate kinase 3-like 1, nuclear gene encoding mitochondrial protein	−13.86	−1.49
2700087H15Rik	RIKEN cDNA 2700087H15 gene	−13.93	−1.54
Grit	RHOGTPase-activating protein	−13.95	−2.23
X99384	cDNA sequence X99384	−13.96	−1.77
Ddx27	DEAD (Asp-Glu-Ala-Asp) box polypeptide 27	−13.97	−2.09
Zfp313	Zinc finger protein 313	−13.98	−1.53
D15Wsu169e	DNA segment, Chr 15, Wayne State University 169, expressed	−14.02	−4.17
Zer1	Zer-1 homologue (*Caenorhabditis elegans*)	−14.03	−2.01
Snapc2	Small nuclear RNA activating complex, polypeptide 2	−14.05	−2.04
Dock1	Dedicator of cytokinesis 1	−14.19	−1.91
Pak4	P21 (CDKN1A)-activated kinase 4	−14.21	−1.51
Arl2	ADP-ribosylation factor-like 2	−14.22	−6.24
Pcolce	Procollagen C-endopeptidase enhancer protein	−14.24	−2.15
1110018G07Rik	RIKEN cDNA 1110018G07 gene	−14.28	−1.61
2610528J11Rik	RIKEN cDNA 2610528J11 gene	−14.29	−2.35
Akp2	Alkaline phosphatase 2, liver	−14.31	−2.72
Mapre1	Microtubule-associated protein, RP/EB family, member 1	−14.35	−1.56
Tmem138	Transmembrane protein 138	−14.36	−2.51
Pacs2	Phosphofurin acidic cluster sorting protein 2	−14.41	−1.70
LOC100047173	PREDICTED: similar to synaptotagmin-like 1	−14.41	−3.34

Table 4 List of genes significantly regulated by PFJ *(Continued)*

Ano10	Anoctamin 10	−14.47	−5.94
Vasn	Vasorin	−14.48	−1.65
Cml4	Camello-like 4	−14.50	−3.02
Clcn3	Chloride channel 3, transcript variant a	−14.50	−1.73
Pik3r3	Phosphatidylinositol 3-kinase, regulatory subunit, polypeptide 3 (p55)	−14.54	−4.60
Timp1	TIMP metallopeptidase inhibitor 1	−14.61	−1.60
Fbxl15	F-box and leucine-rich repeat protein 15	−14.65	−1.59
Npc2	Niemann-Pick disease, type C2	−14.68	−1.60
Mrps33	Mitochondrial ribosomal protein S33, nuclear gene encoding mitochondrial protein, transcript variant 2	−14.73	−1.65
Pgam5	Phosphoglycerate mutase family member 5	−14.73	−1.84
2310005N01Rik	RIKEN cDNA 2310005N01 gene	−14.79	−2.67
Ctdspl	CTD (carboxy-terminal domain, RNA polymerase II, polypeptide A) small phosphatase-like	−14.83	−2.49
LOC100046039	PREDICTED: similar to histone deacetylase HD1	−14.85	−2.29
Gnptab	N-acetylglucosamine-1-phosphate transferase, alpha and beta subunits	−14.93	−1.90
Tbc1d14	TBC1 domain family, member 14	−15.03	−2.88
Cyr61	Cysteine-rich protein 61	−15.07	−4.37
Gdpd1	Glycerophosphodiester phosphodiesterase domain containing 1	−15.11	−1.58
2310022B05Rik	RIKEN cDNA 2310022B05 gene	−15.16	−1.53
Asna1	Arsa arsenite transporter, ATP-binding, homologue 1 (bacterial)	−15.16	−1.66
Tcf4	Transcription factor 4, transcript variant 1	−15.17	−2.10
Vps26b	Vacuolar protein sorting 26 homologue B (yeast)	−15.43	−1.57
Nf2	Neurofibromatosis 2	−15.54	−2.64
LOC192758	Similar to hypothetical protein MGC39650	−15.63	−3.10
Drg2	Developmentally regulated GTP binding protein 2	−15.66	−1.74
Iqgap1	IQ motif containing GTPase activating protein 1	−15.89	−1.73
Nrp1	Neuropilin 1	−16.05	−2.33
Tbc1d13	TBC1 domain family, member 13	−16.13	−3.24
2310003P10Rik	RIKEN cDNA 2310003P10 gene	−16.15	−3.82
Trim28	Tripartite motif protein 28	−16.18	−1.79
Tlr2	Toll-like receptor 2	−16.41	−2.26
0910001L09Rik	RIKEN cDNA 0910001L09 gene	−16.42	−2.15
B930041F14Rik	RIKEN cDNA B930041F14 gene	−16.74	−2.44
Nup93	Nucleoporin 93 kDa	−16.93	−2.22
Lphn1	Latrophilin 1	−17.11	−2.08
Odz4	Odd Oz/ten-m homologue 4 (*Drosophila*)	−17.13	−4.10
Gnai2	Guanine nucleotide binding protein, alpha inhibiting 2	−17.14	−2.08
Cyp4f13	Cytochrome P450, family 4, subfamily f, polypeptide 13	−17.16	−4.76
Aacs	Acetoacetyl-coa synthetase	−17.26	−1.62
Smarca4	SWI/SNF related, matrix associated, actin dependent regulator of chromatin, subfamily a, member 4	−17.42	−1.89

Table 4 List of genes significantly regulated by PFJ *(Continued)*

Gatad2b	GATA zinc finger domain containing 2B	−17.46	−2.31
Actr1b	ARP1 actin-related protein 1 homologue B, centractin beta (yeast)	−17.87	−1.74
Neo1	Neogenin 1	−17.93	−2.00
Meis2	Meis homeobox 2, transcript variant 2	−18.31	−1.91
Serpinh1	Serine (or cysteine) peptidase inhibitor, clade H, member 1	−18.44	−9.72
Cc2d2a	Coiled-coil and C2 domain containing 2A	−18.44	−2.28
Vdac1	Voltage-dependent anion channel 1	−18.88	−1.65
Picalm	Phosphatidylinositol binding clathrin assembly protein	−19.13	−1.73
Ankrd24	Ankyrin repeat domain 24	−19.20	−6.41
Pi4ka	Phosphatidylinositol 4-kinase, catalytic, alpha polypeptide	−19.52	−2.19
Map3k2	Mitogen-activated protein kinase kinase kinase 2	−19.53	−3.51
1700029G01Rik	RIKEN cDNA 1700029G01 gene	−19.78	−2.21
Atn1	Atrophin 1	−21.42	−1.86
Itprip	Inositol 1,4,5-triphosphate receptor interacting protein	−22.26	−6.38
Gadd45g	Growth arrest and DNA-damage-inducible 45 gamma	−23.65	−2.44
Ly6e	Lymphocyte antigen 6 complex, locus E	−23.91	−2.53
Ctcfl	CCCTC-binding factor (zinc finger protein)-like	−27.64	−2.21

source for food supplementation or as a nutraceutical having possible anti-diabetic properties.

PFJ reduced weight gain, adipose tissue, plasma TG and plasma RBG but increased caecum weight

Following the 4-week high-carbohydrate diet challenge in weanling male NRs, the group supplemented with PFJ weighed less and their food intake was significantly lower. However, the carcass (lean mass) and food efficiency tended to be greater for the PFJ group, and they had less adipose tissue. Thus, control rats gained more weight than those in the PFJ group, mostly due to the accumulation of adipose tissue, while PFJ seemed to inhibit appetite and reduce body fat percentage without reducing food efficiency or leading to a decrease in lean body mass. The latter effect is a characteristic of dietary fibres that are fermented by large bowel microbiota [107], and it is noteworthy that the enlarged caeca in rats fed PFJ would be consistent with enhanced fermentation of PFJ components by their large bowel flora. Faster weight gain in male NRs has also been found to enhance T2DM induction in growing rats [15, 21]. As visceral adiposity and hyperlipaemia are two of the risk factors for cardiovascular insults in metabolic syndrome, the reduced body fat percentage and TG levels observed in the PFJ group indicate a beneficial metabolic effect beyond improved blood glucose levels.

The PFJ group also had a significantly lower level of RBG compared to the controls, although no differences were observed in terms of FBG. RBG is an early and more reliable parameter of T2DM than FBG in NRs

[14–16, 21, 85]. This is because the correlations between circulating glucose and different markers of T2DM, such as elevations in HbA1c and hypertension, are stronger for RBG than FBG in NRs. In addition, acute cell and organ damage is best reflected by the degree and duration of postprandial hyperglycaemia, thus rendering RBG the best indicator of such damage [15, 16]. The observation that insulin levels were not significantly different between the two groups ($p > 0.05$) indicates that the improved glucose control was due to mechanisms other than increased insulin secretion, such as reduced intestinal glucose absorption or improved insulin sensitivity. As hyperinsulinaemia is one of the first indicators of insulin resistance and a risk factor for the eventual depletion of pancreatic beta cells, this is a crucial observation for the prevention of T2DM, potentially reducing the need for or delaying the onset of insulin therapy or enabling a reduced dose. PFJ thus exerted beneficial metabolic effects, preventing NRs from overconsumption of calories and achieving improved control of plasma glucose and lipids.

As NRs in the present study were fed ad libitum, at least part of the effects ascribed to PFJ could be due to mild caloric restriction caused by reduced food intake. Nevertheless, caloric restriction in the classical sense typically entails a 20–40 % reduction in food consumption relative to normal intake [64], which was not the case here at 15–20 %. Furthermore, we previously found no reduction in food intake or any difference in PFJ protection in older NRs when given artificially sweetened PFJ, suggesting that PFJ protection against diabetes

Table 5 List of WikiPathways significantly regulated by PFJ

WikiPathway name	No. changed	% changed	Z score	Permuted p
Up-regulated WikiPathways				
Tryptophan metabolism:WP79	6	15.3846	9.4735	0.0000
Aflatoxin B1 metabolism:WP1262	2	40.0000	9.1192	0.0005
Methylation:WP1247	2	28.5714	7.6363	0.0000
Fatty acid omega oxidation:WP33	2	28.5714	7.6363	0.0015
Statin pathway (PharmGKB):WP1	3	16.6667	6.9838	0.0000
Blood clotting cascade:WP460	3	15.7895	6.7763	0.0000
Nuclear receptors in lipid metabolism and toxicity:WP431	3	10.0000	5.2068	0.0005
Complement and coagulation cascades:WP449	4	6.8966	4.7841	0.0000
Urea cycle and metabolism of amino groups:WP426	2	11.1111	4.5187	0.0020
Retinol metabolism:WP1259	3	7.6923	4.4328	0.0005
Metapathway biotransformation:WP1251	5	4.4248	3.9468	0.0000
One-carbon metabolism:WP435	2	8.3333	3.7980	0.0040
Nuclear receptors:WP509	2	5.5556	2.9123	0.0075
Cytochrome P450:WP1274	2	5.2632	2.8039	0.0105
Down-Regulated WikiPathways				
Regulation of actin cytoskeleton:WP523	4	3.0534	3.6287	0.0080
Insulin signalling:WP65	4	2.8169	3.4170	0.0110
Endochondral ossification:WP1270	2	3.3898	2.7401	0.0460
TNF-alpha NF-κβ signalling pathway:WP246	3	2.2222	2.4278	0.0430

development does not depend on reductions in food consumption [16].

In addition, NRs in the PFJ group had heavier caeca ($p < 0.05$) than the controls. This may be attributed to the presence of fermentable dietary fibres in the PFJ extract that resisted upper gut digestion and reached the caecum (the main site of bacterial fermentation in rodents) where they were fermented by the microbiota. However, the bioactive components in PFJ and/or their derived metabolites may have also played a part in the observed caecum enlargement. In the colon, where microbial glucosidases and glucuronidases are active, phenolic glycosides are intensively metabolised and their metabolites also modify colon parameters, such as short-chain fatty acids, amino acids and vitamins [30]. This is in agreement with the results of others, where increased caecal weight was observed in rats fed diets containing polyphenols [2, 37, 53]. Romo-Vaquero et al. [95] also reported that rosemary extract enriched in the bioactive compound carnosic acid caused caecum enlargement in female Zucker rats. The presence of non-digested materials fermented by large bowel microbiota might have caused the enlarged caeca. The same study also reported that the rosemary extract lowered body weights, serum lipids and insulin levels in the rats and partially attributed this to the inhibition of a pre-duodenal butyrate esterase activity [95]. Thus, the lower adipose tissue

content and body weights of the NRs on PFJ may also have been a consequence of the inhibition of specific enzymes in the gut. A pomegranate extract, rich in punicalagin and ellagic acid, also increased caecum size and *Bifidobacterium* in mice [84]. The gut microbiota can modulate host energy metabolism and is thus a significant contributor to the development of obesity and metabolic disorders [130].

Microarray gene expression analysis revealed down-regulation of the insulin-signalling pathway linked to altered insulin availability

Research on the health effects of plant-based foods will benefit from taking a holistic approach to understand the plethora of effects mediated by a range of bioactive metabolites derived from plant consumption. Thus, the combination of different 'omics' profiling techniques in the concept of systems biology, or nutrigenomics as termed in the context of nutrition-related sciences, would be important for this purpose [47]. In the present study, microarrays delineated hepatic gene expression differences between young NRs supplemented with PFJ or not and further confirmed several target genes of interest using real-time qRT-PCR.

In relation to T2DM, the most significant observation from the functional enrichment analysis of the microarray gene expression data was that the insulin-

Table 6 List of gene ontologies (biological processes) significantly regulated by PFJ

GO ID	GO name	No. changed	% changed	Z score	Permuted p
Up-regulated gene ontologies (biological processes)					
GO:0010903	Negative regulation of very-low-density lipoprotein particle remodelling	3	100.0000	26.2353	0.0000
GO:0060192	Negative regulation of lipase activity	4	40.0000	19.0387	0.0000
GO:0033700	Phospholipid efflux	4	33.3333	17.3429	0.0000
GO:0060416	Response to growth hormone stimulus	4	30.7692	16.6448	0.0000
GO:0032488	Cdc42 protein signal transduction	2	50.0000	15.0814	0.0000
GO:0046461	Neutral lipid catabolic process	3	33.3333	15.0179	0.0000
GO:0042157	Lipoprotein metabolic process	5	20.0000	14.8938	0.0000
GO:0007494	Midgut development	3	30.0000	14.2268	0.0000
GO:0048261	Negative regulation of receptor-mediated endocytosis	2	40.0000	13.4602	0.0000
GO:0010915	Regulation of very-low-density lipoprotein particle clearance	2	40.0000	13.4602	0.0000
GO:0071825	Protein-lipid complex subunit organisation	4	19.0476	12.9842	0.0000
GO:0015918	Sterol transport	5	14.2857	12.4800	0.0000
GO:0050995	Negative regulation of lipid catabolic process	3	23.0769	12.4241	0.0005
GO:0030300	Regulation of intestinal cholesterol absorption	2	33.3333	12.2609	0.0000
GO:0034381	Plasma lipoprotein particle clearance	3	21.4286	11.9549	0.0000
GO:0008203	Cholesterol metabolic process	7	9.5890	11.9276	0.0000
GO:0034367	Macromolecular complex remodelling	3	20.0000	11.5328	0.0000
GO:0010873	Positive regulation of cholesterol esterification	2	28.5714	11.3268	0.0000
GO:0018904	Organic ether metabolic process	7	8.6420	11.2675	0.0000
GO:0071941	Nitrogen cycle metabolic process	2	22.2222	9.9459	0.0000
GO:0051055	Negative regulation of lipid biosynthetic process	3	13.6364	9.4265	0.0000
GO:0071320	Cellular response to cyclic adenosine monophosphate	2	20.0000	9.4149	0.0005
GO:0042632	Cholesterol homeostasis	4	10.0000	9.2153	0.0000
GO:0071396	Cellular response to lipid	3	13.0435	9.2059	0.0005
GO:0071383	Cellular response to steroid hormone stimulus	5	6.4935	8.1091	0.0000
GO:0006720	Isoprenoid metabolic process	4	7.0175	7.5752	0.0000
GO:0050817	Coagulation	4	5.8824	6.8498	0.0000
GO:0001101	Response to acid	4	5.7971	6.7922	0.0005
GO:0010243	Response to organic nitrogen	5	4.7170	6.7315	0.0000
GO:0044272	Sulphur compound biosynthetic process	3	7.3171	6.7133	0.0015
GO:0017144	Drug metabolic process	2	10.5263	6.6960	0.0045
GO:0033762	Response to glucagon stimulus	3	6.9767	6.5356	0.0005
GO:0044106	Cellular amine metabolic process	9	2.7692	6.4744	0.0000
GO:0043436	Oxoacid metabolic process	12	2.1053	6.1883	0.0000
GO:0033574	Response to testosterone stimulus	2	9.0909	6.1811	0.0030
GO:0009636	Response to toxin	4	4.7619	6.0507	0.0010
GO:0031100	Organ regeneration	3	5.8824	5.9287	0.0010
GO:0042743	Hydrogen peroxide metabolic process	2	8.3333	5.8913	0.0045
GO:0031667	Response to nutrient levels	7	2.7237	5.6322	0.0000
GO:0051262	Protein tetramerisation	3	5.3571	5.6146	0.0020
GO:0031330	Negative regulation of cellular catabolic process	2	7.1429	5.4051	0.0060
GO:0030193	Regulation of blood coagulation	2	6.8966	5.2990	0.0060

Table 6 List of gene ontologies (biological processes) significantly regulated by PFJ *(Continued)*

GO:0010043	Response to zinc ion	2	6.8966	5.2990	0.0050
GO:0031647	Regulation of protein stability	3	4.8387	5.2867	0.0020
GO:0051384	Response to glucocorticoid stimulus	4	3.3898	4.9035	0.0010
GO:0007623	Circadian rhythm	3	4.2254	4.8711	0.0040
GO:0055114	Oxidation-reduction process	11	1.6129	4.7935	0.0000
GO:0071375	Cellular response to peptide hormone stimulus	4	3.1008	4.6273	0.0035
GO:0006725	Cellular aromatic compound metabolic process	4	2.9851	4.5123	0.0015
GO:0033013	Tetrapyrrole metabolic process	2	5.1282	4.4651	0.0070
GO:0051186	Cofactor metabolic process	5	2.4510	4.4123	0.0005
GO:0033555	Multicellular organismal response to stress	2	4.3478	4.0441	0.0110
GO:0044262	Cellular carbohydrate metabolic process	6	1.8127	3.8583	0.0045
GO:0061061	Muscle structure development	2	3.8462	3.7493	0.0190
GO:0042445	Hormone metabolic process	3	2.7027	3.6494	0.0100
GO:0042493	Response to drug	5	1.8116	3.5138	0.0045
GO:0006730	One-carbon metabolic process	4	1.9802	3.3655	0.0125
GO:0007626	Locomotory behaviour	3	2.3810	3.3384	0.0125
GO:0014070	Response to organic cyclic compound	4	1.9417	3.3146	0.0065
GO:0048513	Organ development	9	1.1704	3.1890	0.0050
GO:0009607	Response to biotic stimulus	6	1.4458	3.1796	0.0090
GO:0009611	Response to wounding	5	1.6026	3.1729	0.0120
GO:0009791	Post-embryonic development	2	2.7778	3.0325	0.0375
GO:0006414	Translational elongation	2	2.6316	2.9216	0.0485
GO:0010466	Negative regulation of peptidase activity	3	1.9868	2.9171	0.0325
GO:0050679	Positive regulation of epithelial cell proliferation	2	2.4096	2.7455	0.0480
GO:0035335	Peptidyl-tyrosine dephosphorylation	2	2.3529	2.6988	0.0380
GO:0034284	Response to monosaccharide stimulus	2	2.3529	2.6988	0.0490
GO:0032989	Cellular component morphogenesis	4	1.4652	2.6156	0.0285
GO:0009967	Positive regulation of signal transduction	5	1.1876	2.3859	0.0305
Down-regulated gene ontologies (biological processes)					
GO:0032006	Regulation of mTOR signalling cascade	2	12.5000	6.1613	0.0040
GO:0031113	Regulation of microtubule polymerisation	2	11.1111	5.7727	0.0070
GO:0001702	Gastrulation with mouth forming second	2	9.0909	5.1559	0.0075
GO:0045216	Cell-cell junction organisation	2	5.2632	3.7231	0.0245
GO:0042632	Cholesterol homeostasis	2	5.0000	3.6045	0.0235
GO:0006793	Phosphorus metabolic process	14	1.4433	3.5098	0.0015
GO:0031214	Biomineral tissue development	2	4.5455	3.3902	0.0280
GO:0002263	Cell activation involved in immune response	2	4.5455	3.3902	0.0320
GO:0042475	Odontogenesis of dentine-containing tooth	2	4.4444	3.3408	0.0315
GO:0032259	Methylation	4	2.5157	3.1405	0.0145
GO:0030155	Regulation of cell adhesion	4	2.4096	3.0318	0.0160
GO:0050790	Regulation of catalytic activity	15	1.2490	3.0295	0.0080
GO:0010243	Response to organic nitrogen	3	2.8302	2.9800	0.0270
GO:0001933	Negative regulation of protein phosphorylation	2	3.6364	2.9179	0.0460
GO:0071841	Cellular component organisation or biogenesis at cellular level	18	1.0508	2.5596	0.0140

Table 6 List of gene ontologies (biological processes) significantly regulated by PFJ *(Continued)*

GO:0019219	Regulation of nucleobase, nucleoside, nucleotide and nucleic acid metabolic process	21	0.9620	2.3612	0.0210
GO:0008219	Cell death	7	1.3514	2.2489	0.0340

signalling pathway was down-regulated in NRs given PFJ, including genes for mitogen-activated protein triple kinases, *Map3k2* and *Map3k11*, phosphatidylinositol kinases, *Pik3r3* and *Pi4ka*, as well as syntaxin binding protein 2 (*Stxbp2*).

Insulin is essential for appropriate tissue development, growth and maintenance of whole body glucose homeostasis. This hormone is secreted by the β cells of the pancreatic islets of Langerhans in response to increased circulating levels of glucose after a meal. Insulin regulates glucose homeostasis by reducing hepatic glucose output and increasing the rate of glucose uptake primarily into striated muscle and adipose tissues. In these tissues, the clearance of circulating glucose depends on the insulin-stimulated translocation of the facilitative glucose transporter 4 (GLUT4) to the cell surface. Insulin also profoundly affects lipid metabolism by increasing lipid synthesis in liver and adipose tissues, as well as attenuating fatty acid release from TG in fat and muscle cells. Insulin resistance occurs when normal circulating concentrations of the hormone are insufficient to dispose of circulating glucose imposed by glucose-rich diets. In fact, insulin rises dramatically in concert with insulin resistance in the early diabetes of NRs fed high-glycaemic load diets, then falls as diabetes progresses [15].

To assure insulin sensitivity, the circulating hormone must bind to an enzyme that activates its functions, in this case the α-subunit of the insulin receptor embedded in the cell membrane. This binding triggers the tyrosine kinase activity in the β-subunit of the insulin receptor, which further causes phosphorylation of two types of enzymes, mitogen-activated protein kinases (MAPKs) and phosphatidylinositol 3-kinases (PI3Ks), which are responsible for expressing the mitogenic and metabolic actions of insulin, respectively [111]. The activation of MAPKs leads to the completion of mitogenic functions such as cell growth and gene expression, while the activation of PI3Ks leads to important metabolic functions such as synthesis of lipids, proteins and glycogen, as well as cell survival and cell proliferation. Most importantly, the PI3K pathway is responsible for the distribution of glucose for essential cell functions.

MAPKs

In our present study, two enzymes involved in the MAPK pathway of insulin signalling, i.e. *Map3k2* and *Map3k11*, were down-regulated in PFJ-supplemented rats. Many studies have causally implicated MAPKs in the development of insulin resistance [96]. Systemic insulin resistance triggers chronic hyperglycaemia, which causes pancreatic β cells to secrete more insulin. In the long term, this adaptation is associated with stress-induced β cell death and leads to insulin deficiency and T2DM. As such, stress mechanisms that trigger insulin resistance are also known to contribute to β cell failure. The majority of studies indicate that prolonged enhanced MAPK signalling is detrimental to insulin sensitivity and β cell function. A growing body of evidence also indicates that MAPKs are involved in physiological metabolic adaptation, the disturbance of which might contribute to metabolic diseases. Thus, although MAPK-dependent signal transduction is required for physiological metabolic adaptation, inappropriate MAPK signalling contributes to the development of T2DM and the metabolic syndrome [41].

GLUT4

By definition, insulin resistance is a defect in signal transduction associated with accumulation of diacylglycerol and ceramides [91, 101]. At present, only one class of downstream signalling molecules is confirmed to be essential for insulin-stimulated glucose uptake and GLUT4 translocation, i.e. the class IA PI3Ks [27]. The GLUT4 vesicle, which is responsible for passive diffusion of glucose, binds to PI3Ks after bringing glucose into the cell. PI3Ks isolate the GLUT4 vesicle from the glucose and send the vesicle back to the cell membrane. The glucose that is isolated is then sent to the mitochondria to produce energy as ATP, and excess glucose is stored in the cell as glycogen, which is increased in NRs with T2DM [21]. The binding of insulin to its receptor on the surface of adipose and muscle cells initiates a signalling cascade that alters the trafficking itinerary of GLUT4 thus releasing it from intracellular stores and delivering it to the cell surface [18, 109]. In the absence of insulin, about 95 % of GLUT4 is confined to intracellular compartments. Insulin stimulation results in GLUT4 redistribution from these intracellular stores to the plasma membrane via alterations in membrane trafficking [18, 109]. This insulin-stimulated translocation of GLUT4 from intracellular sites to the plasma membrane is defective in individuals with insulin resistance and T2DM thus providing an impetus to comprehend how this trafficking pathway is controlled [12, 44].

PI3Ks

Emerging data indicate that the products of class IA PI3Ks act as both membrane anchors and allosteric regulators, serving to localise and activate downstream enzymes and their protein substrates [106]. Several studies have suggested that the interaction of insulin receptor substrate (IRS) proteins with PI3Ks is necessary for the appropriate activation and/or targeting of the enzyme to a critical intracellular site, including its association with GLUT4 vesicles [91]. Class IA PI3Ks play an essential role in insulin stimulation of glucose transport and metabolism and protein and lipid synthesis, as well as cell growth and differentiation [98].

In terms of molecular structure, class IA PI3Ks are heterodimers consisting of one regulatory and one catalytic subunit, each of which occurs in multiple isoforms [118, 119]. Three mammalian genes, *Pik3r1*, *Pik3r2* and *Pik3r3* encode for the p85α (p85α, p50α and p55α isoforms), p85β and p55γ regulatory subunits, respectively. The family of the catalytic subunits includes p110α, p110β, and p110δ [106]. These are the products of three respective genes, *Pik3ca*, *Pik3cb* and *Pik3cd*. The regulatory subunits of class IA PI3Ks appear to play three important functional roles. They confer stability on the catalytic subunits, induce lipid kinase activity upon insulin stimulation [131] and, in the basal state, inhibit the catalytic activity of the p110 subunits to various degrees [116].

The unique structural domains of the PI3K regulatory subunits and their differential abundances in tissues suggest that they are not entirely redundant and may serve unique purposes. Complete disruption of hepatic *Pik3r1* and *Pik3r2* markedly reduces insulin-stimulated PI3K activity, at least in part by destabilising the catalytic subunits [112]. On the other hand, partial loss of the regulatory subunits of PI3Ks increases insulin sensitivity, and this appears to be related to diminished negative feedback to the IRS proteins [40]. For example, mice with a knockout of the full-length p85α exhibit an upregulation of the splice variants p50α and p55α in muscle and fat tissues and have increased insulin sensitivity [114]. In addition, p50α/p55α knockout mice exhibit improved insulin sensitivity, lower fat masses and protection against obesity-induced insulin resistance [23]. However, mice with complete deletion of p85α and its short splice variants p50α and p55α die perinatally with liver necrosis and enlarged muscle fibres [38]. Thus, identifying the precise pathways uniquely mediated by these regulatory subunit isoforms remains an important area for further study.

In the present study, the *Pik3r3* gene encoding for the p55γ regulatory subunit of PI3Ks was down-regulated in NRs given PFJ. p55γ is similar in structure to p55α but is expressed at low levels in most tissues [111]. However, the effect of inhibiting or knocking out p55γ, encoded by the *Pik3r3* gene, on insulin sensitivity has not been conclusively determined. Nevertheless, since rats given PFJ had lower levels of RBG ($p < 0.05$) but similar insulin levels compared to NRs in the control group, the down-regulation of the *Pik3r3* gene and the related hepatic insulin-signalling pathway in general suggests that reduced glucose absorption by PFJ lowered the diabetogenic effects of the high-carbohydrate diet and/or enhanced insulin sensitivity, rather than PFJ acting by increasing insulin secretion. This is in accordance with the physiological parameters, as outlined above. The down-regulation of the insulin-signalling pathway could prove beneficial in the long run, as this would protect the pancreas from overproducing insulin and preserve insulin sensitivity in the related target organs, thereby preventing hyperinsulinaemia and hyperglycaemia.

Down-regulation of hepatic genes involved in fibrotic processes was observed in NRs given PFJ

T2DM and hepatic diseases

T2DM and obesity are risk factors for non-alcoholic fatty liver diseases, which include hepatic steatosis (non-alcoholic fatty liver disease or NAFLD), non-alcoholic steatohepatitis (NASH), fibrosis and cirrhosis. Increased insulin resistance and adiposity contribute to the progression from non-alcoholic steatohepatitis to fibrosis through the development of a pro-fibrotic condition in the liver, including increased hepatocellular death, increased generation of reactive oxygen species and an altered cytokine balance [24]. Liver disease is an important cause of death in T2DM, as T2DM is currently the most common cause of liver disease in the USA, including the hepatocellular carcinoma that results from chronic T2DM [115]. The prevalence of T2DM in cirrhosis is 12.3 to 57 % [117].

Incidentally, hepatic steatosis is the most prevalent early lesions in diabetic NRs and is correlated with advancing T2DM, with hepatomegaly and liver discolouration also present macroscopically [70]. A large proportion of male NRs that reach 1 year of age with T2DM also reveal hepatocellular carcinoma in various stages (Kenneth C. Hayes, Brandeis University, MA, personal communication).

Collagen accumulation and fibrosis

Organ fibrosis including liver fibrosis is characterised by an excessive accumulation of collagen. Mature collagen cross-links in a variety of connective tissues such as bones, tendons, ligaments and cartilages are formed via the hydroxyallysine route. In contrast, collagen in the skin is mainly cross-linked via the allysine route. In organ fibrosis, an increase in cross-links derived from the hydroxyallysine route is found. This change in cross-linking is related to irreversible accumulation of collagen in fibrotic tissues. Collagen containing hydroxyallysine-derived cross-links is more difficult to degrade than collagen containing allysine-derived cross-links. Inhibition of the formation of hydroxyallysine-

Title: Insulin Signaling
Organism: Mus musculus

Glucose Transport — Slc2a4 1.6, Slc2a1 1.0

Insr 2.04, -1.5　Igf1r -4.38

PI 3-Kinase

Pik3ca	1.0	Pik3r1	-1.04
Pik3cb	-2.07	Pik3r2	-1.35
Pik3cd	1.0	Pik3r3	-4.5
Pik3cg	1.0	Pik3r4	1.0
Pik3c2a	-1.54		
Pik3c2g	-1.36		
Pik3c3	1.0		

Insulin Receptor Substrates

Irs1	1.46	Shc1	1.03
Irs2		Shc2	
Irs3	1.0	Shc3	-51.88
Irs4			
Gab1	-2.18		

Ras-MAPK Signaling

Grb2	-1.19	Hras1	1.07
Grb10	-4.66	Raf1	1.48
Grb14	1.61		
		Rrad	1.0
Sos1	1.27	Ras1	-1.41
Sos2		Ras2	2.95

PDK/Akt Signaling

Pdpk1	-1.19	Sgk	-2.9
Akt1	-1.24	Sgk2	1.0
Akt2	1.0	Sgkl	
Gsk3a			
Gsk3b	-1.39		

Tor Signaling — Tsc1, Tsc2, Rheb -1.08, Frap1 -1.32

MEK/MAP Kinases

Mapk1	-1.22	Map3k1	1.0
Mapk3	-2.57	Map3k2	-3.51
Mapk4	1.68	Map3k3	1.29
Mapk6	1.44	Map3k4	1.0
Mapk7	1.0	Map3k5	
Mapk8	1.0	Map3k6	1.0
Mapk9	-1.16	Map3k7	1.0
Mapk10	1.0	Map3k8	1.03
Mapk11	1.12	Map3k9	1.0
Mapk12	-1.14	Map3k10	
Mapk13	-1.18	Map3k11	-1.48
Mapk14	1.59	Map3k12	-2.03
Map2k1	1.0	Map3k13	-1.04
Map2k2	1.26	Map3k14	-1.54
Map2k3	-1.2	Map4k1	
Map2k4	-1.06	Map4k2	-1.95
Map2k5	-1.26	Map4k3	
Map2k6	-1.08	Map4k4	1.2
Map2k7	-1.1	Map4k5	1.0
		Mink1	1.58

Vesicular Trafficking

Flot1	-1.3
Flot2	1.14
Stxbp1	1.0
Stxbp2	-1.68
Stxbp3	-1.42
Stxbp4	-1.71
Vamp2	
Stx4a	3.94
Snap23	1.29
Snap25	1.0
Arf1	
Arf6	1.21
Tbc1d4	1.0
Rhoj	-2.65
Rab4a	1.0
MGI:1345171	1.09
Ehd1	1.0
Ehd2	-5.03
Snx26	1.19
Pscd3	-1.18

Sorbs1	1.0
Cap1	1.0
Cbl	1.0
Cblb	1.0
Cblc	1.0
Crk	-1.11
Rapgef1	1.0
Rhoq	1.0
Kif3a	1.0
Kif5b	1.38
Myo1c	1.14

Transcriptional Regulators & Immediate Early Genes

Foxo1	1.0
Foxo3a	1.0
Elk1	
Srf	-1.46
Egr1	-1.57
Fos	1.27
Jun	1.01

p70 S6 Kinases — Rps6kb1 1.01, Rps6kb2 -1.22

Translation Regulation — Eif4ebp1 1.0, Eif4e 1.0

Metabolic Regulation

Pfkm	-11.24
Pfkl	-1.28
Lipe	1.0
Gys1	-2.03, 1.0
Gys2	2.21
Ppp1cc	1.26
Gyg1	-1.31

Modulators of Insulin Action

Ptprf	1.0	Prkca	1.29
Ptpn1	-1.63	Prkcb1	-1.12
Enpp1	1.0	Prkcd	-1.84
Pten	-1.16, 1.28	Prkch	-1.27
Inppl1	-1.05	Prkci	1.0
Ptpn11	1.0	Prkcq	1.0
Inpp4a	-1.01	Prkcz	-1.5
Mapk8	1.0	Trib3	
Socs1	1.0	Prkaa1	
Socs3	-1.05	Prkaa2	1.0
Ikbkb	1.0		
Xbp1			

p90 Rsk Kinases

Rps6ka1	-1.97
Rps6ka2	
Rps6ka3	1.07
Rps6ka4	1.0
Rps6ka5	1.12
Rps6ka6	1.0

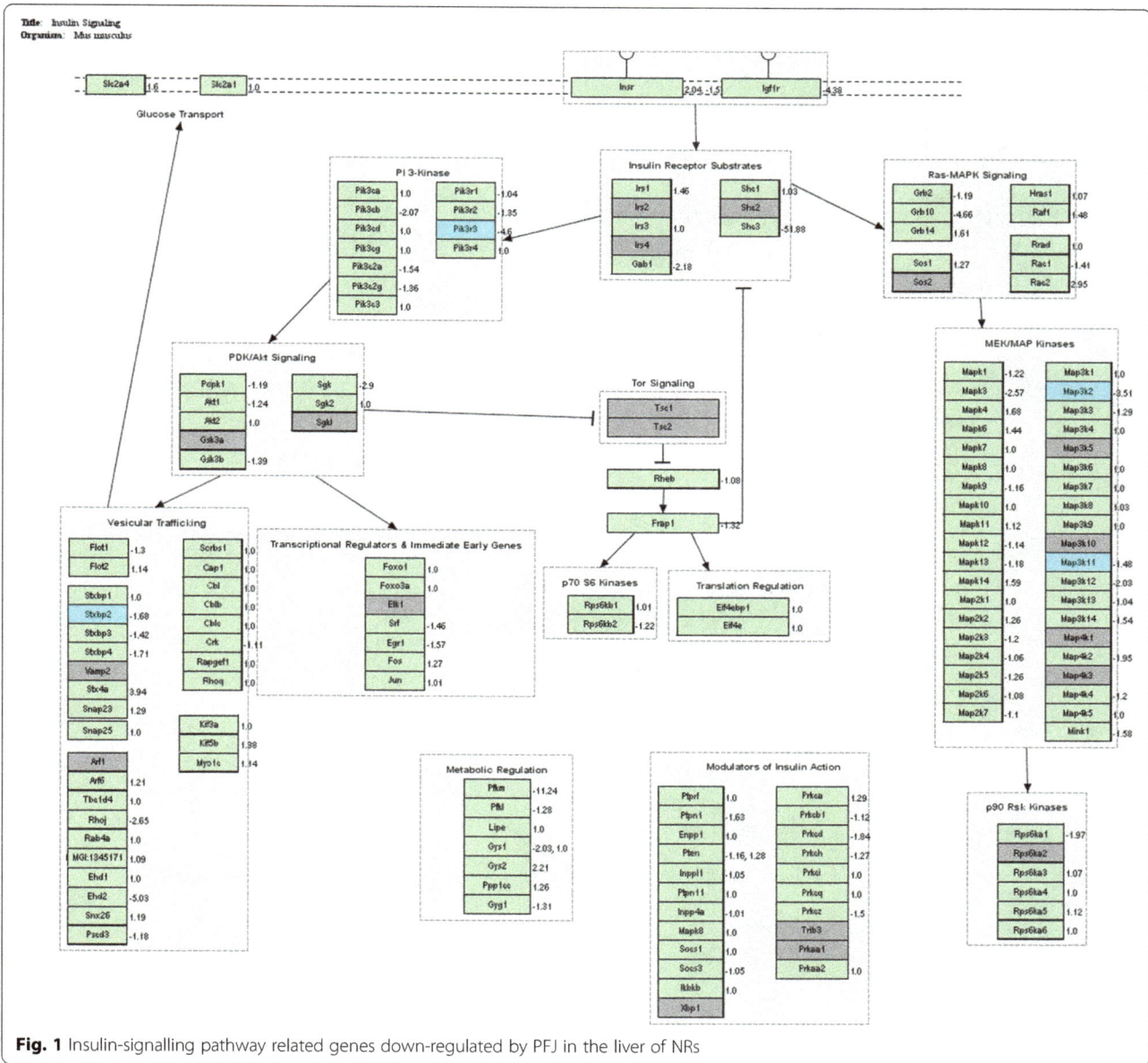

Fig. 1 Insulin-signalling pathway related genes down-regulated by PFJ in the liver of NRs

derived cross-links in fibrosis is therefore likely to result in the formation of collagen that is easier to degrade, thereby preventing unwanted collagen accumulation.

In the present study, two genes involved in fibrotic processes, i.e. *Pcolce* and *Plod2*, were found down-regulated in the PFJ group. The procollagen C-endopeptidase enhancer 1 (*Pcolce*) gene encodes a glyco-protein which binds and drives the enzymatic cleavage of type I procollagen and heightens C-proteinase activity, hence increasing fibrotic processes [108]. The increase in hydroxyallysine-derived cross-links in fibrosis is the result of an overhydroxylation of lysine residues within the collagen telopeptides, a function carried out by the enzyme encoded by procollagen-lysine, 2-oxoglutarate 5-dioxygenase 2 (*Plod2*). *Plod2* is thus involved in fibrotic processes as well [120].

PFJ up-regulated hepatic apolipoprotein genes, especially apolipoprotein A1

Metabolic pathways for the utilisation of carbohydrates and fats are intricately intertwined. In addition to having profound effects on carbohydrate metabolism, insulin also has important effects on lipid metabolism. One of these is to promote the synthesis of fatty acids in the liver when the organ is saturated with glycogen, and these fatty acids are then exported from the liver as lipoproteins, which are

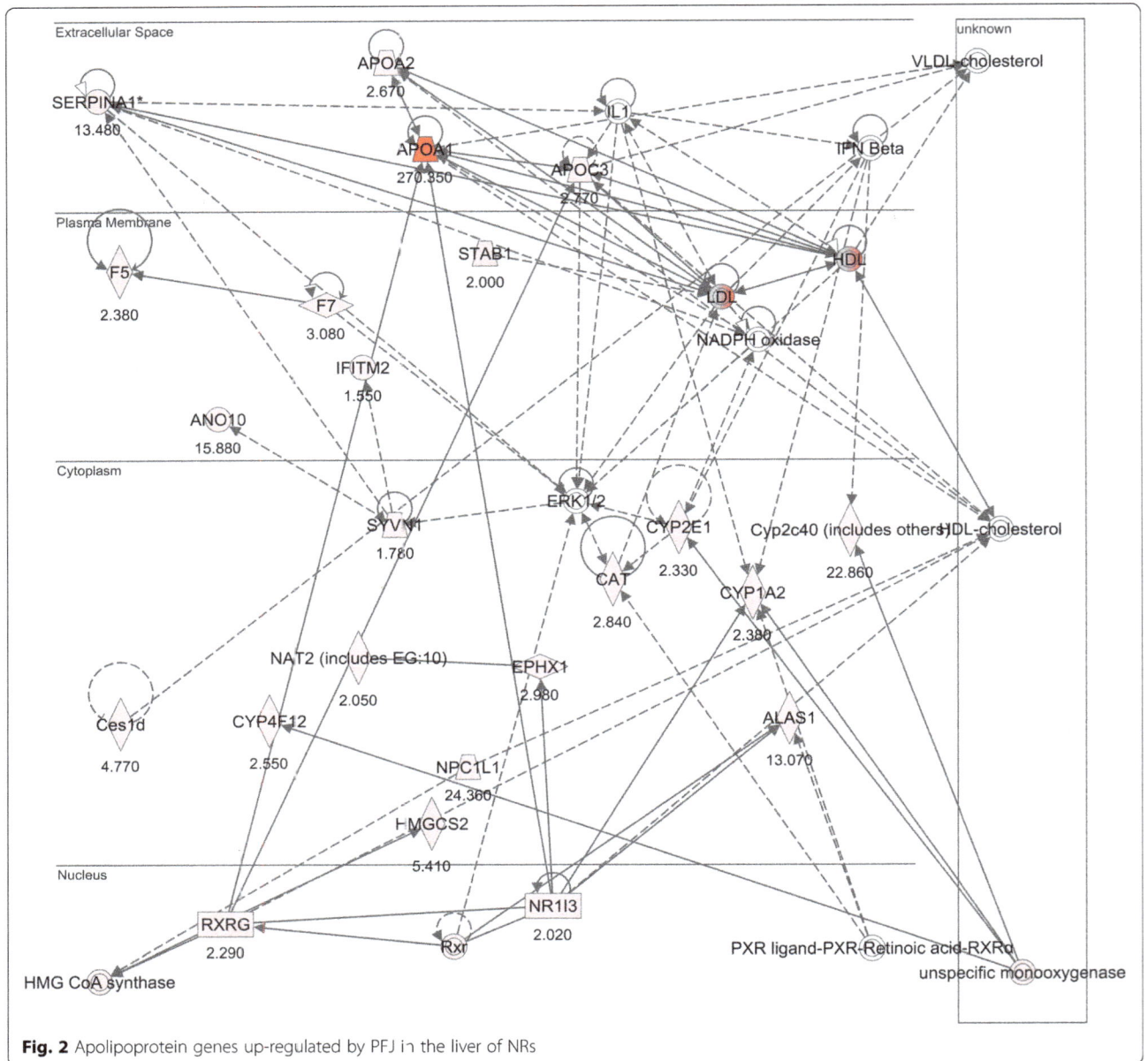

Fig. 2 Apolipoprotein genes up-regulated by PFJ in the liver of NRs

further catabolised in the circulation, eventually yielding free fatty acids for use by other tissues. Insulin resistance and T2DM are associated with plasma lipid and lipoprotein abnormalities, which include reduced high-density lipoproteins (HDL), a predominance of low-density lipoproteins (LDL) and elevated TG levels, also previously described in NRs with T2DM [14]. Increased hepatic secretion of very-low-density lipoproteins (VLDL) and their impaired clearance also appear to be of central importance in the pathophysiology of this diabetic dyslipaemia [62]. In T2DM, increased efflux of free fatty acids from adipose tissues and impaired insulin-mediated skeletal muscle uptake of free fatty acids also increase fatty acid flux to the liver [11, 59]. Epidemiologic studies have

demonstrated a relationship between insulin resistance and plasma free fatty acid levels [93]. In line with this, agents that lower elevated free fatty acids, such as thiazolidinediones, have been shown to improve insulin sensitivity in muscle, liver and adipose tissues [76, 78].

In the present study, genes up-regulated in the livers of NRs given PFJ include those encoding for apolipoproteins. The up-regulation of apolipoprotein genes, including *Apoa1*, *Apoa2*, *Apoc1* and *Apoc3*, suggests an increase in HDL synthesis relative to controls, as all apolipoproteins A1, A2, C1 and C3 are components of HDL. The first step in HDL synthesis involves the secretion of apolipoprotein A1 mainly by the liver and the intestine [132, 133]. Apolipoproteins A1 and A2 are the

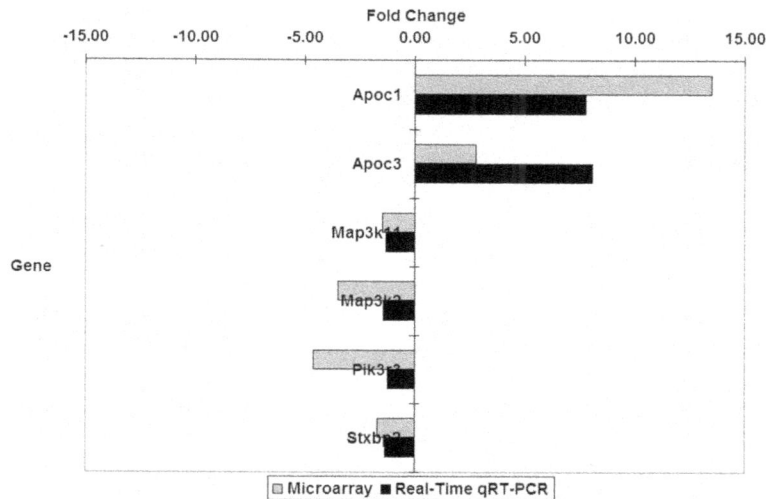

Fig. 3 Gene expression fold changes quantified by microarray and real-time qRT-PCR

main scaffold proteins that determine HDL particle structure [13]. Apolipoprotein A1 levels are reported to be inversely associated with diabetic retinopathy [51]. Apolipoproteins C are constituents of chylomicrons, VLDL and HDL [55]. However, in the fasting state, apolipoproteins C are mainly associated with HDL, whereas in the fed state, they preferentially redistribute to the surface of chylomicrons and VLDL [73]. Apolipoprotein C1 overexpression in transgenic mice has been associated with protection from obesity and insulin resistance [56]. On the contrary, apolipoprotein C3 deficiency has been reported to result in diet-induced obesity and aggravated insulin resistance in mice [31].

Virtually, every lipid and lipoprotein is affected by insulin resistance and T2DM, but the control of hyperglycaemia is unlikely to correct existing dyslipaemia. Although plasma glucose control is important in reducing microvascular complications due to T2DM, lipid management is also essential in these patients to decrease the incidence of cardiovascular events. In the present study, the up-regulation of apolipoproteins important in HDL synthesis appeared beneficial, as evidenced by the significantly lower amounts of plasma TG ($p < 0.05$) and adipose tissues ($p < 0.05$) in NRs given PFJ compared to the control group. Although we did not measure the levels of HDL in the present study, we have previously shown that PFJ increased plasma HDL levels of golden Syrian hamsters fed an atherogenic diet [6]. In line with this, green tea extract rich in phenolic compounds was also previously found to significantly reduce fasting TG and increase HDL in within-group analysis of people with T2DM, in addition to causing a decreasing trend of fasting TG in between-group analysis [69]. The increase in apolipoprotein A1 in these T2DM patients is also comparable with that in HDL after green tea extract supplementation [69].

Phase I and phase II detoxification genes were up-regulated in the livers of NRs given PFJ

Phase I and phase II detoxification enzyme systems are involved in the degradation of xenobiotics. To some extent, phenolic compounds in general may be regarded as xenobiotics by animal cells and are treated as such through interactions with these enzymes [81]. Phase I detoxification in the liver involves the activation of a series of enzymes called the cytochrome P450 mixed-function oxidases. These biotransformation enzymes function by oxidising, reducing or hydrolysing xenobiotics thus creating biotransformed intermediates [90]. Several cytochrome P450 genes involved in phase I detoxification, such as *Cyp1a2*, *Cyp2c67*, *Cyp2e1* and *Cyp4f14*, were up-regulated in NRs given PFJ. This is consistent with our previous observations, whereby cytochrome P450 genes were also up-regulated in mice given PFJ [65]. Conversely, hepatic *Cyp1a2* was found down-regulated in diabetic and insulin resistant New Zealand obese mice [89], while a decrease in hepatic *Cyp2e1* activity was reported in ob/ob mice and fa/fa Zucker rats [34]. *Cyp4f14* plays a role in the inactivation of eicosanoids [60], which could be beneficial in reducing inflammation.

Phase II detoxification enzymes perform conjugation reactions such as acylation, acetylation, glucuronidation, methylation, sulfation and glutathione conjugation, which help to convert biotransformed intermediates into less toxic, water-soluble substances that are easily excreted or eliminated from the body [90]. Incidentally, three antioxidant genes involved in phase II detoxification, i.e. *Ugt2b36*, *Cat* and *Gsto2*, were up-regulated in the livers of NRs given PFJ. *Ugt2b36* (uridine diphosphate glucuronosyltransferase 2 family, polypeptide B36) is a glycosyltransferase enzyme that catalyses the transfer of the glucuronic acid component of uridine diphosphate glucuronic acid to xenobiotics. *Ugt2b36* messenger ribonucleic acid (mRNA) levels were found to decrease in aging mice [39]. *Cat* (catalase) is a very important enzyme which protects cells from oxidative damage, as it catalyses the decomposition of hydrogen peroxide to water and oxygen. Blood catalase activity in T2DM subjects was found decreased when compared to that in non-diabetic controls, and this consequently increased hydrogen peroxide in muscle cells [43]. *Gsto2* (glutathione S-transferase omega-2) is an enzyme involved in glutathione conjugation. Patients with uncontrolled T2DM have severely deficient synthesis of glutathione attributed to limited precursor availability [104]. In addition, insulin administration is known to increase glutathione S-transferase gene expression through the PI3K/AKT/mTOR pathway and decrease intracellular oxidative stress [36].

Real-time qRT-PCR validated the microarray data obtained

In the present study, the directions of fold changes of the target genes obtained from the real-time qRT-PCR technique as quantified by the qBase software [48] were comparable to those obtained from the microarray technique (Fig. 3). However, the magnitudes of fold changes obtained using real-time qRT-PCR were consistently lower than those obtained using microarrays. This has been described as the fold change compression phenomenon, which is caused by various technical microarray limitations, including limited dynamic range, signal saturations and cross hybridisations [127].

Anti-diabetic effects of polyphenols and glucose homeostasis: does PFJ affect glucose absorption, insulin secretion or insulin sensitivity?

In addition to improving insulin production and function, another approach to overcome T2DM is to reduce glucose absorption by inhibiting the activities of digestive enzymes for glucose release/production or those of enterocyte membrane transporters responsible for glucose transport. Phenolic compounds have been reported to influence the apparent glycaemic indices of foods and limit postprandial glucose increases through these mechanisms [129]. For instance, phenolic compounds from certain fruits have been shown to inhibit activities of α-amylase and α-glucosidase [77], and some even have the potential to replace or reduce the dose of acarbose required during clinical trials to improve postprandial glycaemic control in T2DM [10]. Enterocyte membrane transporters responsible for glucose absorption in the small intestine include sodium-dependent glucose transporter 1 (SGLT1) and glucose transporter 2 (GLUT2). SGLT1 is responsible for glucose entrance from the apical side of the intestinal lumen into

enterocytes via active transport, while GLUT2 assists glucose exit from the basolateral side of the intestinal lumen into the hepatic portal vein via facilitated diffusion [102]. Phenolic compounds have also been shown to inhibit these two types of transporters in human intestinal Caco-2 cell lines [54, 74].

We previously suggested that PFJ may slow the rate of glucose absorption, enhance insulin secretion and/or increase insulin sensitivity [16]. The results obtained in the present study indicate that the anti-diabetic effects of PFJ are likely due to mechanisms other than an increase in insulin secretion. This is because plasma insulin was not increased after PFJ supplementation in NRs, and another previous study also revealed that the early problem in NRs was insulin resistance with hyperinsulinaemia, not insulin insufficiency [15]. Nonetheless, it would be useful to conduct an insulin tolerance test on these NRs to further differentiate these two possible mechanisms.

Insulin signalling in relation to longevity and chronic diseases: could the positive health effects of PFJ be attributed to modulation of insulin signalling?

The insulin-signalling pathway is an evolutionarily conserved mechanism of longevity from yeast to humans [7]. Therefore, modulation of this pathway has been suggested as an avenue in extending longevity and battling chronic diseases. Ample genetic evidence demonstrates that mild inhibition of insulin-signalling components (including the insulin receptor, IRS proteins and PI3Ks) or overactivation of forkhead box protein O (FoxO) transcription factors contributes to lifespan extension with improved metabolic profiles [49, 113]. Interestingly, Ayyadevara et al. [3] reported that genetic disruption of insulin-like signalling extended lifespan in the nematode *Caenorhabditis elegans* and to a lesser degree in other taxa including fruit flies and mice. They found remarkable longevity and stress resistance of nematode PI3K-null mutants that lacked the PI3K catalytic subunit [3]. Interestingly, the PI3K pathway has paradoxically two opposite functions, i.e. impairment of its signalling activates FoxO factors and extends lifespan, whereas its overactivity triggers nuclear factor-kappa beta (NF-κβ) signalling and accelerates the aging process. FoxO activation also causes concomitant enhancement of cellular stress resistance and protection, suppression of low-grade inflammation and enhanced mitochondrial biogenesis [121]. NF-κβ signalling has been recognised as one of the targets of PI3K pathway. The NF-κβ system is a pleiotropic factor regulating developmental processes, host defence systems and cellular survival functions [97]. Since the suppression of PI3K signalling can extend lifespan, this implies that excessive and sustained activation of PI3K signalling triggers the aging process.

In addition, there is increasing evidence for an association between obesity, T2DM and cancer. Epidemiologic data suggest that insulin resistance with hyperinsulinaemia, as well as increased insulin and insulin-like growth factor-1 (IGF-1) signalling account for the relationship between these conditions. Besides influencing T2DM, the PI3K pathway itself is also implicated in cancer. PI3K signalling is activated in human cancers via several different mechanisms, including direct mutational activation or amplification of genes encoding key components of the PI3K pathway. Activation of the PI3K pathway results in the activation of protein kinase B or AKT. AKT inhibits apoptosis and stimulates protein synthesis and cell proliferation. The fact that insulin receptor signalling can stimulate protein synthesis and inhibit apoptosis and the fact that IGF-1 receptor signalling enhances cell proliferation explain how hyperinsulinaemia and increased IGF-1 may result in tumour growth. These pathways thus represent an intricate balance, and disruption of this equilibrium may lead to obesity, T2DM and cancer. Uncontrolled signalling through the PI3K pathway also contributes to metastatic cancers [72]. Thus, understanding the intricacies of the PI3K pathway may provide new avenues in terms of extending longevity and overcoming chronic diseases [20].

It is thus exciting to find that PFJ down-regulated insulin signalling in the present study, as this pathway is a potential target for modulation of longevity and chronic diseases. It is also important to note that the *Pik3r3* gene, down-regulated in the livers of NRs given PFJ in the present study, is considered an oncogene important for cell proliferation and tumour growth, as it is overexpressed in certain cancers [126]. It is also interesting, but not surprising, that the gene expression patterns with regards to insulin signalling observed in the present study were not found in previous hepatic transcriptomic analyses of BALB/c mice tested on a low-fat diet [65] (with the exception of up-regulated cytochrome P450 genes), given a high-fat atherogenic diet [67] or injected with myeloma cells [66], as mice are not predisposed to T2DM since they are HDL animals in general and do not easily develop the metabolic syndrome. Nevertheless, we have previously shown that PFJ displayed many beneficial effects on degenerative diseases in various animal models [65–68, 99, 100, 103]. Therefore, from the results obtained in the present study, it would be noteworthy in future studies to investigate whether PFJ confers its positive effects on these diseases by modulating components of the insulin-signalling pathway, especially PI3Ks.

Limitations of study

We acknowledge that a limitation in the present study was that mouse (*Mus musculus*) microarrays and real-time qRT-PCR assays were used to assess the gene

expression changes of the NR (*Arvicanthis niloticus*). However, the application of the NR as a laboratory diurnal rodent for biomedical research applicable to humans is relatively new [94]. Therefore, detailed knowledge of its physiology is still lacking, and its genome has not been sequenced. Accordingly, no commercial whole genome microarrays are currently available for this species. Nevertheless, cross hybridisation studies using microarrays have been conducted previously, such as studies involving hybridising monkey samples to human microarrays [25, 29, 42, 52, 63, 75]. NRs belong to the Muridae family, as do mice and rats [124]. As with the standard laboratory rat, the NR is relatively insensitive to variations in photoperiod and does not hibernate. Compared to the standard laboratory rat however, the NR reaches asymptotic body mass early in life and does not show marked sexual dimorphism [94]. We have previously tried hybridising NR samples to rat (*Rattus norvegicus*) microarrays, but quality control of the hybridisation indicated that the hybridisation was not satisfactory (Vassilis Zannis, Boston University School of Medicine, MA, personal communication). On the other hand, the hybridisation of NR samples to mouse (*Mus musculus*) microarrays carried out in the present study was of high quality, enabling interpretation of the data obtained. Nevertheless, future studies to delve further into the transcriptomic effects of PFJ on NRs would benefit from the various next-generation sequencing technologies and platforms currently available. It would also be interesting to compare the effects of PFJ in different animal models, especially to identify whether species-specific genes are involved.

Another limitation in the present study was that microarray gene expression profiling was not carried out on pancreatic islet β cells, the site for insulin production. Obtaining high-quality and intact RNA from the pancreatic β cells is difficult, however, as the primary function of the pancreas is as an exocrine aid in digestion. The pancreas thus expresses large quantities of proteases, DNases and RNases that initiate an autolytic process almost immediately upon harvest [83]. In addition, some techniques also involve tedious pancreatic cannulation procedures and cause tissue artefacts. However, newer and simpler techniques are emerging, such as the perfusion method using RNase inhibitors [45] and modifications of standard phenol/guanidine thiocyanate lysis reagent protocols [4]. These emerging protocols could be used in future experiments to study the gene expression changes caused by PFJ in the pancreas.

Conclusions

Transcriptomic gene expression analysis using microarrays from the livers of young male NRs supplemented with PFJ to prevent T2DM induction showed that genes related to HDL apolipoproteins and hepatic detoxification were up-regulated, while genes related to insulin signalling and fibrosis were down-regulated. Based on the results obtained, it is more likely that the anti-diabetic effects of PFJ may be due to mechanisms other than an increase in insulin secretion, as the levels of insulin were not increased after PFJ supplementation in NRs, and young NRs have high concentrations of insulin during diabetes induction that suggest insulin resistance is the primary defect [15]. Further studies to investigate whether PFJ confers its positive effects on degenerative diseases by modulating components of the insulin-signalling pathway are also warranted.

Abbreviations

ANOVA: Analysis of variance; cDNA: Complementary deoxyribonucleic acid; cRNA: Complementary ribonucleic acid; Ct: Threshold cycle; En: Energy; FBG: Fasting blood glucose; FoxO: Forkhead box protein O; GAE: Gallic acid equivalent; GLUT2: Glucose transporter 2; GLUT4: Glucose transporter 4; HDL: High-density lipoproteins; IGF-1: Insulin-like growth factor 1; IRS: Insulin receptor substrate; LDL: Low-density lipoproteins; MAPK: Mitogen-activated protein kinase; mRNA: Messenger ribonucleic acid; mTOR: Mammalian target of rapamycin; NF-κβ: Nuclear factor-kappa beta; NR: Nile rat; NTC: Non-template control; PFJ: Palm fruit juice; PI3K: Phosphatidylinositol 3-kinase; qRT-PCR: Quantitative reverse transcription-polymerase chain reaction; RBG: Random blood glucose; SD: Standard deviation; SGLT1: Sodium-dependent glucose transporter 1; T2DM: Type 2 diabetes mellitus; TC: Total cholesterol; TG: Triacylglycerol; VLDL: Very-low-density lipoproteins

Acknowledgements

The authors thank the Director-General of the Malaysian Palm Oil Board for the permission to publish this manuscript. They also thank the support staff of the Phenolics Group in the Malaysian Palm Oil Board for the preparation of PFJ. Fadi Chaabo from Brandeis University is also acknowledged for his assistance with the animal feeding experiments. The authors are also grateful to Karen Lai and Yulia Dushkina from Brandeis University for their technical assistance in the care and handling of the NR breeding colony.

Funding

This research was funded by the Malaysian Palm Oil Board and the Brandeis University Foster Biomedical Research Laboratory funds for research and teaching.

Authors' contributions

SSL carried out the gene expression experiments and analyses, interpreted the gene expression data and drafted the manuscript. JB carried out the animal feeding experiments, performed the animal sample collection and interpreted the animal data. AP performed statistical analyses on the physiological and biochemical parameters of the animal study. KCH designed the animal feeding and helped in the interpretation of the animal data. RS was involved in the preparation of PFJ and helped in the interpretation of the gene expression data. All authors participated in helpful discussions and read as well as approved the final manuscript.

Competing interests

The authors declare that they have no competing interests.

Author details

[1]Malaysian Palm Oil Board, No. 6, Persiaran Institusi, Bandar Baru Bangi, 43000 Kajang, Selangor, Malaysia. [2]Brandeis University, 415 South Street, Waltham, MA 02454, USA.

References

1. Anhe FF, Desjardins Y, Pilon G, Dudonne S, Genovese MI, Lajolo FM, Marette A. Polyphenols and type 2 diabetes: a prospective review. Pharma Nutr. 2013;1:105–14.
2. Aprikian O, Duclos V, Guyot S, Besson C, Manach C, Bernalier A, Morand C, Remesy C, Demigne C. Apple pectin and a polyphenol-rich apple concentrate are more effective together than separately on cecal fermentations and plasma lipids in rats. J Nutr. 2003;133(6):1860–5.
3. Ayyadevara S, Alla R, Thaden JJ, Shmookler Reis RJ. Remarkable longevity and stress resistance of nematode PI3K-null mutants. Aging Cell. 2008;7(1):13–22.
4. Azevedo-Pouly AC, Elgamal OA, Schmittgen TD. RNA isolation from mouse pancreas: a ribonuclease-rich tissue. J Vis Exp. 2014;90:e51779.
5. Bahadoran Z, Mirmiran P, Azizi F. Dietary polyphenols as potential nutraceuticals in management of diabetes: a review. J Diabetes Metab Disord. 2013;12(1):43.
6. Balasundram N, Sundram K, Samman S. Phenolic-rich palm fruit juice raises plasma HDL-C concentrations and improves antioxidant status in Golden Syrian hamsters fed an atherogenic diet. Asia Pac J Clin Nutr. 2005; 14(Suppl):S75.
7. Barbieri M, Bonafe M, Franceschi C, Paolisso G. Insulin/IGF-I-signaling pathway: an evolutionarily conserved mechanism of longevity from yeast to humans. Am J Physiol Endocrinol Metab. 2003;285(5):E1064–1071.
8. Bauer F, Beulens JW, Van der AD, Wijmenga C, Grobbee DE, Spijkerman AM, Van der Schouw YT, Onland-Moret NC. Dietary patterns and the risk of type 2 diabetes in overweight and obese individuals. Eur J Nutr. 2013;52(3):1127–34.
9. Bhupathiraju SN, Tobias DK, Malik VS, Pan A, Hruby A, Manson JE, Willett WC, Hu FB. Glycemic index, glycemic load, and risk of type 2 diabetes: results from 3 large US cohorts and an updated meta-analysis. Am J Clin Nutr. 2014;100(1):218–32.
10. Boath AS, Stewart D, McDougall GJ. Berry components inhibit alpha-glucosidase in vitro: synergies between acarbose and polyphenols from black currant and rowanberry. Food Chem. 2012;135(3):929–36.
11. Boden G. Role of fatty acids in the pathogenesis of insulin resistance and NIDDM. Diabetes. 1997;46(1):3–10.
12. Bogan JS. Regulation of glucose transporter translocation in health and diabetes. Annu Rev Biochem. 2012;81:507–32.
13. Bolanos-Garcia VM, Miguel RN. On the structure and function of apolipoproteins: more than a family of lipid-binding proteins. Prog Biophys Mol Biol. 2003;83(1):47–68.
14. Bolsinger J, Pronczuk A, Hayes KC. Dietary carbohydrate dictates development of type 2 diabetes in the Nile rat. J Nutr Biochem. 2013;24(11):1945–52.
15. Bolsinger J, Pronczuk A, Landstrom M, Auerbach A, Hayes KC. Low glycemic load diets protect against metabolic syndrome and type 2 diabetes mellitus in the Nile rat. J Nutr Biochem. 2016, In press.
16. Bolsinger J, Pronczuk A, Sambanthamurthi R, Hayes KC. Anti-diabetic effects of palm fruit juice in the Nile rat (Arvicanthis niloticus). J Nutr Sci. 2014;3:e5.
17. Bray GA, Lovejoy JC, Smith SR, DeLany JP, Lefevre M, Hwang D, Ryan DH, York DA. The influence of different fats and fatty acids on obesity, insulin resistance and inflammation. J Nutr. 2002;132(9):2488–91.
18. Bryant NJ, Govers R, James DE. Regulated transport of the glucose transporter GLUT4. Nat Rev Mol Cell Biol. 2002;3(4):267–77.
19. Bustin SA, Nolan T. Pitfalls of quantitative real-time reverse-transcription polymerase chain reaction. J Biomol Tech. 2004;15(3):155–66.
20. Cantley LC. The phosphoinositide 3-kinase pathway. Science. 2002; 296(5573):1655–7.
21. Chaabo F, Pronczuk A, Maslova E, Hayes K. Nutritional correlates and dynamics of diabetes in the Nile rat (Arvicanthis niloticus): a novel model for diet-induced type 2 diabetes and the metabolic syndrome. Nutr Metab. 2010;7:29.
22. Che Idris CA, Karupaiah T, Sundram K, Tan YA, Balasundram N, Leow SS, Nasruddin NS, Sambanthamurthi R. Oil palm phenolics and vitamin E reduce atherosclerosis in rabbits. J Funct Foods. 2014;7:541–50.
23. Chen D, Mauvais-Jarvis F, Bluher M, Fisher SJ, Jozsi A, Goodyear LJ, Ueki K, Kahn CR. p50alpha/p55alpha phosphoinositide 3-kinase knockout mice exhibit enhanced insulin sensitivity. Mol Cell Biol. 2004;24(1):320–9.
24. Chiang DJ, Pritchard MT, Nagy LE. Obesity, diabetes mellitus, and liver fibrosis. Am J Physiol Gastrointest Liver Physiol. 2011;300(5):G697–702.
25. Chismar JD, Mondala T, Fox HS, Roberts E, Langford D, Masliah E, Salomon DR, Head SR. Analysis of result variability from high-density oligonucleotide arrays comparing same-species and cross-species hybridizations. Biotechniques. 2002;33(3):516–8. 520, 522 passim.
26. Cuervo A, Valdes L, Salazar N, De los Reyes-Gavilan CG, Ruas-Madiedo P, Gueimonde M, Gonzalez S. Pilot study of diet and microbiota: interactive

associations of fibers and polyphenols with human intestinal bacteria. J Agric Food Chem. 2014;62(23):5330–6.

27. Czech MP, Corvera S. Signaling mechanisms that regulate glucose transport. J Biol Chem. 1999;274(4):1865–8.

28. De Bock M, Derraik JG, Brennan CM, Biggs JB, Morgan PE, Hodgkinson SC, Hofman PL, Cutfield WS. Olive (Olea europaea L.) leaf polyphenols improve insulin sensitivity in middle-aged overweight men: a randomized, placebo-controlled, crossover trial. PLoS One. 2013;8(3):e57622.

29. Dillman 3rd JF, Phillips CS. Comparison of non-human primate and human whole blood tissue gene expression profiles. Toxicol Sci. 2005;87(1):306–14.

30. Duda-Chodak A, Tarko T, Satora P, Sroka P. Interaction of dietary compounds, especially polyphenols, with the intestinal microbiota: a review. Eur J Nutr. 2015;54(3):325–41.

31. Duivenvoorden I, Teusink B, Rensen PC, Romijn JA, Havekes LM, Voshol PJ. Apolipoprotein C3 deficiency results in diet-induced obesity and aggravated insulin resistance in mice. Diabetes. 2005;54(3):664–71.

32. Eckel RH, Alberti KG, Grundy SM, Zimmet PZ. The metabolic syndrome. Lancet. 2010;375(9710):181–3.

33. Edgar R, Domrachev M, Lash AE. Gene Expression Omnibus: NCBI gene expression and hybridization array data repository. Nucleic Acids Res. 2002;30(1):207–10.

34. Enriquez A, Leclercq I, Farrell GC, Robertson G. Altered expression of hepatic CYP2E1 and CYP4A in obese, diabetic ob/ob mice, and fa/fa Zucker rats. Biochem Biophys Res Commun. 1999;255(2):300–6.

35. Eshak ES, Iso H, Mizoue T, Inoue M, Noda M, Tsugane S. Soft drink, 100 % fruit juice, and vegetable juice intakes and risk of diabetes mellitus. Clin Nutr. 2013;32(2):300–8.

36. Franco R, Schoneveld OJ, Pappa A, Panayiotidis MI. The central role of glutathione in the pathophysiology of human diseases. Arch Physiol Biochem. 2007;113(4-5):234–58.

37. Frejnagel S, Juskiewicz J. Dose-dependent effects of polyphenolic extracts from green tea, blue-berried honeysuckle, and chokeberry on rat caecal fermentation processes. Planta Med. 2011;77(9):888–93.

38. Fruman DA, Mauvais-Jarvis F, Pollard DA, Yballe CM, Brazil D, Bronson RT, Kahn CR, Cantley LC. Hypoglycaemia, liver necrosis and perinatal death in mice lacking all isoforms of phosphoinositide 3-kinase p85 alpha. Nat Genet. 2000;26(3):379–82.

39. Fu ZD, Csanaky IL, Klaassen CD. Effects of aging on mRNA profiles for drug-metabolizing enzymes and transporters in livers of male and female mice. Drug Metab Dispos. 2012;40(6):1216–25.

40. Geering B, Cutillas PR, Vanhaesebroeck B. Regulation of class IA PI3Ks: is there a role for monomeric PI3K subunits? Biochem Soc Trans. 2007;35(Pt 2):199–203.

41. Gehart H, Kumpf S, Ittner A, Ricci R. MAPK signalling in cellular metabolism: stress or wellness? EMBO Rep. 2010;11(11):834–40.

42. George MD, Sankaran S, Reay E, Gelli AC, Dandekar S. High-throughput gene expression profiling indicates dysregulation of intestinal cell cycle mediators and growth factors during primary simian immunodeficiency virus infection. Virology. 2003;312(1):84–94.

43. Goth L. Catalase deficiency and type 2 diabetes. Diabetes Care. 2008; 31(12):e93.

44. Graham TE, Kahn BB. Tissue-specific alterations of glucose transport and molecular mechanisms of intertissue communication in obesity and type 2 diabetes. Horm Metab Res. 2007;39(10):717–21.

45. Griffin M, Abu-El-Haija M, Abu-El-Haija M, Rokhlina T, Uc A. Simplified and versatile method for isolation of high-quality RNA from pancreas. Biotechniques. 2012;52(5):332–4.

46. Groop L, Pociot F. Genetics of diabetes—are we missing the genes or the disease? Mol Cell Endocrinol. 2014;382(1):726–39.

47. Hanhineva K, Torronen R, Bondia-Pons I, Pekkinen J, Kolehmainen M, Mykkanen H, Poutanen K. Impact of dietary polyphenols on carbohydrate metabolism. Int J Mol Sci. 2010;11(4):1365–402.

48. Hellemans J, Mortier G, De Paepe A, Speleman F, Vandesompele J. qBase relative quantification framework and software for management and automated analysis of real-time quantitative PCR data. Genome Biol. 2007; 8(2):R19.

49. Holzenberger M, Kappeler L, De Magalhaes FC. IGF-1 signaling and aging. Exp Gerontol. 2004;39(11-12):1761–4.

50. Huang PL. A comprehensive definition for metabolic syndrome. Dis Model Mech. 2009;2(5-6):231–7.

51. Irshad M, Dubey R. Apolipoproteins and their role in different clinical conditions: an overview. Indian J Biochem Biophys. 2005;42(2):73–80.

52. Jacquelin B, Mayau V, Brysbaert G, Regnault B, Diop OM, Arenzana-Seisdedos F, Rogge L, Coppee JY, Barre-Sinoussi F, Benecke A, Muller-Trutwin MC. Long oligonucleotide microarrays for African green monkey gene expression profile analysis. FASEB J. 2007;21(12):3262–71.

53. Johnson IT. Anticarcinogenic effects of diet-related apoptosis in the colorectal mucosa. Food Chem Toxicol. 2002;40(8):1171–8.

54. Johnston K, Sharp P, Clifford M, Morgan L. Dietary polyphenols decrease glucose uptake by human intestinal Caco-2 cells. FEBS Lett. 2005;579(7):1653–7.

55. Jong MC, Hofker MH, Havekes LM. Role of ApoCs in lipoprotein metabolism: functional differences between ApoC1, ApoC2, and ApoC3. Arterioscler Thromb Vasc Biol. 1999;19(3):472–84.

56. Jong MC, Voshol PJ, Muurling M, Dahlmans VE, Romijn JA, Pijl H, Havekes LM. Protection from obesity and insulin resistance in mice overexpressing human apolipoprotein C1. Diabetes. 2001;50(12):2779–85.

57. Kaur J. A comprehensive review on metabolic syndrome. Cardiol Res Pract. 2014; 2014:943162.

58. Kelder T, van Iersel MP, Hanspers K, Kutmon M, Conklin BR, Evelo CT, Pico AR. WikiPathways: building research communities on biological pathways. Nucleic Acids Res. 2012;40(Database issue):D1301–1307.

59. Kelley DE, Simoneau JA. Impaired free fatty acid utilization by skeletal muscle in non-insulin-dependent diabetes mellitus. J Clin Invest. 1994;94(6):2349–56.

60. Kikuta Y, Kasyu H, Kusunose E, Kusunose M. Expression and catalytic activity of mouse leukotriene B4 omega-hydroxylase, CYP4F14. Arch Biochem Biophys. 2000;383(2):225–32.

61. Kim M, Kim J. The effects of green tea on obesity and type 2 diabetes. Diabetes Metab J. 2013;37(3):173–5.

62. Krauss RM. Lipids and lipoproteins in patients with type 2 diabetes. Diabetes Care. 2004;27(6):1496–504.

63. Lachance PE, Chaudhuri A. Microarray analysis of developmental plasticity in monkey primary visual cortex. J Neurochem. 2004;88(6):1455–69.

64. Lee C, Longo V (2016) Dietary restriction with and without caloric restriction for healthy aging. F1000Res 5.

65. Leow SS, Sekaran SD, Sundram K, Tan YA, Sambanthamurthi R. Differential transcriptomic profiles effected by oil palm phenolics indicate novel health outcomes. BMC Genomics. 2011;12:432.

66. Leow SS, Sekaran SD, Sundram K, Tan YA, Sambanthamurthi R. Gene expression changes in spleens and livers of tumour-bearing mice suggest delayed inflammation and attenuated cachexia in response to oil palm phenolics. J Nutrigenet Nutrigenomics. 2013a;6(6):305-326.

67. Leow SS, Sekaran SD, Sundram K, Tan YA, Sambanthamurthi R. Oil palm phenolics attenuate changes caused by an atherogenic diet in mice. Eur J Nutr. 2013b;52(2):443-456.

68. Leow SS, Sekaran SD, Tan YA, Sundram K, Sambanthamurthi R. Oil palm phenolics confer neuroprotective effects involving cognitive and motor functions in mice. Nutr Neurosci. 2013c;16(5):207-217.

69. Liu CY, Huang CJ, Huang LH, Chen IJ, Chiu JP, Hsu CH. Effects of green tea extract on insulin resistance and glucagon-like peptide 1 in patients with type 2 diabetes and lipid abnormalities: a randomized, double-blinded, and placebo-controlled trial. PLoS One. 2014;9(3), e91163.

70. Lyons J, Brown F, Remillard DE, Bolsinger J, Hayes KC. Pathology of the Nile rat developing type 2 diabetes [abstract]. Faseb J. 2013;27(Meeting Abstract Supplement):874.813.

71. Lyssenko V, Jonsson A, Almgren P, Pulizzi N, Isomaa B, Tuomi T, Berglund G, Altshuler D, Nilsson P, Groop L. Clinical risk factors, DNA variants, and the development of type 2 diabetes. N Engl J Med. 2008;359(21):2220–32.

72. Maehama T, Dixon JE. PTEN: a tumour suppressor that functions as a phospholipid phosphatase. Trends Cell Biol. 1999;9(4):125–8.

73. Mahley RW, Innerarity TL, Rall Jr SC, Weisgraber KH. Plasma lipoproteins: apolipoprotein structure and function. J Lipid Res. 1984;25(12):1277–94.

74. Manzano S, Williamson G. Polyphenols and phenolic acids from strawberry and apple decrease glucose uptake and transport by human intestinal Caco-2 cells. Mol Nutr Food Res. 2010;54(12):1773–80.

75. Marvanova M, Menager J, Bezard E, Bontrop RE, Pradier L, Wong G. Microarray analysis of nonhuman primates: validation of experimental models in neurological disorders. FASEB J. 2003;17(8):929–31.

76. Mayerson AB, Hundal RS, Dufour S, Lebon V, Befroy D, Cline GW, Enocksson S, Inzucchi SE, Shulman GI, Petersen KF. The effects of rosiglitazone on insulin sensitivity, lipolysis, and hepatic and skeletal

muscle triglyceride content in patients with type 2 diabetes. Diabetes. 2002;51(3):797–802.

77. McDougall GJ, Shpiro F, Dobson P, Smith P, Blake A, Stewart D. Different polyphenolic components of soft fruits inhibit alpha-amylase and alpha-glucosidase. J Agric Food Chem. 2005;53(7):2760–6.

78. Miyazaki Y, Mahankali A, Matsuda M, Mahankali S, Hardies J, Cusi K, Mandarino LJ, DeFronzo RA. Effect of pioglitazone on abdominal fat distribution and insulin sensitivity in type 2 diabetic patients. J Clin Endocrinol Metab. 2002;87(6):2784–91.

79. Moco S, Martin FP, Rezzi S. Metabolomics view on gut microbiome modulation by polyphenol-rich foods. J Proteome Res. 2012;11(10):4781–90.

80. Morimoto A, Ohno Y, Tatsumi Y, Mizuno S, Watanabe S. Effects of healthy dietary pattern and other lifestyle factors on incidence of diabetes in a rural Japanese population. Asia Pac J Clin Nutr. 2012;21(4):601–8.

81. Moskaug JO, Carlsen H, Myhrstad MC Blomhoff R. Polyphenols and glutathione synthesis regulation. Am J Clin Nutr. 2005;81(1 Suppl):277S–83S.

82. Movahed A, Nabipour I, Lieben Louis X, Thandapilly SJ, Yu L, Kalantarhormozi M, Rekabpour SJ, Netticadan T. Antihyperglycemic effects of short term resveratrol supplementation in type 2 diabetic patients. Evid Based Complement Alternat Med. 2013;2013:851267.

83. Mullin AE, Soukatcheva G, Verchere CB, Chantler JK. Application of in situ ductal perfusion to facilitate isolation of high-quality RNA from mouse pancreas. Biotechniques. 2006;40(5):617–21.

84. Neyrinck AM, Van Hee VF, Bindels LB, De Backer F, Cani PD, Delzenne NM. Polyphenol-rich extract of pomegranate peel alleviates tissue inflammation and hypercholesterolaemia in high-fat diet-induced obese mice: potential implication of the gut microbiota. Br J Nutr. 2013;109(5):802–9.

85. Noda K, Melhorn MI, Zandi S, Frimmel S, Tayyari F, Hisatomi T, Almulki L, Pronczuk A, Hayes KC, Hafezi-Moghadam A. An animal model of spontaneous metabolic syndrome: Nile grass rat. Faseb J. 2010;24(7):2443–53.

86. Nolan T, Hands RE, Bustin SA. Quantification of mRNA using real-time RT-PCR. Nat Protoc. 2006;1(3):1559–82.

87. Olokoba AB, Obateru OA, Olokoba LB. Type 2 diabetes mellitus: a review of current trends. Oman Med J. 2012;27(4):269–73.

88. Osman HF, Eshak MG, El-Sherbiny EM, Bayoumi MM. Biochemical and genetic evaluation of pomegranate impact on diabetes mellitus induced by alloxan in female rats. Life Sci J. 2012;9(3):1543–53.

89. Pass GJ, Becker W, Kluge R, Linnartz K, Plum L, Giesen K, Joost HG. Effect of hyperinsulinemia and type 2 diabetes-like hyperglycemia on expression of hepatic cytochrome p450 and glutathione s-transferase isoforms in a New Zealand obese-derived mouse backcross population. J Pharmacol Exp Ther. 2002;302(2):442–50.

90. Percival M. Phytonutrients and detoxification. Clin Nutr Insights. 1997;5(2):1–4.

91. Pessin JE, Saltiel AR. Signaling pathways in insulin action: molecular targets of insulin resistance. J Clin Invest. 2000;106(2):165–9.

92. Pico AR, Kelder T, van Iersel MP, Hanspers K, Conklin BR, Evelo C. WikiPathways: pathway editing for the people. PLoS Biol. 2008;6(7):e184.

93. Reaven GM, Chen YD. Role of abnormal free fatty acid metabolism in the development of non-insulin-dependent diabetes mellitus. Am J Med. 1988; 85(5A):106–12.

94. Refinetti R. The Nile grass rat as a laboratory animal. Lab Anim (NY). 2004; 33(9):54–7.

95. Romo-Vaquero M, Selma MV, Larrosa M, Obiol M, García-Villalba R, Gonzalez-Barrio R, Issaly N, Flanagan J, Roller M, Tomas-Barberan FA, Garcia-Conesa MT. A rosemary extract rich in carnosic acid selectively modulates caecum microbiota and inhibits beta-glucosidase activity, altering fiber and short chain fatty acids fecal excretion in lean and obese female rats. PLoS One. 2014;9(4):e94687.

96. Sabio G, Davis RJ. cJun NH2-terminal kinase 1 (JNK1): roles in metabolic regulation of insulin resistance. Trends Biochem Sci. 2010;35(9):490–6.

97. Salminen A, Kaarniranta K. Insulin/IGF-1 paradox of aging: regulation via AKT/IKK/NF-kappaB signaling. Cell Signal. 2010;22(4):573–7.

98. Saltiel AR, Kahn CR. Insulin signalling and the regulation of glucose and lipid metabolism. Nature. 2001;414(6865):799–806.

99. Sambanthamurthi R, Tan YA, Sundram K, Abeywardena M, Sambandan TG, Rha C, Sinskey AJ, Subramaniam K, Leow SS, Hayes KC, Wahid MB. Oil palm vegetation liquor: a new source of phenolic bioactives. Br J Nutr. 2011a; 106(11):1655-1663.

100. Sambanthamurthi R, Tan YA, Sundram K, Hayes KC, Abeywardena M, Leow SS, Sekaran SD, Sambandan TG, Rha C, Sinskey AJ, Subramaniam K, Fairus S,

Wahid MB. Positive outcomes of oil palm phenolics on degenerative diseases in animal models. Br J Nutr. 2011b;106(11):1664-1675.

101. Samuel VT, Shulman GI. Mechanisms for insulin resistance: common threads and missing links. Cell. 2012;148(5):852–71.

102. Scheepers A, Joost HG, Schurmann A. The glucose transporter families SGLT and GLUT: molecular basis of normal and aberrant function. JPEN J Parenter Enteral Nutr. 2004;28(5):364–71.

103. Sekaran SD, Leow SS, Abobaker N, Tee KK, Sundram K, Sambanthamurthi R, Wahid MB. Effects of oil palm phenolics on tumor cells in vitro and in vivo. Afr J Food Sci. 2010;4(8):495–502.

104. Sekhar RV, McKay SV, Patel SG, Guthikonda AP, Reddy VT, Balasubramanyam A, Jahoor F. Glutathione synthesis is diminished in patients with uncontrolled diabetes and restored by dietary supplementation with cysteine and glycine. Diabetes Care. 2011;34(1):162–7.

105. Shen J, Goyal A, Sperling L. The emerging epidemic of obesity, diabetes, and the metabolic syndrome in china. Cardiol Res Pract. 2012;2012:178675.

106. Shepherd PR, Withers DJ, Siddle K. Phosphoinositide 3-kinase: the key switch mechanism in insulin signalling. Biochem J. 1998;333(Pt 3):471–90.

107. Slavin J. Fiber and prebiotics: mechanisms and health benefits. Nutrients. 2013;5(4):1417–35.

108. Steiglitz BM, Kreider JM, Frankenburg EP, Pappano WN, Hoffman GG, Meganck JA, Liang X, Hook M, Birk DE, Goldstein SA, Greenspan DS. Procollagen C proteinase enhancer 1 genes are important determinants of the mechanical properties and geometry of bone and the ultrastructure of connective tissues. Mol Cell Biol. 2006;26(1):238–49.

109. Stockli J, Fazakerley DJ, James DE. GLUT4 exocytosis. J Cell Sci. 2011;124(Pt 24):4147–59.

110. Szkudelski T, Szkudelska K. Anti-diabetic effects of resveratrol. Ann N Y Acad Sci. 2011;1215:34–9.

111. Taniguchi CM, Emanuelli B, Kahn CR. Critical nodes in signalling pathways: insights into insulin action. Nat Rev Mol Cell Biol. 2006a;7(2):85-96.

112. Taniguchi CM, Kondo T, Sajan M, Luo J, Bronson R, Asano T, Farese R, Cantley LC, Kahn CR. Divergent regulation of hepatic glucose and lipid metabolism by phosphoinositide 3-kinase via Akt and PKClambda/zeta. Cell Metab. 2006b;3(5):343-353.

113. Tatar M, Bartke A, Antebi A. The endocrine regulation of aging by insulin-like signals. Science. 2003;299(5611):1346–51.

114. Terauchi Y, Tsuji Y, Satoh S, Minoura H, Murakami K, Okuno A, Inukai K, Asano T, Kaburagi Y, Ueki K, Nakajima H, Hanafusa T, Matsuzawa Y, Sekihara H, Yin Y, Barrett JC, Oda H, Ishikawa T, Akanuma Y, Komuro I, Suzuki M, Yamamura K, Kodama T, Suzuki H, Yamamura K, Kodama T, Suzuki H, Koyasu S, Aizawa S, Tobe K, Fukui Y, Yazaki Y, Kadowaki T. Increased insulin sensitivity and hypoglycaemia in mice lacking the p85 alpha subunit of phosphoinositide 3-kinase. Nat Genet. 1999;21(2):230–5.

115. Tolman KG, Fonseca V, Dalpiaz A, Tan MH. Spectrum of liver disease in type 2 diabetes and management of patients with diabetes and liver disease. Diabetes Care. 2007;30(3):734–43.

116. Tozzo E, Gnudi L, Kahn BB. Amelioration of insulin resistance in streptozotocin diabetic mice by transgenic overexpression of GLUT4 driven by an adipose-specific promoter. Endocrinology. 1997;138(4):1604–11.

117. Trombetta M, Spiazzi G, Zoppini G, Muggeo M. Review article: type 2 diabetes and chronic liver disease in the Verona diabetes study. Aliment Pharmacol Ther. 2005;22 Suppl 2:24–7.

118. Ueki K, Algenstaedt P, Mauvais-Jarvis F, Kahn CR. Positive and negative regulation of phosphoinositide 3-kinase-dependent signaling pathways by three different gene products of the p85alpha regulatory subunit. Mol Cell Biol. 2000;20(21):8035–46.

119. Ueki K, Fruman DA, Yballe CM, Fasshauer M, Klein J, Asano T, Cantley LC, Kahn CR. Positive and negative roles of p85 alpha and p85 beta regulatory subunits of phosphoinositide 3-kinase in insulin signaling. J Biol Chem. 2003;278(48):48453–66.

120. van der Slot AJ, Zuurmond AM, Bardoel AF, Wijmenga C, Pruijs HE, Sillence DO, Brinckmann J, Abraham DJ, Black CM, Verzijl N, DeGroot J, Hanemaaijer R, TeKoppele JM, Huizinga TW, Bank RA. Identification of PLOD2 as telopeptide lysyl hydroxylase, an important enzyme in fibrosis. J Biol Chem. 2003;278(42):40967–72.

121. van Heemst D. Insulin, IGF-1 and longevity. Aging Dis. 2010;1(2):147–57.

122. van Iersel MP, Kelder T, Pico AR, Hanspers K, Coort S, Conklin BR, Evelo C. Presenting and exploring biological pathways with PathVisio. BMC Bioinformatics. 2008;9:399.

123. Vandesompele J, De Preter K, Pattyn F, Poppe B, Van Roy N, De Paepe A, Speleman F. Accurate normalization of real-time quantitative RT-PCR data by geometric averaging of multiple internal control genes. Genome Biol. 2002;3(7):RESEARCH0034.

124. Volobouev VT, Ducroz JF, Aniskin VM, Britton-Davidian J, Castiglia R, Dobigny G, Granjon L, Lombard M, Corti M, Sicard B, Capanna E. Chromosomal characterization of Arvicanthis species (Rodentia, Murinae) from western and central Africa: implications for taxonomy. Cytogenet Genome Res. 2002;96(1-4):250–60.

125. Wainstein J, Ganz T, Boaz M, Bar Dayan Y, Dolev E, Kerem Z, Madar Z. Olive leaf extract as a hypoglycemic agent in both human diabetic subjects and in rats. J Med Food. 2012;15(7):605–10.

126. Wang G, Yang X, Li C, Cao X, Luo X, Hu J. PIK3R3 induces epithelial-to-mesenchymal transition and promotes metastasis in colorectal cancer. Mol Cancer Ther. 2014;13(7):1837–47.

127. Wang Y, Barbacioru C, Hyland F, Xiao W, Hunkapiller KL, Blake J, Chan F, Gonzalez C, Zhang L, Samaha RR. Large scale real-time PCR validation on gene expression measurements from two commercial long-oligonucleotide microarrays. BMC Genomics. 2006;7:59.

128. Wang YW, Sun GD, Sun J, Liu SJ, Wang J, Xu XH, Miao LN. Spontaneous type 2 diabetic rodent models. J Diab Res. 2013;2013:401723.

129. Williamson G. Possible effects of dietary polyphenols on sugar absorption and digestion. Mol Nutr Food Res. 2013;57(1):48–57.

130. Wu GD, Chen J, Hoffmann C, Bittinger K, Chen YY, Keilbaugh SA, Bewtra M, Knights D, Walters WA, Knight R, Sinha R, Gilroy E, Gupta K, Baldassano R, Nessel L, Li H, Bushman FD, Lewis JD. Linking long-term dietary patterns with gut microbial enterotypes. Science. 2011;334(6052):105–8.

131. Yu J, Zhang Y, McIlroy J, Rordorf-Nikolic T, Orr GA, Backer JM. Regulation of the p85/p110 phosphatidylinositol 3'-kinase: stabilization and inhibition of the p110alpha catalytic subunit by the p85 regulatory subunit. Mol Cell Biol. 1998;18(3):1379–87.

132. Zannis VI, Cole FS, Jackson CL, Kurnit DM, Karathanasis SK. Distribution of apolipoprotein A-I, C-II, C-III, and E mRNA in fetal human tissues. Time-dependent induction of apolipoprotein E mRNA by cultures of human monocyte-macrophages. Biochemistry. 1985;24(16):4450–5.

133. Zannis VI, Fotakis P, Koukos G, Kardassis D, Ehnholm C, Jauhiainen M, Chroni A. HDL biogenesis, remodeling, and catabolism. Handb Exp Pharmacol. 2015;224:53–111.

9

Ancestors' dietary patterns and environments could drive positive selection in genes involved in micronutrient metabolism—the case of cofactor transporters

Silvia Parolo[1†], Sébastien Lacroix[1†], Jim Kaput[2] and Marie-Pier Scott-Boyer[1*]

Abstract

Background: During evolution, humans colonized different ecological niches and adopted a variety of subsistence strategies that gave rise to diverse selective pressures acting across the genome. Environmentally induced selection of vitamin, mineral, or other cofactor transporters could influence micronutrient-requiring molecular reactions and contribute to inter-individual variability in response to foods and nutritional interventions.

Methods: A comprehensive list of genes coding for transporters of cofactors or their precursors was built using data mining procedures from the HGDP dataset and then explored to detect evidence of positive genetic selection. This dataset was chosen since it comprises several genetically diverse worldwide populations whom ancestries have evolved in different environments and thus lived following various nutritional habits and lifestyles.

Results: We identified 312 cofactor transporter (CT) genes involved in between-cell or sub-cellular compartment distribution of 28 cofactors derived from dietary intake. Twenty-four SNPs distributed across 14 CT genes separated populations into continental and intra-continental groups such as African hunter-gatherers and farmers, and between Native American sub-populations. Notably, four SNPs were located in *SLC24A3* with one being a known eQTL of the NCKX3 protein.

Conclusions: These findings could support the importance of considering individual's genetic makeup along with their metabolic profile when tailoring personalized dietary interventions for optimizing health.

Keywords: Positive selection, Cofactor transport, Inter-individual variability, Ancestry, Dietary habits, Biological response

Background

Diet and food availability shaped genetic variation in humans and left distinct adaptation signals among geographically and culturally diverse populations [1–3]. Lactase persistence in adults is the prime example of food-based positive selection. Cattle domestication after the Neolithic transition provided access to dairy products and the advantages of an additional source of calories, calcium, protein, and other nutrients [4]. The ability to utilize this nutrient dense food resulted in a strong positive selective pressure on a variant of the lactase-phlorizin hydrolase gene (*LCT*) responsible for lactose metabolism in the small intestine [5, 6]. Other genetic changes can also be selected by food availability. For example, the number of copies of the salivary amylase gene may reflect adaptation to starch-rich diets and with consequences for modern health as amylase copy number variations may be negatively associated with body mass index [7–9]. Positive adaptation signals have also been described for *FADS2*, which codes for an enzyme involved in long-chain polyunsaturated fatty acid synthesis. A variant of *FADS2* was associated with higher

* Correspondence: scottboyer@cosbi.eu
†Equal contributors
[1]The Microsoft Research, University of Trento Centre for Computational Systems Biology (COSBI), piazza Manifattura 1, 38068 Rovereto, TN, Italy
Full list of author information is available at the end of the article

mRNA expression in vegan individuals [10] which have diets typically low in long chain unsaturated fatty acids. Positive selection has also been demonstrated for genes coding for transporters of zinc, an important cofactor of several enzymes and DNA-binding proteins [11, 12].

The objective of this study was to identify variants showing signs of positive selection in genes coding for cofactor transporters (hereafter referred to as CT and listed in Additional file 1: Table S1). We posit that adaptation to different ecological niches may also select for other genes involved in nutrient transport and metabolism, especially those that affect multiple cellular and biochemical processes such as cofactors or their micronutrient precursors. Cofactor transporter genes may be more susceptible to being influenced by different environments and nutritional habits because of their importance in nutrient absorption and subsequent tissue distribution.

To fulfill this objective, genetic differentiation of CT-associated variants were analyzed using data from the Human Genome Diversity Project (HGDP), a dataset chosen because it includes multiple world populations representative of a variety of environments and ancestral nutritional habits [1, 13, 14]. Using an approached based on principal component analysis (PCA) [15–17], 24 variants in 14 CT genes with signals of positive selection that could contribute to various disease risks and response to nutritional intervention observed between individuals with different genetic makeup were identified.

Results

Identification of proteins involved in cofactor transport

Public databases (i.e., NCBI PubMed, UniProt, and OMIM databases) were searched for proteins involved in the transport of cofactors (or their nutrient precursors) between cells or sub-cellular compartments. CTs are a subset of proteins that transport other nutrients such as essential fatty acids or amino acids. At least one transporter was identified for 28 of 43 nutrient-derived cofactors [18] (see the "Methods" section for further details and Additional file 1: Table S1 for full list of cofactors and corresponding transporters). Some of the fat-soluble cofactors such as pyrroloquinoline quinone (PQQ), topaquinone, qbiquinone (CoQ), menaquinone (Vitamin K), and lipoic acid diffuse freely across membranes and are transported in lipoproteins in the blood. Other cofactors, such as biopterin, tetrahydrobiopterin (BH4), molybdopterin (MPT), and S-adenosyl-L-homocysteine (SAH), are synthesized in cells and used locally and as such do not require transporters. Fe-S complex, heme-thiolate, inositol hexaphosphate, and dipyrromethane circulate as part of hemoglobin in red blood cells. The gene coding for the pyridoxal phosphate (vitamin B_6) transporter has not yet been identified [19].

A total of 312 proteins are involved in the transport of cofactors with 39 able to transport more than one cofactor. The transporters with affinity to the most cofactors are the cation transporters CNNM2 (cyclin and CBS domain divalent metal cation transport mediator 2) and NIPAL1 (non-imprinted in Prader-Willi-like domain containing 1) that mediate the trans-membrane movement of five divalent cations—cobalt, copper, iron, magnesium, and manganese.

Cofactor transporters genetic diversity

Genotype data from HGDP was used to study the genetic differentiation in genes coding for CTs. The final sample set included 940 individuals from 53 populations using the quality control criteria described in the "Methods" section. Genetic variation in CT genes was summarized by PCA. During the computation, smartpca removed 27 subjects belonging to Papuan and Melanesian populations because their PC values exceeded 6 standard deviations from population and were deemed as outliers. Nine hundred thirteen individuals were thus included in the following analyses. The percentage of explained variance of each PC is shown in Additional file 2: Figure S1. First three PCs were sufficient to separate the populations into their corresponding continental groups using the genetic variants in CT genes. In particular, PC1 separated African populations from all others, PC2 described a gradient from East Asia to Middle East and Europe, and PC3 divided Native American populations from the others (Fig. 1 and Additional file 3: Figure S2). The subsequent PCs described intra-continental genetic differences. In particular, PC5 and PC6 separated the traditional African hunter-gatherer groups (San, Mbuty Pygmy, and Biaka Pygmy) from the African populations that adopted the agricultural, sedentary lifestyle hereafter referred to as farmers (Bantu from South Africa, Bantu from Kenya, Yoruba, and Mandenka) (Additional file 4: Figure S3). The grouping of subjects observed in the PCA of transporters was similar to the results of PCA performed using genome-wide genotype data (Additional file 5: Figure S4).

Positively selected SNPs and genes

A methodology based on PCA loadings was used to identify loci under positive selection. This method does not require a priori separation of individuals by population and is thus beneficial with datasets such as the HGDP composed of individuals representing a large spectrum of genetic diversity (see the "Discussion" and "Methods" sections for further details). This method was first tested on the entire genome-wide dataset (Additional file 6: Table S2). The relevance of these findings was evaluated by further looking in the literature for the top 10 loci of each of the first ten PCs. All these loci spanned a region that included a SNP with a q value < 0.05, with the exception of the SNPs related to PC1, PC2, and 1 SNP associated to PC6 (rs11682328) that did not exceed this threshold. Sixty-one of these 100 loci corresponded to

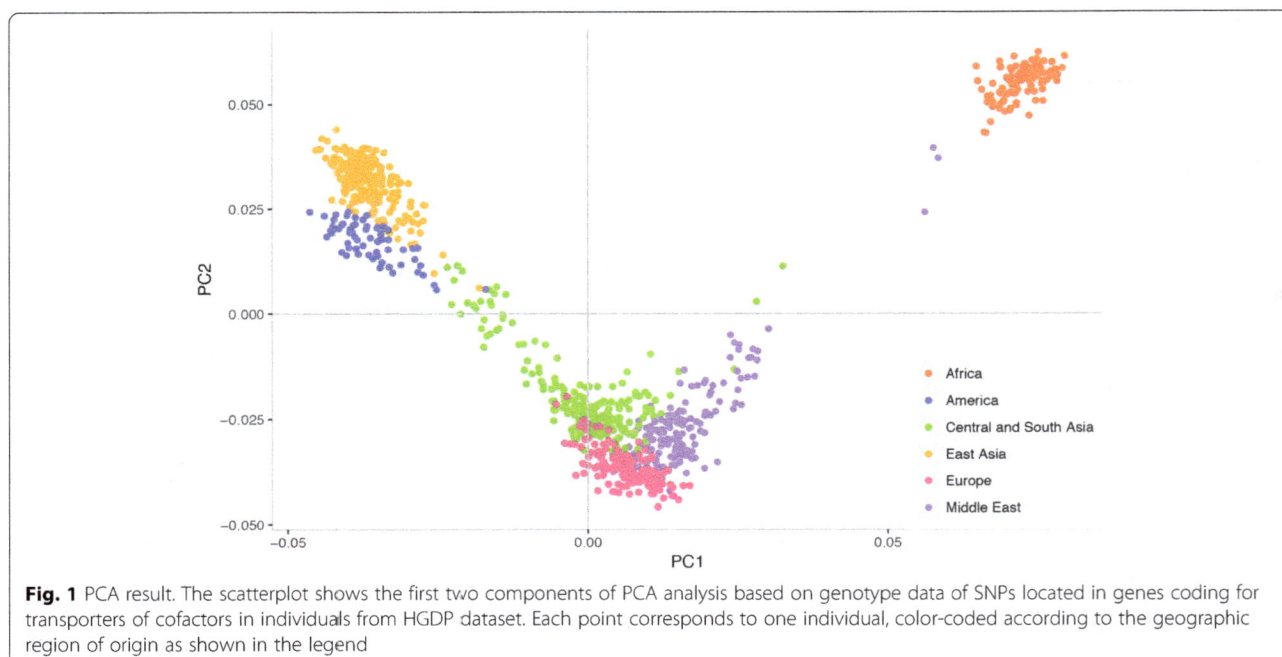

Fig. 1 PCA result. The scatterplot shows the first two components of PCA analysis based on genotype data of SNPs located in genes coding for transporters of cofactors in individuals from HGDP dataset. Each point corresponds to one individual, color-coded according to the geographic region of origin as shown in the legend

Table 1 Positively selected SNPs within cofactor transporter genes

Genes	Official gene name	Cofactors	Tissue enrichment[a]	Chr	PC	SNPs
CACNA1A	Calcium voltage-gated channel subunit alpha1 A	Ca	Tissue enhanced: cerebral cortex; stomach	19	PC3	rs7254771 (0.03)
CACNB4	Calcium voltage-gated channel auxiliary subunit beta 4	Ca	Tissue enhanced: cerebral cortex	2	PC5	rs16830593 (0.007); rs11902858 (0.02)
HPX	Hemopexin	Fe	Tissue enriched: liver	11	PC5	rs16913549 (0.01)
KCNB2	Potassium voltage-gated channel subfamily B member 2	K	Tissue enhanced: cerebral cortex; spleen	8	PC5	rs7833062 (0.04); rs6996335 (0.02)
KCNH5	Potassium voltage-gated channel subfamily H member 5	K	Tissue enhanced: adrenal gland; cerebral cortex	14	PC5	rs8019319 (0.007)
KCNH7	Potassium voltage-gated channel subfamily H member 7	K	Tissue enriched: cerebral cortex	2	PC3; PC5	rs6753132 (0.05); rs6708255 (0.007); rs7588788 (0.07)
KCNK13	Potassium two pore domain channel subfamily K member 13	K	Tissue enhanced: testis	14	PC3	rs3861656 (0.025); rs4462529 (0.025); rs17223880 (0.025)
LRP2	LDL receptor related protein 2	D3	Group enriched: kidney; placenta; thyroid gland	2	PC5	rs16856593 (0.004)
RYR2	Ryanodine receptor 2	Ca	Tissue enriched: heart muscle	1	PC5	rs12087761 (0.011)
SLC11A2	Solute carrier family 11 member 2	Co	Expressed in all	12	PC5	rs12312876 (2.70E-08)
SLC24A3	Solute carrier family 24 member 3	K,Ca	Mixed	20	PC5	rs10485588 (0.04); rs16980447 (0.03); rs6112335 (0.02); rs6035421 (0.02)
SLC25A26	Solute carrier family 25 member 26	SAM	Expressed in all	3	PC3	rs17044224 (0.03); rs1471476 (0.03);
SLCO1A2	Solute carrier organic anion transporter family member 1A2	GSH	Group enriched: cerebral cortex; liver; lung; salivary gland	12	PC5	rs2199685 (0.03)
TRPM4	Transient receptor potential cation channel subfamily M member 4	Ca	Mixed	19	PC5	rs8104571 (0.0008)

Ca calcium, *Co* cobalt, *Chr* chromosome, *D3* vitamin D$_3$, *Fe* iron, *K* potassium, *GSH* Glutathione, *PC* principal component, *SAM* S-Adenosylmethionine
[a]Tissue enrichment category from Human Protein Atlas among the following categories: (i) Tissue enriched: mRNA levels in one tissue at least five times higher than all other tissues, (ii) Group enriched: mRNA levels of a group of 2 to 7 tissues at least five times those of all other tissues, (iii) Tissue enhanced: mRNA levels in a particular tissue at least five times the average level in all tissues, (iv) Expressed in all: mRNA detected in all tissues, (v) Mixed: detected in fewer than 32 tissues but not elevated in any tissue, or (vi) Not detected. Tissue(s) where protein is enriched in cases of Tissue enriched, enhanced or group enhanced is listed

genes previously described as being positively selected in the dbPSHP database [20] (Additional file 7: Table S3) such as, *OCA2/HERC2*, *SLC24A5*, and *EDAR* [21, 22]. The workflow was then applied to the CT dataset. Twenty-four SNPs corresponding to 14 CT genes differentiated along the first five PCs (i.e., PC3 and PC5) (Table 1). The SNPs showing evidences of positive selection in the subsequent PCs are reported in Additional file 8: Table S4. Positive selection in CTs was also evaluated using the integrated Haplotype Score (iHS) selection metrics calculated in HGDP [23] and grouping SNPs at the gene level. Most of the genes previously identified using the PCA workflow, with the exception of *CACNA1A*, *HPX*, *SLC11A2* *SLCO1A2*, and *TRPM4*, showed evidence of positive selection in at least one population or group of populations using this method (detailed in the Additional file 9: Note 1).

Functional annotation and linkage disequilibrium patterns of positively selected SNPs

SNPs showing signs of positive selection were annotated using Ensembl transcript to investigate their functional consequences within or flanking each gene. None were found in exons (Additional file 10: Table S5). However, four SNPs (rs16830593 in *CACNB4*, rs1471476 and rs17044224 in *SLC25A26*, and rs10485588 in *SLC24A3*) were identified as significant cis-eQTLs from the GTeX eQTL database [24] (Table 2). Moreover, an additional SNP in *SLC24A3* (rs16980447) showed a nominal *p* value < 0.05 but was not significant after FDR correction. *SLC24A3* SNPs were found to be associated with its expression level in blood cells while the *CACNB4* variant was associated with its gene expression level in skin exposed to sun. *SLC25A26* SNPs were cis-eQTL in the heart and adipose tissue. Two SNPs, rs3861656 in *KCNK13* andrs16830593 in *CACNB4*, are likely to affect transcription factor binding (RegulomeDB variant classification of 2b and 2c, respectively) (Additional file 11: Table S6).

Proxy SNPs using the Yoruba population from the 1000 Genomes database were used to investigate whether non-mapped functional SNPs were in linkage disequilibrium (LD) with SNPs differentiated in African populations (related to PC5). No non-synonymous SNPs were found among those in LD with the differentiated SNPs (*R*-square > 0.8). However, two missense SNPs were identified as proxy SNPs (rs6757850 correlated with *KCNH7* SNP rs6708255 and rs7588788 and rs114005357 correlated with *SLC11A2* SNP rs12312876) when lowering the *R*-square threshold to 0.4. Similar analysis was not possible for Native American populations since no sequencing data from a different dataset was available to evaluate LD. For what concern PC5, we observed that the clustering of African populations in two groups corresponded to one of the two subsistence strategies traditionally adopted by these populations, namely being primarily farmers or hunter-gatherers. The best candidate gene related to PC5 is *SLC24A3* since it contains four SNPs showing evidences of positive selection, one of which also being a strong eQTL in GTeX database. The African genetic variation in the *SLC24A3* region was further examined by estimating haplotypes to better evaluate the difference in allele frequencies of *SLC24A3* region between the previously identified groups of farmers and hunter-gatherers. The most common haplotype is characterized by the SNP alleles ACAG shared by both farmers and hunter-gatherers. Notably, some haplotypes were restricted to only one sub-group (Fig. 2b). Specifically, the haplotype GTAG was separated from the network core by rs10485588 (A [red in Fig. 3] and G [blue in Fig. 3], the ancestral and derived alleles, respectively), the putative eQTL SNP, which is found predominantly in farmer populations (with the exception of two Biaka Pygmies individuals) (Fig. 3). The haplotype with the alternative alleles for those SNPs (i.e., ACGA) is completely absent among farmers.

Discussion

Positive selection of genes coding for proteins involved in cofactor transport between cells or sub-cellular compartments was found by comparing genotypes of populations from the HGDP. This dataset is particularly interesting

Table 2 Significant eQTL from positively selected cofactor transporter SNPs

PC	SNP	Gene	Official gene name	Tissue	Cofactors	Effect size	*p* value
3	rs1471476	SLC25A26	Solute Carrier Family 25 (Mitochondrial Carrier; Phosphate Carrier), Member 26	Heart—left ventricle	SAH	− 0.49	1.4E−06
3	rs17044224	SLC25A26	Solute Carrier Family 25 (Mitochondrial Carrier; Phosphate Carrier), Member 26	Adipose—subcutaneous	SAH	− 0.32	4.9E−05
3	rs17044224	SLC25A26	Solute Carrier Family 25 (Mitochondrial Carrier; Phosphate Carrier), Member 26	Heart—left Ventricle	SAH	− 0.5	5.0E−07
5	rs10485588	SLC24A3	Solute carrier family 24 (sodium/potassium/calcium exchanger), member 3	Whole blood	K, Ca	0.74	1.9E−08
5	rs16830593	CACNB4	Calcium Channel Voltage-Dependent Subunit Beta 4	Skin—sun exposed (lower leg)	Ca	− 0.82	6.6E−05

From GTeX eQTL database
Ca calcium, *K* potassium, *SAH* S-Adenosyl-L-homocysteine, *PC* principal component

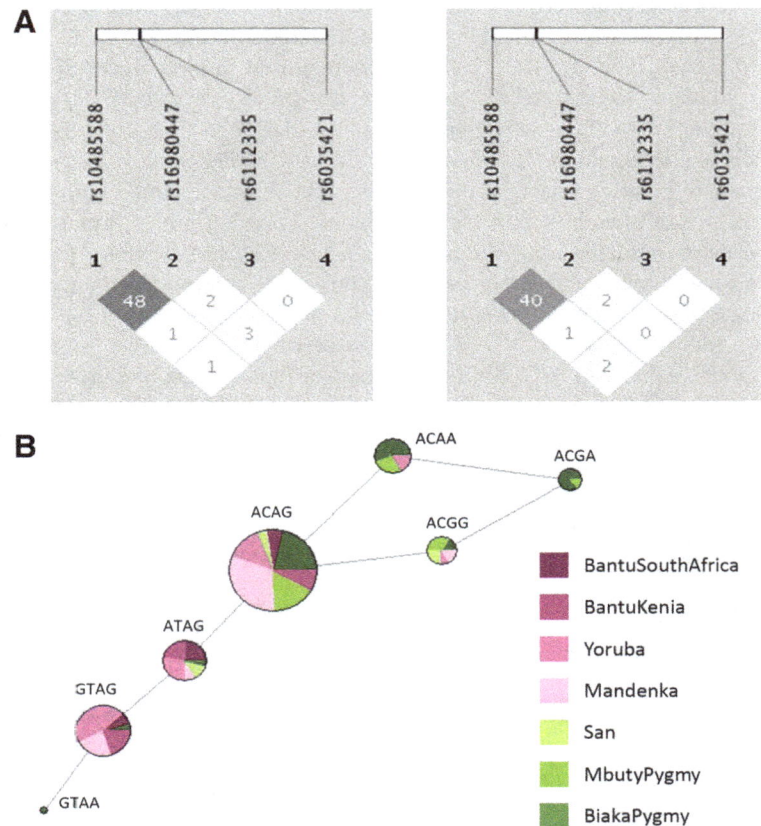

Fig. 2 Linkage disequilibrium plots and haplotype network of *SLC24A3* regions in African populations. **a** Visualization of LD between the genetic variants in *SLC24A3* regions bearing signals of positive selection. LD was calculated using r^2 parameter separately in African populations of farmers and hunter-gatherers. Squares shaded according to strength of LD. **b** Haplotype network analysis of *SLC24A3* regions. Each circle represents a haplotype that is color-coded according to the population in which it is present. Circle sizes are proportional to the haplotype frequency and each line corresponds to one mutational step

since it includes genotypes from several genetically diverse worldwide populations, whom ancestries have evolved in different environments and thus been exposed to diets of varying nutritional composition (i.e., hunter-gatherers and farmers). Cofactor transporters are of particular interest as they regulate the tissue and sub-cellular bioavailability of micronutrient-derived cofactors and are more likely to be influenced by different nutritional habits from ancient populations originating from regions with varying climates [1] and soil composition [25]. Cofactor-requiring biological processes participate in normal and pathophysiological processes that could contribute to between-population differences in disease incidence and response to nutritional interventions and diets [18, 26]. However, other selective forces may have contributed to the evolution and distribution of CT variants among populations.

The PCA-based approach followed here associated the population-specific alleles to a specific PC and thus a specific ancestry gradient. Contrarily to F_{ST} statistic, a popular measure of positive selection based on

population differentiation [27], it does not require a priori definition of populations or groups of populations [16]. We thus considered it more suitable for the HGDP dataset, which contains several populations and some of them not being genetically well separated from one another. Moreover, since the PCA-based approach identifies outlier SNPs for each principal component, it is less likely to identify variants that underwent random genetic drift since such phenomenon should similarly affect all variants in a population.

The signals of positive selection identified here were derived mainly from two PCs, namely PC3 and PC5. The gradient described is intra-continental and is due to the difference in allele frequencies across the Native Americans and Africans populations, respectively. PC5 separated African hunter-gatherers from farmers, two populations that traditionally based their subsistence on different diets and identified *SLC24A3* as being positively selected. *SLC24A3* encodes for the potassium-dependent Na+/Ca2+ exchanger type 3 protein (NCKX3), an

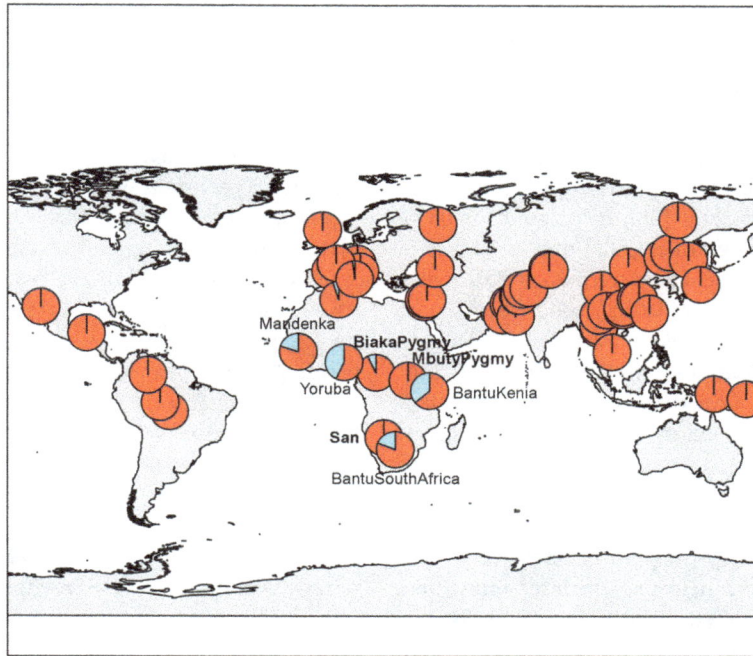

Fig. 3 Spatial frequency distribution of rs10485588 alleles. Each pie chart corresponds to one HGDP population and is positioned on the map according to the latitude and longitude data used by Rosenberg et al. [44]. Pie charts are colored according to the frequency of the common, ancestral A (red) and the derived G (light blue) alleles. Note that among the African populations, hunter-gatherers are written in bold

important regulator of intracellular calcium homeostasis. This gene is expressed most abundantly in the brain but also found in the aorta, uterus, intestine, and skeletal muscle with low expression in other tissues [28].

Polymorphisms in *SLC24A3* have been associated with salt-sensitive vasoconstriction and hypertension [29], while the expression of NCKX3 protein was linked to preeclampsia (i.e., pregnancy complicated by high blood pressure) [30]). Selection of these variants in hunter-gatherers may be due to diverse, animal-based, diets that were low in sodium chloride and high in potassium salt intake compared with the diet adopted after the Neolithic transition [31]. Indeed, this transition took place at the end of the most recent ice age and coincided with the advent of agriculture which was characterized by increases in plant-based at the expense of animal-based ingredients and where salt became an important commodity. Adaptation to such dietary pattern must have induced genetic adaptation in many genes involved in nutrient metabolism and may partly explain modern-day phenotypes, as that observed recently with the FADS gene [10, 32]. Namely, individuals with varying admixture from hunter-gatherers to farmers, such as modern Europeans [33], have different risks of cardiovascular disease, hypertension, stroke, kidney stones, and osteoporosis (e.g., [34]) compared to African-Americans (e.g., [35]), which could be mediated by their different metabolic response to various dietary minerals. In fact, a short-term intervention with a hunter-gatherer, or Paleolithic, diet

improved glucose homeostasis and lipid profiles in modern-day Americans living with type II diabetes [36]. The opposite is also possible to envision. Namely, transitioning from a hunter-gatherer to a post-Neolithic diet could induce metabolic alterations that, in longer-terms, would increase cardiovascular and other chronic disease risks.

Limitations were inevitably present in the study and should be considered when interpreting observations. First, the HGDP dataset, obtained using the DNA chip technology, does not allow studying rare variants that would instead be detected using newer technology such as the next generation sequencing. Moreover, each population in the dataset is represented by a small sample and could be the reason of not having extremely significant results. In fact, even if all the SNPs reported in the manuscript were significant after FDR correction, only one met the genome-wide significance threshold of $p < 5 \times 10^{-8}$, rs12312876 ($p = 2.70 \times 10^{-8}$). This issue could be overcome using 1000 Genomes dataset; however, the populations included in that project do not cover the spectrum of human genetic differentiation that would be necessary to study the selective pressure exerted by diet. In fact, even close populations such as the African farmers and hunter-gatherers, not present in 1000 Genomes, could have been affected by different environmental factors. Another important limitation is the lack of direct information on dietary habits of reference populations that prevent any conclusion about the driving force of the adaptation. For what concern the analysis, the method we chose allowed us not to split the dataset in separate populations and thus has been the methodology of choice. However, if we had the possibility of using larger sample sizes for the population of interest, it would have been interesting to apply other selection metrics such as the haplotype-based methods such as iHS [37] and XP-EHH [38], calculated for each population instead of groups of populations, or the XP-CLR method [39], which uses allele frequency differentiation between populations to detect selective sweeps. The availability of sequencing data would allow to test also other methods, such as the population branch statistic (PBS), which was successful in identifying genes involved in adaptation to high altitude from exome sequencing data [40].

Conclusion

Genetic variation in cofactor transporters may be of use clinically to investigate and help explain inter-individual variability in response to dietary interventions [18]. Indeed, individual CT SNP distribution, reflective of their genetic backgrounds, could influence the expression or activity of these important mediators of micronutrient-derived cofactor ADME and biological effect. Thus, our findings support the importance of considering an individual's genetic makeup along with their metabolic profiles (e.g., homeostatic measures of vitamin levels for instance) when tailoring and analyzing responses to personalized dietary interventions aimed at optimizing health.

Methods

Cofactor and transporter identification

NCBI PubMed (http://www.ncbi.nlm.nih.gov/pubmed), UniProt (http://www.uniprot.org/), and OMIM (http://www.omim.org/) databases were searched for transporters of cofactors [18]. The cofactor name and their synonyms with the addition of the word "transport" or "transporter" were used for the PubMed search. For instance, combinations of one of the following vitamin C synonyms "vitamin C", "vit C", "ascorbic acid", and "ascorbate" AND "transporter" were searched to identify vitamin C transporters. The transporters identified from NCBI PubMed were verified on the UniProt database for their involvement in the transport of other cofactors.

Tissue-specific expression of CTs was evaluated using data extracted from the Human Protein Atlas database, which classifies proteins into the following categories: (i) Tissue enriched: mRNA levels in one tissue at least five times higher than all other tissues, (ii) group enriched: mRNA levels of a group of 2 to 7 tissues at least five times those of all other tissues, (iii) tissue enhanced: mRNA levels in a particular tissue at least five times the average level in all tissues, (iv) expressed in all: mRNA

detected in all tissues, (v) mixed: detected in fewer than 32 tissues but not elevated in any tissue, or (vi) not detected (resulting tissue-specific information can be found in Additional file 1: Table S1) [41].

Genetic variation data

The genotype data were obtained from the HGDP–CEPH panel, a resource that captures a significant proportion of human genetic diversity. The genotypes were obtained with the Illumina BeadStation technology for 1043 individuals, were downloaded from http://www.hagsc.org/hgdp/files.html, and were pre-processed at the SNP and individual levels using PLINK v1.07 [42]. Before the quality control procedure, 660,918 SNPs were available. Sixteen thousand six hundred fifty non-autosomal SNPs and 1248 SNPs with a genotyping rate less than 0.95 and 12,085 SNPs with a minor allele frequency less than 0.01 were excluded for a total of 630,935 remaining SNPs (of which 8960 SNPs for CT genes). Additionally, 103 related individuals from both first- and second-degree relative pairs, as described in Rosenberg, 2006 [43], were also discarded. The assignment of individuals to populations was performed using the table downloaded from the Rosenberg Lab website http://rosenberglab.stanford.edu/data/rosenberg2006ahg/SampleInformation.txt, as published in Rosenberg, 2006 [43]. According to this data the HGDP individuals were assigned to 53 populations. The geographic coordinates were downloaded from the same web source (https://web.stanford.edu/group/rosenberglab/data/rosenbergEtAl2005/rosenbergEtAl2005.coordinates.txt), and they have been previously used in Rosenberg et al. [44].

Principal component analysis

Principal component analysis was performed with smartpca tool of the EIGENSOFT package v6.0.1 [45] using the default settings that allow the removal of individuals detected as outliers during the computation. A preliminary PCA on the genome-wide data was used as an additional quality control step to detect the presence of outliers or individuals not grouped with their geographic region of origin, and we did not detect any issue. Next, we used PCA to evaluate the population stratification both at genome-wide level and on CT genes only. The pattern of differentiation in CT genes was investigated on a subset of 8960 SNPs located in CT genes [46, 47].

Selection statistic

Statistical analyses were performed with R 3.1.2 (R Foundation for Statistical Computing, Vienna, Austria; http://www.r-project.org/) unless otherwise specified. Our analysis was designed to identify SNPs with signal of positive selection on the basis of outlier detection from principal component analysis. Such PCA-based approaches were recently successful in identifying genetic loci under adaptive selection [15–17]. The main advantage of this approach over other methods like F_{ST} statistic is that it assesses genetic differentiation along gradients without requiring a priori clustering of the individuals by population. Starting from the SNP weights (loadings) obtained from the smartpca output, the selection statistics D^2 was calculated and it corresponds to the squared loading of each SNP [15, 16]. The discrepancy between the empirical distribution and the theoretical one was determined, and the pchisq R function was used to associate a p value to each SNP. p values obtained were corrected for multiple testing using the R package q value, which controls for false discovery rate (FDR) [48]. q value significance threshold of 0.05 was used. To evaluate the results obtained applying the selection statistic to the genome-wide HGDP dataset, the top ten SNPs were extracted for the first ten PCs (100 total SNPs). A genomic region spanning 200 kb around each SNP was identified and genes annotated using the Bioconductor annotation package TxDb.Hsapiens.UCSC.hg18.knownGene. The comparison of results with literature was done using the data from dbPSHP, a database which contains information about genes and genomic regions from curated publications about positive selection in different human populations [20].

Linkage disequilibrium and haplotype analysis

The identification of the proxy SNPs of each significant variant associated to PC5 was performed using the genotype data of 1000 genomes Yoruba population. The analysis was carried out using the online tool LDlink (https://analysis-tools.nci.nih.gov/LDlink/?tab=home). We submitted the significant SNPs identified, and for each of them, we retrieved a list of proxy variants located –/+ 500 Kb of the query variant with a pairwise R^2 value greater than 0.01.

The pattern of LD in *SLC24A3* gene was estimated using Haploview v4.2. The haplotype phase was inferred using fastPHASE v1.4.8. The input files were created using PLINK, and the tool was run using these parameters: 25 iterations of the EM algorithm (C parameter) and 200 as the number of the number of haplotypes sampled from the "posterior" distribution obtained from a particular random start of the EM algorithm (H parameter). To build the haplotype network, we used the indiv.out file which contains estimates which attempt to minimize individual error. The haplotype network was produced by Network 4.2.0.1 using the median-joining algorithm [49].

Functional annotation

The impact of SNPs on protein function was examined using the Ensembl Variant Effect Predictor tool (http://www.ensembl.org/Homo_sapiens/Tools/VEP/), using the GRCh38.p7 human assembly. The regulatory potential of the SNPs was investigated using the RegulomeDB,

Version 1.1 [50]. The data from GTEx database V6 [24] (http://www.gtexportal.org/home/) were used to investigate the presence of correlations between the SNPs and tissue-specific gene expression levels (i.e., eQTL).

Additional files

Additional file 1: Table S1. List of all proteins identified as transporters of cofactors.

Additional file 2: Figure S1. Scree plot from PCA. This chart shows the eigenvalues associated with each PC.

Additional file 3: Figure S2. PCA analysis for PC3 and PC4. The two scatter plots show the grouping of individuals according to PC1/PC3 and PC1/PC4.

Additional file 4: Figure S3. PCA analysis for PC5, 6, and 8. Principal components showing positive selection between African sub-populations of Hunter-gatherers and Farmers (PC5/6) and between Native Americans (PC5/8).

Additional file 5: Figure S4. PCA analysis of entire HGDP dataset. The scatter plots show the grouping of individuals according to PC1 and PC2 using all the autosomal SNPs.

Additional file 6: Table S2. Analysis of positive selection using the GWAS dataset and literature comparison.

Additional file 7: Table S3. SNP functional annotation.

Additional file 8: Table S4. Regulome DB annotation.

Additional file 9: Note 1.

Additional file 10: Table S5. SNP functional annotation

Additional file 11: Table S6. Regulome DB annotation.

Abbreviations
CT: Cofactor transporter; HGDP: Human genome diversity project; IHS: Integrated haplotype score; PC: Principal components; PCA: Principal component analysis

Acknowledgements
The authors would like to acknowledge the contribution of Dr. Laura Caberlotto in the initial data mining.

Funding
This research project was funded by the Nestlé Institute of Health Science.

Authors' contributions
MPSB and JK conceived and designed the study. SP and MPSB performed the analyses. SL interpreted the results and drafted the manuscript. All authors have read and approved the final manuscript.

Competing interests
Jim Kaput works for the Nestlé Institute of Health Sciences. The other authors declare that they have no competing interests.

Author details
[1]The Microsoft Research, University of Trento Centre for Computational Systems Biology (COSBI), piazza Manifattura 1, 38068 Rovereto, TN, Italy. [2]Vydiant, Inc, Gold River, CA, USA.

References

1. Hancock AM, Witonsky DB, Ehler E, Alkorta-Aranburu G, Beall C, Gebremedhin A, et al. Human adaptations to diet, subsistence, and ecoregion are due to subtle shifts in allele frequency. Proc Natl Acad Sci. 2010;107(Supplement_2):8924–30.

2. Ye K, Gu Z. Recent advances in understanding the role of nutrition in human genome evolution. Adv Nutr An Int Rev J. 2011;2:486–96.

3. Fumagalli M, Moltke I, Grarup N, Racimo F, Bjerregaard P, Jørgensen ME, et al. Greenlandic Inuit show genetic signatures of diet and climate adaptation. Science. 2015;349:1343–7.

4. Ingram CJE, Mulcare CA, Itan Y, Thomas MG, Swallow DM. Lactose digestion and the evolutionary genetics of lactase persistence. Hum Genet. 2009;124:579–91.

5. Bersaglieri T, Sabeti PC, Patterson N, Vanderploeg T, Schaffner SF, Drake JA, et al. Genetic signatures of strong recent positive selection at the lactase gene. Am J Hum Genet. 2004;74:1111–20.

6. Tishkoff SA, Reed FA, Ranciaro A, Voight BF, Babbitt CC, Silverman JS, et al. Convergent adaptation of human lactase persistence in Africa and Europe. Nat Genet. 2007;39:31–40.

7. Perry GH, Dominy NJ, Claw KG, Lee AS, Fiegler H, Redon R, et al. Diet and the evolution of human amylase gene copy number variation. Nat Genet. 2007;39:1256–60.

8. Santos JL, Saus E, Smalley SV, Cataldo LR, Alberti G, Parada J, et al. Copy number polymorphism of the salivary amylase gene: implications in human nutrition research. J Nutrigenet Nutrigenomics. 2012;5:117–31.

9. Carpenter D, Dhar S, Mitchell LM, Fu B, Tyson J, Shwan NAA, et al. Obesity, starch digestion and amylase: association between copy number variants at human salivary (AMY1) and pancreatic (AMY2) amylase genes. Hum Mol Genet. 2015;24:3472–80.

10. Kothapalli KSD, Ye K, Gadgil MS, Carlson SE, O'Brien KO, Zhang JY, et al. Positive selection on a regulatory insertion-deletion polymorphism in FADS2 influences apparent endogenous synthesis of arachidonic acid. Mol Biol Evol. 2016;33:1726–39.

11. Zhang C, Li J, Tian L, Lu D, Yuan K, Yuan Y, et al. Differential natural selection of human zinc transporter genes between African and non-African populations. Sci Rep. 2015;5:9658.

12. Engelken J, Carnero-Montoro E, Pybus M, Andrews GK, Lalueza-Fox C, Comas D, et al. Extreme population differences in the human zinc transporter ZIP4 (SLC39A4) are explained by positive selection in Sub-Saharan Africa. PLoS Genet. 2014;10:e1004128.

13. Cann HM, de Toma C, Cazes L, Legrand M-F, Morel V, Piouffre L, et al. A human genome diversity cell line panel. Science. 2002;296:261–2.

14. Cavalli-Sforza LL. Opinion: the Human Genome Diversity Project: past, present and future. Nat Rev Genet. 2005;6:333–40.

15. Galinsky KJ, Bhatia G, Loh P-R, Georgiev S, Mukherjee S, Patterson NJ, et al. Fast principal-component analysis reveals convergent evolution of ADH1B in Europe and East Asia. Am J Hum Genet. 2016;98:456–72.

16. Duforet-Frebourg N, Luu K, Laval G, Bazin E, Blum MGB. Detecting genomic signatures of natural selection with principal component analysis: application to the 1000 Genomes data. Mol Biol Evol. 2016;33:1082–93.

17. Chen G-B, Lee SH, Zhu Z-X, Benyamin B, Robinson MR. EigenGWAS: finding loci under selection through genome-wide association studies of eigenvectors in structured populations. Heredity (Edinb). 2016;117:51–61.

18. Scott-Boyer MP, Lacroix S, Scotti M, Morine MJ, Kaput J, Priami C. A network analysis of cofactor-protein interactions for analyzing associations between human nutrition and diseases. Sci Rep. 2016;6:19633.

19. Albersen M, Bosma M, Knoers NVVAM, de Ruiter BHB, Diekman EF, de Ruijter J, et al. The intestine plays a substantial role in human vitamin B6 metabolism: a Caco-2 cell model. PLoS One. 2013;8:e54113.

20. Li MJ, Wang LY, Xia Z, Wong MP, Sham PC, Wang J. dbPSHP: a database of recent positive selection across human populations. Nucleic Acids Res. 2014;42(Database issue):D910-6.

21. Sturm RA. Molecular genetics of human pigmentation diversity. Hum Mol Genet. 2009;18:R9–17.

22. Tan J, Yang Y, Tang K, Sabeti PC, Jin L, Wang S. The adaptive variant EDARV370A is associated with straight hair in East Asians. Hum Genet. 2013;132:1187–91.

23. Pickrell JK, Coop G, Novembre J, Kudaravalli S, Li JZ, Absher D, et al. Signals of recent positive selection in a worldwide sample of human populations. Genome Res. 2009;19:826–37.

24. GTEx Consortium TGte, Welter D, MacArthur J, Morales J, Burdett T, Hall P, et al. Human genomics. The Genotype-Tissue Expression (GTEx) pilot analysis: multitissue gene regulation in humans. Science. 2015;348:648–60.

25. Adrogué HJ, Madias NE. Sodium and potassium in the pathogenesis of hypertension. N Engl J Med. 2007;356:1966–78.

26. Ames BN. Low micronutrient intake may accelerate the degenerative diseases of aging through allocation of scarce micronutrients by triage. Proc Natl Acad Sci. 2006;103:17589–94.

27. Holsinger KE, Weir BS. Genetics in geographically structured populations: defining, estimating and interpreting FST. Nat Rev Genet. 2009;10:639–50.

28. Visser F, Valsecchi V, Annunziato L, Lytton J. Exchangers NCKX2, NCKX3, and NCKX4: identification of Thr-551 as a key residue in defining the apparent K(+) affinity of NCKX2. J Biol Chem. 2007;282:4453–62.

29. Citterio L, Simonini M, Zagato L, Salvi E, Delli Carpini S, Lanzani C, et al. Genes involved in vasoconstriction and vasodilation system affect salt-sensitive hypertension. PLoS One. 2011;6:e19620.

30. Yang H, Kim T-H, An B-S, Choi K-C, Lee H-H, Kim J-M, et al. Differential expression of calcium transport channels in placenta primary cells and tissues derived from preeclamptic placenta. Mol Cell Endocrinol. 2013;367:21–30.

31. Frassetto LA, Schloetter M, Mietus-Synder M, Morris RC, Sebastian A. Metabolic and physiologic improvements from consuming a paleolithic, hunter-gatherer type diet. Eur J Clin Nutr. 2009;63:947–55.

32. Hunter-gatherers to farmers. http://www.historyworld.net/wrldhis/PlainTextHistories.asp?ParagraphID=ayj. Accessed 18 Sept 2017.

33. Callaway E. Ancient European genomes reveal jumbled ancestry. Nature. 2014; https://doi.org/10.1038/nature.2014.14456.

34. Ramos E, Rotimi C. The A's, G's, C's, and T's of health disparities. BMC Med Genet. 2009;2:29.

35. Helgadottir A, Manolescu A, Helgason A, Thorleifsson G, Thorsteinsdottir U, Gudbjartsson DF, et al. A variant of the gene encoding leukotriene A4 hydrolase confers ethnicity-specific risk of myocardial infarction. Nat Genet. 2006;38:68–74.

36. Masharani U, Sherchan P, Schloetter M, Stratford S, Xiao A, Sebastian A, et al. Metabolic and physiologic effects from consuming a hunter-gatherer (Paleolithic)-type diet in type 2 diabetes. Eur J Clin Nutr. 2015;69:944–8.

37. Voight BF, Kudaravalli S, Wen X, Pritchard JK. A map of recent positive selection in the human genome. PLoS Biol. 2006;4:e72.

38. Sabeti PC, Varilly P, Fry B, Lohmueller J, Hostetter E, Cotsapas C, et al. Genome-wide detection and characterization of positive selection in human populations. Nature. 2007;449:913–8.

39. Chen H, Patterson N, Reich D. Population differentiation as a test for selective sweeps. Genome Res. 2010;20:393–402.

40. Yi X, Liang Y, Huerta-Sanchez E, Jin X, Cuo ZXP, Pool JE, et al. Sequencing of 50 human exomes reveals adaptation to high altitude. Science. 2010;80:329.

41. Uhlén M, Fagerberg L, Hallström BM, Lindskog C, Oksvold P, Mardinoglu A, et al. Proteomics. Tissue-based map of the human proteome. Science. 2015;347. https://doi.org/10.1126/science.1260419.

42. Purcell S, Neale B, Todd-Brown K, Thomas L, Ferreira MAR, Bender D, et al. PLINK: a tool set for whole-genome association and population-based linkage analyses. Am J Hum Genet. 2007;81:559–75.

43. Rosenberg NA. Standardized subsets of the HGDP-CEPH Human Genome Diversity Cell Line Panel, accounting for atypical and duplicated samples and pairs of close relatives. Ann Hum Genet. 2006;70(Pt 6):841–7.

44. Rosenberg NA, Mahajan S, Ramachandran S, Zhao C, Pritchard JK, Feldman MW. Clines, clusters, and the effect of study design on the inference of human population structure. PLoS Genet. 2005;1:e70.

45. Patterson N, Price AL, Reich D. Population structure and eigenanalysis. PLoS Genet. 2006;2:e190.

46. Cavalli-Sforza LL, Menozzi P, Piazza A. The History and Geography of Human Genes. New Jersey: Princeton University Press; 1994.

47. Price AL, Zaitlen NA, Reich D, Patterson N. New approaches to population stratification in genome-wide association studies. Nat Rev Genet. 2010;11:459–63.

48. Storey JD. False discovery rates. In: International Encyclopedia of Statistical Science. Miodrag Lovric, editor. Berlin: Springer-Verlag; 2011.

49. Bandelt HJ, Forster P, Röhl A. Median-joining networks for inferring intraspecific phylogenies. Mol Biol Evol. 1999;16:37–48.

50. Boyle AP, Hong EL, Hariharan M, Cheng Y, Schaub MA, Kasowski M, et al. Annotation of functional variation in personal genomes using RegulomeDB. Genome Res. 2012;22:1790–7.

10

Fatty acid extract from CLA-enriched egg yolks can mediate transcriptome reprogramming of MCF-7 cancer cells to prevent their growth and proliferation

Aneta A. Koronowicz[1*], Paula Banks[1], Dominik Domagała[1], Adam Master[2], Teresa Leszczyńska[1], Ewelina Piasna[1], Mariola Marynowska[1] and Piotr Laidler[3]

Abstract

Background: Our previous study showed that fatty acids extract obtained from CLA-enriched egg yolks (EFA-CLA) suppressed the viability of MCF-7 cancer cell line more effectively than extract from non-enriched egg yolks (EFA). In this study, we analysed the effect of EFA-CLA and EFA on transcriptome profile of MCF-7 cells by applying the whole Human Genome Microarray technology.

Results: We found that EFA-CLA and EFA treated cells differentially regulated genes involved in cancer development and progression. EFA-CLA, compared to EFA, positively increased the mRNA expression of *TSC2* and *PTEN* tumor suppressors as well as decreased the expression of *NOTCH1*, *AGPS*, *GNA12*, *STAT3*, *UCP2*, *HIGD2A*, *HIF1A*, *PPKAR1A* oncogenes.

Conclusions: We show for the first time that EFA-CLA can regulate genes engaged in AKT/mTOR pathway and inhibiting cell cycle progression. The observed results are most likely achieved by the combined effect of both: incorporated CLA isomers and other fatty acids in eggs organically modified through hens' diet. Our results suggest that CLA-enriched eggs could be easily available food products with a potential of a cancer chemopreventive agent.

Keywords: AKT/mTOR pathway, CLA-enriched egg yolks, DNA microarray, Cancer chemoprevention, MCF-7 cancer cells, Transcriptome, SFA/MUFA

Introduction

Conjugated linoleic acid (CLA) term includes several isomers of linoleic acid (18:2), naturally present in ruminant and dairy products, due to the activity of the rumen microflora [25, 30]. In numerous studies, CLA was shown to have several beneficial properties on human health. Researchers examined its effect on stimulating the immune system [1], reducing cancerogenesis [32, 52], atherogenesis [34], diabetes, and obesity [54]. However, most of the available literature was focused on the activity of isolated, pure substances. In addition,

according to available data, the consumable quantities of naturally occurring CLA are relatively too low to effectively impact human health [27]. The recommended effective dose of CLA was estimated at least 1.5–3.5 g/day [13], while natural ruminant products contain between 1.2 and 12.5 mg per gram of fat [25, 30, 47, 78] and in poultry CLA concentration remains relatively low, at 0.6 to 0.9 mg per gram of fat [13]. Enhancing CLA concentration in food products such as eggs, chosen dairy products/yogurts, and meat could then become an alternative to synthetic CLA supplements. Indeed, studies have shown an easy incorporation of CLA into eggs of chickens by diet fortification [11, 65, 74] and that CLA-enriched eggs meet the requirements of functional food [24].

* Correspondence: aneta.koronowicz@gmail.com
[1]Department of Human Nutrition, Faculty of Food Technology, University of Agriculture, Krakow, Poland
Full list of author information is available at the end of the article

Little is known about the effect of fatty acids (FA) from CLA-enriched food products on cancer cells [16, 46]. Our previous study showed that FA extracts obtained from CLA-enriched egg yolks (EFA-CLA) suppressed the viability of MCF-7 cancer cell line more effectively than the extracts from non-enriched egg yolks (EFA) [32]. To analyze the potential molecular mechanism, we decided to compare the effects of both extracts on MCF-7 cells transcriptome profile.

The whole-genome DNA microarray technology has become a very powerful tool to analyze global gene expression profiles, and in multiple studies, it has been shown to be an effective method for detecting genomic variation of closely related samples. Finally, we identified and analyzed differently expressed genes based on family, molecular functions, biological processes, cellular components, or pathways. As suggested in this article, relationships between studied genes require a confirmation at protein level; nevertheless, the microarray results are a valuable and multi-faceted source of information for other scientists and a foundation for further in vivo research [67].

Methods

Hens' and eggs' management

The Animal Ethics Committee of the National Institute of Animal Production (Poland) approved all experiments involving animals (approval number: 851/2011). All applicable international, national, and/or institutional guidelines for the care and use of animals were followed.

Forty-eight *Isa Brown* laying hens (26 weeks old) were housed in a controlled room under 14/10 h light/dark cycle, given free access to water and commercial starter diet ('DJ' feed). After a 1-week adaptation period, an equal number of hens was randomly allocated to the control or experimental group for 4 months of the experiment. Diets (Additional file 1: Table S1) were calculated to provide 2700 kcal/kg and 17 % crude protein. The 0.75 % dietary CLA (TONALIN FFA 80, BASF Company, Germany) concentration was based on previously determined formula [24] and contained 80 % CLA in 50:50 ratio for *cis-9,trans-11* and *trans-10,cis-12* isomers. Eggs were collected daily for the period of 10 weeks and stored at 4 °C. Yolks were separated from albumen, homogenized with rotary homogenizer, and frozen at −20 °C. Samples were then lyophilized (Martin Christ Model Alpha 1–4, Germany) and again stored at −20 °C. The total dry matter was determined by oven drying method [3] and the total fat content was determined by Soxhlet method (Soxtec Avanti's 2050 Auto Extraction Unit, Tecator Foss, Sweden) using petroleum ether as a solvent [23].

Fatty acids extraction and GC/MS analysis

Lipids from control and CLA-enriched yolks were extracted by using modified Folch method [22]. One gram per liter of butylated hydroxytoluen (BHT) was used as an antioxidant. Briefly, after overnight incubation with chloroform/methanol (2:1) solution, samples were filtrated and mixed with 4 mL of 0.88 % sodium chloride solution to obtain phase separation. Chloroform lipids layer was then carefully dried under nitrogen. Ten milligrams of each lipid extract was subjected to saponification (20 min, 60 °C) with 0.5 M KOH/methanol followed by methylation with 14 % (*v/v*) BF3/methanol (15 min, 60 °C) and extraction with hexane. The obtained fatty acid methyl esters (FAME) were analyzed by GC/MS (Additional file 2: Table S2). The profile of EFA-CLA and EFA was expressed as percentage (%) of relative area, obtained by area normalization (FA peak area relative to chromatogram total area). For the treatment, lipid extracts were subjected to the basic hydrolysis (0.5 M KOH, 60 °C, 15 min) and extracted with hexane. The free fatty acids were then dissolved in ethanol at the stock concentration 1 g/mL and stored under nitrogen in the temperature of −20 °C.

Cell culture and treatment

Human breast adenocarcinoma cell line MCF-7 (ATCC* HTB22™) was purchased from the American Type Culture Collection. Cells were cultured according to the manufacturer's procedure. Cells were seeded in culture plates (BD Biosciences) for 24 h. After that time, growing medium was replaced by a medium containing (a) fatty acid extract from CLA-enriched egg yolks (EFA-CLA) and (b) fatty acids extract from non-enriched egg yolks (EFA), both at the concentration of 0.5 mg/mL. We used (c) cell cultures only in growth medium (empty control (EC)) and (d) cell cultures treated with only a solvent of fatty acids (ET-ethanol) at final concentration 0.1 %, as a negative control (NC).

Cell proliferation

Cell proliferation was determined with 5′-bromo-2′-deoxy-uridine (BrdU) Labeling and Detection Kit III (Roche), according to manufacturer's instruction.

Microarray analysis of gene expression profile

Whole Human Genome Microarrays containing about 50 000 probes (Agilent Technologies, USA) were used to establish the expression profile of each tested sample. Total RNA was isolated from cells using RNA isolation kit (A&A Biotechnology, Poland). RNA quantity was measured with NanoDrop (NanoDrop Technologies, USA). The analysis of its quality and integrity was performed with BioAnalyzer (Agilent, USA). Only samples with RNA integrity number (RIN) ≥8.0 were included in the analysis which was performed using SurePrint G3 Human Gene Expression 8x60K v2 Microarray. Each slide contained eight microarrays representing about 50

000 probe sets. The Low Input Quick Amp Labeling Kit, two-color (Agilent, USA) was used to amplify and label target RNA to generate complementary RNA (cRNA) for oligo microarrays used in gene expression profiling. The experiment was performed using a common reference design, where the common reference was a pool of equal amounts of RNA from control cells. On each of two-color microarrays, 300 ng of cRNA from the pool (labeled Cy3) and 300 ng of cRNA (labeled Cy5) were hybridized. In total, 12 microarrays were run—three for each experimental group. Microarray hybridization was performed with the Gene Expression Hybridization Kit (Agilent Technologies, USA), according to the manufacturer's protocols. RNA Spike In Kit (Agilent Technologies, USA) was used as an internal control. Acquisition and analysis of hybridization intensities were performed using the Agilent DNA microarray scanner. Data were extracted and background was subtracted using standard procedures contained in the Agilent Feature Extraction (FE) Software version 10.7.3.1. FE performs Lowess normalization. Samples underwent quality control and the results showed that each sample had a similar QC metric profile. The next step was filtering probe sets by flags to remove poor quality probes (absent flags). Microarray data were deposited at the Gene Expression Omnibus data repository under the number GSE65397 and followed MIAME requirements. To identify signaling pathways and gene functions, the microarray data were analyzed using Panther Classification System—an online database.

RT and real-time PCR analysis

Reverse transcription was performed using 1 μg of total RNA isolated from the cells by using the Maxima first Strand cDNA Synthesis kit for RT-qPCR (Thermo Scientific). A quantitative verification of genes was performed using the CFX96 Touch™ Real-Time PCR Detection System instrument (Bio-Rad), utilizing the SYBR Green Precision Melt Supermix kit (Bio-Rad). Conditions of individual PCR reactions were optimized for given pair of oligonucleotide primers (Additional file 3: Table S3). Basic conditions were as follows: 95 °C for 10 min, 45 PCR cycles at 95 °C, 15 s; 59 °C, 15 s; 72 °C, 15 s, followed by melting curve analysis (65–97 °C with 0.11 °C ramp rate and five acquisitions per 1 °C). Results were normalized using at least two reference genes (*GAPDH*, *HPRT1*, *ACTB*, or *HSP90AB1*) and were calculated using the $2^{-\Delta\Delta C}T$ method [39].

Statistical analysis

Each treatment included three replicates and the experiment was repeated three times. Statistical analysis for microarrays was performed using Gene Spring 12.6.1 software (Agilent, USA). Statistical significance of the differences was evaluated using a one-way ANOVA and Tukey's HSD Post hoc test ($p < 0.05$). A multiple testing correction was performed using Benjamini and Hochberg false discovery rate (FDR) <5 %. Other experiments were assessed by Student's *t* tests.

Results

Bird performance and egg composition

There were no significant differences in egg production between hens as well as egg characteristics [33]. Fatty acid profile in CLA-enriched egg yolks was significantly affected by dietary CLA fortification (Fig. 1). Both CLA isomers were found incorporated into the yolk, and their concentration did not reflect their initial proportion in the experimental diets (Additional file 1: Table S1), with the preference for the *cis-9,trans-11* isomer. Compared to the control, feeding with 0.75 % of dietary CLA significantly increased ($p < 0.001$) total SFA concentration at the expenses of MUFA ($p < 0.001$) (Fig. 1 and [33]).

Cell proliferation

EFA-CLA extract at a concentration of 0.5 mg/mL suppressed MCF-7 cell proliferation more effectively than the extract from non-enriched egg yolks. Specifically, treatment with EFA-CLA reduced the cell proliferation by approximately 40 % compared to the negative control, while EFA reached 20 % (Fig. 2). Moreover, this effect was weaker for estrogen-negative MDA-MB-231 (Additional file 4: Figure S12) and not observed for a non-tumorigenic MCF-10A cell line (Fig. 3).

Effect of applied treatments on MCF-7 cell line transcriptome profile

The analysis was performed on 1589 transcripts, of which 160 were differently expressed between EFA-CLA and EFA studied groups (Fig. 4 and Additional file 5: Table S4). We omitted 21 genes, which could have been directly affected by the solvent (ET) leaving 139 genes (Additional file 6: Table S10). Further analysis showed 69 transcripts shared by all three comparison groups: EFA-CLA vs. EFA, NC vs. EFA-CLA, and NC vs. EFA and 36 transcripts shared by EFA-CLA vs. EFA and NC vs. EFA. We determined 34 transcripts unique only to EFA-CLA vs. EFA. Among those, 11 were uncharacterized in available databases. Finally, we identified 18 (underlined) that, according to the available data, can be linked to cancer development and/or progression and which are involved in important cellular processes including regulation of cell cycle, apoptosis, or cell metabolism (Table 1). For those, the differences in expression between EFA and NC were statistically insignificant (Additional file 7: Table S5).

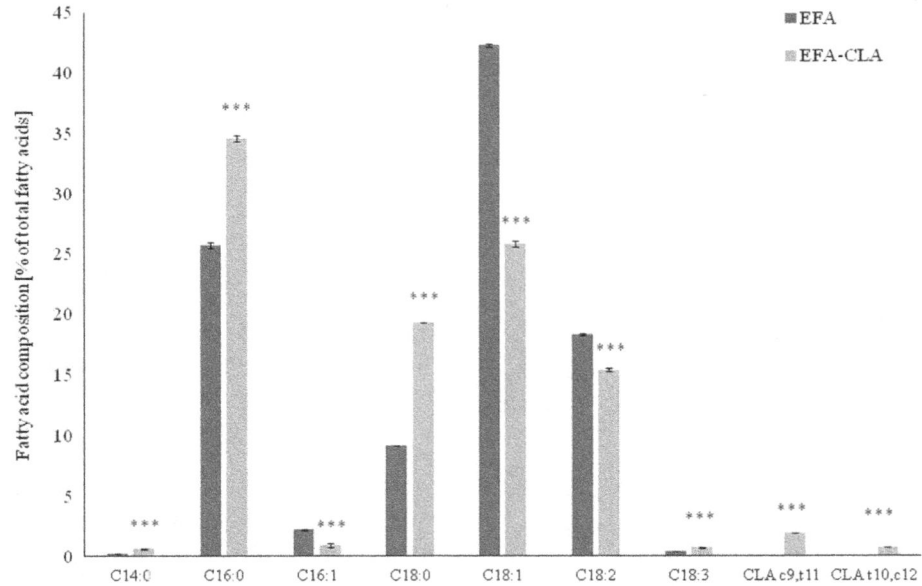

Fig. 1 Effect of dietary CLA on relative (%) fatty acids composition of egg yolks. Statistical significance of treatment: *p < 0.05; **p < 0.01; ***p < 0.001

Real-time PCR

To validate microarray data, we selected eight random genes from EFA-CLA vs. EFA comparison group: *NOTCH1*, *HIGD2A*, *PPKAR1A*, *UPC2*, *NAP1L1*, *CAMSAP2*, *PPP2R5E*, and *TSC2* (*p* < 0.05, Table 2). Our analysis showed a significant decrease in the messenger RNA (mRNA) expression of *NOTCH1*, *HIGD2A*, *PPKAR1A*, and *UCP2* and an increase in the expression of *CAMSAP2*, *PPP2R5E*, and *TSC2* genes due to the EFA-CLA treatment. Interestingly, only RT-qPCR results

for *NAP1L1* exhibited changes in the opposite direction than the microarray.

GO molecular complete analysis

Next, we examined the Gene Ontology (GO) for EFA-CLA vs. EFA differently regulated genes, using Panther Classification System. Results obtained from analysis of the signaling pathways, biological processes, molecular functions, and protein classes are presented in supplementary material (Additional file 8: Table S6, Additional file 9:

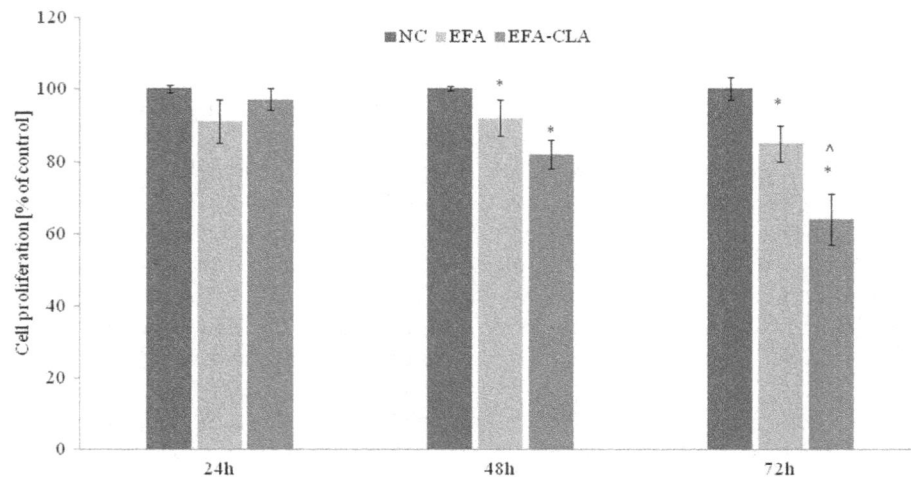

Fig. 2 Effect of EFA-CLA on MCF-7 cells proliferation. Values are expressed as means ± SEM for the *N* ≥ 9, standarized to NC as 100 %. Statistical significance was based on Student's *t* test *p < 0.05 vs. NC and ^p < 0.05 vs. EFA

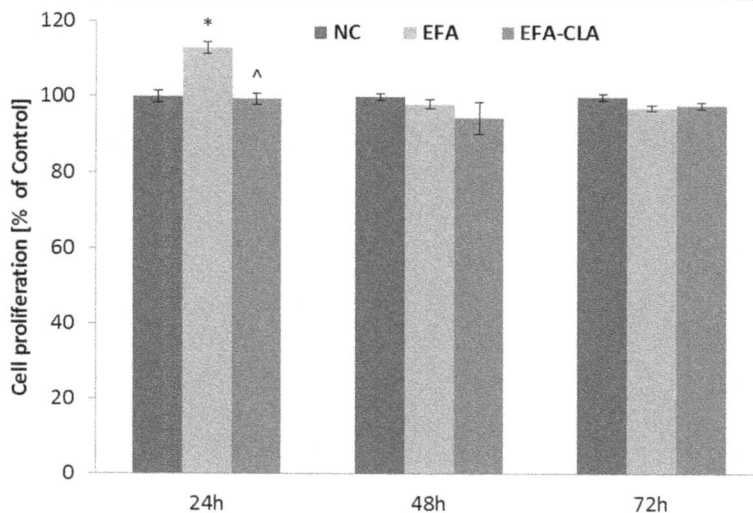

Fig. 3 Effect of EFA-CLA on MCF-10A cells proliferation. Values are expressed as means ± SEM for the $N \geq 9$, standarized to NC as 100 %. Statistical significance was based on Student's t test $*p < 0.05$ vs. NC and $^\wedge p < 0.05$ vs. EFA

Table S7, Additional file 10: Table S8, and Additional file 11: Table S9).

Effect of EFA-CLA on oncogenic pathways

In addition to signaling pathways listed in Additional file 8: Table S6, we aimed to study the connections between all the transcripts from Table 1, especially in terms of oncogenic pathways (Fig. 5) [79]. Our results showed that EFA-CLA treatment affected the downstream genes of the mammalian target of rapamycin (mTOR) signaling pathway. The increased mRNA expression of *PTEN*, *PPP2R5E*, and *TSC2* and decreased expression of *GNA12*, *UPC2*,

AGPS, *ANAX5A*, and *HIF1A*, together with observed reduced proliferation of MCF-7, suggest that EFA-CLA negatively regulates AKT/mTOR pathway.

Discussion

Breast cancer is one of the most common malignancies among women [21]; however, despite extensive research, the cellular processes that lead to carcinogenesis have not yet been fully explained. In the current research, we chose the estrogen receptor-positive (ER+) MCF-7 breast cancer cell line—the most studied cellular model of breast cancer [26, 59, 73].

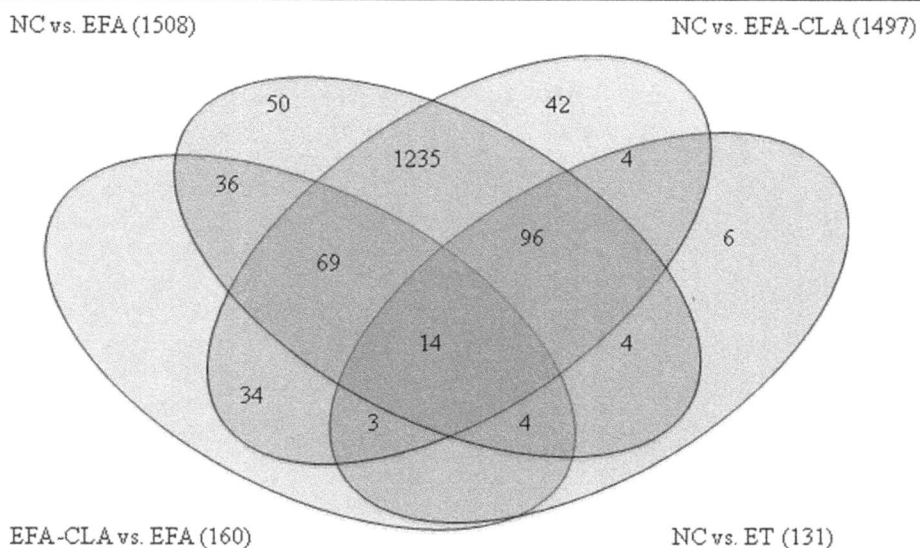

Fig. 4 Analysis of differently expressed transcripts between experimental groups

Table 1 The list of the differently regulated EFA-CLA vs. EFA specific transcripts in MCF-7 cell line

Gene Symbol	Adjusted p values	FC value	Gene name
NOTCH1	0.0146	−2.63	Notch homolog 1, translocation-associated
AGPS	0.0424	−2.19	Alkylglycerone phosphate synthase
GNA12	0.0009	−1.56	Guanine nucleotide binding protein (G protein) alpha 12
HIF1A	0.0134	−1.56	Hypoxia inducible factor 1, alpha subunit (basic helix-loop-helix transcription factor)
STAT3	0.0038	−1.32	Signal transducer and activator of transcription 3 (acute-phase response factor)
UCP2	0.0083	−1.29	Uncoupling protein 2 (mitochondrial, proton carrier)
HIGD2A	0.0089	−1.27	HIG1 hypoxia inducible domain family, member 2A
WASH1	0.0038	−1.27	WAS protein family homolog 1
BIN3	0.0477	−1.16	Bridging integrator 3
PRKAR1A	0.0462	−1.14	Protein kinase, cAMP-dependent, regulatory, type I, alpha
NDUFB11	0.0105	−1.13	NADH dehydrogenase (ubiquinone) 1 beta subcomplex, 11, 17.3 kDa
ANXA5	0.031	−1.05	Annexin A5
SMS	0.0399	1.08	Spermine synthase
PPP2R5E	0.0009	1.13	Protein phosphatase 2, regulatory subunit B', epsilon isoform
NAP1L1	0.0335	1.14	Nucleosome assembly protein 1-like 1
PTEN	0.0382	1.15	Phosphatidylinositol 3,4,5-trisphosphate 3-phosphatase and dual-specificity protein phosphatase PTEN
LOC646214	0.0213	1.16	p21 protein (Cdc42/Rac)-activated kinase 2 pseudogene
LMCD1	0.0067	1.21	LIM and cysteine-rich domains 1
CAMSAP2	0.0174	1.23	Calmodulin regulated spectrin-associated protein family, member 2
TSC2	0.0177	1.26	Tuberous sclerosis 2
FLJ45139	0.0406	1.33	FLJ45139 protein
CHSY3	0.0359	1.72	Chondroitin sulfate synthase 3
OVOS	0.0403	1.72	Ovostatin
SCD	0.19	−1.18[NS]	Stearoyl-CoA desaturase (delta-9-desaturase)

Statistical significance of treatment: $p < 0.05$; NS $p > 0.05$; bolded genes are to be associated with cancer

Table 2 The validation of microarray results with RT-qPCR in MCF-7 cell line (EFA-CLA vs. EFA)

Gene symbol	Adjusted p values	FC value RT-qPCR	FC value Microarray	Gene name
NOTCH1	0.0022	−2.02	−2.63	Notch homolog 1, translocation-associated
HIGD2A	0.0121	−1.75	−1.27	HIG1 hypoxia inducible domain family, member 2A
PRKAR1A	0.0047	−1.58	−1.14	Protein kinase, cAMP-dependent, regulatory, type I, alpha
UCP2	0.0023	−1.53	−1.29	Uncoupling protein 2 (mitochondrial, proton carrier)
NAP1L1	0.0023	−1.37	1.17	Nucleosome assembly protein 1-like 1
CAMSAP2	0.0031	1.57	1.23	Calmodulin regulated spectrin-associated protein family, member 2
PPP2R5E	0.0035	1.72	1.13	Protein phosphatase 2, regulatory subunit B', epsilon isoform
TSC2	0.0001	1.85	1.26	Tuberous sclerosis 2

Statistical significance of treatment: $p < 0.05$

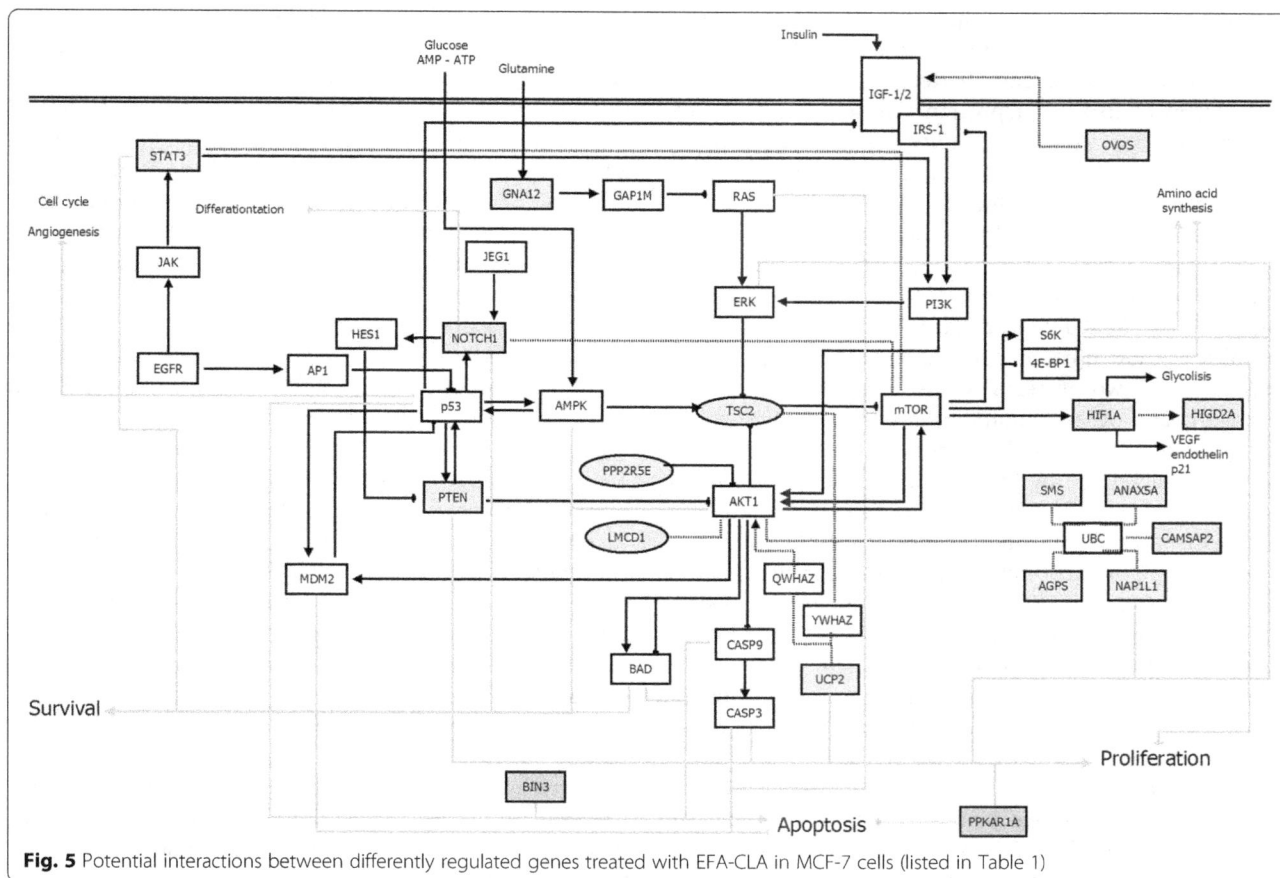

Fig. 5 Potential interactions between differently regulated genes treated with EFA-CLA in MCF-7 cells (listed in Table 1)

One of the main reasons behind our choice is that the (ER+) breast cancers are the most frequently diagnosed breast cancer subtype.

CLA is an extensively studied compound, and research findings showed a variety of possible beneficial effects of dietary CLA on human health. In addition, some of the molecular aspects of CLA mechanisms of action have been already described, and to our knowledge, Murphy et al. [50] applied microarray technique to show the effects of CLA isomers on the global gene expression using Caco-2 cells. However, most of published results are based on studying pure, isolated isomers which may not reflect the effect of a food product naturally enriched in CLA. Thus, our research would be the first to address the effects of the extract from CLA-enriched egg yolks on a breast cancer cell model in a wide spectrum of the whole human genome.

Our previous experiments showed that EFA-CLA extract suppressed the viability of MCF-7 breast cancer cell line more effectively than extract from non-enriched egg yolks [32]. Our current study supports those findings not only for estrogen receptor-positive MCF- 7 but also for estrogen receptor-negative MDA-MB-231; however, the EFA-CLA effect was most notable for MCF-7 (Fig. 2

and Additional file 4: Figure S12), which we proposed to be associated with affected mTOR signaling pathway [8]. In addition, we also performed experiments on commercially available and described as a non-tumorigenic MCF-10A cell line (ATCC). Interestingly, we did not observe a decreased proliferation in that cell line after treatment with tested fatty acids (Fig. 3). Some authors recommend caution when using MCF-10A cell line as non-transformed human breast epithelial cells in carcinogenesis research. They point out their potential for morphological and phenotypic transformation [56]. However, it should be noted that, to some extent, this could be due to the modification of the cell line microenvironment, including culture conditions, presence of serum, and used medium [53, 76].

In the present manuscript, we discuss selected genes, which expression differs the most between cells treated with FA from CLA-enriched and non-enriched egg yolks (Table 1), specifically, in terms of their potential significance in the neoplastic process. Based on a scheme of the interactions between those genes (Fig. 5), we pointed the anti-proliferative and pro-apoptotic properties of EFA-CLA, specifically through the regulation of AKT/ mTOR signaling pathway. mTOR interacts with several proteins and forms two distinct complexes named mTOR complex 1 (mTORC1) and 2 (mTORC2) of which mTORC1 is currently better characterized. mTOR is a central controller of protein synthesis, cell growth, cell proliferation, and cell viability [37]. Several components of the PI3K/PTEN/AKT/mTOR pathway (Fig. 5) are frequently mutated in human cancers.

Most notably, our results showed that treatment of MCF-7 cells with EFA-CLA (compared to EFA) increased the mRNA expression of known tumor suppressors, such as *TSC2, PTEN, PPP2R5E,* and *LMCD1.* TSC2 complex is a key upstream regulator of mTORC1, and it constitutes of two proteins, TSC1 and TSC2, that interacts with each other. Mutations in either of them result in the development of the tuberous sclerosis complex (TSC), characterized by the growth of benign tumors in multiple vital organs [29]. Reduced expression of TSC2 was determined in the invasive breast cancer compared to normal mammary epithelium [45]. Another mTOR pathway inhibitor, PTEN, was also found up-regulated. *PTEN* is a p53-regulated tumor suppressor, which transcription can be enhanced by p53 protein—acting as a transcription factor. Although our microarrays did not show statistically significant change in TP53 mRNA expression in the EFA-CLA cells vs. EFA group, additional Western blot analysis clearly showed an accumulation of p53 at the protein levels in the EFA-CLA treated cells (data not shown). *PTEN* is one of the most frequently mutated genes in various human cancers [9, 17, 70], including breast cancers, and is linked to aggressive tumors [64]. Information on *PPP2R5E* is limited, but it has been suggested as a potential negative regulator of PI3K/AKT signaling (2016). It has been also found to act as a tumor suppressor in breast cancer [19] and gastric cancer cells [38].

During our analysis, we have also found other genes potentially associated with PI3K/AKT/mTOR pathway, which were down-regulated in cells: *AGPS, ANXA5, STAT3, NOTCH1, PRKAR1A,* and *HIF1A* (Table 1), after the treatment with EFA-CLA. Whether observed decrease in gene expression is the cause or the result of inhibition of AKT/mTOR pathway requires further study. Zhu et al. [77] showed that phosphorylation of AKT1 in glioma and hepatic carcinoma cell lines was reduced simultaneously with *AGPS* silencing, whereas Benjamin et al. [6] showed that silencing of *AGPS* in breast cancer (including MCF-7) and melanoma cells manifested in a life-time reduction of cancer cells viability, tumor growth, and invasiveness. Although we did not find a direct link between *ANXA5* and AKT/mTOR pathway (Fig. 5), its up-regulation may be a predictive factor for tumor stage and clinical outcome of colorectal cancer [71]. ANXA5 has been also found in a group of pro-apoptotic genes [48]. These data may suggest that the

expression of ANXA5 could be dependent on the expression profile of other superior genes being a part of anti-tumor response of cells. In our study, we show a significant down-regulation of *STAT3* and *NOTCH1* gene under the influence of EFA-CLA. Phosphorylated STAT3 is being observed in nearly 70 % of human cancers. Acting as an oncoprotein, it is constitutively activated in many primary human tumors, being activated by a number of different cytokines as well as oncoproteins, i.e., Src and Ras. NOTCH1 is associated with PI3K and PI3K-dependent activation of AKT1. It has been shown to play a role in growth, proliferation, and inhibition of apoptosis [10, 58]. It has been also reported that Hes1, NOTCH1's downstream target protein, negatively regulates *PTEN* expression [51]. A fly model of tumorigenesis induced by NOTCH1 showed a synergism of NOTCH1 signaling and PI3K/AKT pathway, suggesting that the interplay between these two signaling pathways was conserved during the evolution process.

PRKAR1A has been found to be down-regulated in MCF-7 cells, due to the treatment with EFA-CLA. Information about *PRKAR1A* in available literature is ambiguous. Some studies have shown its up-regulation in many tumors, including breast cancer [7, 40, 41], suggesting its role in cell cycle regulation, growth, and/or proliferation. Other studies have pointed its tumor suppressing properties in osteosarcoma [49] and follicular thyroid cancer [55]. Due to EFA-CLA treatment, we determined a reduction in the mRNA expression of *UCP2,* which belongs to the family of mitochondrial carriers. Significant amount of studies is available on *UCP2,* but its functions are still under debate. It has been recently proposed to control routing of mitochondrial substrates [20, 69]. The overexpression of UCP2 has been shown in various tumors, including breast cancer [44]. Some data reveal that up-regulation of UCP2 may facilitate an increased chemoresistance as well as cancer adaptation to oxidative stress via mitochondrial suppression of reactive oxygen species (ROS) [4, 15, 18]. Sayeed et al. [60] have shown that *UCP2* gene silencing rapidly led to the induction of apoptosis and differentiation in breast cancer cells, concurrent with reduced cell survival and proliferation. These results may be supported by numerous studies reporting evidences suggesting a correlation between oxidative stress and breast cancer, due to mitochondrial dysfunction [57]. Being the source of ROS, mitochondria are particularly exposed to potential oxidative DNA damage. Several studies have determined a higher rate of mitochondrial DNA (mtDNA) mutations in breast tumor tissue, specifically, they identified somatic mutations in the D-loop region as, probably, the major factor leading to decreased mtDNA level in breast tumors and indicating a poor prognosis [36]. Recent results have shown that a reduced number of mtDNA copy may be involved in cancer development and/or progression [66, 75] and mtDNA content might be potentially used as a tool to predict prognosis. Interestingly, in our unpublished studies on prostate cancer cells and melanoma, we determined a significant increase in the levels of mtDNA when treating with EFA-CLA extracts (compared to EFA).

We also determined a down-regulation of *HIGD2A*, a subunit of the cytochrome C oxidase (COX, complex IV). However, little is known about its mechanism of action. A study presented by An et al. [2] on *HIGD1A*, another member of *HIG1* gene family, showed that expression of *HIGD1A* is directly dependent on binding of HIF-1α to HRE (hypoxia-response element) site at −32 bp in the *HIG1D1A* promoter. Transfecting RAW264.7 cell line with *HIGD1A* under hypoxia condition promoted cell survival, whereas silencing the endogenous gene with siRNA resulted in hypoxia-induced apoptosis. The authors have proposed the inhibition of cytochrome C release and the reduction of caspases as a potential mechanism. They also obtained similar results for *HIGD2A*. It should be noted that similarity between *HIG1* gene family members might have influenced obtained microarray results as probe specificity for gene isoforms is limited [35]. Interestingly, in our unpublished results on prostate cancer cells and melanoma, we determined a down-regulation of HIF-1α, after treatment with EFA-CLA. In our present study, we also observed down-regulation of HIF-1α in MCF-7 cells after EFA-CLA treatment, which is a positive signal confirming the anti-proliferative activity of EFA-CLA in the AKT/mTOR pathway (Fig. 5). HIF-1α is responsible for the activation of transcription of various genes, such as *VEGF*, *EDN1*, or *CDKN1A*, which are involved in cell cycle regulation, neovascularization, and metastasis [62]. Overexpression of HIF-1α correlates with an advanced tumor stage and poor survival [63, 68]. Majumder et al. [43] have demonstrated that the expansion of AKT-driven prostate epithelial cells requires mTOR-dependent survival signaling and activation of HIF-1α.

Finally, our results showed a down-regulation of *GNA12* mRNA expression after the treatment with EFA-CLA. Although we did not find a direct association with mTOR, *GNA12* has been found to participate in oncogenesis and metastasis in pathological conditions [28]. Kim et al. [31]), while studying breast cancer cells, proposed that *GNA12* up-regulates the activity of matrix metalloproteinase (MMP)-2 via p53-dependent manner and promotes malignant phenotypic conversion of this cancer cells. A recent study supported those findings [12]. Their results also show that *GNA12* stimulates the expression and activity of tumor promoting cytokines IL-6 and IL-8 and MMP-2 via binding and activation of NF-kB.

Although in current manuscript we focused on differences between the CLA-enriched (CLA-EFA) and non-enriched egg (EFAs), attached data (database GSE65397) suggest that EFAs can change the gene expression profile as well; however, they are unable to suppress the cell proliferation as efficiently as CLA-EFA can. The analysis of MCF-7 transcriptomes revealed that some of the observed changes may not be solely caused by CLA isomers present in the pool of other fatty acids identified in the enriched egg yolk. As shown in Fig. 1, the incorporation of CLA was accompanied by significant changes in the general FA profile of egg yolk. The most notable was an increase in total SFA concentration at the expense of MUFA. Our calculations showed that the altered SFA/MUFA ratio can affect the expression of some genes including *HIGD2A* and *SMS* (Additional file 12: Table S11) suggesting that the changed FA ratio in EFA-CLA extract could be responsible, at least in part, for the specific response of the cancer cells (Fig 2). It seems therefore that our functional products, obtained through the process of modification of hens' diet, may show specific features determined by both the presence of CLA and altered SFA/MUFA ratio. This may also suggest that CLA-enriched eggs cannot be simply replaced with a synthetic CLA supplements.

Although available literature on effects of CLA on other FAs is limited, some authors have shown that treatment of cells with synthetic CLA increased the SFA/MUFA ratio in cell culture [14, 72]. As potential explanation, authors suggested that CLA could reduce the expression of SCD gene, which is responsible for conversion of SFA into MUFA. Interestingly, overexpression of SCD was associated with increased cancer cell proliferation, both in vitro for breast, prostate and lung cancer cells as well as in vivo [5, 14]. Our results showed a decreasing tendency for SCD mRNA for EFA-CLA vs. EFA treatment groups (Table 1); however, these results were statistically non-significant. Nevertheless, comparison with the negative control revealed a significant reduction in SCD expression for EFA-CLA at the level of transcription (Additional file 7: Table S5). It should be noticed, however, that the SCD mRNA levels does not necessarily correspond with this enzyme activity that has been shown by Choi et al. [14] for both MDA-MB- 231 and MCF-7 cells treated with synthetic *cis-9*, *trans-11* and *trans-10*, *cis-12* CLA isomers. *SCD* has been also reported to be involved in mTOR pathway. Scaglia and Igal [61] have showed that the down-regulation of *SCD* reduces the activity of AKT in A549 cell line (SCD-ablated A549 cells). In addition, Luyimbazi et al. [42] have observed an increase in SCD protein expression when using activators of mTOR pathway in both MCF-7 (ER+) and MDA-MB-231 (ER−) cell lines, while the use of selective mTOR inhibitors showed an opposite effect. All these data may suggest that the observed decrease in MCF-7 proliferation in the presence of EFA-CLA could result from down-regulation of AKT/mTOR signaling pathway and reduced expression of SCD and other genes involved in mTOR pathway (database GSE65397). However, the role of CLA, other egg FAs, and the altered SFA/MUFA ratio in mTOR-dependent down-regulation of cell proliferation needs further studies.

Although some of our results may require to be confirmed at protein levels, the microarrays are a valuable and multi-faceted source of information and may explain the adequacy of further in vivo research, according to 3R principles (replacement, reduction, and refinement).

Conclusions

In summary, our study presents the first evidence that the fatty acids extracts from CLA-enriched egg yolks (EFA-CLA) can affect transcriptome of MCF-7 cancer cells and inhibit their proliferation. We found this effect to be accompanied by changes in gene expression associated with down-regulation of AKT/mTOR signaling pathway. EFA-CLA increased expression of TSC2 and PTEN tumor suppressors as well as decreased the expression of oncogenes including NOTCH1, AGPS, GNA12, STAT3, UCP2, HIGD2A, HIF1A, and PPKAR1A. The observed results are most likely achieved by the combined effect of both incorporated CLA isomers and other fatty acids in eggs organically modified through hens' diet. It seems, therefore, that in contrast to synthetic CLA supplements, CLA-enriched eggs with an altered SFA/MUFA ratio could be easily available food products with a potential of a cancer chemopreventive agent. Although this concept needs further in vivo studies, it is clear that our microarray-derived results are a rich source of information on pathways in which fatty acids from CLA-enriched egg yolks can modify the response of the cancer cells at the level of transcription.

Additional files

Additional file 1: S1. Composition of hens' experimental diets (%).

Additional file 2: S2. FAME analysis GC/MS conditions.

Additional file 3: S3. Nucleotide sequences of primers. ACTB, actin, beta; CAMSAP2, calmodulin regulated spectrin-associated protein family, member 2; GAPDH, glyceraldehyde-3-phosphate dehydrogenase; HIGD2A, HIG1 hypoxia inducible domain family, member 2A; HFRT1, hypoxanthine phosphoribosyltransferase 1; HSP90AB1, heat shock protein 90 kDa alpha (cytosolic); NAP1L1, nucleosome assembly protein 1-like 1; NOTCH1, Notch homolog 1, translocation-associated; PPKAR1A, protein kinase, cAMP-dependent, regulatory, type I, alpha; PPP2R5E,protein phosphatase 2, regulatory subunit B', epsilon isoform; TSC2, tuberous sclerosis 2; UCP2 uncoupling protein 2 (mitochondrial, proton carrier).

Additional file 4: S12. Effect of EFA-CLA on MDA-MB-231 cells proliferation. The assay was performed using BrdU test (Roche). Values are expressed as means ± SEM for the $N \geq 9$, standarized to NC as 100 %. Statistical significance was based on Student's t test *$p < 0.05$ vs. NC and ^$p < 0.05$ vs. EF.

Additional file 5: S4. Analysis of differently expressed transcripts between experimental groups in MCF-7 cell line. Tukey's HSD post hoc test ($p < 0.05$);

underlining determined different transcripts between the compared groups; italics determined a common transcripts between the compared groups; bold determined all the analyzed transcripts.

Additional file 6: S10. The list of the differently regulated EFA-CLA vs. EFA specific transcripts in MCF-7 cell line (without genes, which expression could directly be affected by the ET solvent). Statistical significance of treatment: $p < 0.05$.

Additional file 7: S5. The list of the differently regulated EFA vs. NC specific transcripts in MCF-7 cell line. *$p < 0.05$ for EFA vs. NC; NC, negative control; NS $p > 0.05$

Additional file 8: S6. Pathways based on EFA-CLA vs. EFA specific genes differently regulated in MCF-7 cell line. Statistical significance of treatment: $p < 0.05$.

Additional file 9: S7. Table GO biological processes based on EFA-CLA vs. EFA specific genes differently regulated in MCF-7 cell line. Statistical significance of treatment: $p < 0.05$.

Additional file 10: S8. GO molecular functions based on EFA-CLA vs. EFA specific genes differently regulated in MCF-7 cell line. Statistical significance of treatment: $p < 0.05$.

Additional file 11: S9. Protein classes based on EFA-CLA vs. EFA specific genes differently regulated in MCF-7 cell line. Statistical significance of treatment: $p < 0.05$.

Additional file 12: S11. Calculated effects of altered FA and SFA/MUFA (S/M) ratio on gene expression profile in MCF-7 cells. *potential role of SFA/MUFA ratio in the regulation of gene expression. Abbreviations: c9. t11CLA—cis-9.trans-11-CLA; t10. c12CLA—trans-10.cis-12-CLA. S/M. changed SFA/MUFA ratio.

Abbreviations

AKT, protein kinase B; BF3, boron trifulouride; BHT, butylated hydroxytoluen; BrdU, 5'-bromo-2'-deoxy-uridine; CLA, conjugated linoleic acid; COX, cytochrome C oxidase; DNA, deoxyribonucleic acid; EC, empty control; EFA, fatty acids extract from non-enriched egg yolks; EFA-CLA, fatty acids extract from CLA-enriched egg yolks; FA, fatty acids; FAME, fatty acid methyl esters; FC, fold change; GC/MS, gas chrmoatography/mass spectrometry; GO, Gene Ontology; HRE, hypoxia-response element; KOH, potassium hydroxide; MCF-7, human breast adenocarcinoma cell line; mtDNA, mitochondrial DNA; mTOR, mammalian target of rapamycin; NC, negative control; QC, quality control; RNA, ribonucleic acid; ROS, reactive oxygen species; siRNA, small interfering RNA

Funding

This work was supported by the Polish National Science Center (grant number 2011/03/B/NZ9/01423) "Conjugated linoleic acid (CLA)-induced transcriptional activation of PPAR-an investigation of molecular mechanisms of putative anticancer action of fatty acids of CLA-enriched egg yolks."

Authors' contributions

AAK, AM, and PL made substantial contributions to the conception and design of experiments. DD, EP, MM, and AAK participated in performing the experiments. AAK and AM participated in the analysis and interpretation of data. AAK and PB participated in drafting the article. PL and AM participated in critically revising article for its important intellectual content. TL gave the final approval of the version to be submitted and any revised version. All authors read and approved the final manuscript.

Competing interests

The authors declare that they have no competing interests.

Author details

[1]Department of Human Nutrition, Faculty of Food Technology, University of Agriculture, Krakow, Poland. [2]Department of Biochemistry and Molecular Biology, Medical Centre for Postgraduate Education, Warsaw, Poland. [3]Department of Medical Biochemistry, Jagiellonian University Medical College, Krakow, Poland.

Reference

1. Albers R, Van der Wielen RPJ, Brink EJ, Hendrix HF, Dorovska-Taran VN, Mohede IC. Effects of cis-9, trans-11 and trans-10, cis-12 conjugated linoleic acid (CLA) isomers on immune function in healthy men. Eur J Clin Nutr. 2003;57(4):595–603.

2. An HJ, Shin H, Jo SG, Kim YJ, Lee JO, Paik SG, et al. The survival effect of mitochondrial Higd-1a is associated with suppression of cytochrome C release and prevention of caspase activation. Biochim Biophys Acta. 2011;1813(12):2088–98.

3. AOAC. Official methods of analysis. 18th ed. Gaintersburg: Association of Offcial Analitical Chemists International; 2006.

4. Baffy G, Derdak Z, Robson SC. Mitochondrial recoupling: a novel therapeutic strategy for cancer? Br J Cancer. 2011;105(4):469–74.

5. Belkaid A, Duguay SR, Ouellette RJ, Surette ME. 17β-estradiol induces stearoyl-CoA desaturase-1 expression in estrogen receptor-positive breast cancer cells. BMC Cancer. 2015;29(15):440.

6. Benjamin DI, Cozzo A, Ji X, Roberts LS, Louie SM, Mulvihill MM, et al. Ether lipid generating enzyme AGPS alters the balance of structural and signaling lipids to fuel cancer pathogenicity. Proc Natl Acad Sci U S A. 2013;110(37):14912–7.

7. Beristain AG, Molyneux SD, Joshi PA, Pomroy NC, Di Grappa MA, Chang M, et al. PKA signaling drives mammary tumorigenesis through Src. Oncogene. 2015;34(9):1160–73.

8. Boulay A, Rudloff J, Ye J, Zumstein-Macker S, O'Reilly T, Evans DB, Chen S, Lane HA. Dual inhibition of mTOR and estrogen receptor signaling in vitro induces cell death in models of breast cancer. Clin Cancer Res. 2005;11(14):5319–28.

9. Bose S, Crane A, Hibshoosh H, Mansukhani M, Sandweis L, Parsons R. Reduced expression of PTEN correlates with breast cancer progression. Hum Pathol. 2002;33(4):405–9.

10. Calzavara E, Chiaramonte R, Cesana D, Basile A, Sherbet GV, Comi P. Reciprocal regulation of Notch and PI3K/Akt signalling in T-ALL cells in vitro. J Cell Biochem. 2008;103(5):1405–12.

11. Chamruspollert M, Sell JL. Transfer of dietary conjugated linoleic acid to egg yolks of chickens. Poult Sci. 1999;78(8):1138–50.

12. Chia CY, Kumari U, Casey PJ. Breast cancer cell invasion mediated by Gα12 signaling involves expression of interleukins-6 and -8, and matrix metalloproteinase-2. J Mol Signal. 2014;9:6.

13. Chin SF, Liu W, Storkson JM, Ha YL, Pariza MW. Dietary sources of conjugated dienoic isomers of linoleic acid, a newly recognized class of anticarcinogens. J Food Comp Anal. 1992;5(3):185–97.

14. Choi Y, Park Y, Storkson JM, Pariza MW, Ntambi JM. Inhibition of stearoyl-CoA desaturase activity by the cis-9, trans-11 isomer and the trans-10, cis-12 isomer of conjugated linoleic acid in MDA-MB- 231 and MCF-7 human breast cancer cells. Biochem Biophys Res Commun. 2002;294(4):785–90.

15. Dalla Pozza E, Fiorini C, Dando I, Menegazzi M, Sgarbossa A, Constanzo C, et al. Role of mitochondrial uncoupling protein 2 in cancer cell resistance to gemcitabine. Biochim Biophys Acta. 2012;1823(10):1856–63.

16. De la Torre A, Debiton E, Juanéda P, Durand D, Chardigny J-M, Barthomeuf C, et al. Beef conjugated linoleic acid isomers reduce human cancer cell growth even when associated with other beef fatty acids. Br J Nutr. 2006;95(2):346–52.

17. Deocampo ND, Huang H, Tindall DJ. The role of PTEN in the progression and survival of prostate cancer. Minerva Endocrinol. 2003;28(2):145–53.

18. Derdak Z, Mark NM, Beldi G, Robson SC, Wands JR, Baffy G. The mitochondrial uncoupling protein-2 promotes chemoresistance in cancer cells. Cancer Res. 2008;68(8):2813–9.

19. Dupont WD, Breyer JP, Bradley KM, Schuyler PA, Plummer WD, Sanders ME, et al. Protein phosphatase 2A subunit gene haplotypes and proliferative breast disease modify breast cancer risk. Cancer. 2010;116(1):8–19.

20. Esteves P, Pecqueur C, Ransy C, Esnous C, Lenoir V, Bouillaud F, et al. Mitochondrial retrograde signaling mediated by UCP2 inhibits cancer cell proliferation and tumorigenesis. Cancer Res. 2014;74(14):3971–82.

21. Ferlay J, Soerjomataram I, Ervik M, Dikshit R, Eser S, Mathers C, Rebelo M, Parkin DM, Forman D, Bray F, GLOBOCAN 2012 v1.0, Cancer incidence and morality worldwide: IARC Cancer Base No. 11 [Internet]. Lyon, France: International Agency for Research on Cancer; 2013. Available from: http://globocan.iarc.fr/. Accessed 16 Jan 2015.

22. Folch J, Lees M, Sloane-Stanley GH. A simple method for the isolation and purification of total lipids from animal tissues. J Biol Chem. 1957;226(1):497–509.

23. Fortuna T, Juszczak L, Sobolewska-Zielińska J. Basis for food analysis. A script for laboratory classes at the University of Agriculture in Krakow. Krakow: Publishing House of the University of Agriculture in Krakow; 2003.

24. Franczyk-Żarów M, Kostogrys RB, Szymczyk B, Jawień J, Gajda M, Cichocki T, et al. Functional effects of eggs, naturally enriched with conjugated linoleic acid, on the blood lipid profile, development of atherosclerosis and composition of atherosclerotic plaque in apolipoprotein E and low-density lipoprotein receptor double-knockout mice (apoE/LDLR−/−). Br J Nutr. 2008;99(1):49–58.

25. Griinari JM, Bauman DE. Biosynthesis of conjugated linoleic acid and its incorporation into meat and milk in ruminants. In: Yurawecz MP, Mossoba MM, Kramer JKG, Pariza MW, Nelson GJ, editors. Advances in conjugated linoleic acid research, vol. 1. Champaign, IL: AOSC Press; 1999. p. 180–200.

26. Holliday DL, Speirs V. Choosing the right cell line for breast cancer research. Breast Cancer Res. 2011;13(4):215. doi:10.1186/bcr2889.

27. Ip C, Scimeca JA, Thompson HJ. Conjugated linoleic acid. A powerful anticarcinogen from animal fat sources. Cancer. 1994;74(3 Suppl):1050–4.

28. Juneja J, Casey PJ. Role of G12 proteins in oncogenesis and metastasis. Br J Pharmacol. 2009;158(1):32–40.

29. Kang YJ, Lu MK, Guan KL. The TSC1 and TSC2 tumor suppressors are required for proper ER stress response and protect cells from ER stress-induced apoptosis. Cell Death Differ. 2011;18(1):133–44.

30. Kepler CR, Hirons KP, McNeill JJ, Tove SB. Intermediates and products of the biohydrogenation of linoleic acid by Butyrivibrio fibrisolvens. J Biol Chem. 1966;241:1350–4.

31. Kim ES, Jeong JB, Kim S, Lee KM, Ko E, Noh DY, et al. The G12 family proteins upregulate matrix metalloproteinase-2 via p53 leading to human breast cell invasion. Breast Cancer Res Treat. 2010;124(1):49–61.

32. Koronowicz A, Dulińska-Litewka J, Pisulewski P, Laidler P. Effect of conjugated linoleic acid isomers on proliferation of mammary cancer cells. Rocz Panstw Zakl Hig. 2009;60(3):261–7.

33. Koronowicz A, Banks P, Szymczyk B, Leszczyńska T, Master A, Piasna E, Szczepański W, Domagała D, Kopeć A, Piątkowska E & Laidler P (2016): Dietary conjugated linoleic acid affects blood parameters, liver morphology and expression of selected hepatic genes in laying hens, British Poultry Science, DOI:10.1080/00071668.2016.1192280.

34. Kostogrys RB, Franczyk-Żarów M, Maślak E, Gajda M, Mateuszuk Ł, Chłopicki S. Effects of margarine supplemented with T10C12 and C9T11 CLA on atherosclerosis and steatosis in apoE/LDLR−/−mice. J Nutr Health Aging. 2012;16(5):482–90.

35. Kothapalli R, Yoder SJ, Mane S, et al. Microarray results: how accurate are they? BMC Bioinformatics. 2002;3:22.

36. Kuo SJ, Chen M, Ma GC, Chen ST, Chang SP, Lin WY, et al. Number of somatic mutations in the mitochondrial D-loop region indicates poor prognosis in breast cancer, independent of TP53 mutation. Cancer Genet Cytogenet. 2010;201(2):94–101.

37. Laplante M, Sabatini DM. mTOR signaling in growth control and disease. Cell. 2012;149(2):274–93.

38. Liu X, Liu Q, Fan Y, Wang S, Liu X, Zhu L, et al. Downregulation of PPP2R5E expression by miR-23a suppresses apoptosis to facilitate the growth of gastric cancer cells. FEBS Lett. 2014;588(17):3160–9.

39. Livak KJ, Schmittgen TD. Analysis of relative gene expression data using real-time quantitative PCR and the 2(−delta delta C(T)) method. Methods. 2001;25(4):402–8.

40. Loilome W, Juntana S, Namwat N, Bhudhisawasdi V, Puapairoj A, Sripa B, et al. PRKAR1A is overexpressed and represents a possible therapeutic target in human cholangiocarcinoma. Int J Cancer. 2011;129(1):34–44.

41. Loilome W, Juntana S, Pinitsoontorn C, Namwat N, Tassaneeyakul W, Yongvanit P. Suppression of PRKAR1A expression enhances anti-proliferative and apoptotic effects of protein kinase inhibitors and chemotherapeutic drugs on cholangiocarcinoma cells. Asian Pac J Cancer Prev. 2012;13(Suppl):143–7.

42. Luyimbazi D, Akcakanat A, McAuliffe PF, Zhang L, Singh G, Gonzalez-Angulo AM, Chen H, Do K-A, Zheng Y, Hung M-C, Mills GB, Meric-Bernstam F. Rapamycin regulates stearoyl CoA desaturase 1 expression in breast cancer. Mol Cancer Ther. 2010;9(10):2770–84.

43. Majumder PK, Febbo PG, Bikoff R, Berger R, Xue Q, McMahon LM, et al. (2004) mTOR inhibition reverses Akt-dependent prostate intraepithelial neoplasia through regulation of apoptotic and HIF-1-dependent pathways. Nat Med. 2004;10(6):594–601.

44. Maraghechi N, Ghaffarpour M, Tehrani GA. Overexpression of UCP2 is associated with tumor progression in Iranian breast cancer patients. Cancer Res. 2014;74(19 Supplement):4325.

45. Mehta MS, Vazquez A, Kulkarni DA, Kerrigan JE, Atwal G, Metsugi S, et al. Polymorphic variants in TSC1 and TSC2 and their association with breast cancer phenotypes. Breast Cancer Res Treat. 2011;125(3):861–8.

46. Miller A, Stanton C, Murphy J, Devery R. Conjugated linoleic acid (CLA)-enriched milk fat inhibits growth and modulates CLA-responsive biomarkers in MCF-7 and SW480 human cancer cell lines. Br J Nutr. 2003;90(5):877–85.

47. Mir PS, McAllister TA, Scott S, Alhaus J, Baron V, McCartney D, et al. Conjugated linoleic acid-enriched beef production. Am J Clin Nutr. 2004; 79(6 Suppl):1207S–11S.

48. Mitra S, Khaidakov M, Lu J, Ayyadevara S, Szwedo J, Wang XW, et al. Prior exposure to oxidized low-density lipoprotein limits apoptosis in subsequent generations of endothelial cells by altering promoter methylation. Am J Physiol Heart Circ Physiol. 2011;301(2):H506–13.

49. Molyneux SD, Di Grappa MA, Beristain AG, McKee TD, Wai DH, Pederova J, et al. Prkar1a is an osteosarcoma tumor suppressor that defines a molecular subclass in mice. J Clin Invest. 2010;120(9):3310.

50. Murphy EF, Hooiveld GJ, Muller M, Calogero RA, Cashman KD. Conjugated linoleic acid alters global gene expression in human intestinal-like Caco-2 cells in an isomer-specific manner. J Nutr. 2007;137(11):2359–65.

51. Palomero T, Sulis ML, Cortina M, Real PJ, Barnes K, Ciofani M, et al. Mutational loss of PTEN induces resistance to NOTCH1 inhibition in T-cell leukemia. Nat Med. 2007;13(10):1203–10.

52. Pariza MW, Ha YL. Conjugated dienoic derivatives of linoleic acid: a new class of anticarcinogens. Med Onco Tumor Pharmacother. 1990;7(2–3):169–71.

53. Park S-B, Kim B, Bae H, Lee H, Lee S, Choi EH, et al. Differential epigenetic effects of atmospheric cold plasma on MCF-7 and MDA-MB-231 breast cancer cells. PLoS ONE. 2015;10(5):e0129931. doi:10.1371/journal.pone.0129931.

54. Park Y, Albright KJ, Liu W, Storkson JM, Cook ME, Pariza MW. Effect of conjugated linoleic acid on body composition in mice. Lipids. 1997;32(8):853–8.

55. Pringle DR, Vasko VV, Yu L, Manchanda PK, Lee AA, Zhang X. Follicular thyroid cancers demonstrate dual activation of PKA and mTOR as modeled by thyroid-specific deletion of Prkar1a and Pten in mice. J Clin Endocrinol Metab. 2014;99(5):E804–12.

56. Qu Y, Han B, Yu Y, Yao W, Bose S, Karlan BY, et al. Evaluation of MCF10A as a reliable model for normal human mammary epithelial cells. PLoS ONE. 2015;10(7):e0131285. doi:10.1371/journal.pone.0131285.

57. Rohan TE, Wong LJ, Wang T, Haines J, Kabat GC (2010) Do alterations in mitochondrial DNA play a role in breast carcinogenesis? J Oncol 11 pages. doi:10.1155/2010/604304.

58. Sade H, Krishna S, Sarin A. The anti-apoptotic effect of Notch-1 requires p56lck-dependent, Akt/PKB-mediated signaling in T cells. J Biol Chem. 2004;279(4):2937–44.

59. Savanur MA, Eligar SM, Pujari R, Chen C, Mahajan P, Borges A, et al. Sclerotium rolfsii lectin induces stronger inhibition of proliferation in human breast cancer cells than normal human mammary epithelial cells by induction of cell apoptosis. PLoS ONE. 2014;9(11):e110107. doi:10.1371/journal.pone.0110107.

60. Sayeed A, Meng Z, Luciani G, Chen L-C, Bennington JL, Dairkee SH. Negative regulation of UCP2 by TGFβ signaling characterizes low and intermediate-grade primary breast cancer. Cell Death Dis. 2010;1(7):e53.

61. Scaglia N, Igal RA. Inhibition of stearoyl-CoA desaturase 1 expression in human lung adenocarcinoma cells impairs tumorigenesis. Int J Oncol. 2008;33(4):839–50.

62. Semenza GL. Signal transduction to hypoxia-inducible factor 1. Biochem Pharmacol. 2002;64(5–6):993–8.

63. Shibaji T, Nagao M, Ikeda N, Kanehiro H, Hisanaga M, Ko S, et al. Prognostic significance of HIF-1 alpha overexpression in human pancreatic cancer. Anticancer Res. 2003;23(6C):4721–7.

64. Song MS, Salmena L, Pandolfi PP. The functions and regulation of the PTEN tumor suppressor. Nat Rev Mol Cell Biol. 2012;13(5):283–96.

65. Szymczyk B, Pisulewski PM. Effects of dietary conjugated linoleic acid on fatty acid composition and cholesterol content of hen egg yolks. Br J Nutr. 2003;90(1):93–9.

66. Thyagarajan B, Wang R, Nelson H, Barcelo H, Koh WP, Yuan JM. Mitochondrial DNA copy number is associated with breast cancer risk. PLoS One. 2013;8(6):e65968.

67. Törnqvist E, Annas A, Granath B, Jalkesten E, Cotgreave I, Öberg M. Strategic focus on 3R principles reveals major reductions in the use of animals in pharmaceutical toxicity testing. PLoS One. 2014;9(7):e101638. doi:10.1371/journal.pone.0101638.

68. Vaupel P. The role of hypoxia-induced factors in tumor progression. Oncologist. 2004;9 Suppl 5:10–7.

69. Vozza A, Parisi G, De Leonardis F, Lasorsa FM, Castegna A, Amorese D, et al. UCP2 transports C4 metabolites out of mitochondria, regulating glucose and glutamine oxidation. Proc Natl Acad Sci U S A. 2014;111(3):960–5.

70. Wang Q, Wang X, Evers BM. Induction of cIAP-2 in human colon cancer cells through PKCδ/NF-kB. J Biol Chem. 2003;278(51):51091–9.

71. Xue G, Hao LQ, Ding FX, Mei Q, Huang JJ, Fu CG, et al. Expression of annexin a5 is associated with higher tumor stage and poor prognosis in colorectal adenocarcinomas. J Clin Gastroenterol. 2009;43(9):831–7.

72. Yamasaki M, Yanagita T. Adipocyte response to conjugated linoleic acid. Obes Res Clin Pract. 2013;7(4):e235–42.

73. Yao P-L, Morales JL, Zhu B, Kang B-H, Gonzalez FJ, Peters JM. Activation of peroxisome proliferator-activated receptor-β/δ (PPARβ/δ) inhibits human breast cancer cell line tumorigenicity. Mol Cancer Ther. 2014;13(4):1008–17.

74. Yin JD, Shang XG, Li DF, Wang FL, Guan YF, Wang ZY. Effects of dietary conjugated linoleic acid on the fatty acid profile and cholesterol content of egg yolks from different breeds of layers. Poult Sci. 2008;87(2):284–90.

75. Yu M, Zhou Y, Shi Y, Ning L, Yang Y, Wei X, et al. Reduced mitochondrial DNA copy number is correlated with tumor progression and prognosis in Chinese breast cancer patients. IUBMB Life. 2007;59(7):450–7.

76. Yusuf R, Frenkel K. Morphologic transformation of human breast epithelial cells MCF-10A: dependence on an oxidative microenvironment and estrogen/epidermal growth factor receptors. Cancer Cell Int. 2010;10:30. doi:10.1186/1475-2867-10-30.

77. Zhu Y, Liu A, Zhang X, Qi L, Zhang L, Xue J, et al. The effect of benzyl isothiocyanate and its computer-aided design derivants targeting alkylglycerone phosphate synthase on the inhibition of human glioma U87MG cell line. Tumor Biol. 2015;36(5):3499–509.

78. Zlatanos SN, Laskaridis K, Sagredos A. Conjugated linoleic acid content of human plasma. Lipids Health Dis. 2008;7:34.

79. PI3K-Akt signaling pathway. http://www.genome.jp/dbget-bin/www_bget?map04151. Accessed 28 April 2016.

11

Differences in genome-wide gene expression response in peripheral blood mononuclear cells between young and old men upon caloric restriction

I. P. G. Van Bussel[1], A. Jolink-Stoppelenburg[1], C. P. G. M. De Groot[1], M. R. Müller[1,2] and L. A. Afman[1,3*]

Abstract

Background: Caloric restriction (CR) is considered to increase lifespan and to prevent various age-related diseases in different nonhuman organisms. Only a limited number of CR studies have been performed on humans, and results put CR as a beneficial tool to decrease risk factors in several age-related diseases. The question remains at what age CR should be implemented to be most effective with respect to healthy aging. The aim of our study was to elucidate the role of age in the transcriptional response to a completely controlled 30 % CR diet on immune cells, as immune response is affected during aging. Ten healthy young men, aged 20–28, and nine healthy old men, aged 64–85, were subjected to a 2-week weight maintenance diet, followed by 3 weeks of 30 % CR. Before and after 30 % CR, the whole genome gene expression in peripheral blood mononuclear cells (PBMCs) was assessed.

Results: Expression of 554 genes showed a different response between young and old men upon CR. Gene set enrichment analysis revealed a downregulation of gene sets involved in the immune response in young but not in old men. At baseline, immune response-related genes were higher expressed in old compared to young men. Upstream regulator analyses revealed that most potential regulators were controlling the immune response.

Conclusions: Based on the gene expression data, we theorise that a short period of CR is not effective in old men regarding immune-related pathways while it is effective in young men.

Keywords: Age, Caloric restriction, Gene expression, Microarray, Peripheral blood mononuclear cells

Background

Caloric restriction (CR), the restriction of food intake without malnutrition, increases longevity in *Caenorhabditis elegans* [31], *Saccharomyces cerevisiae* [18], and rodents [32]. In addition to longevity, CR minimises the age-related dysfunction of organs [19] and lowers risks of several age-related diseases, for example, cancer in rats and mice [22], and age-related aorta sclerosis in rats

[4]. CR studies in primates led to less conclusive results. CR did increase longevity in monkeys at the Wisconsin National Primate Research Centre [6] but did not increase longevity in monkeys at the National Institute of Aging [20]. Factors such as genetics, husbandry, or dietary composition are perhaps more relevant for longevity in these primate studies than the number of calories [20]. Despite contrasting longevity results, both studies documented beneficial health effects of CR, including improved immune function and improved glucose homeostasis [20]. The limited number of studies investigating the effect of a CR diet in humans is, because of long life expectancy [27], solely directed at beneficial health effects and not at longevity [15]. For example, 6 years of CR decreased risk factors for atherosclerosis

* Correspondence: lydia.afman@wur.nl
[1]Division of Human Nutrition, Wageningen University, Bomenweg 2, 6703 HD Wageningen, The Netherlands
[3]Division of Human Nutrition, Wageningen University & Research centre, PO BOX 8129, NL-6700 EV Wageningen, The Netherlands
Full list of author information is available at the end of the article

in humans [11] and 1 year of CR decreased risk factors for coronary heart disease in humans [12]. Also, aging processes seem to be altered by CR: the gene expression profiles from skeletal muscles from humans of the CR Society showed a closer relationship to the gene expression profiles of young subjects than to those of age-matched subjects [21]. The preventive or retardative effect of CR on age-associated changes in gene expression has also been shown in the muscle, brain, heart, and adipose tissue from other species [23].

Mechanisms underlying beneficial effects of CR remain largely unclear. To understand these mechanisms, genes and molecular pathways involved in the effects of CR on longevity and healthy aging have been investigated. Overall, the effects of CR are characterised by the downregulated expression of genes involved in growth hormone signalling and genes involved in immune response [25]. In contrast, aging is characterised by the upregulated expression of genes involved in immune response [10]. The opposing effects of CR and aging on the immune response might be one potential lead for the beneficial effects of CR on healthy aging. In this regard, immune cells, such as peripheral blood mononuclear cells (PBMCs), are an interesting target to study in humans [13, 25]. PBMCs are easily accessible and circulate in the blood [2], exposing them to metabolites, hormones, chemokines, or cytokine from tissues such as the liver and adipose tissue [3], which make them relevant to study. So far, most human CR studies have been executed in middle-aged subjects; the question remains at what age CR should be implemented to be most effective with respect to healthy aging. To approach this question, we aimed to elucidate the effect of age in the response to CR by comparing whole genome gene expression response to 3 weeks of 30 % CR in PBMCs from old and young men.

Results

Baseline characteristics for ten young and nine old men of which high quality microarrays were present are summarised in Table 1. Besides the lower body mass index

Table 1 Baseline characteristics of young ($n = 10$) and old ($n = 9$) men of whom microarray analysis on PBMCs was performed. Data represent mean and (SD) or median and [range]

	Young men	Old men	P value
Age (year)	24 [20, 28]	70 [64 85]	4.37E−09
Height (m)	1.78 (0.06)	1.77 (0.04)	5.26E−01
Weight (kg)	71.1 (8.52)	76.7 (7.4)	1.28E−01
Body mass index (kg/m²)	22.4 (2.3)	24.6 (2.0)	3.08E−02
Glucose (mmol/L)	4.5 [3.7, 5.1]	5.2 [4.8, 5.5]	5.17E−04
Haemoglobin (g/L)	9.4 (0.4)	9.3 (0.4)	5.69E−01
Haematocrit (%)	45 (2)	44 (2)	5.46E−1

(BMI, $P = 0.04$) and lower fasting glucose level ($P < 0.001$) in old compared to young men, no differences were observed.

Three weeks of CR resulted in a decrease in body weight and BMI in both groups (Table 2). Age had no effect on weight ($P = 0.18$) or BMI change ($P = 0.18$).

Effect on gene expression: old versus young
At baseline, before 30 % CR, 696 genes were significantly differently expressed between old and young men (Fig. 1a). To identify the effect of age on CR-induced gene expression changes, responses to CR were compared between old and young men (Fig. 1b). A total of 554 genes showed a significantly different expression response between old and young men.

Effect of CR on gene expression: pathway analysis
Gene Set Enrichment Analysis (GSEA) was used to identify pathways in which gene expression was differentially regulated by age, at baseline, or in response to CR. Before the start of the 30 % CR diet, the expression of genes involved in immune response was higher in old compared to young men and the expression of genes involved in RNA processing was lower in old compared to young men (Table 3). Upon 3 weeks of 30 % CR, the expression of genes involved in immune response and glucose metabolism was downregulated in young men only, whereas the expression of genes involved in olfactory signalling was downregulated in old men only.

Upstream regulator analysis
Ingenuity Pathway Analysis (IPA) Upstream Regulator Analysis is a tool to find transcription regulators that may explain the observed gene expression. To identify these upstream regulators of genes that had a different expression before CR between old and young, or had a changed expression upon CR, we performed IPA Upstream Regulator Analysis. The regulators that were predicted to be affected at baseline and upon CR are listed in Additional file 1: Table S1. This list shows immune-related upstream regulators, interferon lambda 1 (INFL1), interferon alpha 2 (IFNA2), and interferon gamma (IFNG), that were predicted to be significantly higher in old compared to young before intervention. IFNA2 and IFNG were inhibited upon CR in young men, but not in old men. To identify correlation between the genes predicted to be regulated, we selected all significantly changed genes targeted by the predicted transcriptional regulators upon CR and created correlation heat maps of the significant changes in expression of these genes for young men (Fig. 2 (A1)) and old men (Fig. 2 (A2)). For young men, 57 unique genes were affected by the six identified transcriptional regulators, i.e. IFNA2, IFNG,

Table 2 Body weight and body mass index of young and old men before and upon 3 weeks of 30 % CR and significance (*P* value). Data represent mean with (SD)

		Before CR	Upon CR	P value
Weight (kg)	Young (*n* = 10)	71.1 (8.5)	68.7 (8.6)	2.87E−05
	Old (*n* = 9)	76.7 (7.4)	74.9 (7.4)	6.53E−05
Body mass index (kg/m²)	Young (*n* = 10)	22.4 (2.3)	21.6 (2.3)	3.64E−05
	Old 9 (*n* = 9)	24.6 (2.0)	24.0 (2.0)	4.21E−05

eukaryotic translation initiation factor 2-alpha kinase 2 (EIF2AK2), mitogen-activated protein kinase 1 (MAPK1), glyceraldehyde-2-phosphate dehydrogenase (GAPDH), and transglutaminase 2 (TGM2) (Additional file 1: Table S1). These genes showed a distinct correlation in young men (Fig 2 (A1)) which was less strong or absent in old men (Fig 2 (A2)). Contrary for old men, many genes regulated by the upstream regulators were overlapping: 15 potential upstream regulators

(Additional file 1: Table S1) were predicted to affect 17 unique genes, and no specific correlation pattern for old could be identified (Fig. 2 (B)).

Younger transcriptional profile upon CR

To identify if old men were able to obtain, at least for a subset of genes, a younger gene expression profile upon CR, the following approach was used: selection of genes with a different expression between old and young before CR resulting in 696 genes (Fig. 3); 96 of these genes also showed a significant different response upon CR between old and young men (Fig. 3); 55 of these genes had a changed expression in old men only. Figure 4 shows a heat map of the gene expression per subject and illustrates the different expressed genes at baseline and the change towards a young profile in old men, as is shown by the third part of the heat map where no significant expression differences between old and young upon CR were present.

Discussion

We aimed to investigate the potential relevance of age at which CR should be implemented to be most effective on gene expression changes of pathways important for healthy aging. To achieve this, we compared the gene expression changes in PBMCs of old men with the gene expression changes in PBMCs of young men upon 3 weeks of 30 % CR.

Three weeks of CR resulted in a downregulated expression of genes involved in immune response and glucose metabolism in young but not in old men. Effects

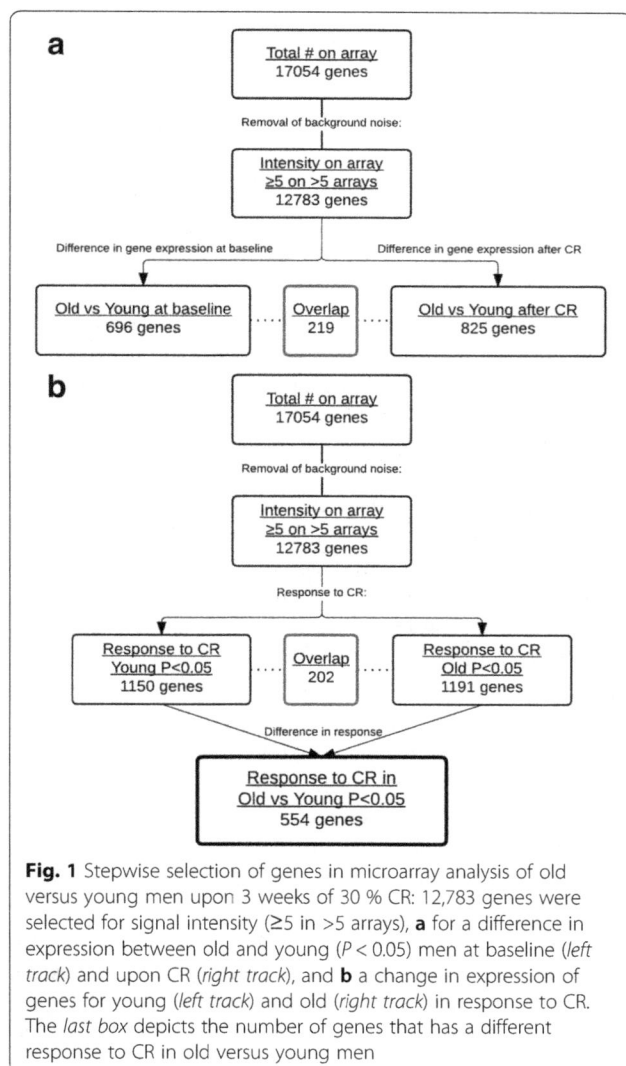

Fig. 1 Stepwise selection of genes in microarray analysis of old versus young men upon 3 weeks of 30 % CR: 12,783 genes were selected for signal intensity (≥5 in >5 arrays), **a** for a difference in expression between old and young (*P* < 0.05) men at baseline (*left track*) and upon CR (*right track*), and **b** a change in expression of genes for young (*left track*) and old (*right track*) in response to CR. The *last box* depicts the number of genes that has a different response to CR in old versus young men

Table 3 Pathways changed in PBMC gene expression profiles of young and old men before and upon 3 weeks of 30 % CR

Pathway	Baseline (old vs young)	Young men	Old men
RNA processing	↓	↑	↑
Cell cycle	–	↑/↓[a]	↑/–[a]
Oxidative stress	–	↓	↓
Immune response	↑	↓	–
Glucose metabolism	–	↓	–
Olfactory signalling	–	–	↓

↓ downregulated, ↑ upregulated, – no change
[a] Part of gene sets classified under these pathways were upregulated, whereas others where downregulated

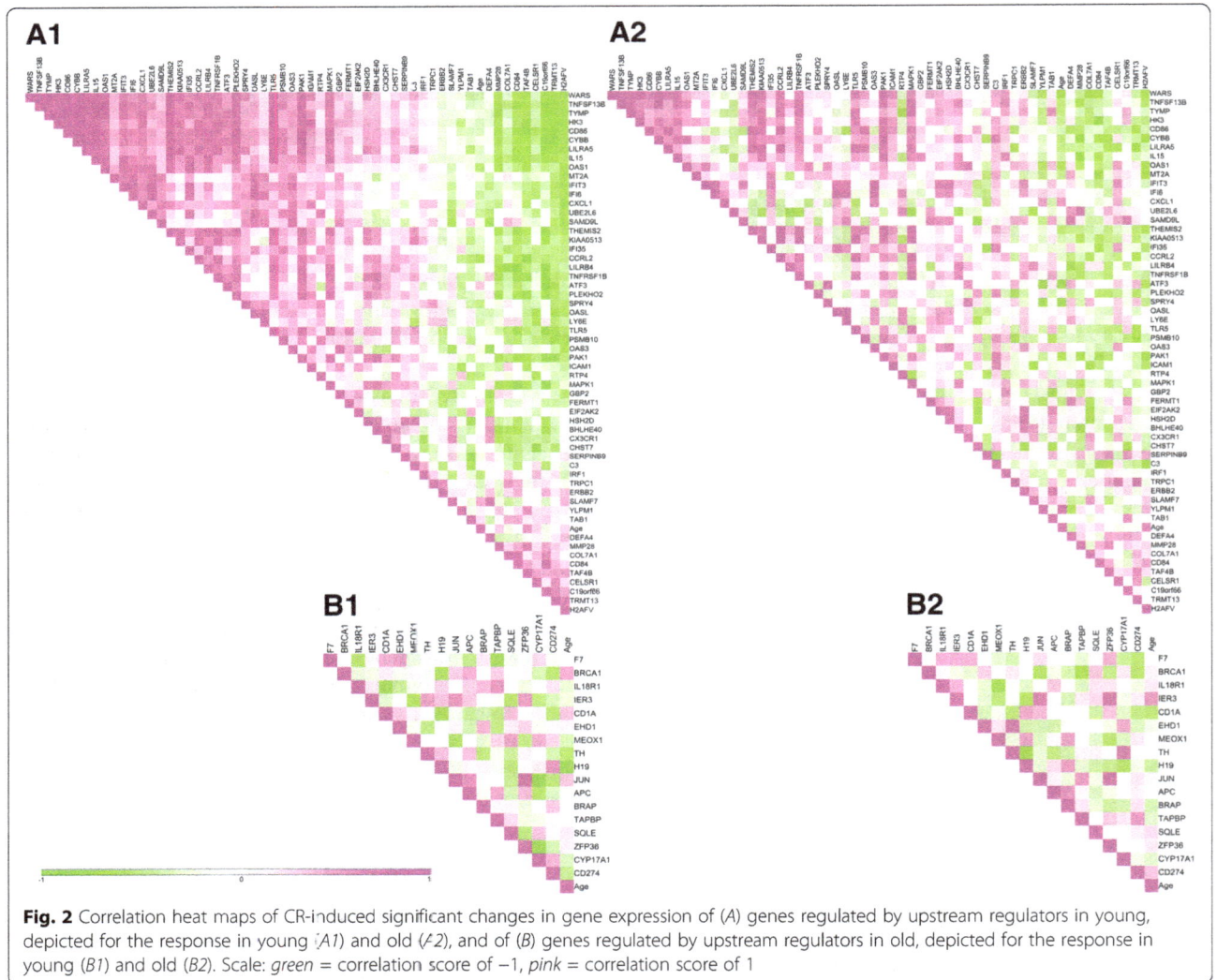

Fig. 2 Correlation heat maps of CR-induced significant changes in gene expression of (A) genes regulated by upstream regulators in young, depicted for the response in young (A1) and old (A2), and of (B) genes regulated by upstream regulators in old, depicted for the response in young (B1) and old (B2). Scale: green = correlation score of −1, pink = correlation score of 1

of CR on immune response-related gene expression have been shown before; 8 weeks of CR in middle-aged obese men downregulated the expression of genes involved in immune response in PBMCs [7]. The response of these middle-aged obese men is similar to the response of young men in our study. One reason why we do not see the response in old men might be due to 'immunosenescence' [24], known to take place in elderly individuals above 65 years of age. Immunosenescence means the loss of immune functions and is characterised by an increase in the expression of inflammation- and immune response-related genes [10]. Although the overlap between the genes in this paper and in the current study is minimal, we also observed an increase in gene expression and a predicted activation of transcriptional regulators involved in immune pathways, i.e. IFNA2 and IFNG, in old men at baseline when compared to young. Upon CR, a decreased activation of IFNA2 and IFNG was only observed in young men. MAPK1 was activated

upon CR. MAPK1 represses the expression of IFNG-induced genes via DNA-binding [16]. An increase in MAPK1 might have affected the decrease in IFNG-induced genes. The potential immunosenescence present at baseline may be the reason why we do not see a response on immune-related pathways upon CR in the old men. This is further illustrated by the correlation heat maps of immune-related genes in which high correlations are observed between gene expression responses in young men and far less pronounced effects are observed in old men. Old men seem to have lost the ability to change gene expression in immune response upon CR. This inability to change expression might be due to a potential advanced aging-related state of epigenetics, keeping the DNA structure in a more rigid structure and making it less likely to change gene expression. Either 3 weeks of 30 % CR is not sufficient to reduce the higher gene expression of immune-related genes in old men or the age-related potential epigenetic changes are

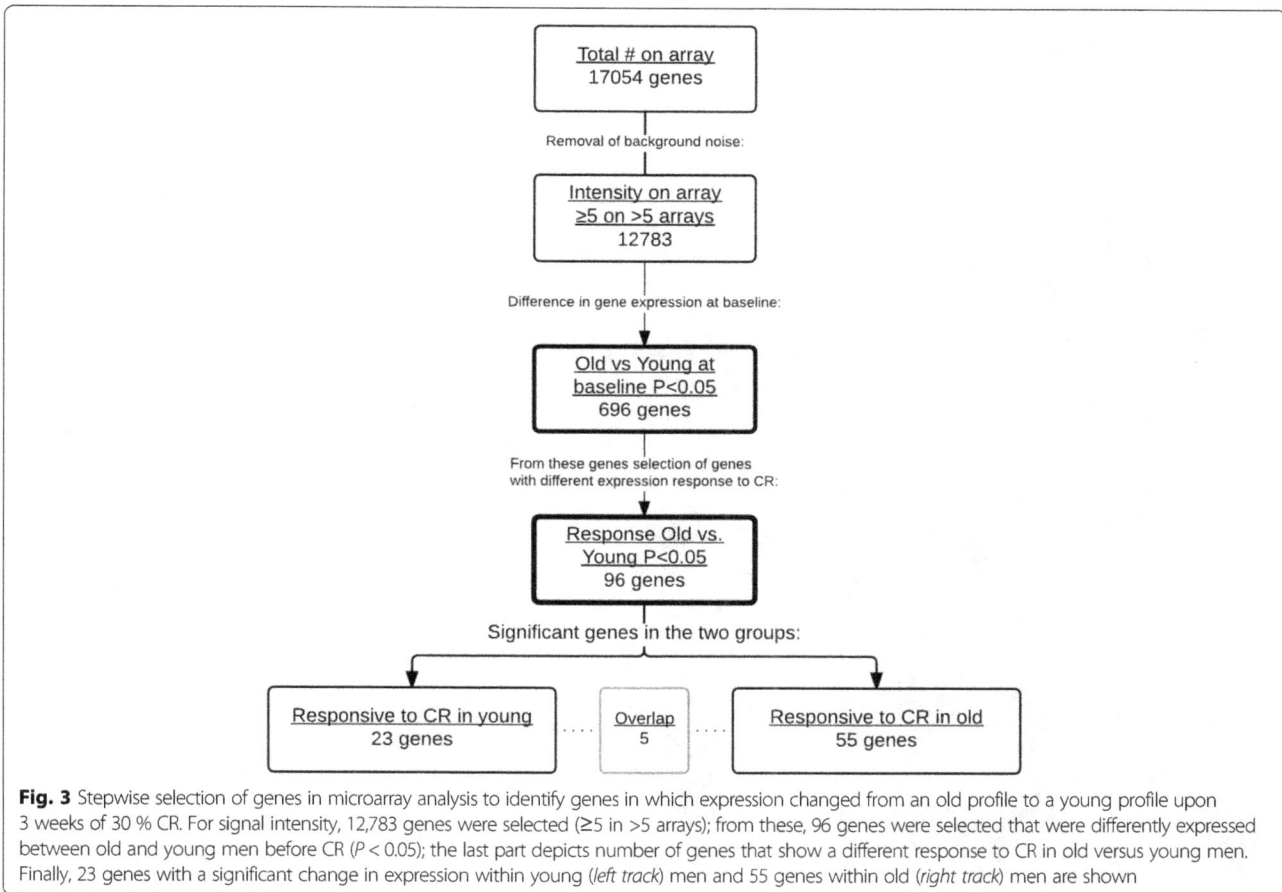

Fig. 3 Stepwise selection of genes in microarray analysis to identify genes in which expression changed from an old profile to a young profile upon 3 weeks of 30 % CR. For signal intensity, 12,783 genes were selected (≥5 in >5 arrays); from these, 96 genes were selected that were differently expressed between old and young men before CR (P < 0.05); the last part depicts number of genes that show a different response to CR in old versus young men. Finally, 23 genes with a significant change in expression within young (*left track*) men and 55 genes within old (*right track*) men are shown

too strong to overcome with CR and CR should be started at an earlier age. Three weeks of CR also resulted in a downregulated expression of genes involved in glucose metabolism in young men only. We did not find a difference in the expression of genes involved in glucose metabolism at baseline between old and young men, even though aging is known to have a diminishing effect on adequate glucose metabolism [9]. Aging might, however, have played a role in the nonresponsive effect of our short-term CR on glucose metabolism-related pathways in old men.

The decreased expression of genes related to olfactory signalling pathways in old men has not been described in the literature. However, other studies in fruit flies have been done in which the absence of odorants from nutrients affected the expression of odorant-binding proteins [26]. In addition, it has been described before in yeast that CR has an increasing effect on the expression of genes involved in RNA processing [5] as seen in our study for both young and old men.

Although old men did not respond with the same changes on immune response and glucose metabolism, many genes did show a change in expression upon CR. We identified a group of genes that changed from an 'old' expression level towards a 'young' expression level upon

CR. This was in line with the finding that the expression of genes from the skeletal muscle tissue of middle-aged subjects of the Caloric Restriction Society matched closer to gene expression profiles of younger subjects than to gene expression profiles of age-matched controls [21]. We could, however, not find any clear signalling route, pathway, or network for these genes.

It should be mentioned that both baseline differences and differences in gene expression changes between young and old can be due to different subpopulations of immune cells in the PBMCs between the groups. During aging, involution of the thymus, responsible for production of naïve T cells, leads to a shift in the T cell population [14]. Unfortunately, we did not have the opportunity to determine PBMC subpopulations. Furthermore, a period of 3 weeks of CR is short and might not have been long enough to induce changes in the gene expression of old men. A strength of our study design is the completely controlled dietary run-in period of 2 weeks and the completely controlled dietary 30 % CR intervention of 3 weeks which excludes a potential effect of habitual diet differences between the young and old men on gene expression differences at baseline and on gene expression response upon CR.

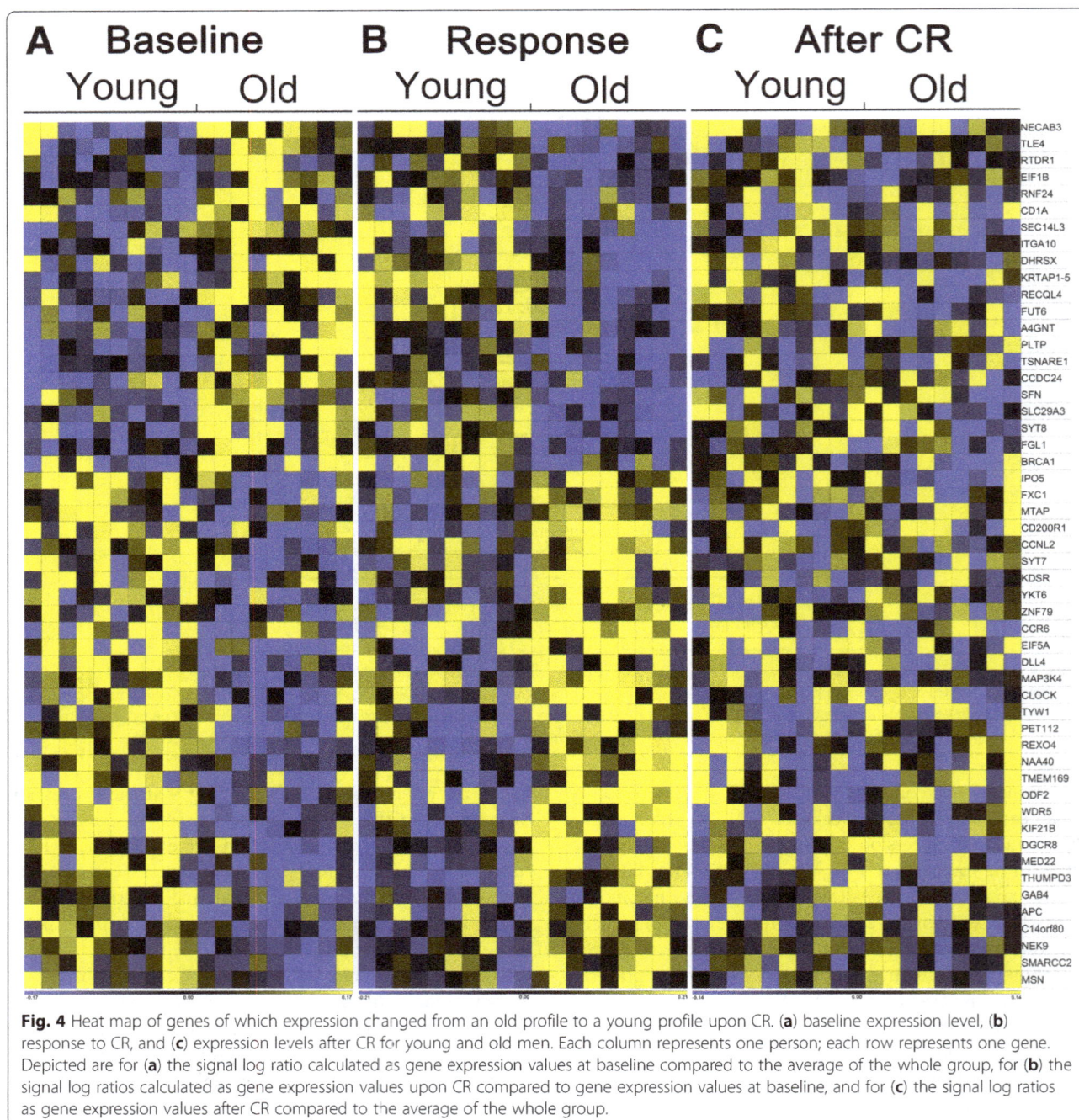

Fig. 4 Heat map of genes of which expression changed from an old profile to a young profile upon CR. (**a**) baseline expression level, (**b**) response to CR, and (**c**) expression levels after CR for young and old men. Each column represents one person; each row represents one gene. Depicted are for (**a**) the signal log ratio calculated as gene expression values at baseline compared to the average of the whole group, for (**b**) the signal log ratios calculated as gene expression values upon CR compared to gene expression values at baseline, and for (**c**) the signal log ratios as gene expression values after CR compared to the average of the whole group.

Conclusions

In our study, the expression of genes involved in immune response pathways was higher in old compared to young men at baseline. Three-week 30 % CR did not affect this higher immune-related gene expression in old men whereas it did reduce immune-related gene expression in young men. Due to our small sample size, we cannot draw solid conclusions about the relevance of age on the effect of CR on gene expression changes of

pathways important for healthy aging. We hypothesise based on immune-related gene expression changes in men that for a short period of 30 % CR a young onset has more potential benefit than an old onset.

Methods
Study population and eligibility criteria
Our study population was a subgroup of participants who participated in a previously reported controlled-feeding

trial [34]. Male Caucasian participants were recruited, by publishing advertisements in local newspapers and by sending out general e-mails to an e-mail list of persons who had indicated their interest in participating in studies of our university, at Wageningen University (The Netherlands), in October 2007 till January 2008, and followed up until the 15th of March 2008. Participants were excluded based on the following criteria: body mass index (BMI, kg/m^2) less than 20 or higher than 30, adherence to a weight-reduction or medically prescribed diet, dementia (Mini-Mental State Examination score <21), diabetes, anaemia, gastrointestinal disorders, use of drugs known to interfere with energy balance, or a history of medical or surgical events known to affect the study outcome. Participants were divided based on their age into young (20–40 years) and old (65–85 years) men. Based on these criteria, 15 young and 17 old men were included in the original study at Wageningen University (The Netherlands) [34]. Microarray analyses were performed on high-quality PBMC RNA of ten young men, age range 20–28 years, and nine old men, age range 64–85 years (Fig. 5).

Each of the participants was informed about the design and purpose of the study, and each of the participants provided written informed consent. The Medical Ethical Committee of Wageningen University (The Netherlands) approved the study. This clinical study was registered with ClinicalTrials.gov as NCT00561145.

Study design

The original study consisted of three subsequent phases as described previously [34] and was all carried out at the Division of Human Nutrition of Wageningen University (The Netherlands). Only samples collected after phases 1 and 2 are the subject of the current paper. Phase 1 (days 1–14): controlled dietary intervention in which each of the participants had to remain weight stable. Each of the participants was provided with a diet containing approximately 90 % of their estimated total daily energy requirement. The remaining 10 % was chosen from a list of choice items. In phase 2 (days 15–35): each of the participants was provided with a diet containing 70 % of the energy consumed during the last 3 days of phase 1. Composition of the diets was determined as described in [34]. Blood samples were taken at the end of phase 1, before CR, and at the end of phase 2, after CR.

PBMC RNA isolation and microarray processing

PBMCs were isolated from whole blood using BD Vacutainer® Cell Preparation Tubes™ according to the manufacturer's instructions. Total RNA was isolated from PBMC samples using TRIzol reagent (Invitrogen, Breda, The Netherlands) and purified using Qiagen RNeasy Micro Kit (Qiagen, Venlo, The Netherlands). RNA integrity was checked with Agilent 2100 Bioanalyzer (Agilent Technologies, Amstelveen, The Netherlands). Total RNA (500 ng/sample) was labelled using a one-cycle cDNA labelling kit (MessageAmpTM II-Biotin Enhanced Kit; Ambion Inc., Nieuwerkerk aan de IJssel, The Netherlands) and hybridised to human whole genome GeneChip arrays encoding 17,054 genes, designed by the European Nutrigenomics Organization and manufactured by Affymetrix (Santa Clara, CA). Sample labelling, hybridization to chips, and image scanning were performed according to the manufacturer's instructions.

Microarray data analysis

Quality control was performed and fulfilled the criteria for array hybridisation suggested by the Tumor Analysis Best Practices Working Group [30].

Microarrays were analysed using reorganised oligonucleotide probes as described by Dai et al. [8]. All individual probes for a gene were combined, allowing the

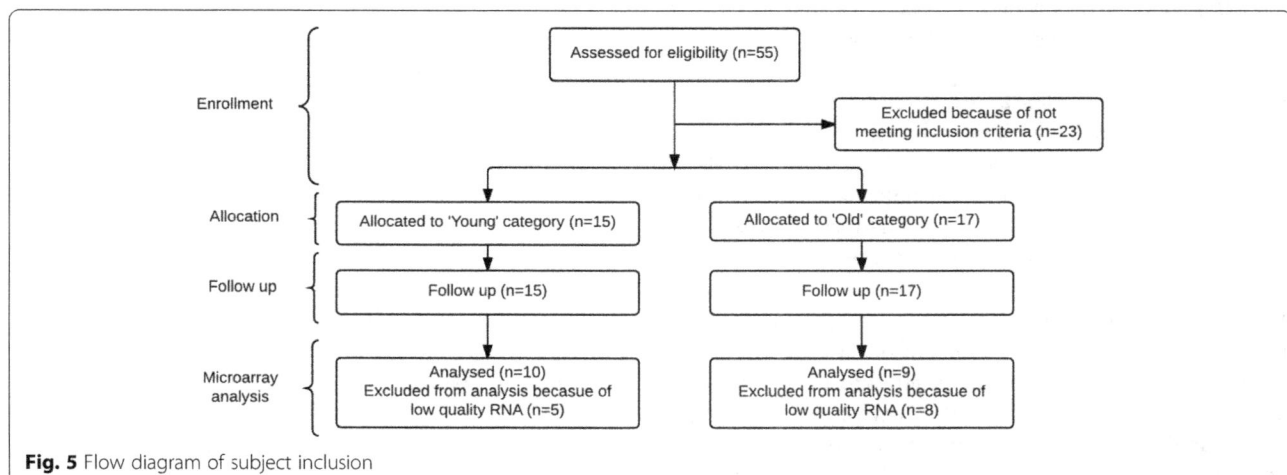

Fig. 5 Flow diagram of subject inclusion

possibility to detect overall transcription activity on the basis of latest genome and transcriptome information, rather than on the basis of Affymetrix probe set annotation. Expression values were calculated with the Robust Multi-array Average (RMA) method and quantile normalised [1, 17]. Only probe sets with normalised signals >5 on ≥5 arrays were defined as expressed and selected for analysis. This normalisation level was chosen because of a low microarray intensity level, due to the use of expired microarrays. It has, however, been shown that microarray data generated by microarrays more than 4 years past the manufacturer's expiration date had lower signal intensities but were highly specific and consistent with those from unexpired microarrays [33]. We used microarrays within 2 years of the expiry date.

Individual genes were defined as changed when comparison of the average normalised signal intensities showed a P value <0.05 in a two-tailed paired t test with Bayesian correction (Limma) [29]. Filtered data were analysed with Gene Set Enrichment Analysis (GSEA; GSEA/MSigDB website v3.87 released April 4, 2013). Significantly regulated gene sets were defined with a false discovery rate of <0.25. Gene sets were visualised and clustered using Cytoscape [28], which enabled the identification of clusters of gene sets. Ingenuity Pathway Analysis version 8.5 (Ingenuity Systems, Redwood City, CA) was also used for pathway analysis and upstream regulator analysis, but because of similar results, only GSEA results are displayed. Ingenuity Pathway Analysis has been performed based on findings from human experiments.

For upstream regulator analysis at baseline, genes with a significant different expression at baseline were included (P < 0.05). For young, genes with a significant different response upon CR in young were included ($P < 0.05$), and for old, genes with a significant different response upon CR in old were included ($P < 0.05$). For correlation heat maps, target genes of the upstream regulators were included if they also had a significantly different response between old and young ($P < 0.05$) upon CR. Array data have been submitted to Gene Expression Omnibus under accession number GSE63117.

Statistical analysis of clinical measurements

The statistical package SPSS (version 15.0; SPSS Inc, Chicago, IL) was used for analysis of the following data: expression changes within age groups were determined by paired t tests, and differential changes between age groups were determined by unpaired t tests.

Availability of supporting data

The data set supporting the results of this article is available in the Gene Expression Omnibus repository, under accession number GSE63117, at http://www.ncbi.nlm.nih.gov/geo/. Additional data can be found in supplemental files. Additional file 2 contains the Quality Control report,

Additional file 3 contains gene expression analysis, Additional file 4 contains GSEA outputs, and Additional file 5 contains IPA outputs.

Additional files

Additional file 1: Table S1. Predicted upstream regulators. Predicted difference before CR between old and young, in the response of young, the response in old, and the difference upon CR between old and young.

Additional file 2: Complete quality control report of microarrays.

Additional file 3: Gene expression file with expression analysis (A) baseline, (B) response to intervention in old men compared to response to intervention in young men, and (C) genes in old towards a young expression profile.

Additional file 4: Gene Set Enrichment Analysis outputs for (A) old men compared to young men before intervention, (B) response to intervention in young men, (C) response to intervention in old men, and (D) response to intervention in old men compared to response to intervention in young men.

Additional file 5: Ingenuity Pathway Analysis Upstream regulators output used for Additional file 1: Table S1 (A) baseline, (B) response to intervention in young men, and (C) response to intervention in old men.

Abbreviations

BMI: body mass index; CR: caloric restriction; GSEA: Gene Set Enrichment Analysis; PBMCs: peripheral blood mononuclear cells; RMA: Robust Multi-Array Average.

Competing interests

The authors declare that they have no competing interests.

Authors' contributions

CPGMG conceived and designed the experiments. JAS and IPGB performed the experiments. IPGB and LAA analysed the data. IPGB wrote the paper. MM and LAA critically revised the manuscript for important intellectual content. All authors read and approved the final manuscript.

Acknowledgements

We thank the participants, Mechteld Grootte-Bromhaar, Jenny Jansen, the nurses, and dieticians, for their practical work during the study. Furthermore, we thank Philip de Groot and Mark Boekschoten for helping with microarray analysis.

Author details

[1]Division of Human Nutrition, Wageningen University, Bomenweg 2, 6703 HD Wageningen, The Netherlands. [2]Current Address: Norwich Medical School, University of East Anglia, Norwich NR4 7TJ, UK. [3]Division of Human Nutrition, Wageningen University & Research centre, PO BOX 8129, NL-6700 EV Wageningen, The Netherlands.

References

1. Bolstad BM, Irizarry RA, Astrand M, Speed TP. A comparison of normalization methods for high density oligonucleotide array data based on variance and bias. Bioinformatics. 2003;19(2):185–93.
2. Bouwens M, Afman LA, Muller M. Fasting induces changes in peripheral blood mononuclear cell gene expression profiles related to increases in fatty acid beta-oxidation: functional role of peroxisome proliferator activated receptor alpha in human peripheral blood mononuclear cells. Am J Clin Nutr. 2007;86(5):1515–23.
3. Caimari A, Oliver P, Keijer J, Palou A. Peripheral blood mononuclear cells as a model to study the response of energy homeostasis-related genes to

acute changes in feeding conditions. OMICS. 2010;14(2):129–41. doi:10.1089/omi.2009.0092.

4. Castello L, Froio T, Cavallini G, Biasi F, Sapino A, Leonarduzzi G, et al. Calorie restriction protects against age-related rat aorta sclerosis. FASEB J. 2005; 19(13):1863–5. doi:10.1096/fj.04-2864fje.

5. Choi KM, Kwon YY, Lee CK. Characterization of global gene expression during assurance of lifespan extension by caloric restriction in budding yeast. Exp Gerontol. 2013;48(12):1455–68. doi:10.1016/j.exger.2013.10.001.

6. Colman RJ, Anderson RM, Johnson SC, Kastman EK, Kosmatka KJ, Beasley TM, et al. Caloric restriction delays disease onset and mortality in rhesus monkeys. Science. 2009;325(5937):201–4. doi:10.1126/science.1173635.

7. Crujeiras AB, Parra D, Milagro FI, Goyenechea E, Larrarte E, Margareto J, et al. Differential expression of oxidative stress and inflammation related genes in peripheral blood mononuclear cells in response to a low-calorie diet: a nutrigenomics study. OMICS. 2008;12(4):251–61. doi:10.1089/omi.2008.0001.

8. Dai M, Wang P, Boyd AD, Kostov G, Athey B, Jones EG, et al. Evolving gene/ transcript definitions significantly alter the interpretation of GeneChip data. Nucleic Acids Res. 2005;33(20):e175. doi:10.1093/nar/gni179.

9. Davidson MB. The effect of aging on carbohydrate metabolism: a review of the English literature and a practical approach to the diagnosis of diabetes mellitus in the elderly. Metab Clin Exp. 1979;28(6):688–705.

10. de Magalhaes JP, Curado J, Church GM. Meta-analysis of age-related gene expression profiles identifies common signatures of aging. Bioinformatics. 2009;25(7):875–81. doi:10.1093/bioinformatics/btp073.

11. Fontana L, Meyer TE, Klein S, Holloszy JO. Long-term calorie restriction is highly effective in reducing the risk for atherosclerosis in humans. Proc Natl Acad Sci U S A. 2004;101(17):6659–63. doi:10.1073/pnas.0308291101.

12. Fontana L, Villareal DT, Weiss EP, Racette SB, Steger-May K, Klein S, et al. Calorie restriction or exercise: effects on coronary heart disease risk factors. A randomized, controlled trial. Am J Physiol Endocrinol Metab. 2007;293(1): E197–202. doi:10.1152/ajpendo.00102.2007.

13. Gerbase-DeLima M, Liu RK, Cheney KE, Mickey R, Walford RL. Immune function and survival in a long-lived mouse strain subjected to undernutrition. Gerontologia. 1975;21(4):184–202.

14. Gruver AL, Hudson LL, Sempowski GD. Immunosenescence of ageing. J Pathol. 2007;211(2):144–56. doi:10.1002/path.2104.

15. Holloszy JO, Fontana L. Caloric restriction in humans. Exp Gerontol. 2007; 42(8):709–12. doi:10.1016/j.exger.2007.03.009.

16. Hu S, Xie Z, Onishi A, Yu X, Jiang L, Lin J, et al. Profiling the human protein-DNA interactome reveals ERK2 as a transcriptional repressor of interferon signaling. Cell. 2009;139(3):610–22. doi:10.1016/j.cell.2009.08.037.

17. Irizarry RA, Bolstad BM, Collin F, Cope LM, Hobbs B, Speed TP. Summaries of Affymetrix GeneChip probe level data. Nucleic Acids Res. 2003;31(4):e15.

18. Jiang JC, Jaruga E, Repnevskaya MV, Jazwinski SM. An intervention resembling caloric restriction prolongs life span and retards aging in yeast. FASEB J. 2000;14(14):2135–7. doi:10.1096/fj.00-0242fje.

19. Masoro EJ. Overview of caloric restriction and ageing. Mech Ageing Dev. 2005;126(9):913–22. doi:10.1016/j.mad.2005.03.012.

20. Mattison JA, Roth GS, Beasley TM, Tilmont EM, Handy AM, Herbert RL, et al. Impact of caloric restriction on health and survival in rhesus monkeys from the NIA study. Nature. 2012. doi:10.1038/nature11432.

21. Mercken EM, Crosby SD. Lamming DW, Jebailey L, Krzysik-Walker S, Villareal D, et al. Calorie restriction in humans inhibits the PI3K/AKT pathway and induces a younger transcription profile. Aging Cell. 2013. doi:10.1111/acel.12088.

22. Pallavi R, Giorgio M, Pelicci PG. Insights into the beneficial effect of caloric/ dietary restriction for a healthy and prolonged life. Front Physiol. 2012;3:318. doi:10.3389/fphys.2012.00318.

23. Park SK, Prolla TA. Lessons learned from gene expression profile studies of aging and caloric restriction. Ageing Res Rev. 2005;4(1):55–65. doi:10.1016/j.arr.2004.09.003.

24. Pawelec G. Immunosenescence comes of age. Symposium on aging research in immunology: the impact of genomics. EMBO Rep. 2007;8(3):220–3. doi:10.1038/sj.embor.7400922.

25. Plank M, Wuttke D, van Dam S, Clarke SA, de Magalhaes JP. A meta-analysis of caloric restriction gene expression profiles to infer common signatures and regulatory mechanisms. Mol Biosyst. 2012;8(4):1339–49. doi:10.1039/c2mb05255e.

26. Pletcher SD. The modulation of lifespan by perceptual systems. Ann N Y Acad Sci. 2009;1170:693–7. doi:10.1111/j.1749-6632.2009.04926.x.

27. Ribaric S. Diet and aging. Oxidative Med Cell Longev. 2012;2012:741468. doi:10.1155/2012/741468.

28. Shannon P, Markiel A, Ozier O, Baliga NS, Wang JT, Ramage D, et al. Cytoscape: a software environment for integrated models of biomolecular interaction networks. Genome Res. 2003;13(11):2498–504. doi:10.1101/gr. 1239303.

29. Smyth GK. Linear models and empirical Bayes methods for assessing differential expression in microarray experiments. Stat Appl Genet Mol Biol. 2004;3:Article3. doi:10.2202/1544-6115.1027.

30. Tumor Analysis Best Practices Working G. Expression profiling—best practices for data generation and interpretation in clinical trials. Nat Rev Genet. 2004;5(3):229–37. doi:10.1038/nrg1297.

31. Walker G, Houthoofd K, Vanfleteren JR, Gems D. Dietary restriction in C. elegans: from rate-of-living effects to nutrient sensing pathways. Mech Ageing Dev. 2005;126(9):929–37. doi:10.1016/j.mad.2005.03.014.

32. Weindruch R, Sohal RS. Seminars in medicine of the Beth Israel Deaconess Medical Center. Caloric intake and aging. N Engl J Med. 1997;337(14):986–94. doi:10.1056/NEJM199710023371407.

33. Wen Z, Wang C, Shi Q, Huang Y, Su Z, Hong H, et al. Evaluation of gene expression data generated from expired Affymetrix GeneChip(R) microarrays using MAQC reference RNA samples. BMC Bioinformatics. 2010;11 Suppl 6: S10. doi:10.1186/1471-2105-11-S6-S10.

34. Winkels RM, Jolink-Stoppelenburg A, de Graaf K, Siebelink E, Mars M, de Groot L. Energy intake compensation after 3 weeks of restricted energy intake in young and elderly men. J Am Med Dir Assoc. 2011;12(4):277–86. doi:10.1016/j.jamda.2010.08.011.

12

Ranges of phenotypic flexibility in healthy subjects

T. J. van den Broek, G. C. M. Bakker, C. M. Rubingh, S. Bijlsma, J. H. M. Stroeve, B. van Ommen, M. J. van Erk and S. Wopereis*

Abstract

Background: A key feature of metabolic health is the ability to adapt upon dietary perturbations. A systemic review defined an optimal nutritional challenge test, the "PhenFlex test" (PFT). Recently, it has been shown that the PFT enables the quantification of all relevant metabolic processes involved in maintaining or regaining homeostasis of metabolic health. Furthermore, it was demonstrated that quantification of PFT response was more sensitive as compared to fasting markers in demonstrating reduced phenotypic flexibility in metabolically impaired type 2 diabetes subjects.

Methods: This study aims to demonstrate that quantification of PFT response can discriminate between different states of health within the healthy range of the population. Therefore, 100 healthy subjects were enrolled (50 males, 50 females) ranging in age (young, middle, old) and body fat percentage (low, medium, high), assuming variation in phenotypic flexibility. Biomarkers were selected to quantify main processes which characterize phenotypic flexibility in response to PFT: flexibility in glucose, lipid, amino acid and vitamin metabolism, and metabolic stress. Individual phenotypic flexibility was visualized using the "health space" by representing the four processes on the health space axes. By quantifying and presenting the study subjects in this space, individual phenotypic flexibility was visualized.

Results: Using the "health space" visualization, differences between groups as well as within groups from the healthy range of the population can be easily and intuitively assessed. The health space showed a different adaptation to the metabolic PhenFlex test in the extremes of the recruited population; persons of young age with low to normal fat percentage had a markedly different position in the health space as compared to persons from old age with normal to high fat percentage.

Conclusion: The results of the metabolic PhenFlex test in conjunction with the health space reliably assessed health on an individual basis. This quantification can be used in the future for personalized health quantification and advice.

Keywords: Metabolic health, Personalized health, Nutritional challenge, Data visualization, Challenge test

Background

In this paper, we present a comprehensive strategy with the ultimate goal of quantifying and visualizing (personal) health across a range of healthy phenotypes from the general population. We reach this goal by using a nutritional challenge test as a procedure of health assessment, coupled to a novel statistical visualization method.

A crucial aspect of health is the ability to maintain homeostasis under a large variety of continuously changing environmental conditions. Viewing health as a function of the resilience to daily stressors makes measuring phenotypic flexibility a necessary part of the quantification of health [1].

A pivotal part of the strategy presented here is the ability to assess this resilience in human subjects. Measuring the response to a (nutritional) challenge allows to quantify the metabolic ability of an individual to deal with a copious meal, and as such to assess metabolic health. Previously, it was shown that quantification of challenge-response significantly contributes to demonstrating health effects of food and nutrition in dietary intervention studies [2–4]. A standardized optimal nutritional challenge test was defined after the performance of a systematic literature review [5], which was named the "PhenFlex test" (PFT). Recently, this "PhenFlex test" was characterized,

* Correspondence: suzan.wopereis@tno.nl
TNO, Utrechtseweg 48, 3704 HE Zeist, The Netherlands

where 132 parameters were quantified during the 8-h response time course, that report on 26 metabolic processes distributed over seven organs (gut, liver, adipose, pancreas, vasculature, muscle, kidney) and systemic stress [6]. It showed that the adaptive capacities of the most relevant metabolic processes can be modulated by PFT. Furthermore, it was demonstrated that the PFT and defined new biomarkers are reliable in discriminating metabolically impaired subjects with type 2 diabetes from healthy subjects, since it was a more sensitive, early, and meaningful measure than the corresponding overnight fasting measure [6]. For these reasons, the quantification of the response after a (nutritional) challenge may be a good alternative for the "classic (i.e., overnight fasting) biomarkers" in nutritional and health sciences. A major remaining challenge in this field is the accurate assessment of the effect of food and nutrition on the health status of individuals, particularly in healthy subjects. Current methods used in nutritional research stem mainly from pharmaceutical and medical research, which traditionally focus on (effects from treatment on) disease, evaluating overnight fasting concentrations of certain (surrogate) biomarkers reflecting disease symptoms. This results in current nutritional science attempting to demonstrate nutritional health effects by using these surrogate or disease-related markers. Nutrition does not interact with a specific target like most drugs, but instead interacts simultaneously on a number of metabolic pathways and functions. Furthermore, the magnitude of nutritional effects is often much lower than that of commonly observed for drugs [7, 8]. Because lifestyle and nutritional interventions in many cases enhance processes that restore or maintain homeostasis, we posit that the assessment of resilience is essential for determining the impact of these interventions on health [9]. To do so, it is important to characterize the response to PFT in the healthy range of the population, ranging from an optimal towards a suboptimal response to the PFT as a measure of health.

The current study aimed to assess the ability of PFT to quantify flexibility in the healthy range of the population and whether it is possible to discriminate between optimal and suboptimal flexibility and therefore evaluated PFT response in 100 healthy male and female volunteers. We hypothesized that male and female subjects of higher age (60–70 years of age) and normal to high body fat percentage would respond differently to PFT as compared to young subjects (20–30 years of age) with a low to normal body fat percentage. Furthermore, we hypothesized that increasing adiposity (in terms of body fat percentage) would decrease phenotypic flexibility resulting in a higher metabolic age. The study is part of a larger endeavor, aiming to develop a set of standardized tools to substantiate health effects of dietary interventions [6]. Standardization of the nutritional challenge is important in generating a solid base of comparable evidence. Only with the use of a standardized challenge test, study results will be comparable and interpretable across studies. The parameters measured during the 8-h response PFT time course cover flexibility in glucose, lipid, and amino acid and vitamin metabolism as well as metabolic stress. A large section of the parameters within this selection is obtained by applying metabolic profiling, which allows for the simultaneous measurement of the challenge response for a large contingent of parameters at once and has been applied extensively in nutrition and health research [10–13]. All of the biochemical parameters measured in this study were also quantified in the previous study, allowing for the integration of both studies permitting the comparison of PFT response of the healthy range of the male population with the PFT response from 20 type 2 diabetic male subjects. To evaluate PFT responses, a statistical visualization methodology called "health space" was applied as described earlier by Bouwman et al. [14].

Concretely, we use the PFT challenge, administered to 100 healthy individuals from a range of phenotypes, together with the application of the health space modeling technique to assess and visualize phenotypic flexibility as a measure of health. The emphasis in this study lies on the visualization and comparison of phenotypic flexibility in a range of healthy phenotypes, reflecting the general population. We show that PFT challenge with the biomarker subset and health space visualization tool form a nutrition research toolbox that can be used for readily interpretable substantiation of health effects from interventions as well as for personalized health quantification and advice.

Methods

Subjects

The study was conducted at the Center for Human Drug Research (CHDR) in Leiden, the Netherlands. Study participants were recruited from the CHDR volunteer database and via study-specific advertisements in local media and over the internet. All subjects gave written informed consent, and the study was approved by the Independent Ethics Committee of Leiden University Medical Center (LUMC), the Netherlands. The study was conducted according to the principles of the Helsinki Declaration and in accordance with the Dutch Medical Research in Human Subjects Act (WMO). The study was performed in compliance with good clinical practice (GCP). The trial was retrospectively registered on 12 May 2017 with ID: ISRCTN10600261.

This was a single-center, explorative, open-label study among 100 healthy subjects (50 males, 50 females). All subjects were aged between 19 and 71 years and were equally assigned to ten groups based on combinations of the three phenotypic characteristics: age, body fat percentage, and gender. The groups present in the study are outlined in Table 1. Body adiposity was determined using bioelectrical impedance analysis using an Inbody 720 body composition analyzer (Biospace Co., Ltd., Korea), and subjects were grouped according to body fat percentage qualifiers (low, normal and high) as seen in the last column of Table 1. All of the groups mentioned in Table 1 contain ten individuals, for a total of 100 subjects. Phenotypic groups 1 and 6 were selected to represent "optimal phenotypic flexibility" as it is commonly perceived, while groups 5 and 10 were selected to represent "reduced phenotypic flexibility." These will be referred to as the two reference groups. The two reference groups were used for the creation of the health space model representing the two extremes of phenotypic flexibility. The other individuals were grouped according to a combination of age and adiposity, representing a range of healthy phenotypes as commonly found in the general population. These will be referred to as "healthy range of phenotypes" and were used for evaluation of PhenFlex challenge test response and its ability to discriminate between different states of health.

Design

All subjects were given the PhenFlex test (PFT) in the morning after an overnight fast (≥ 10 h). On study days before the first blood draw, a cannula was placed and blood samples were taken at $t = 0$ (fasting) and six time-points ($t = 0.5$, $t = 1$, $t = 2$, $t = 4$, $t = 6$, and $t = 8$ h) after consumption of the PFT. Subjects were not allowed to eat or drink until the last blood sampling, except from drinking water. Subjects were instructed to eat the same meal on the evening before the study day. Subjects were instructed to refrain from heavy physical activity/sports, alcohol, paracetamol, NSAIDs (i.e., ibuprofen, aspirin) starting 24 h before each study day.

PhenFlex challenge

The 400 mL beverage consisted of a mixture of 12.40% (w/w) palm olein, 17.25% (w/w) dextrose, 4.13% (w/w) Protifar® (Nutricia), 0.10% (w/w) vanilla flavor, 0.12% (w/w) trisodium citrate, 0.08% (w/w) sodium hydroxide, and 66.12% (w/w) water. This resulted in a drink of 3950 kJ/ 950 kCal with a macronutrient composition of 60 g fat (of which 39% saturated fatty acids, 47% monounsaturated fatty acids, 14% polyunsaturated fatty acids), 75 g glucose, 5 g polysaccharides, and 20 g protein (analyzed by TNO Triskelion BV). The food-grade production of the beverage took place at the NIZO food research processing center in accordance with HACCP principles.

Metabolic plasma parameters

Blood samples were collected in tubes containing clot activator for serum or in ice-chilled tubes containing Li-heparin or ethylenediaminetetraacetic acid (K_2EDTA) as an anticoagulant for plasma and whole blood. In addition to K_2EDTA, aprotinin was added to tubes for glucose-related parameters. After centrifugation (for 15 min at approximately $2000 \times g$ at approximately 4 °C within 30 min after collection), plasma and serum samples were stored at ≤ -20 °C for clinical chemistry and ≤ -70 °C for all other parameters. The following parameters were measured at 0 h (fasting) and six post-prandial time-points (0.5, 1, 2, 4, 6, and 8 h): clinical chemistry in serum—total cholesterol, HDL-cholesterol, LDL-cholesterol, triglycerides, nonesterified free fatty acids (NEFA), glucose,

Table 1 Phenotypic groups of participants included in the study

Gender	Age (years)	Group nr.	Phenotypic group	Body fat %	
Male	20–29	1	Reference group "optimal phenotypic flexibility"	Low to normal	< 20%
	30–59	2	Healthy range of phenotypes	Low	30–39 years < 8% 40–59 years < 11%
		3		Normal	30–39 years 8–20% 40–59 years 11–22%
		4		High	30–39 years > 20% 40–59 years > 22%
	60–70	5	Reference group "reduced phenotypic flexibility"	Normal to high	> 20%
Female	20–29	6	Reference group "optimal phenotypic flexibility"	Low to normal	< 30%
	30–59	7	Healthy range of phenotypes	Low	30–39 years < 21% 40–59 years < 23%
		8		Normal	30–39 years 21–33% 40–59 years 23–34%
		9		High	30–39 years > 33% 40–59 years > 34%
	60–70	10	Reference group "reduced phenotypic flexibility"	Normal to high	> 30%

gamma-glutamyltransferase (GGT), ALAT, aspartate-aminotransferase (ASAT), alkaline phosphatase (ALP), albumin, and creatinine; glucose-related parameters—glucagon, insulin, and C-peptide in plasma by enzyme-linked immunosorbent assay (ELISA). Finally, GC metabolomics has been performed for the assessment of endogenous plasma metabolites by GCMS technology, where only a selection of a total of $n = 26$ amino acids and derivatives and ketone bodies were included according to the method described by Koek et al. [15]. All parameters were analyzed by TNO Triskelion BV.

Indexes and summations

The Matsuda index was calculated according to Matsuda et al. (Eq. 1) [16].

$$\frac{10000}{\sqrt{(\text{fasting insulin (mU/L)}) \times (\text{mean insulin (mU/L)}) \times (\text{mean glucose (mg/dL)})}} \tag{1}$$

The hepatic insulin resistance index (HIRI) was calculated by the validated method of Matsuda et al. (Eq. 2).

$$\text{fasting insulin (mU/L)} \times \text{fasting glucose (mg/dL)} \tag{2}$$

The concentration of non-essential amino acids was calculated as the sum of alanine, glutamine, glycine, proline, serine, and tyrosine. The concentration of aromatic amino acids (AAA) was calculated as the sum of phenylalanine, tyrosine, and tryptophan. The amount of branched-chain amino acids (BCAA) was calculated as the sum of isoleucine, leucine, and valine. Fisher's ratio was defined as BCAA to AAA ratio [17]. We also calculated the phenylalanine hydroxylase activity index which is the concentration of tyrosine divided by the concentration of phenylalanine [18]. Finally, also the vitamin C index was calculated as concentration of proline divided by the concentration of hydroxyproline [19].

Questionnaires

Apart from biomarkers derived from the blood, several questionnaires were administered: the State-Trait Anxiety Inventory (STAI), the short questionnaire to assess health-enhancing physical activity (SQUASH), and the food frequency questionnaire (FFQ) as well as screening questionnaires concerning disease, allergy, smoking, drug/alcohol, and sleep history and status, as well as education level and subjective evaluation of weight.

Area under the curve calculations

For all parameters measured during the dietary challenge, incremental areas under or over the baseline were calculated using the first measurement (0 h) as a reference. The term area under the curve (AUC) refers to both values, which were delineated as negative AUC (AUC–) and positive AUC (AUC+).

Questionnaire features

The inclusion of questionnaires in the health space model required conversion of answers into numerical values. Using each questionnaire question as a separate feature leads to sparse features; to prevent this, it was decided to summarize questionnaires to several constructed features. The feature "allergy" was composed of the questions: allergy for food or food components, allergy for iodine, allergy for latex, allergy for any medication, allergy for plasters, and any other allergy. The feature "disease" was composed of the questions to history of the following: cardiovascular disorder, gastrointestinal disorder, head/eyes/nose/throat disorder, hematological disorder, hepatic disorder, immunological disorder, endocrine/metabolic disorder, musculoskeletal disorder, neurological disorder, psychiatric disorder, pulmonary disorder, dermatological disorder, urogenital disorder, or any other disorder. This was done by setting the constructed feature value to 1 when any of the underlying questions reported positively and 0 when negative. Smoking, sleeping disorder, body weight perception, night-shift, and education level answers were converted to numerical values. Zero or 1 values were used for polar questions, while leveled answers were converted to – 1/0/1. Reported sleep hours were converted to numerical values. After the conversion, these questionnaire answers were used as features.

Health space analysis

To evaluate PFT responses, a statistical visualization methodology called "health space" was applied, described earlier by Bouwman et al. [14]. In the current approach, we have adapted this methodology to use two reference groups to define the health space. This means that the health space was constructed to reflect differences between subjects from the reference group with "optimal phenotypic flexibility" and subjects from the reference group with "reduced phenotypic flexibility." Having this predefined health space allowed for the visualization of individuals from "the healthy range of phenotypes," so that their position in this space reflects their health status. The positioning of the healthy range of individuals in the health space is based on the regression values of the health space model, and since the health space is defined according to the difference between the two reference groups, the individuals' health status is visualized on a spectrum ranging from one reference group to the other.

Axes were defined as four processes which characterize phenotypic flexibility, named (1) flexibility in glucose, (2) lipid, (3) amino acid and vitamin metabolism, and (4) metabolic stress. The first three axes represented metabolic components of phenotypic flexibility, while the fourth represented a measure of metabolic stress on the system as a whole. All measured parameters related to glucose metabolism and carbohydrate intake, lipid metabolism and fat intake, and amino acid metabolism and protein and vitamin intake were used for the axes named flexibility in glucose-, lipid-, amino acid and vitamin metabolism, respectively. The axis on metabolic stress was composed of parameters indicative for metabolic stress such as risk factors, injury markers, and well-being. Axes were not defined to be independent, since features were shared across axes. The metabolic stress axis had overlap with all other axes. The categories contain features from several types of data, namely clinical chemistry, metabolomics, anthropometry, several compound indices, and questionnaire answers. In order to utilize the data obtained during the challenge test in an interpretable way, the 0 h and the AUC– and AUC+ were used for plasma parameters. Subsequently, model performance and assessment of model overfitting with the selected features were evaluated according to the error rate. The error rate was defined as the misclassification rate of the two reference groups per axis of the health space model. For the model training, the "optimal phenotypic flexibility" reference group (aged 20–29, fat percentage low to normal) and the "reduced phenotypic flexibility" reference group (aged 60–70, fat percentage normal to high) were used. The model was trained to discriminate between these two reference groups using a separate tenfold double cross-validated (DCV) PLS-DA model for each of the four axes using their respective features. In this way, the model is repeated ten times in such a way that each individual has a 90% chance of being in the training or in the cross-validation set. In the DCV procedure, the model error was estimated independently of the model complexity and reported as a misclassification rate of the two reference groups per axis of the health space model and was calculated as the average percentage of individuals of the cross-validation set that is wrongly classified in each of the ten DCV-PLS-DA subtests. Since the health space model was composed of four different axes, four different error rates were being calculated. These error rates can be used to determine how relevant a biological process is for the separation of the two reference groups. In all analyses, all features were scaled to mean 0 and variance of 1. In every cross-validation step, the regression value for each parameter is saved (this equals the contribution of each biological compound to the model). Using these values, relative standard deviations (RSDs) of the regression value can be determined for each parameter. The order of magnitude of the RSD values gives an impression of the stability of the parameter for the importance of the discrimination between the reference groups in the axis and hence the

relevance to the health space model. An instable parameter (having a high RSD value) may be of biological importance but acts as noise in the health space model. The RSD values were used as variable selection criterion. Parameters with high RSD values (200, 100, or 50%) were removed from the dataset, and the model was built again. In statistics, this approach of variable selection is called jackknifing.

All features used for each axis after jackknifing of the first health space are listed in Table 2. In the output of the health space model, the relative absolute regression vector values indicate relative importance of the respective feature on an axis.

GCMS-based features from the subjects in this study were combined with the same GCMS features from subjects of [6] in the second health space. Due to the combination of GCMS results, the two study outcomes had to be aligned for the creation of this health space, as this GCMS method produced relative concentrations. To do this, GCMS-based features were centered and normalized around a common value. Features from both groups were normalized separately around the means of their respective healthy controls. Because questionnaires were not available for the subjects in the second study, all questionnaire-related features had to be omitted in this instance. For the training of this model, the same reference groups were used as in the original health space.

After model training, all individuals were assigned values for each axis according to the regression vectors provided by the trained model. The resulting four values per individual represent coordinates on the four predefined axes of the health space model. The same eapproach was taken for the health space that combines data from two different studies. All axes are biologically and statistically interdependent and can be directly visualized in a 4D space. Model output includes error rates indicative of model performance.

FlexScore

The FlexScore is a summarized ranking of subjects based on the preselected features. These preselected features were based on markers of which a higher or lower response to the PFT had a biological meaning in the sense that these could be interpreted as either beneficial or detrimental to health. Each subject was assigned a rank by summating all feature ranks for the subject. It is structured so that a higher score means less flexibility and vice versa. Additional file 1: Table S1 presents an overview of all features used for ranking.

For all features except Matsuda index, disposition index, and 3-hydroxybutanoic acid, rankings were made by ordering subjects from small to large values. For the remaining three features, subjects were ordered by values from large to small, as a small value for these

Table 2 The selected features for the four axes of the health space

Glucose	Coefficients	Lipid	Coefficients	AA and Vit	Coefficients	Metabolic stress	Coefficients
C-peptide (AUCp)	0.062	LDL (t0)	0.060	D-Glutamic acid (t0)	0.054	LDL (t0)	0.060
Total carbohydrates (Q)	− 0.060	Body fat %	0.059	L-Tyrosine (t0)	0.040	Cholesterol (t0)	0.059
Polysaccharides (Q)	− 0.058	Cholesterol (t0)	0.059	L-Isoleucine (AUCp)	0.040	Systolic blood pressure	0.055
Glucose (t0)	0.055	Waist circumference	0.055	Vitamin C index	0.038	Current weight (Q)	0.046
4-Methyl-2-oxovaleric-acid (t0)	− 0.052	BMI	0.055	Fisher ratio	− 0.036	GGTP (t0)	0.041
3-Methyl-2-oxo-valeric-acid (t0)	− 0.049	Systolic blood pressure	0.054	Iron index	− 0.035	Diastolic blood pressure	0.041
Insulin (AUCp)	0.045	Diastolic blood pressure	0.040	L-Phenylalanine (AUCp)	0.035	Triglyceride (AUCp)	0.040
Matsuda index	− 0.045	Triglyceride (AUCp)	0.040	L-Leucine (AUCp)	0.035	Triglyceride (t0)	0.038
L-Isoleucine (AUCp)	0.045	Triglyceride (t0)	0.038	Albumin (t0)	− 0.034	Education (Q)	− 0.038
Mono- and disaccharides (Q)	− 0.044	Body weight	0.037	D-Glutamic acid (AUCn)	− 0.033	Glucose (t0)	0.037
Hepatic insulin resistance (HC)	0.041	Waist-hip ratio	0.037	Vitamin B6 (Q)	− 0.033	L-Tyrosine (t0)	0.031
Glucose (AUCp)	0.040	Triglyceride (AUCn)	0.028	Phenylalanine hydroxylase activity index	0.033	Matsuda index	− 0.031
L-Leucine (AUCp)	0.039	Total fat (Q)	− 0.023	AAA	0.032	Alcohol (Q)	− 0.029
3-Methyl-2-oxo-valeric-acid (AUCn)	0.032	3-Hydroxybutanoic acid (AUCp)	− 0.016	Vitamin B1 (Q)	− 0.031	Triglyceride (AUCn)	0.029
Glucagon (AUCp)	0.030			Albumin (AUCn)	0.029	Fisher ratio	− 0.028
L-Valine (AUCp)	0.029			L-Lysine (t0)	0.029	Glucose (AUCp)	0.027
4-Methyl-2-oxovaleric-acid (AUCn)	0.026			L-Methionine (t0)	− 0.027	L-Phenylalanine (AUCp)	0.027
Glucagon (AUCn)	0.024			L-Valine (AUCp)	0.026	Albumin (t0)	− 0.026
				Creatinine (AUCn)	0.025	Smoking (Q)	− 0.024
				L-Tyrosine (AUCp)	0.025	Allergy (Q)	− 0.024
				L-Ornithine (t0)	0.025	Albumin (AUCn)	0.023
				Vitamin B2 (Q)	− 0.024	Glucose (AUCn)	− 0.022
				Glycine (AUCp)	− 0.023	ALP (t0)	0.021
				L-Serine (AUCp)	− 0.022	L-Tyrosine (AUCp)	0.019
				Glycine (AUCn)	− 0.021	4-oxoproline (AUCp)	− 0.018
				Total protein (Q)	− 0.021		
				Folic acid (Q)	− 0.021		
				L-Valine (AUCn)	0.021		
				Threonine (AUCp)	− 0.020		
				Albumin (AUCp)	0.019		
				L-Leucine (AUCn)	0.018		
				L-Phenylalanine (AUCn)	0.018		
				L-Serine (t0)	− 0.018		
				L-Proline (AUCn)	0.016		
				L-Tyrosine (AUCn)	0.016		
				L-Asparagine (t0)	− 0.015		
				L-Asparagine (AUCp)	− 0.015		
				Nonessential AA	0.014		

Coefficients represent relative weights for the features, indicating importance for separation of reference groups. AUCp refers to positive part of AUC, AUCn to negative part of AUC, t0 to fasting measurements, and Q to questionnaire features is associated with improved flexibility. This means that the FlexScore is a knowledge-based scoring system that provides an unbiased scoring of phenotypic flexibility, which was used to validate the health space model.

Visualization of data

For the health space visualization, the axis scores of each individual were transformed into a JavaScript Object Notation (JSON) data structure. The JSON data format is a language-independent data exchange format specified by the RFC 7159 standard.

For the FlexScore visualization, the scores as well as the additional data for each subject were transformed into a JSON data structure as well. The JSON data structures were interpreted and manipulated for visualization using CanvasXPress (version 7.8, by Isaac Neuhaus, distributed under GNU GPLv3). CanvasXPress provides an interactive HTML5/JavaScript interface for easy data exploration and visualization. Correlations were visualized by CanvasXPress, Spearman's rank correlation coefficients, and associated p values are provided by R (version 3.1.2 by the R Foundation for Statistical Computing, distributed under GNU GPLv3 with the Hmisc package, version 3.14-6 by Frank E. Harrell Jr.).

Results

Young and leaner subjects showed higher phenotypic flexibility in all health domains when compared to elderly subjects with higher adiposity

To investigate if male and female subjects of higher age (60–70 years of age) and normal to high body fat percentage would respond differently to PFT as compared to young subjects (20–30 years of age) with low to normal body fat percentage, we used the health space methodology. After training and optimizing the health space model using "optimal phenotypic flexibility" (20–29 years, low-normal fat percentage, see also Table 1) and "reduced phenotypic flexibility" (60–70 years, normal-high fat percentage, see also Table 1) reference groups, the two groups were seen to be well separated on all four axes of the health space (Fig. 1). The reduced phenotypic flexibility subjects center around a value of 1 for each of the axes, while the optimal phenotypic flexibility subjects center around 0. For the classification of the two reference groups used in this health space model error rates, which is the misclassification rate of the two reference groups per axis of the health space model after tenfold double cross-validation, were 13, 8, 23, and 3% for the glucose, lipid, amino acids and vitamin, and metabolic stress axes, respectively. After feature selection, 18 out of 46, 14 out of 32, 38 out of 75, and 25 out of 71 parameters, respectively, were

important for separating the two reference groups for the glucose, lipid, amino acids and vitamin, and metabolic stress axes (Table 2).

For the axis representing flexibility in glucose metabolism, out of 18 included features, the positive AUC for C-peptide was the most important determinant for reference group separation, which increased in the "reduced phenotypic flexibility" group. Furthermore, results from the Dutch language FFQ were important for the glucose axis; total carbohydrates as well as polysaccharide intake were the second and third most important features for determining separation that decreased in the "reduced phenotypic flexibility" group. As the importance further declines, features which serve as common biomarkers in type 2 diabetes mellitus (T2D) appear (4-methyl-2-oxovaleric acid, 3-methyl-2-oxovaleric acid, fasting glucose, Matsuda index, and positive AUC for insulin) that all have higher concentrations in the "reduced phenotypic flexibility" group.

On the axis representing flexibility in lipid metabolism, fasting LDL and total fasting cholesterol were important determinants for reference group separation, as well as systolic and diastolic blood pressure, together with anthropomorphic features such as percentage body fat, waist circumference, and BMI. These are well-established clinical markers of metabolic syndrome as defined by the World Health Organization [20] and showed elevated concentrations in the "reduced phenotypic flexibility" as compared to the "optimal phenotypic flexibility" reference group.

The amino acid and vitamin flexibility axis used 38 features to create reference group separation, by far the most of any of the axes. While each of these features represents only a small contribution to the reference group separation, fasting glutamic acid is with some distance the most important feature. L-tyrosine, positive AUC of L-isoleucine, vitamin C index, and Fischer's ratio are the following topmost important features. All features' values are higher in the "reduced phenotypic flexibility" reference group, apart from Fischer's ratio which is opposite.

The axis representing metabolic stress shared some of its most distinguishing features with the lipid axis. Here, fasting LDL, total cholesterol, and systolic blood pressure were the most important features together with self-reported satisfaction with body weight for separation of the two reference groups. Because these axes shared features, the behavior of the subjects along the lipid and metabolic stress axes is likely to be similar.

To evaluate if the observed separation between the two reference groups with the health space

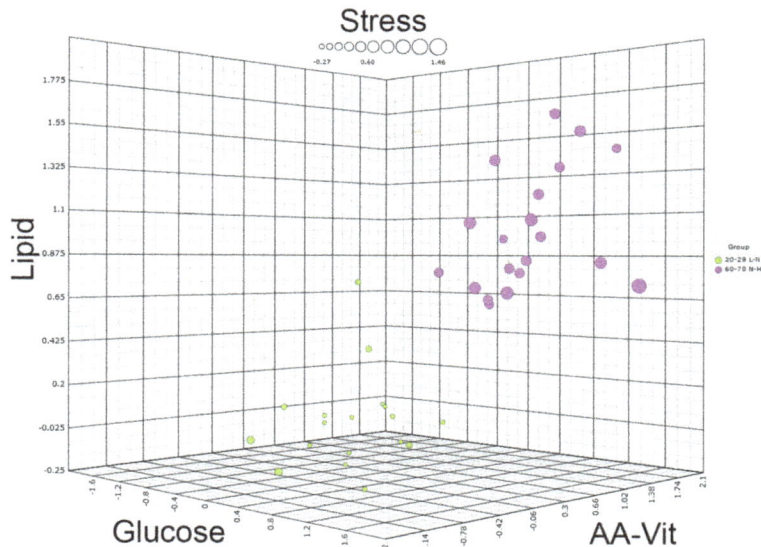

Fig. 1 Overview of the reference groups in the main health space, with both sexes included. Three spatial axes are labeled for the domain they represent. "AA-Vit" stands for amino acids and vitamins. Groups labeled using their respective age intervals as well as their body fat percentage intervals, L for low, N for normal, and H for high. The dot size represents the "metabolic stress" axis of the health space

methodology is reliable, different clinical markers (BMI and waist circumference; total, HDL, and LDL cholesterol; fasting glucose and 2 h glucose; systolic and diastolic blood pressure; and triglycerides) were being evaluated. All, except for HDL, were found to be significantly different (Fig. 2 and Table 3). In response to PFT persons of young age with low to normal fat percentage could be well discriminated from persons of higher age with normal to high fat percentage using the health space methodology.

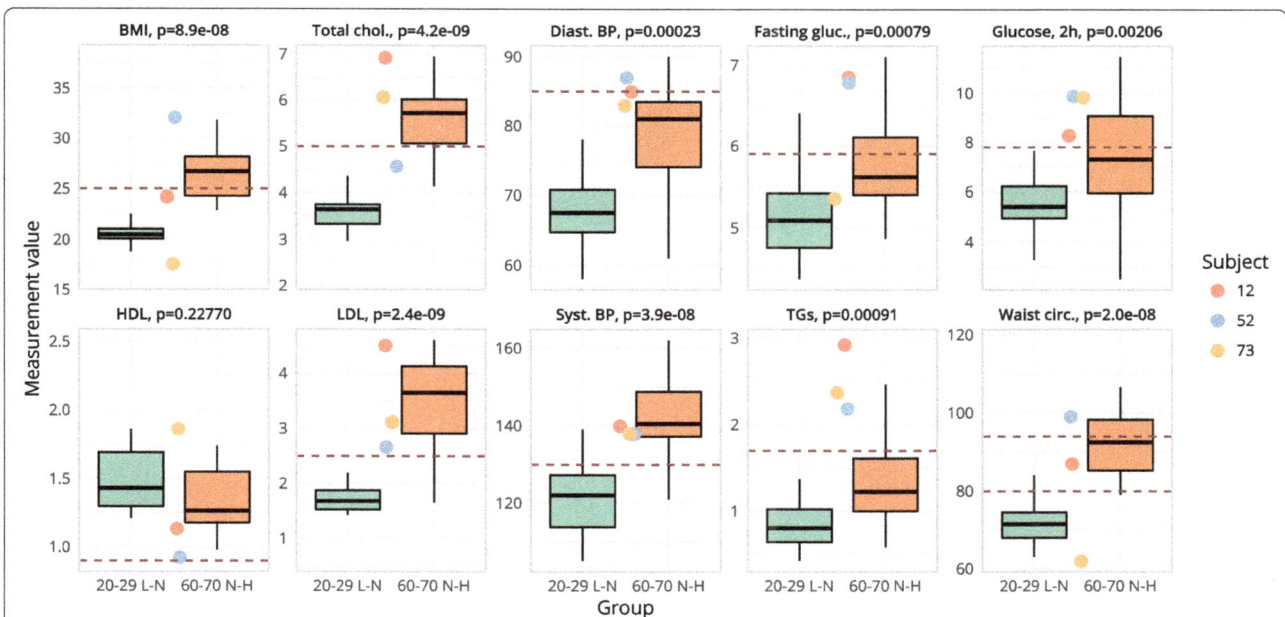

Fig. 2 Boxplots for the two reference groups "optimal phenotypic flexibility" (green) and "reduced phenotypic flexibility" (red) as well as the values of the three outlier subjects (subjects 12, 52, and 73 shown in a red, blue, and yellow circle, respectively). Box shows the 25 to 75% interquartile range; whiskers indicate the maximum and minimum non-outlier values. Crossbar indicates the median values. Horizontal dotted line indicates cut-off values; levels above this line indicate abnormal clinical values. In waist, the lower dotted line represents cut-off values for female and the upper dotted line represents cut-off values for male; p indicates statistical significance after t test

Table 3 This table shows the mean (SD) values for the two reference groups "optimal phenotypic flexibility" (20–29 L to N) and "reduced phenotypic flexibility" (60–70 N to H) as well as the values of the three outlier subjects (subjects 12, 52, and 73)

Marker (unit)	20–29 L to N	60–70 N to H	Subject 12	Subject 52	Subject 73
BMI (kg/m2)[***]	20.61 (2)	27 (3.6)	24.2	32.1	17.6
Cholesterol (mmol/L)[***]	3.56 (0.5)	5.51 (0.9)	6.9	4.6	6.1
LDL (mmol/L)[***]	1.7 (0.4)	3.48 (0.8)	4.5	2.6	3.1
Glucose (mmol/L)[***]	5.11 (0.5)	5.73 (0.6)	6.8	6.8	5.4
HDL (mmol/L)	1.49 (0.2)	1.38 (0.3)	1.1	0.9	1.9
TG (mmol/L)[***]	0.82 (0.3)	1.43 (0.7)	2.9	2.2	2.4
Waist (cm)[***]	72.55 (7.7)	93.02 (10.1)	87	99	62
Sys. BP (mmHg)[***]	120.9 (9.1)	142.15 (10.4)	140	138	138
Dia. BP (mmHg)[***]	68.7 (6.5)	78.15 (8.1)	85	87	83
Glucose, 2 h (mmol/L)[***]	5.57 (1.2)	7.33 (2)	8.3	9.9	9.8

Indicated is the statistical significance level of the difference between the reference groups (***$p < 0.005$)

Increasing body fat percentage is associated with a reduced resilience

To investigate if increasing adiposity (in terms of body fat percentage) would decrease phenotypic flexibility, we visualized male and female subjects from the "healthy range of phenotypes" in the health space model trained on the two reference groups. Figure 3 shows that most of the subjects in the age range of 30–59 years were distributed in between the "optimal" and "reduced phenotypic flexibility" reference groups on all four axes of the health space. From the pattern of distribution, we observed that subjects from the healthy range of phenotypes with a low fat percentage had partly overlapping

and partly reduced resilience when comparing to the "optimal phenotypic flexibility" reference group. The subjects from the healthy range of phenotypes with a normal fat percentage had little overlap with the "optimal" nor "reduced phenotypic flexibility" reference groups and were located in the middle of the health space, in between the two reference groups. The subjects from the healthy range of phenotypes with a high fat percentage were considerably different as compared to the "optimal phenotypic flexibility" reference group and overlapped with the "reduced phenotypic flexibility" reference group who were of higher age. In response to PFT persons from the healthy range of

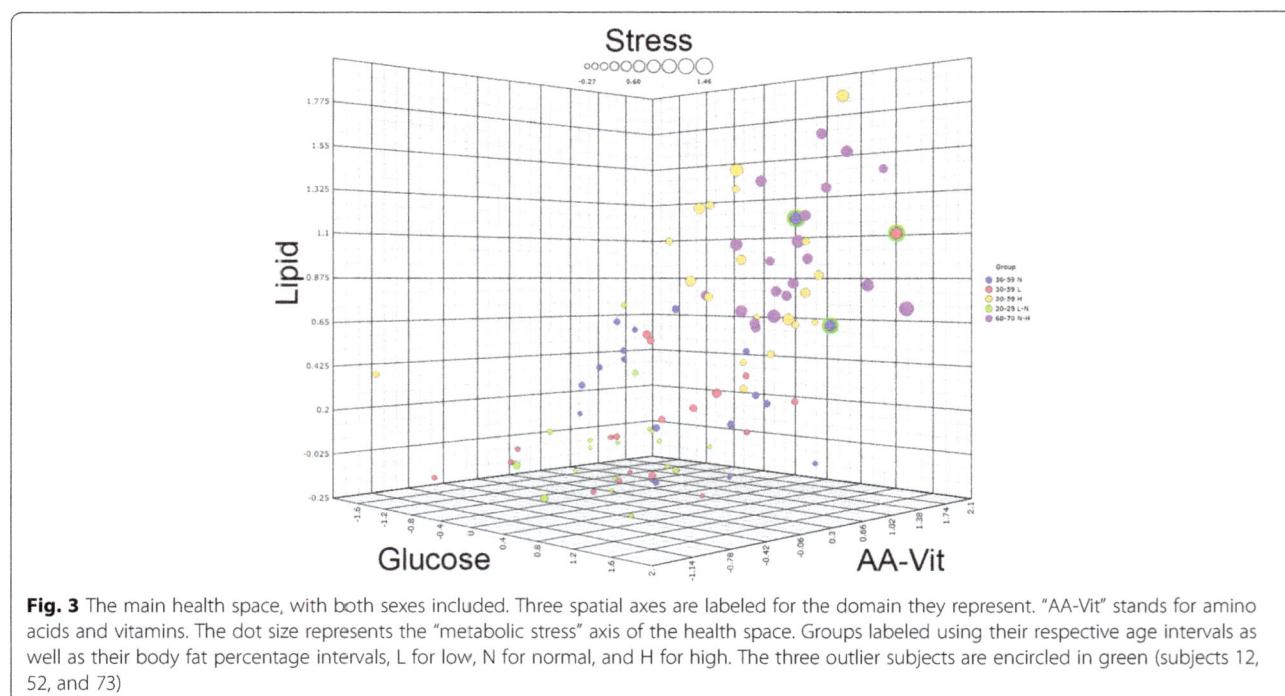

Fig. 3 The main health space, with both sexes included. Three spatial axes are labeled for the domain they represent. "AA-Vit" stands for amino acids and vitamins. The dot size represents the "metabolic stress" axis of the health space. Groups labeled using their respective age intervals as well as their body fat percentage intervals, L for low, N for normal, and H for high. The three outlier subjects are encircled in green (subjects 12, 52, and 73)

phenotypes (aged 30–59 years) with increasing fat percentage showed reduced resilience using the health space methodology.

Male type 2 diabetics showed reduced flexibility compared to healthy males, especially in the domains of glucose metabolism and metabolic stress

To investigate if metabolically impaired subjects with type 2 diabetes could be discriminated from subjects with reduced phenotypic flexibility as well as from subjects from the "healthy range of phenotypes" with this health space model, data from male type 2 diabetics (T2D) were integrated with data from healthy males. Figure 4 shows a second health space which was created using the original male subjects from the healthy ranges study combined with data of subjects from a previous study using the same PFT and similar analytical platforms [6]. In this study, two groups were evaluated: male T2D and healthy controls. In order to project these subjects into a health space, only common features were used. After training and optimizing of the health space model using again males from the original two reference groups ("optimal" and "reduced phenotypic flexibility"), the maximum error rates were 10, 10, 15, and 0% for the glucose, lipid, amino acids and vitamin, and metabolic stress axes, respectively. Subsequently, this optimized health space model was used to visualize data from the healthy males and male T2D from the previous study. It was observed that the 20 healthy males (age range 30–55 with a mean average from 42 ± 7 and BMI range 20–25 with a mean average from 23 ± 1.5) from this previous study was positioned between the two reference groups, similar to the healthy range of male phenotypes with a normal fat percentage. It was clearly observed that 20 male T2D had a different position in the health space as compared to all groups from the healthy range of phenotypes, especially in the domain of glucose metabolism and metabolic stress. Together, these data showed that male T2D in response to PFT showed reduced flexibility compared to healthy males, especially in the domains of glucose metabolism and metabolic stress.

FlexScore validates that health space model reflect individual phenotypic flexibility

To investigate if the health space model provides a biological valid representation of individual phenotypic flexibility as a measure of health, we wanted to test the individual health space representation against an independent and unbiased score of phenotypic flexibility. Therefore, a so-called FlexScore was calculated for the 100 subjects from the original study. The FlexScore was based on preselected features of which a higher or lower response to the PFT had a biological meaning in the sense that these could be interpreted as either beneficial or detrimental to health. A higher FlexScore indicated a lower overall phenotypic flexibility.

When evaluating the FlexScores per phenotypic group (Table 1), it becomes apparent that a separation of groups was present in the FlexScores, similar to as what

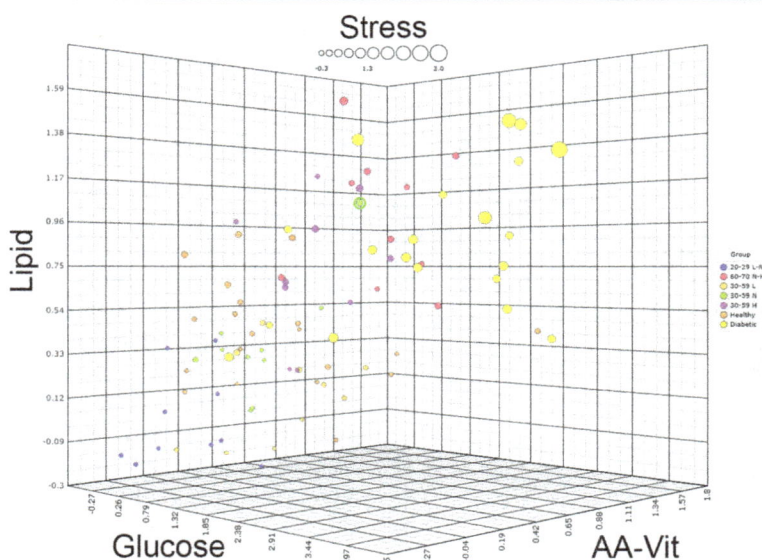

Fig. 4 The combined health space including subjects from two different studies. Three spatial axes are labeled for the domain they represent. "AA-Vit" stands for amino acids and vitamins. The dot size represents the "metabolic stress" axis of the health space. Groups labeled using their respective age intervals as well as their body fat percentage intervals, L for low, N for normal, and H for high. The male outlier (subject 12) from the first health space is again encircled in green

was observed in the health space model (Fig. 5). Again, the optimal phenotypic flexibility reference group (age 20–29 with a low to normal fat percentage) and the reduced phenotypic flexibility group (age 60–70 with a normal to high fat percentage) had the lowest and highest average FlexScores, respectively, (1539, SD = 199 and 1863, SD = 184). The three intermediate groups from the healthy range of phenotypes appeared each with an increasing FlexScore in proportion to their respective phenotypes (low fat percentage 1580, SD = 271; normal fat percentage 1655, SD = 248; high fat percentage 1696, SD = 175). The FlexScore showed a pattern that was remarkably similar to that observed in the health space. These FlexScore results substantiated, in an objective way, the findings from the health space.

Phenotypic flexibility in conjunction with the health space is a reliable measure for individual health

To investigate how reliable the outcome of the health space model was as a measure for personalized health, we investigated the PFT biomarker response of the individual data of the so-called outlier subjects. Figure 3 shows outlier subjects (12, 52, and 73) that did not follow the general pattern seen for increasing age and body fat percentage. Figure 2 and Table 3 show the values for ten clinical parameters for the two reference groups as well as for these three outlier subjects.

Subject 52 is a female subject from the healthy range of phenotypes with a low body fat percentage that was visualized among subjects of the reference group with reduced phenotypic flexibility. This subject appeared to be the least flexible of all subjects in the amino acids and vitamin domain and among the least flexible for the other axes. A closer look at the biomarkers allowed for a

clinical view of the health status for this particular individual when comparing her PFT responses to the two reference groups. The 59-year-old female subject had a high BMI and waist circumference despite a low fat percentage (subject 52, Figs. 2 and 3). This indicated the retention of fluids, perhaps in the form of edema. Fasting glucose, C-peptide, and ketones as well as glucose and glucagon PFT response indicated insulin resistance. Furthermore, the triglyceride and cholesterol PFT responses were above average when compared to the reference group with reduced phenotypic flexibility. Possible reduced liver functioning can be deduced by looking at Fischer's ratio, which showed worse values as compared to the reference group with reduced phenotypic flexibility. More evidence for liver damage in this subject came from extreme PFT responses of ASAT and GGT, two features that were measured but not used in the construction of the health space model.

Also, two other subjects from the healthy range of phenotypes (subjects 12 and 73, Figs. 2 and 3) can be seen among the least flexible subjects which were not expected based by their age or fat percentage. Subject 12 was a 47-year-old male who showed a CVD risk phenotype with high total cholesterol and LDL, and high fasting triglycerides as well as elevated triglyceride PFT response, high ALP, and high GGT, despite a normal fat percentage and BMI when comparing his data to the reference group with reduced phenotypic flexibility. This clinical signature indicated possible liver steatosis. Furthermore, the data of this subject indicated impaired amino acid metabolism, shown by glutamic acid, tyrosine, methionine, and serine PFT response profiles. Furthermore, insulin sensitivity in this subject was decreased as indicated by fasting glucose, C-peptide, and Matsuda index as well as glucose and glucagon responses.

The third outlier, subject 73, was a 53-year-old male with a very low BMI and waist circumference. The response of the clinical parameters projected this individual among the subjects from the reference group with reduced phenotypic flexibility. His biomarker data indicated impaired lipid metabolism and visceral fattening. Elevated fasting cholesterol and triacylglycerol as well as triacylglycerol PFT response and diastolic blood pressure indicated disturbed lipid metabolism as do decreased 3-hydroxybutanoic acid and total ketone bodies. Liver steatosis is indicated by elevated ALP and the Fisher index. Furthermore, in this subject, glucose showed prediabetes, as indicated by glucose, C-peptide and glucagon responses, and the Matsuda index.

Interestingly, these three outlying subjects appeared to have extreme values for several non-clinical parameters, even when compared to T2D average values from data of a previous study [6]. All three subjects showed

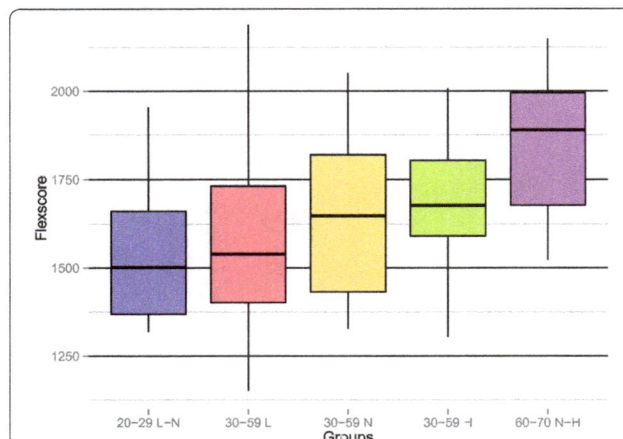

Fig. 5 FlexScore distribution per study group. Box shows the interquartile range (IQR) with the median. The line indicates the range of observations within the ± 1.5 × IQR. Groups labeling used the respective age intervals as well as their body fat percentage intervals, L for low, N for normal, and H for high

extreme values for 4-oxoproline (non-contributing). More specifically, subject 73 showed similarities to the T2D group for the triglyceride PFT response as well as for the ketone body feature. Subject 12 showed values more extreme than the average for the T2D group for fasting C-peptide, PFT glucose, and the PFT triglyceride response. For this same subject, the ASAT response is extreme and much higher as compared to the T2D group average. We refer to the supplementary for graphs showing several key parameters of these outlier subjects plotted against the values for the most flexible and least flexible reference groups. Based on the individual biomarker data of the three outlier subjects, it was shown that health space model outcomes provided a reliable measure for individual health.

Discussion

In the current study, we showed that using the PFT and the analysis and visualization of predefined biomarker panels enabled the discrimination between different states of health. Within the healthy range of the population, it was possible to separate between subjects with optimal and suboptimal phenotypic flexibility since persons of young age with low to normal fat percentage had a markedly different position in the health space as compared to persons from old age with normal to high fat percentage in all four health domains which were glucose metabolism, lipid metabolism, amino acids and vitamins, and metabolic stress. This was also confirmed when evaluating a subset of clinical markers (BMI and waist circumference; total, HDL, and LDL cholesterol; fasting glucose and 2 h glucose; systolic and diastolic blood pressure; and triglycerides) that all showed significantly different values between the two reference groups except for HDL. Furthermore, it was shown that with increasing adiposity in terms of fat percentage, subjects decreased phenotypic flexibility. The health space including the 100 healthy subjects of both sexes showed that the individual phenotypic flexibility scores fall within a convex range, reaching from most flexible to least flexible. The general pattern within this data indicated a relationship between age and adiposity and the resulting phenotypic flexibility score on each of the four defined axes. This relationship between age, adiposity, and phenotypic flexibility was also observed in the unbiased FlexScore. In addition, the clinical marker subset for the three outlier subjects showed that multiple markers had values outside the normal range confirming their outlier position in the health space. Finally, this study showed that using the PFT and the analysis and visualization of predefined biomarker panels also enabled the discrimination between subjects from the healthy range of the population from diseased subjects with T2D. T2D male subjects had higher values for all of the four defined axes. In this health space, the glucose axis showed the largest overall range with [− 0.65 to 3.38] and [− 0.26 to 4.29]

for healthy and T2D subjects, respectively. Perhaps surprisingly, of all axes, it was the metabolic stress axis with the largest range difference between groups; healthy subjects' stress axis values range from − 0.3 to 1.53, while in the T2D group this ranges from 1.12 to 2.95. It can thus be concluded that these T2D subjects showed a reduced phenotypic flexibility in comparison with the most inflexible healthy individuals, even those of high age, especially for glucose metabolism and metabolic stress. Together, these results indicated that phenotypic flexibility as quantified by using the health space model appeared to be a reliable representation of individual health.

As a follow-up, the quantification of the metabolic PhenFlex test in conjunction with the health space methodology can be used to assess the effects of (nutritional) interventions on (individual) health. By applying PFT at various stages in the experiment and measuring and visualizing the biomarker responses according to the health space concept, one can assess health effects that occur by the (nutritional) intervention. In a parallel or crossover designed intervention study, the ideal behavior of the study groups would be that individuals from the control or placebo group occupy the same area of the health space, at the start and the end of the intervention period. The individuals from the intervention group would be expected to occupy the same area as would the control subjects at the start of the study, while they would move away from their starting position towards the "optimal health" reference group after the intervention period.

The aforementioned uses of the health space methodology concern group-wise comparisons. However, tracking changes for one individual across multiple occasions is one of the strengths of the health space approach. Because individuals are visualized within the health space in relation to the selected reference groups, it is possible to determine improvement or deterioration of individual health status, associated to time and/or treatment. The visual nature of the method enables intuitive display and tracking of individual health status. In personalized health, this can serve as both a personal feedback method and a way to determine and address areas of health in which changes are occurring, for targeted advice and interventions.

Several publications using a challenge test show that it has been difficult to show and interpret changes in health status as judged by changes in challenge-response induced by a nutritional intervention, especially for the less known nutrigenomics based biomarkers [2, 21, 22]. Our used approach would be able to facilitate accurate quantification of health changes as well as allow for intuitive interpretation of the results on a group and individual subject level simultaneously. This was shown for example by the description of the three outlier subjects.

By putting their individual data in the context of PFT responses from the two reference groups, but also in the context of T2D responses, it was possible to provide an interpretation if the direction of the PFT biomarker response was beneficial or disadvantageous.

For one of the outlier subjects (subject 12), none of the features used for the generation of the health space appeared to be a true outlier. This means that an additive combination of features placed this subject among the least flexible. Without a composite-based biomarker model of health status, the highly decreased phenotypic flexibility of this subject would not be apparent. This subject is a prime example of the added value of the PFT biomarker response quantification in conjunction with health space visualization.

Conclusions

The current study aimed to assess the ability of PFT to quantify flexibility in the healthy range of the population and whether it is possible to discriminate between optimal and suboptimal flexibility and therefore evaluated PFT response in 100 healthy male and female volunteers. We conclude that the results of the metabolic PFT in conjunction with the health space reliably assessed health on an individual basis. In response to PFT persons of young age with low to normal fat percentage could be well discriminated from persons of higher age with normal to high fat percentage using the health space methodology. Furthermore, in response to PFT persons from the healthy range of phenotypes (aged 30–59 years) with increasing fat percentage showed reduced resilience using the health space methodology. Finally, male T2D in response to PFT showed reduced flexibility compared to the full healthy range of males, especially in the domains of glucose metabolism and metabolic stress. The results from the work shown here may provide a toolbox for the quantification and interpretation of the effect of (nutritional) intervention studies on health status by quantifying phenotypic flexibility, be it in groups or for individuals. The use of this toolbox on an individual level opens up the possibilities for personal health diagnosis. Such a detailed and accurate personal health diagnosis can be used as a starting point for the generation of personalized health advices.

Abbreviations

AAA: Aromatic amino acids; ALAT: Alanine-aminotransferase; ALP: Alkaline phosphatase; ASAT: Aspartate-aminotransferase; AUC: Area under the curve; BCAA: Branched-chain amino acids; CCMO: Central Committee for Medical Research; CHDR: Centre for Human Drug Research; CVD: Cardiovascular disease; DCV: Tenfold double cross-validated; ELISA: Enzyme-linked immunosorbent assay; FFQ: Food frequency questionnaire; GCMS: Gas chromatography-mass spectrometry; GCP: Good clinical practice; GGT: Gamma-glutamyltransferase; HACCP: Hazard analysis and critical control point; HDL: High-density lipoprotein; HIRI: Hepatic insulin resistance index; JSON: JavaScript Object Notation; kCal: Kilocalorie; kJ: Kilojoule; LDL: Low-density lipoprotein; LUMC: Leiden University Medical Centre; NEFA: Nonesterified fatty acids; NSAID: Nonsteroidal anti-inflammatory drugs; PFT: PhenFlex test; RSD: Relative standard deviation; SQUASH: The short questionnaire to assess health-enhancing physical activity; STAI: The state-trait anxiety inventory; T2DM: Type 2 diabetes mellitus; w/w: Mass/mass; WMO: Wet medisch-wetenschappelijk onderzoek met mensen (Dutch medical research in Humans act); Y: Year

Acknowledgements
The authors thank the volunteers for participating in the study and acknowledge Jacobus Burggraaf and coworkers from CHDR for conducting the clinical study. Furthermore, we thank Femke Hoevenaars for the final editing of the manuscript. The critical advice and evaluation of results from the study by Christian Drevon, Hannelore Daniel, and Michael Müller are very much appreciated.

Funding
This research was sponsored by TNO roadmap Nutrition and Health and co-funded by Abbott Nutrition, Danisco-DuPont, DSM, FrieslandCampina, and Nestlé. Furthermore, the research was supported by the NutriTech project (financed by the European Commission in the 7th Framework Programme FP7, Grant agreement no: 289511). The funders of the study had no role in the study design, the data collection, analysis and interpretation, or the preparation of the manuscript.

Authors' contributions
ADS, GB, BvO, MvE, and SW designed the research. AD and GB conducted the research. TvdB, AD, and SW analyzed and interpreted the data. CMR and SB performed the statistical analysis. Finally, TvdB and SW wrote the manuscript. AD, BvO, and MvE reviewed the manuscript, and all authors read and approved the final manuscript.

Competing interests
The authors declare that they have no competing interests.

References
1. Huber M, Knottnerus JA, Green L, van der Horst H, Jadad AR, Kromhout D, et al. How should we define health? BMJ. 2011;343:d4163. Available from: http://www.bmj.com/content/343/bmj.d4163. [cited 2014 Aug 10].
2. Bakker GC, van Erk MJ, Pellis L, Wopereis S, Rubingh CM, Cnubben NH, et al. An antiinflammatory dietary mix modulates inflammation and oxidative and metabolic stress in overweight men: a nutrigenomics approach. Am J Clin Nutr. 2010;91:1044–59. Available from: http://www.ncbi.nlm.nih.gov/pubmed/20181810. [cited 2015 May 27]. American Society for Nutrition.
3. Esser D, Mars M, Oosterink E, Stalmach A, Muller M, Afman LA. Dark chocolate consumption improves leukocyte adhesion factors and vascular function in overweight men. FASEB J. 2014;28:1464–73. Available from: http://www.ncbi.nlm.nih.gov/pubmed/24302679. [cited 2017 Oct 30]
4. Cruz-Teno C, Pérez-Martínez P, Delgado-Lista J, Yubero-Serrano EM, García-Ríos A, Marín C, et al. Dietary fat modifies the postprandial inflammatory state in subjects with metabolic syndrome: the LIPGENE study. Mol Nutr Food Res. 2012;56:854–65. Available from: http://www.ncbi.nlm.nih.gov/pubmed/22707261. [cited 2017 Oct 30]
5. Stroeve JHM, van Wietmarschen H, Kremer BHA, van Ommen B, Wopereis S. Phenotypic flexibility as a measure of health: the optimal nutritional stress response test. Genes Nutr. 2015;10:459. Available from: https://www.ncbi.nlm.nih.gov/pubmed/25896408. [cited 2015 Jun 22]
6. Wopereis S, Stroeve JHM, Stafleu A, Bakker GC, Burggraaf J, van Erk MJ, et al. Multi-parameter comparison of a standardized mixed meal tolerance test in healthy and type 2 diabetic subjects: the PhenFlex challenge. Genes Nutr. 2017;(29)12:21. https://www.ncbi.nlm.nih.gov/pubmed/28861127.
7. van Ommen B, Fairweather-Tait S, Freidig A, Kardinaal A, Scalbert A, Wopereis S. A network biology model of micronutrient related health. Br J Nutr. 2008;99(Suppl 3):S72–80. Available from: http://www.ncbi.nlm.nih.gov/pubmed/18598592. [cited 2015 Mar 17]

8.   Heaney RP. Nutrients, endpoints, and the problem of proof. J Nutr. 2008;
      138:1591–5. Available from: http://www.ncbi.nlm.nih.gov/pubmed/
      18716155. [cited 2015 Mar 17]

9.   van Ommen B, van den Broek T, de Hoogh I, van Erk M, van Someren E,
      Rouhani-Rankouhi T, et al. Systems biology of personalized nutrition. Nutr
      Rev. 2017. Available from: https://academic.oup.com/nutritionreviews/
      article/75/8/579/4056663. [cited 2017 Aug 18].

10. Elliott R, Pico C, Dommels Y, Wybranska I, Hesketh J, Keijer J. Nutrigenomic
      approaches for benefit-risk analysis of foods and food components: defining
      markers of health. Br J Nutr. 2007;98:1095–100. Available from: http://www.
      ncbi.nlm.nih.gov/pubmed/17678571. [cited 2015 Mar 17]

11. Kussmann M, Raymond F, Affolter M. OMICS-driven biomarker discovery in
      nutrition and health. J Biotechnol. 2006;124:758–87. Available from: http://
      www.ncbi.nlm.nih.gov/pubmed/16600411. [cited 2015 Mar 17]

12. van Ommen B, Keijer J, Kleemann R, Elliott R, Drevon CA, McArdle H, et al.
      The challenges for molecular nutrition research 2: quantification of the
      nutritional phenotype. Genes Nutr. 2008;3:51–9. Available from: http://www.
      pubmedcentral.nih.gov/articlerender.fcgi?artid=2467450&tool=
      pmcentrez&rendertype=abstract. [cited 2015 Mar 17]

13. Scalbert A, Brennan L, Fiehn O, Hankemeier T, Kristal BS, van Ommen B,
      et al. Mass-spectrometry-based metabolomics: limitations and
      recommendations for future progress with particular focus on nutrition
      research. Metabolomics. 2009;5:435–58. Available from: https://www.ncbi.
      nlm.nih.gov/pmc/articles/PMC2794347/. [cited 2015 Jan 6]

14. Bouwman J, Vogels JT, Wopereis S, Rubingh CM, Bijlsma S, van Ommen B.
      Visualization and identification of health space, based on personalized
      molecular phenotype and treatment response to relevant underlying
      biological processes. BMC Med Genet. 2012;5:1. Available from: https://www.
      biomedcentral.com/1755-8794/5/1. [cited 2015 Feb 22]

15. Koek MM, Jellema RH, van der Greef J, Tas AC, Hankemeier T. Quantitative
      metabolomics based on gas chromatography mass spectrometry: status
      and perspectives. Metabolomics. 2011;7:307–28. Available from: https://
      www.ncbi.nlm.nih.gov/pmc/articles/PMC3155681/. [cited 2014 Dec 22]

16. Matsuda M, DeFronzo RA. Insulin sensitivity indices obtained from oral glucose
      tolerance testing: comparison with the euglycemic insulin clamp. Diabetes Care.
      1999;22:1462–70. Available from: http://www.ncbi.nlm.nih.gov/pubmed/
      10480510. [cited 2016 Nov 15]

17. Fischer JE, Rosen HM, Ebeid AM, James JH, Keane JM, Soeters PB. The effect
      of normalization of plasma amino acids on hepatic encephalopathy in man.
      Surgery. 1976;80:77–91. Available from: http://www.ncbi.nlm.nih.gov/
      pubmed/818729. [cited 2016 Nov 15]

18. Regier DS, Greene CL. Phenylalanine Hydroxylase Deficiency [Internet].
      GeneReviews(®). 1993. Available from: http://www.ncbi.nlm.nih.gov/
      pubmed/20301677. [cited 2016 Nov 15].

19. Bates CJ. Vitamin C deficiency in guinea pigs: changes in urinary excretion
      of proline, hydroxyproline and total amino nitrogen. Int J Vitam Nutr Res.
      1979;49:152–9. Available from: http://www.ncbi.nlm.nih.gov/pubmed/
      468470. [cited 2016 Nov 15]

20. Alberti KG, Zimmet PZ. Definition, diagnosis and classification of diabetes
      mellitus and its complications. Part 1: diagnosis and classification of
      diabetes mellitus provisional report of a WHO consultation. Diabet Med.
      1998;15:539–53. Available from: http://www.ncbi.nlm.nih.gov/pubmed/
      9686693. [cited 2014 Sep 1]

21. Pellis L, van Erk MJ, van Ommen B, Bakker GCM, Hendriks HFJ, Cnubben NHP,
      et al. Plasma metabolomics and proteomics profiling after a postprandial
      challenge reveal subtle diet effects on human metabolic status. Metabolomics.
      2012;8:347–59. Available from: https://www.ncbi.nlm.nih.gov/pmc/articles/
      PMC3291817/. [cited 2015 Mar 17]

22. Kardinaal AFM, van Erk MJ, Dutman AE, Stroeve JHM, Van De Steeg E,
      Bijlsma S, et al. Quantifying phenotypic flexibility as the response to a high-
      fat challenge test in different states of metabolic health. FASEB J. 2015;29:
      4600–13. Available from: http://www.ncbi.nlm.nih.gov/pubmed/26198450.
      [cited 2015 Oct 1]

13

The effect of maternal undernutrition on the rat placental transcriptome

Zoe Daniel[1], Angelina Swali[1], Richard Emes[2,3] and Simon C Langley-Evans[1*]

Abstract

Background: Fetal exposure to a maternal low protein diet during rat pregnancy is associated with hypertension, renal dysfunction and metabolic disturbance in adult life. These effects are present when dietary manipulations target only the first half of pregnancy. It was hypothesised that early gestation protein restriction would impact upon placental gene expression and that this may give clues to the mechanism which links maternal diet to later consequences.

Methods: Pregnant rats were fed control or a low protein diet from conception to day 13 gestation. Placentas were collected and RNA sequencing performed using the Illumina platform.

Results: Protein restriction down-regulated 67 genes and up-regulated 24 genes in the placenta. Ingenuity pathway analysis showed significant enrichment in pathways related to cholesterol and lipoprotein transport and metabolism, including atherosclerosis signalling, clathrin-mediated endocytosis, LXR/RXR and FXR/RXR activation. Genes at the centre of these processes included the apolipoproteins ApoB, ApoA2 and ApoC2, microsomal triglyceride transfer protein (Mttp), the clathrin-endocytosis receptor cubilin, the transcription factor retinol binding protein 4 (Rbp4) and transerythrin (Ttr; a retinol and thyroid hormone transporter). Real-time PCR measurements largely confirmed the findings of RNASeq and indicated that the impact of protein restriction was often striking (cubilin up-regulated 32-fold, apoC2 up-regulated 17.6-fold). The findings show that gene expression in specific pathways is modulated by maternal protein restriction in the day-13 rat placenta.

Conclusions: Changes in cholesterol transport may contribute to altered tissue development in the fetus and hence programme risk of disease in later life.

Keywords: Placenta, Transcriptome, Pregnancy, Protein restriction, Undernutrition, Cholesterol

Background

The causes of chronic diseases of adulthood are complex. In addition to influences of adult lifestyle, such as dietary pattern, physical activity and the consumption of alcohol and smoking, the environment experienced during infancy and fetal life plays a critical role in establishing adult metabolic and cardiovascular phenotypes [1]. Early life exposure to poor nutrition (both under- and over-nutrition) can programme aspects of adult anatomy, physiology and metabolism [2, 3]. Risk of cardiovascular and metabolic disorders that emerge later in life may therefore already in place even before birth. Epidemiological studies which show relationships between proxy markers of poor nutrition in pregnancy and diseases including cardiovascular disease, type-2 diabetes and chronic kidney disease are supported by observations in animals [2, 4–6]. Manipulating either overall food supply or dietary composition such that one or more nutrients is limiting during pregnancy leads to permanent changes in organ structure and establishes a predisposition to ageing-related insulin resistance, cardiovascular dysfunction and renal disease [1].

* Correspondence: Simon.Langley-Evans@nottingham.ac.uk
[1]School of Biosciences, University of Nottingham, Sutton Bonington, Loughborough LE12 5RD, UK
Full list of author information is available at the end of the article

We previously showed that exposure of the developing rat fetus to maternal undernutrition (both protein restriction and iron deficiency) up to day 13 gestation (full-term is 22 days) induced changes in renal morphology that may underpin the development of hypertension in later life [7]. These effects were associated with a number of changes in the expression of genes and proteins in the day 13 embryo, which were clustered around regulation of the cell cycle, the cytoskeleton and formation of clathrin vesicles [7, 8]. Whilst these processes within the embryo can be envisaged as contributing to remodelling of tissues and therefore permanent changes in the physiology of the animal, leading to later disease [9], they do not give an indication of what initiates these changes in response to maternal diet.

The placenta has long been recognised as having an important role in nutritional programming of later disease [10] either through dietary modulation of placentally derived hormones, dietary modulation of the placental transport of hormones [11] or variation in the delivery of key substrates to the developing fetus [12]. As such, it may be at the centre of the response to maternal undernutrition and the transfer of signals of adverse conditions from mother to fetus. Placental functions will vary with stage of development and the demands of the fetus. In this study, we have focused on the day-13 rat placenta. At this point, full development of the organ has not been completed, but all five basic placental layers are in place (myometrium, deciduum, giant trophoblasts, trophospongium and labyrinth; [13]. The tissue is rich in blood cells and glycogen cells but has not yet developed invasive vessels [13]. In the rat, maximum placental weight is not reached until day 16. We hypothesised that the established but immature placenta would show differential patterns of gene expression in response to maternal protein restriction. These patterns may give important clues as to how maternal nutrition at this stage of development may have long-term consequences for the fetus.

Methods

This paper reports data from analysis of placentas collected in our previously published study of gene and protein expression in day-13 rat embryos [7]. Female virgin Wistar rats (Harlan, UK) were subjected to a 12 h light (08:00–20:00)-dark (20:00–08:00) cycle at a temperature of 20–22 °C with ad libitum access to food and water. At a weight of approximately 180–200 g, females were mated with stud males. After conception, determined by the presence of a semen plug on the cage floor, females were single-housed and animals were fed either a control 18 % (*w*/*w*) casein protein diet (control protein (CP)) or a 9 % (*w*/*w*) casein (low protein (LP)) diet until day 13 gestation (*n* = 8 per group). The LP diet was isocaloric relative to the control (see Additional file 1: Table S1 for composition of diets). To achieve a 50 % reduction in protein content of the LP diet, an additional 9 % carbohydrate was added.

We have previously discussed the relative contributions of protein, carbohydrate and lipids to programming effects of the diet in detail [14–16]. During pregnancy, the animals were weighed and food intake was recorded daily. All animal work was performed under licence from the Home Office (UK) and complied with the Animals (Scientific Procedures) Act (1986). The project was approved by the University of Nottingham, Animal Ethics Committee.

On day 13 of gestation the rats were culled by CO_2 asphyxia and cervical dislocation. Individual embryos and placentas were harvested. Tails were removed from embryos to establish sex. Tissues were snap frozen in liquid nitrogen and stored at –80 °C. PCR was used to verify presence or absence of the sex determining region-Y (SRY) gene in lysed embryo tail tissue [7]. This study used placenta only from male embryos and to generate the RNA samples for RNASeq analysis three placentas from the same litter were pooled. Only male embryos were selected to remove complications of sex from the analysis. Previous work has shown that the impact of maternal undernutrition upon long-term health of offspring is greater in males than in females [17–19]. Overall six samples per group were used for the analysis, with each sample representing three placentas associated with male embryos from a separate litter (18 placentas, 6 litters per group).

High-quality RNA was prepared from frozen tissue using Roche High Pure Tissue Kit according to the manufacturer's instructions. Samples of high-quality RNA (RIN >6.0) were sent to Oxford Gene Technology (Begbrooke, Oxfordshire, UK) for polyA-enriched RNA sequencing using the Illumina TruSeq RNA sample prep kit v2 (Illumina, Little Chesterford, Essex, UK). With this kit, total RNA was captured using olido-dT coated magnetic beads and messenger RNA (mRNA) was fragmented and randomly primed. First strand complementary DNA (cDNA) was initiated from random primers, followed by second strand synthesis. After end repair, phosphorylation and A-tailing, adapter ligation and PCR amplification was performed to prepare the library for sequencing.

Sequencing was performed on the Illumina HiSeq2000 platform using TruSeq v3 chemistry. Read files (Fastq) were generated from the sequencing platform via the manufacturer's proprietary software, and read level QC metrics were generated by FastQC http://www.bioinformatics.babraham.ac.uk/projects/fastqc/). Reads were processed through the Tuxedo suite [20] and mapped to their location using Bowtie version 2.o2 (http://bowtie-bio.sourceforge.net/index.shtml). Cufflinks v2.1.1 (http://cole-trapnell-lab.github.io/cufflinks/) was used to perform transcript assembly, abundance estimation and differential expression for the samples. RNASeq alignment metrics

Table 1 Differentially expressed genes in rat placenta at d13 gestation

Gene ID	Locus	Expression (control)	Expression (LP)	Fold–change (log2)	Q value
Actg2	4:117732482-117747006	71.49	2.48	−4.85	0.00922
Gzmf	15:34696237-34707618	103.92	4.98	−4.38	0.00922
Gzmb	15:35195449-35198468	384.48	20.68	−4.22	0.00922
Nkg7	1:93813122-93814188	146.90	8.65	−4.09	0.00922
Prf1	20:28658366-28663866	171.89	10.39	−4.05	0.00922
Ccl5	10:71605790-71610330	59.82	4.15	−3.85	0.00922
Zbtb32	1:85635283-85637589	7.78	0.57	−3.77	0.04862
Asb2	6:127609501-127645492	5.26	0.46	−3.53	0.00922
Lama2	1:18203478-18885460	4.48	0.40	−3.49	0.00922
Cd96	11:56183624-56258356	11.16	1.03	−3.43	0.01702
MYH11_RAT	10:666714-776052	8.22	0.77	−3.42	0.00922
Rgs1	13:58121190-58125514	12.73	1.29	−3.31	0.00922
Ptprcap	1:206738734-206740893	13.28	1.57	−3.08	0.04148
LOC305103	13:88606173-88611105	120.74	14.38	−3.07	0.00922
D4ADB8_RAT	8:21210583-21221026	9.83	1.18	−3.06	0.00922
Cdh17	5:26047159-26099164	3.75	0.46	−3.02	0.02304
E9PSV0_RAT	20:4300723-4315876	10.67	1.34	−2.99	0.00922
Igfbp6	7:140885375-140890043	228.66	28.85	−2.99	0.00922
Col6a6	8:110793848-110892578	5.48	0.69	−2.98	0.00922
ADH1_RAT	2:235799456-235811584	69.42	9.27	−2.90	0.00922
Mcpt9	15:34541881-34544835	26.43	3.53	−2.90	0.00922
Lck	5:148707506-148718296	15.93	2.21	−2.85	0.00922
C1s	4:160736132-160748150	22.95	3.25	−2.82	0.00922
Pla1a	11:64099836-64137355	12.63	1.79	−2.82	0.00922
Sep1	1:186474714-186478580	11.10	1.58	−2.82	0.00922
COBA1_RAT	2:209996818-210193378	12.61	1.92	−2.71	0.02304
C1r	4:160712581-160729361	29.45	4.56	−2.69	0.00922
Q3MIE5_RAT	10:19207498-19660353	2.64	0.41	−2.67	0.00922
CLM8_RAT	10:104775859-104788927	15.09	2.50	−2.59	0.01702
Phf11	15:38444406-38477945	27.05	4.56	−2.57	0.00922
Sfrp4	17:53121424-53131513	42.94	7.23	−2.57	0.00922
Cytip	3:39893892-39921114	6.66	1.17	−2.50	0.02304
Rac2	7:116520065-116532482	38.51	6.90	−2.48	0.00922
C1qb	5:155647525-155653074	13.93	2.52	−2.47	0.02873
Coro1a	1:185852741-185857715	40.30	7.80	−2.37	0.00922
Aldh1a2	8:75692098-75771159	6.41	1.26	−2.35	0.00922
Pla2g2a	5:157654785-157657360	19.90	3.90	−2.35	0.02304
Smoc2	1:53165791-53295122	3.31	0.68	−2.29	0.04862
Rab27a	8:77798829-77861089	8.05	1.73	−2.22	0.00922
Serping1	3:67968807-67978102	39.91	8.61	−2.21	0.00922
D3ZXA0_RAT	15:38372728-38391822	21.10	4.62	−2.19	0.00922
RGD1565772	1:67630583-67648373	4.21	0.94	−2.17	0.00922
Rgs2	13:57890948-57894465	30.51	6.87	−2.15	0.00922
Psmb8	20:4786263-4739173	43.92	10.48	−2.07	0.00922

Table 1 Differentially expressed genes in rat placenta at d13 gestation *(Continued)*

TagIn	8:48902208-48907693	99.68	23.75	−2.07	0.00922
C1qc	5:155656104-155659430	13.41	3.31	−2.02	0.04502
Prelp	13:46801474-46943977	12.67	3.13	−2.02	0.00922
LOC100365668	10:38109857-38110205	120.96	30.50	−1.99	0.00922
Fst	2:46542245-46550678	60.50	15.49	−1.97	0.00922
Ptprc	13:51246163-51357995	11.13	2.93	−1.93	0.00922
Selplg	12:43842267-43843560	11.84	3.10	−1.93	0.04862
Angpt4	3:142249114-142282307	14.42	4.07	−1.82	0.04502
Itgal	1:186561794-186598905	4.37	1.26	−1.80	0.02873
Fcer1g	13:87119465-87123902	78.98	23.70	−1.74	0.00922
Plek	14:97841598-97875052	18.70	5.63	−1.73	0.00922
Ccdc88b	1:209520223-209536201	3.50	1.06	−1.72	0.04502
Ifitm3	1:201198666-201199807	153.46	48.97	−1.65	0.01702
Pcolce	12:19672504-19678821	53.84	18.12	−1.57	0.04862
Plcg2	19:47875571-47947573	5.87	2.12	−1.47	0.03500
Prl8a7	17:44148436-44154238	43.87	15.87	−1.47	0.00922
Bgn	X:159380548-159391521	29.57	11.81	−1.32	0.02873
Cgm4	1:77441012-77453814	15.02	6.04	−1.31	0.02304
Pmp22	10:49305834-49335864	30.24	12.39	−1.29	0.03500
Laptm5	5:149775895-149797951	70.71	29.18	−1.28	0.02304
Mmp12	8:4249934-4328865	53.39	26.46	−1.01	0.04502
Ifitm2	1:201134356-201135537	141.63	72.01	−0.98	0.02873
Prl7b1	17:43783361-43791538	96.93	51.16	−0.92	0.04502
Sod3	14:63381447-63387180	7.22	20.37	1.50	0.00922
Tf	8:108196748-108244545	62.61	188.51	1.59	0.02304
Gpc3	X:139192114-139393977	9.56	30.69	1.68	0.00922
Ccdc37	4:124661801-124671607	5.76	18.58	1.69	0.00922
Cldn2	X:127538684-127549018	1.66	5.37	1.69	0.04862
Pcdh24	17:15937976-15962796	1.80	6.02	1.74	0.02873
Muc13	11:68772164-68794880	3.41	11.77	1.79	0.00922
Fgg	2:174727311-174734592	11.29	41.76	1.89	0.00922
Creb3l3	7:10106524-10114955	3.23	12.04	1.90	0.01702
Mttp	2:235613709-235654848	2.33	9.12	1.97	0.00922
Serpinf2	10:62748115-62756200	3.56	14.05	1.98	0.00922
Serpina1	6:127998618-128021719	4.90	20.49	2.06	0.01702
Fmo1	13:78503769-78536359	6.70	28.40	2.08	0.00922
Maob	X:17553528-17657839	6.15	26.17	2.09	0.00922
Rbp4	1:242443797-242450998	83.56	362.99	2.12	0.00922
Tdh	15:42758307-42771849	4.69	21.22	2.18	0.00922
Ttr	18:12406550-12413680	135.68	616.60	2.18	0.00922
Vil1	9:73748631-73776345	1.11	5.07	2.19	0.04502
Apoa4	8:49233139-49233436	61.26	291.64	2.25	0.00922
Apob	6:31508011-31556597	9.20	43.86	2.25	0.00922
Apoa2	13:87114733-87116372	70.35	335.96	2.26	0.00922

Table 1 Differentially expressed genes in rat placenta at d13 gestation *(Continued)*

Spp2	9:87297051-87316545	16.85	80.97	2.26	0.00922
Apoc2	1:78979033-78980136	42.59	241.21	2.50	0.00922
Cubn	17:87655812-87772079	0.96	6.33	2.72	0.00922

n = 6 per group

were generated using Picard tools (http://broadinstitute. github.io/picard/).

RNASeq was carried out on 12 samples with an average of 12279507 paired end reads per sample. A total of 11.63 gigabases of sequence data were read and aligned at high quality. The number of mapped reads per sample ranged from 3081828 to 17579532, and the proportion of mapped reads exceeded 99 % across all samples. The percentage of high-quality aligned bases was in excess of 98.5 and >96.5 % of reads were aligned in pairs.

Data was analysed using Cufflinks v2.1.1. A one-sided *t* test was used to determine the significant changes in gene expression (*P* value), and a Benjamini-Hochberg correction for multiple testing was also used (*q* value) as reported by Trapnell et al. [21]. Selection of genes identified as differentially expressed in the protein restricted group was based upon false discovery rate adjusted *q* values <0.05 (unadjusted *P* < 0.0005). Pathways and networks of interacting proteins enriched for differentially expressed genes were identified using ingenuity pathway analysis. Statistical enrichment is calculated by a right tailed Fisher's exact test (IPA, QIAGEN Redwood City www.qiagen.com/ingenuity).

To further explore the differential expression data, we performed quantitative real-time PCR for 13 genes that were differentially expressed according to the RNASeq analysis. These included seven genes in the main pathways showing enrichment in the ingenuity analysis (ApoA2, ApoC2, Ttr, Fgg, Actg2, serpin G1 and Rbp4); Cubn and Mttp, which have functions closely related to those enriched pathways; and four genes that were shown to be differentially expressed in the protein restricted condition (Vil1, Gpc3, Muc13, Prf1). The PCR measurements were performed on the same RNA samples that were originally analysed through RNASeq. Total RNA (500 ng) was reverse transcribed using a cDNA synthesis kit (RevertAid RT Reverse Transcription Kit, Thermo Fisher) with random primers. Real-time PCR primers were designed using Primer Express software (version 1.5; Applied Biosystems) from the RNA sequence, checked using BLAST (National Center for Biotechnology Information) and were purchased from Sigma (UK). The primer sequences for these analyses are presented in Additional file 2: Table S2. Real-time PCR was performed on a Lightcycler 480 (Roche, Burgess Hill, UK) using the 384 well format. Each reaction contained 5 μl of cDNA with the following reagents: 7.5 μl SYBR green master mix (Roche), 0.45 μl forward and

reverse primers (final concentration 0.3 μM each) and 1.6 μl RNase-free H_2O. Samples were pre-incubated at 95 C for 5 min followed by 45 PCR amplification cycles (de-naturation, 95 C for 10 s; annealing, 60 C for 15 s; elongation, 72 C for 15 s). Transcript abundance was determined using a standard curve generated from serial dilutions of a pool of cDNA made from all samples. Expression was normalised against the expression of cyclophilin, which was shown to be unaffected by maternal diet in the RNASeq analysis and subsequently by PCR. The primer sequences for these analyses are presented in Additional file 2: Table S2. Data from real-time PCR measurements was tested using independent samples *t* tests. Ten of the targets were shown to be differentially expressed in the protein restricted group, confirming the RNASeq analysis.

Results

The RNASeq analysis revealed differential expression of 91 genes in the day 13 rat placenta in response to maternal protein restriction. Of these, 24 were up-regulated and 67 were down-regulated. The full list of differentially expressed genes is provided in Table 1, and

Table 2 Pathways significantly influenced by maternal protein restriction in the day 13 rat placenta

Pathway	*P* value ($\log_{10}$)	Differentially expressed genes in pathway
Acute-phase signalling	11	C1R, C4A/C4B, Serpin G1, TTr, TF, C1S, ApoA2, Serpin A1, Serpin F2, Fgg, Rbp4
FXR/RXR activation	10.9	C4A/C4B, TTr, ApoB, TF, ApoA2, Serpin A1, ApoC2, Serpoin G2, Mttp, Rbp4
LXR/RXR activation	9.59	C4A/C4B, Ttr, ApoB, TF, ApoA2, ApoC2, Serpin A1, Serpin F, Rbp4
Atherosclerosis signalling	6.72	ApoB, ApoA2, ApocC2, Serpin A1, Pla2g2A, Selpg, Rbp4
Clathrin-mediated endocytosis	5.55	ApoB, RF, ApoA2, ApoC2, Serpin A1, Actg2, Rbp4
IL12 signalling in macrophages	4.08	ApoB, ApoA2, ApoC2, Serpin A1, Rbp4
Coagulation system	3.66	Serpin A1 Serpin F2, Fgg
Nitric oxide and ROS production in macrophages	3.47	ApoB, ApoA2, ApoC2, Serpin A1, Rbp4

The table shows ingenuity canonical pathways with significant enrichment in comparison of control and low protein exposed placentas the full transcriptome analysis is available in Additional file 3: Table S3.

Analysis of the data set using ingenuity pathway analysis identified 19 pathways that were significantly affected by maternal protein restriction with $P < 0.01$. A more stringent cut-off of $P < 0.001$ identified eight significantly affected pathways (Table 2). The top six pathways (acute-phase response signalling, FXR/RXR activation, liver X receptor (LXR)/retinoid X receptor (RXR) activation, complement system, atherosclerosis signalling, clathrin-mediated endocytosis signalling) were closely related functionally, with a strong focus on cholesterol uptake and efflux across the placenta. Figure 1 shows heat maps for the genes involved in the functionally interesting enriched pathways. A relatively small number of genes contributed to the enrichment noted for all of these pathways (Ttr, ApoA2, ApoB. ApoC2, Fgg, Rbp4, Serpin A1, Serpin F2 and Serpin G1).

To validate the observations made using RNASeq analysis, quantitative real-time PCR was performed to explore the expression of 13 genes in two selection groups. The first group comprised genes that were differentially expressed with protein restriction and deemed functionally significant (associated with cholesterol transport) based upon the Ingenuity analysis (Ttr, ApoA2, ApoC2, Rbp4, Fgg, Actg2). The second group were genes that were differentially expressed but not associated with the pathways identified by Ingenuity (Muc13, Vil1, Gpc3, Cubn, Mttp). It should be noted that Cubn has a role in the uptake of high-density

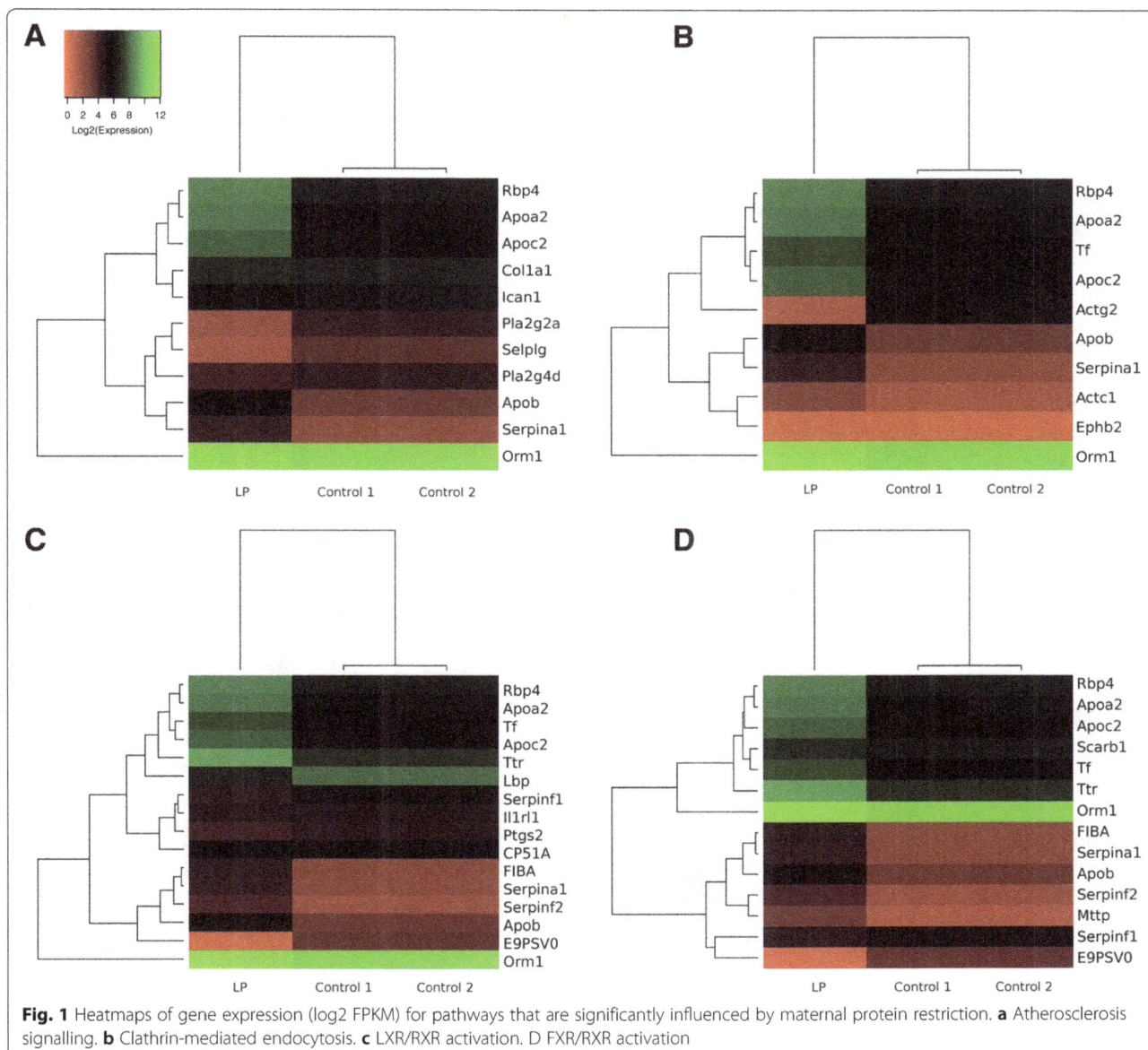

Fig. 1 Heatmaps of gene expression (log2 FPKM) for pathways that are significantly influenced by maternal protein restriction. **a** Atherosclerosis signalling. **b** Clathrin-mediated endocytosis. **c** LXR/RXR activation. D FXR/RXR activation

lipoprotein (HDL)-cholesterol by the placenta and that Mttp has a role in the packaging of cholesterol and lipid into low-density lipoprotein (LDL). Figures 2 and 3 show the data from the PCR analyses of these genes and Table 3 compares the fold-change in expression noted in the RNASeq analysis. The majority of genes in the validation set were strongly over-expressed in placentas from protein restricted pregnancies compared to controls, with a minimum of 4.53-fold (Gpc3) and maximum 41.35-fold (Fgg) up-regulation noted in this set. PCR analysis of three genes did not reproduce the statistically significant effects of protein restriction that

were shown by RNASeq (Actg2, SerpinG1 and Prf1; Fig. 4). The PCR analysis generally detected a greater degree of up-regulation in the validation set than was noted with RNASeq (Table 3).

Discussion

In this experiment, we tested the hypothesis that maternal protein restriction would impact upon gene expression in the day-13 rat placenta. The data showed that this was in fact the case and that although the number of genes affected was small, the nutritional insult had a major impact upon expression of genes associated with

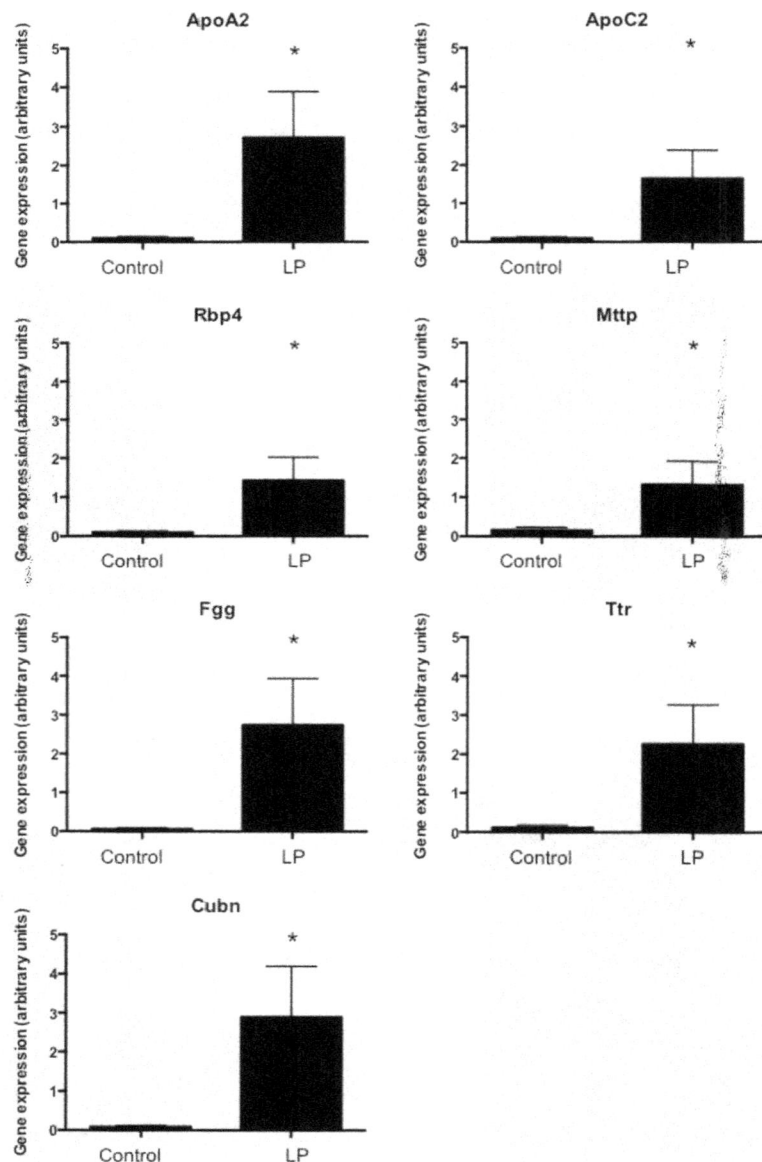

Fig. 2 Expression of genes related to enriched pathways. Real-time qualitative PCR was used to validate the differential expression of seven genes related to canonical pathways identified by ingenuity as significantly influenced by maternal protein restriction. Expression was normalised to cyclophilin mRNA expression and *$P < 0.05$ between groups. $n = 6$ per group

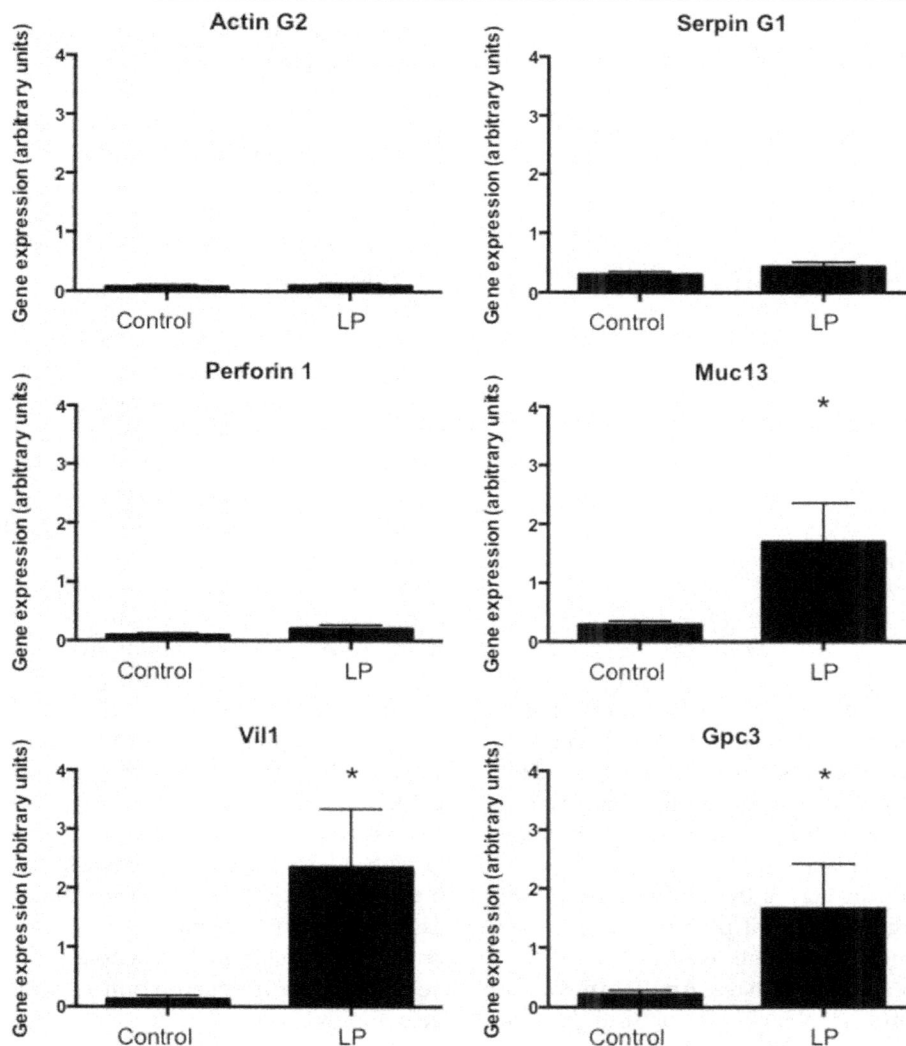

Fig. 3 Expression of genes unrelated to enriched pathways. Real-time qualitative PCR was used to validate the differential expression of six genes related to canonical pathways identified by ingenuity as significantly influenced by maternal protein restriction. Expression was normalised to cyclophilin mRNA expression. *$P < 0.05$ between groups. $n = 6$ per group

cholesterol transport processes within the tissue. The expression of genes involved in the uptake of cholesterol by the placenta from HDL- LDL- and very low-density lipoprotein (VLDL)-cholesterol (ApoA2, ApoB, ApoC2, Cubn), the formation of clathrin-coated pits in which VLDL- and LDL-cholesterol receptors are located (Tf, Orm1, ApoA2, ApoC2, Actg2, Rbp4), the regulation of cholesterol efflux (Ttr, Tf, Orm1, Serpin F1, Rbp4, Mttp, Fgg, Serpin F2, Serpin A1) and the efflux from the placenta as LDL-cholesterol (ApoB, Mttp) were generally up-regulated by maternal undernutrition. Importantly, we have confirmed that the effects of maternal protein restriction during the first half of pregnancy may be mediated through changes in placental function.

Previous studies suggest that placental structure and organisation may be influenced by maternal protein restriction in both rats and mice [22–24]. These diet-related changes appear to be related to differential expression of adhesion molecules (beta catenin and vascular endothelial cadherin) and impaired cell proliferation. These processes appeared to be largely unaffected in the present study (although cadherin Cdh17 was down-regulated by protein restriction) and the discrepancies may stem from species differences or differences in stage of gestation at which samples were collected.

Functionally, placentas from protein-restricted rodents are known to differ in terms of materno-fetal steroid

Table 3 Comparison of fold-change in gene expression between RNASeq and real-time PCR

Gene	Log$_2$ fold-change RNA Seq	Log$_2$ fold-change RNA PCR
Actg2	−4.85***	0.28
Apo A2	2.26***	4.79*
Apo C2	2.52***	4.14*
Cubn	2.71***	5.01*
Fgg	1.88***	5.37*
Gpc3	1.68***	2.18*
Mttp	1.97***	3.14*
Muc13	1.79***	2.71*
Prf1	−4.04***	1.68
Rbp4	2.11***	3.85*
Serpin G1	−2.21***	0.69
Ttr	2.18***	3.52*
Vil1	2.19***	3.41*

Significant differences were noted between control and low protein exposed placentas within each analytical approach (*$P < 0.05$, ***$P < 0.001$)

exchange [11] and transport of fatty acids and amino acids [12, 25, 26]. Whilst specific genes related to these functions have been previously identified as being sensitive to protein restriction, none were found to be differentially expressed in the current study. This is most likely explained by our study concentrating on day-13 rather than later stage placentas.

Cholesterol transport across the placenta is complex and involves a large number of proteins [27]. Cholesterol reaches the placenta in the form of LDL- VLDL- and HDL-cholesterol, which have ApoB, ApoC2 and ApoA2 respectively as their key structural proteins. LDL- and VLDL-cholesterol are taken up by their respective receptors which are located in clathrin-coated pits on trophoblasts. HDL-cholesterol can be taken up by SR-B1 (scavenger receptor class B member 1) or by binding to proteins such as megalin and cubilin. The latter two are multifunctional receptors which mediate uptake of material by endocytosis [28, 29]. Once taken up by trophoblasts, cholesterol is hydrolysed to cholesterol esters. Export from trophoblasts is in the form of either LDL-cholesterol or HDL-cholesterol. LDL-cholesterol is formed through placental expression of apoB and the action of microsomal triglyceride transfer protein (Mttp). HDL-cholesterol can be formed through complexing of lipids and cholesterol with a range of different apolipoproteins (ApoA1, ApoE, ApoA4, ApoC1, ApoC4; [27]). These are synthesised in response to LXR/RXR activation [30]. ApoA1 synthesis is also influenced by FXR/RXR activation [31]. Cholesterol efflux for formation of HDL-cholesterol complexes is dependent upon a range of ATP binding cassette proteins

(AbcA1, AbcG1, AbcG5, AbcG8, [27]), which are downstream targets of FXR/RXR activation [32]. The present study has shown that almost all of these processes are sensitive to maternal protein restriction, and importantly, we have found that the only significant enrichment of pathways within our dataset lies in these processes. If there are any strong drivers of nutritional programming through the placenta at this stage of development, then cholesterol must play a key role.

The uptake of cholesterol by the embryo and fetus is critical for normal development [27], and defects of endogenous cholesterol synthesis are known to be lethal [33]. Cholesterol will also play an important role in placental function as it is the precursor for all steroid hormone synthesis. Disturbances of placental transport or endogenous fetal synthesis can have a number of effects on growth, cell proliferation, metabolism and the organisation of tissues [27, 34]. Low maternal cholesterol is associated with lower birth weight and microcephaly in humans [35], and women who have growth retarded infants have been found to have lower circulating cholesterol [36]. Optimal cholesterol transport to the fetus is therefore likely to have a positive impact upon development, and it is known that some of the effects are mediated through the cell cycle [37, 38]. However, some animal studies suggest that excessive cholesterol may also have a negative impact on growth. Bhasin et al. [39] reported that hypercholesterolaemia in pregnant LDL receptor knockout mice was associated with intrauterine growth retardation. The relationship between fetal cholesterol and the normal development and organisation of tissues may therefore be complex.

It is known that hypercholesterolaemia during pregnancy is associated with adverse health outcomes in the longer term. In humans, there is evidence that maternal hypercholesterolaemia is associated with the development of fatty streaks in fetal arteries [40], and cholestasis during pregnancy is associated with programming of an overweight, insulin-resistant phenotype in humans [41]. Animal studies have shown greater atherosclerosis in offspring of hypercholesterolaemic mothers [42, 43]. Previous work from our laboratory showed that in the ApoE*3 Leiden mouse, a transgenic rodent which has a predisposition to atherosclerosis, maternal protein restriction during fetal development increased atherosclerotic lesion size in adult life [44]. As atherosclerosis in this mouse is related to the degree of cholesterol exposure, it may be that intrauterine exposure to higher than normal cholesterol transport across the placenta may contribute to the adult disease phenotype. Induction of cholestasis using cholic acid in mouse pregnancy produces the same

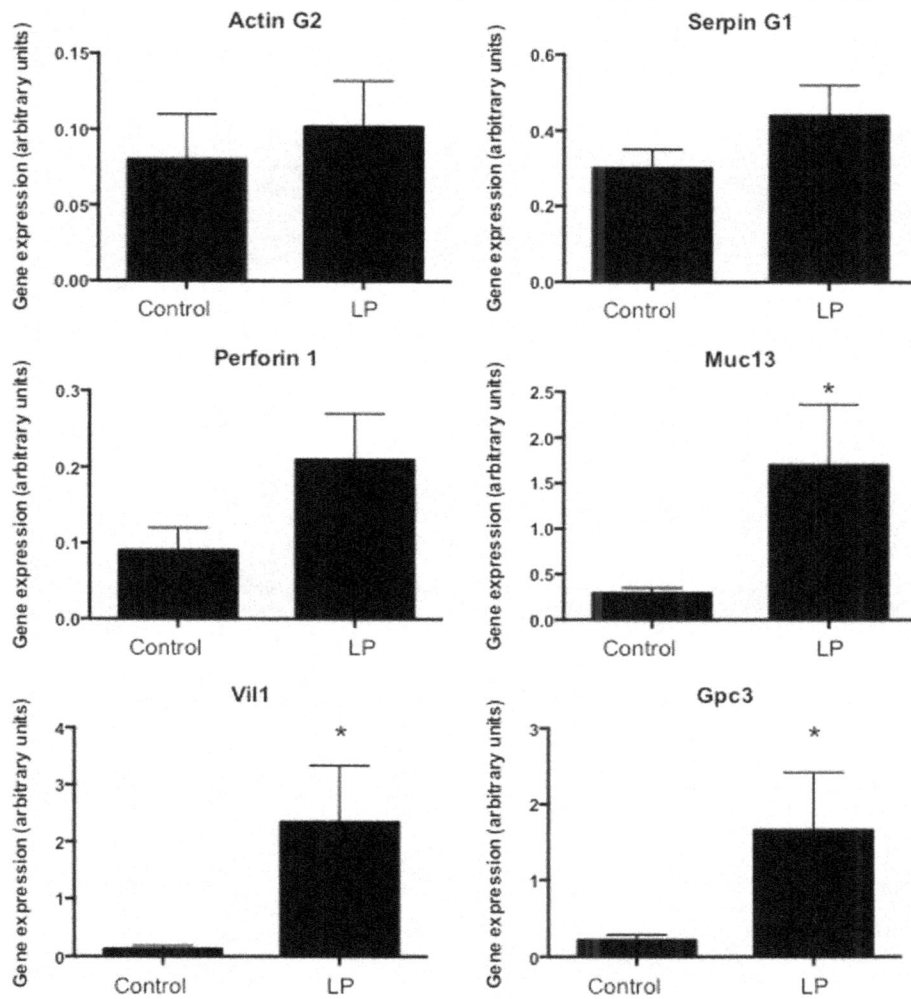

Fig. 4 PCR analysis of three genes

phenotype as in seen in humans [41] and is associated with greater cholesterol efflux from the placenta.

This study was an initial exploratory study to establish whether the placental transcriptome was significantly impacted by maternal protein restriction and to determine whether any observed effects were isolated to discrete processes within the tissue. One limitation of the study is that the whole placenta was used to generate the RNA, with no distinction between the maternal and fetal placental tissue. In the absence of any direct measurements of cholesterol transport or measurement of the genes of interest at the level of protein, assumptions are being made about the processes of cholesterol uptake and efflux being sensitive to maternal undernutrition. These measurements will be a priority for future studies, as will confirmation that placentas associated with female embryos respond in the same way as those from males.

Conclusions

Current thinking about the mechanisms which link maternal nutritional status and long-term health in offspring is largely focused upon lasting epigenetic changes within the fetal genome [45]. This study has highlighted placental function as being modulated by maternal undernutrition and reinforces the alternative concept that programming of fetal development and long-term health may be a product of dysregulation of nutrient transfer across the placenta. Further studies are needed to evaluate cholesterol transport across the placenta in protein-restricted pregnancies and to determine the impact of cholesterol on fetal gene expression, epigenetic regulation of gene expression and tissue morphology. This analysis of the placental transcriptome at the point where the placenta is not fully mature has supported the hypothesis that maternal undernutrition impacts upon placental function. The findings of this study will provide a platform for further investigation of processes within placenta that may be important new mechanistic targets or biomarkers that indicate nutritional programming of disease.

Abbreviations
Actg2: Actin G2; Apo A4: Apolipoprotein A4; Apo B: Apolipoprotein B; ApoC2: Apolipoprotein C2; ApoE: Apolipoprotein E; CP: Control protein; Cubn: Cublin; Fgg: Fibrinogen gamma chain; FXR: Farnesoid X receptor; Gpc3: Glypican 3; HDL: High-density lipoprotein; Igf2: Insulin-like growth factor 2; LDL: Low-density lipoprotein; LP: Low protein; LXR: Liver X receptor; Mttp: Microsomal triglyceride transfer protein; Muc13: Mucin 13; PCR: Polymerase chain reaction; Prf1: Perforin 1; Rbp4: Retinol binding protein 4; RXR: Retinoid X receptor; Ttr: Transthyretin; Vil1: Villin 1; VLDL: Very low-density lipoprotein; Wnt2: Wingless-type MMTV integration site family, member 2

Acknowledgements
The authors gratefully acknowledge Dr Sarah McMullen, Professor Harry McArdle and Dr Lorraine Gambling who contributed to the original experimental design for the animal experiment. Dr Samantha Ware performed analysis of the energy and protein content of the diets.

Funding
This work was supported by the Biotechnology and Biological Sciences Research Council [grant number BB/F005245/1], the Rosetrees Trust and the Stoneygate Trust.

Authors' contributions
SLE designed the experiment and was responsible for data analysis. RE carried out bioinformatics analysis, AS performed the animal experiment and ZD was responsible for the preparation of samples for RNASeq and the PCR analyses. All authors contributed to the preparation of the manuscript. All authors read and approved the final manuscript.

Competing interests
The authors declare that they have no competing interests.

Author details
[1]School of Biosciences, University of Nottingham, Sutton Bonington, Loughborough LE12 5RD, UK. [2]School of Veterinary Medicine and Science, University of Nottingham, Sutton Bonington, Loughborough, UK. [3]Advanced

Data Analysis Centre, University of Nottingham, Sutton Bonington, Loughborough, UK.

References
1. Langley-Evans SC. Nutrition in early life and the programming of adult disease: a review. J Hum Nutr Diet. 2015;28 Suppl 1:1–14.
2. Barker DJ, Bull AR, Osmond C, Simmonds SJ. Fetal and placental size and risk of hypertension in adult life. BMJ. 1990;301:259–62.
3. Eriksson JG, Forsen TJ, Osmond C, Barker DJ. Pathways of infant and childhood growth that lead to type 2 diabetes. Diabetes Care. 2003;26:3006–10.
4. Hales CN, Barker DJ, Clark PM, Cox LJ, Fall C, Osmond C, Winter PD. Fetal and infant growth and impaired glucose tolerance at age 64. BMJ. 1991;303:1019–22.
5. Hoy WE, Hughson MD, Bertram JF, Douglas-Denton R, Amann K. Nephron number, hypertension, renal disease, and renal failure. J Am Soc Nephrol. 2005;16:2557–64.
6. Langley-Evans SC, Welham SJ, Jackson AA. Fetal exposure to a maternal low protein diet impairs nephrogenesis and promotes hypertension in the rat. Life Sci. 1999;64:965–74.
7. Swali A, McMullen S, Hayes H, Gambling L, McArdle HJ, Langley-Evans SC. Cell cycle regulation and cytoskeletal remodelling are critical processes in the nutritional programming of embryonic development. PLoS One. 2011;6:e23189.
8. Swali A, McMullen S, Hayes H, Gambling L, McArdle HJ, Langley-Evans SC. Processes underlying the nutritional programming of embryonic development by iron deficiency in the rat. PLoS One. 2012;7:e48133.
9. Langley-Evans SC. Fetal programming of CVD and renal disease: animal models and mechanistic considerations. Proc Nutr Soc. 2013;72:317–25.
10. Burton GJ, Fowden AL. Review: the placenta and developmental programming: balancing fetal nutrient demands with maternal resource allocation. Placenta. 2012;33(Suppl):S23–27.
11. Langley-Evans SC, Phillips GJ, Benediktsson R, Gardner DS, Edwards CR, Jackson AA, Seckl JR. Protein intake in pregnancy, placental glucocorticoid metabolism and the programming of hypertension in the rat. Placenta. 1996;17:169–72.
12. Jansson N, Pettersson J, Haafiz A, Ericsson A, Palmberg I, Tranberg M, Ganapathy V, Powell TL, Jansson T. Down-regulation of placental transport of amino acids precedes the development of intrauterine growth restriction in rats fed a low protein diet. J Physiol. 2006;576:935–46.
13. de Rijk EP, van Esch E, Flik G. Pregnancy dating in the rat: placental morphology and maternal blood parameters. Toxicol Pathol. 2002;30:271–82.
14. Langley SC, Jackson AA. Increased systolic blood pressure in adult rats induced by fetal exposure to maternal low protein diets. Clin Sci (Lond). 1994;86:217–22.
15. Langley-Evans SC, Phillips GJ, Jackson AA. In utero exposure to maternal low protein diets induces hypertension in weanling rats, independently of maternal blood pressure changes. Clin Nutr. 1994;13:319–24.
16. Langley-Evans SC. Critical differences between two low protein diet protocols in the programming of hypertension in the rat. Int J Food Sci Nutr. 2000;51:11–7.
17. McMullen S, Langley-Evans SC (2005a) Maternal low-protein diet in rat pregnancy programs blood pressure through sex-specific mechanisms. Am J Physiol Regul Integr Comp Physiol 288:R85-90
18. McMullen S, Langley-Evans SC (2005b) Sex-specific effects of prenatal low-protein and carbenoxolone exposure on renal angiotensin receptor expression in rats. Hypertension 46:1374-1380
19. Sugden MC, Holness MJ. Gender-specific programming of insulin secretion and action. J Endocrinol. 2002;75:757–67.
20. Trapnell C, Roberts A, Goff L, Pertea G, Kim D, Kelley DR, Pimentel H, Salzberg SL, Rinn JL, Pachter L. Differential gene and transcript expression analysis of RNA-seq experiments with TopHat and Cufflinks. Nat Protoc. 2012;7:562–78.
21. Trapnell C, Williams BA, Pertea G, Mortazavi A, Kwan G, van Baren MJ, Salzberg SL, Wold BJ, Pachter L. Transcript assembly and quantification by RNA-Seq reveals unannotated transcripts and isoform switching during cell differentiation. Nat Biotechnol. 2010;28:511–5.
22. Gao H, Yallampalli U, Yallampalli C. Gestational protein restriction affects trophoblast differentiation. Front Biosci. 2013;5:591–601.
23. Rebelato HJ, Esquisatto MA, de Sousa Righi EF, Catisti R. Gestational protein restriction alters cell proliferation in rat placenta. J Mol Histol. 2016;47:203–11.
24. Rutland CS, Latunde-Dada AO, Thorpe A, Plant R, Langley-Evans S, Leach L. Effect of gestational nutrition on vascular integrity in the murine placenta. Placenta. 2007;28:734–42.
25. Nüsken E, Gellhaus A, Kühnel E, Swoboda I, Wohlfarth M, Vohlen C, Schneider H, Dötsch J, Nüsken KD. Increased rat placental fatty acid, but decreased amino acid and glucose transporters potentially modify intrauterine programming. J Cell Biochem. 2016;117:1594–603.
26. Rosario FJ, Jansson N, Kanai Y, Prasad PD, Powell TL, Jansson T. Maternal protein restriction in the rat inhibits placental insulin, mTOR, and STAT3 signaling and down-regulates placental amino acid transporters. Endocrinology. 2011;152:1119–29.
27. Woollett LA. Review: transport of maternal cholesterol to the fetal circulation. Placenta. 2011;32 Suppl 2:S218–221.
28. Barth JL, Argraves WS. Cubilin and megalin: partners in lipoprotein and vitamin metabolism. Trends Cardiovasc Med. 2001;11:26–31.
29. Willnow TE, Nykjaer A. Cellular uptake of steroid carrier proteins—mechanisms and implications. Mol Cell Endocrinol. 2010;316:93–102.
30. Zhu R, Ou Z, Ruan X, Gong J. Role of liver X receptors in cholesterol efflux and inflammatory signaling (review). Mol Med Rep. 2012;5:895–900.
31. Claudel T, Sturm E, Duez H, Torra IP, Sirvent A, Kosykh V, Fruchart JC, Dallongeville J, Hum DW, Kuipers F, Staels B. Bile acid-activated nuclear receptor FXR suppresses apolipoprotein A-I transcription via a negative FXR response element. J Clin Invest. 2002;109:961 71.
32. de Aguiar Vallim TQ, Tarling EJ, Kim T, Civelek M, Baldán Á, Esau C, Edwards PA. MicroRNA-144 regulates hepatic ATP binding cassette transporter A1 and plasma high-density lipoprotein after activation of the nuclear receptor farnesoid X receptor. Circ Res. 2013;112:1602–12.

33. Porter FD. Human malformation syndromes due to inborn errors of cholesterol synthesis. Curr Opin Pediatr. 2003;15:607–13.

34. Haas D, Morgenthaler J, Lacbawan F, Long B, Runz H, Garbade SF, Zschocke J, Kelley RI, Okun JG, Hoffmann GF, Muenke M. Abnormal sterol metabolism in holoprosencephaly: studies in cultured lymphoblasts. J Med Genet. 2007;44:298–305.

35. Edison RJ, Berg K, Remaley A, Kelley R, Rotimi C, Stevenson RE, Muenke M. Adverse birth outcome among mothers with low serum cholesterol. Pediatrics. 2007;120:723–33.

36. Wadsack C, Tabano S, Maier A, Hiden U, Alvino G, Cozzi V, Huttinger M, Schneider WJ, Lang U, Cetin I, Desoye G. Intrauterine growth restriction (IUGR) is associated with alterations in placental lipoprotein receptors and maternal lipoprotein composition. Am J Physiol. 2007;292:E476–84.

37. Fernández C, Martín M, Gómez-Coronado D, Lasunción MA. Effects of distal cholesterol biosynthesis inhibitors on cell proliferation and cell cycle progression. J Lipid Res. 2005;46:920–9.

38. Singh P, Saxena R, Srinivas G, Pande G, Chattopadhyay A. Cholesterol biosynthesis and homeostasis in regulation of the cell cycle. PLoS One. 2013;8:e58833.

39. Bhasin KK, van Nas A, Martin LJ, Davis RC, Devaskar SU, Lusis AJ. Maternal low-protein diet or hypercholesterolemia reduces circulating essential amino acids and leads to intrauterine growth restriction. Diabetes. 2009;58:559–66.

40. Palinski W, Napoli C. The fetal origins of atherosclerosis: maternal hypercholesterolemia, and cholesterol-lowering or antioxidant treatment during pregnancy influence in utero programming and postnatal susceptibility to atherogenesis. FASEB J. 2002;16:1348–60.

41. Papacleovoulou G, Abu-Hayyeh S, Nikolopoulou E, Briz O, Owen BM, Nikolova V, Ovadia C, Huang X, Vaarasmaki M, Baumann M, Jansen E, Albrecht C, Jarvelin MR, Marin JJ, Knisely AS, Williamson C. Maternal cholestasis during pregnancy programs metabolic disease in offspring. J Clin Invest. 2013;123:3172–81.

42. Goharkhay N, Sbrana E, Gamble PK, Tamayo EH, Betancourt A, Villarreal K, Hankins GD, Saade GR, Longo M. Characterization of a murine model of fetal programming of atherosclerosis. Am J Obstet Gynecol. 2007;197(416):e1–5.

43. Napoli C, de Nigris F, Welch JS, Calara FB, Stuart RO, Glass CK, Palinski W. Maternal hypercholesterolemia during pregnancy promotes early atherogenesis in LDL receptor-deficient mice and alters aortic gene expression determined by microarray. Circulation. 2002;105:1360–7.

44. Yates Z, Tarling EJ, Langley-Evans SC, Salter AM. Maternal undernutrition programmes atherosclerosis in the ApoE*3-Leiden mouse. Br J Nutr. 2009;101:1185–94.

45. Burdge GC, Lillycrop KA. Nutrition, epigenetics, and developmental plasticity: implications for understanding human disease. Annu Rev Nutr. 2010;30:315–39.

14

Dibutyryl-cAMP affecting fat deposition of finishing pigs by decreasing the inflammatory system related to insulin sensitive or lipolysis

Xianyong Ma[1,2,3,4,5], Wei Fang[1,2,3,4,5], Zongyong Jiang[1,2,3,4,5*], Li Wang[1,2,3,4,5], Xuefen Yang[1,2,3,4,5] and Kaiguo Gao[1,2,3,4,5]

Abstract

Background: The mechanism of db-cAMP regulating fat deposition and improving lean percentage is unclear and needs to be further studied.

Methods: Eighteen 100-day-old Duroc × Landrance × Large White barrows (49.75 ± 0.75 kg) were used for experiment 1, and 15 eighteen 135-day-old barrows (78.34 ± 1.22 kg) were used for experiment 2 to investigate the effects of dietary dibutyryl-cAMP (db-cAMP) on fat deposition in finishing pigs. Pigs were fed with a corn-soybean meal-based diet supplemented with 0 cr 15 mg/kg db-cAMP, and both experiments lasted 35 days, respectively.

Results: The results showed that db-cAMP decreased the backfat thickness, backfat percentage, and diameter of backfat cells without changing the growth performance or carcass characteristics in both experiments, and this effect was more marked in experiment 1 than in experiment 2; db-cAMP enhanced the activity of the growth hormone–insulin-like growth factor-1 (GH-IGF-1) axis and pro-opiomelanocortin (POMC) system in both experiments, which suppressed the accumulation of backfat deposition; microarray analysis showed that db-cAMP suppressed the inflammatory system within the adipose tissue related to insulin sensitivity, which also reduced fat synthesis.

Conclusions: In summary, the effect of db-cAMP on suppressing fat synthesis and accumulation is better in the earlier phase than in the later phase of finishing pigs, and db-cAMP plays this function by increasing the activity of the GH-IGF-1 axis and POMC system, while decreasing the inflammatory system within the adipose tissue related to insulin sensitive or lipolysis.

Keywords: Backfat thickness, Adipocyte cell, Gene microarray, Inflammatory system, Endocrine system

Background

Dibutyryl cAMP (db-cAMP), an orally active cell-permeant derivative of cAMP, has the same functions as endogenous cAMP, the latter playing a crucial role of signal transduction in numerous biological activities, such as regulating cell growth, enzyme activities, lipolysis, and gene expression [31, 38]. In recent years, dietary db-cAMP has been used in the pig production with beneficial effect on increasing the content of lean meat and decreasing fat in pig carcasses [39]. Our previous work [38] also showed that db-cAMP increased the lean percentage and decreased the backfat thickness, while it did not affect the growth performance or meat quality, indicating that db-cAMP may have potential for producing more lean meat as a feed additive in pig production. Some reports indicated that db-cAMP decreased the size of adipocytes, inhibited fat deposition in adipocytes, and reduced proliferation and differentiation of the preadipocytes [21, 38]. As cAMP is well-known for many hormones mediating signal transduction, and promoting lipolysis through adenylyl cyclase-cAMP-protein kinase pathway [4, 6], it seemed likely that exogenous db-cAMP

* Correspondence: jiangz28@qq.com
[1]Institute of Animal Science, Guangdong Academy of Agricultural Sciences, 510640 Guangzhou, China
[2]The Key Laboratory of Animal Nutrition and Feed Science (South China) of Ministry of Agriculture, 510640 Guangzhou, China
Full list of author information is available at the end of the article

also played functions through the endocrine and cell signaling pathway. Exogenous supplementation with cAMP or db-cAMP to anterior pituitary cells promoted the secretion of growth hormone [30] which is known to stimulate lean-tissue growth and inhibit adipose tissue growth [5]. Db-cAMP also increased the expression of beta-adrenoceptors and activated endogenous adenylate cyclase [7]. In addition, cAMP inhibited expression of genes such as *fatty acid synthase* (*FAS*) and *malate dehydrogenase* (*MDH*) in fat cells in vitro [11]. However, the mechanism of db-cAMP regulating fat deposition and improving lean percentage needs to be further studied. The present research has investigated the effect of dietary db-cAMP on concentrations of relevant hormones, metabolic indices, and gene expression profiles in backfat adipocytes of pigs to better understand the functional mechanisms of its action.

Methods
Pigs and diets
Eighteen 100-day-old Duroc × Landrance × Large White barrows (49.75 ± 0.75 kg) were used for experiment 1, and eighteen 135-day-old barrows (78.34 ± 1.22 kg) were used for experiment 2, each experiment lasting for 35 days and treated at the same condition. Other than for balancing on the basis of weight and ancestry, pigs were randomly assigned to 2 groups, controls, or supplemented with db-cAMP. Each treatment consisted of three replicate pens, each with three pigs. All pigs were housed in the animal facilities of the Institute of Animal Science in the Guangdong Academy of Agricultural Sciences. Pigs were fed with a corn-soybean meal-based diet (Table 1, meeting requirements for finishing pigs according to NRC (1998), without (as controls) or with

15 mg/kg db-cAMP (98 % purity, Hangzhou Meiya Biotechnology Co, Ltd, Hangzhou, China) as described by Wang et al. [38] (note: experiment 1 stands for the earlier phase of fattening pigs; experiment 2 stands for the later phase of fattening pigs).

Feeding and slaughter procedure
Pigs were weighed at the end of the experiment, and feed consumed was recorded daily for each replicate to determine average daily gain (ADG), average daily feed intake (ADFI), and feed to gain (F:G). At the end of each experiment, pigs were fasted for 14 h, blood sampled, then immediately electro-stunned, and exsanguinated. All aspects of the experiment including transport and slaughtering procedures were carried out in accordance with the Chinese guidelines [29] and approved by Animal Ethical Committee of Institute of Animal Science, Guangdong Academy of Agricultural Sciences. Carcasses were weighed and split in the median plane. The dressing percentage, lean percentage, and fat percentage were measured using one side of the individual carcass. Backfat thickness was measured on the midline over the first, tenth, and last rib and cross-sectional area. The longissimus muscle area was measured at the junction of thoracic and lumbar vertebrae, by tracing onto sulfate paper followed by planimetry.

Sample collection
Blood was collected from the anterior vena cava using vacuum tubes (no anticoagulant), allowed to clot at room temperature for 120 min, and centrifuged for 5 min at 3000 × g at 4 °C, and serum was stored at −20 °C. Samples of longissimus muscle over the ninth to tenth ribs were immediately obtained and frozen in liquid N_2 for

Table 1 Composition and nutrient levels of the basal diets for two stages of finishing pigs

Item	Experiment 1	Experiment 2	Chemical composition	Experiment 1	Experiment 2
Corn	67.700	69.300	Digestible energy (MJ/kg)	13.39	13.27
Soybean	25.900	20.700	Crude protein (%)	17.04	15.57
Wheat bran	3.645	7.645	Calcium (%)	0.66	0.55
Salt	0.370	0.370	Available energy (%)	0.24	0.19
Dicalcium Phosphate	0.900	0.600	Lysine (%)	0.97	0.85
Limestone	1.000	0.900	Methionine (%)	0.25	0.23
Lysine.HCl	0.130	0.130	Methionine + cysteine (%)	0.52	0.48
Mineral mix[a]	0.100	0.100			
Vitamin mix[b]	0.040	0.040			
Chloride choline (50 %)	0.100	0.100			
Antimildew agent	0.100	0.100			
Antioxidant agent	0.015	0.015			
Total	100.00	100.00			

[a]supplied 8 mg Cu (CuSO₄.5H₂O); 60 mg Fe (FeSO₄.7H₂O); 60 mg Zn (ZnSO₄. H₂O); 35 mg Mn (MnO); 0.35 mg I (KI); 0.3 mg Se (NaSeO₃) per kg of diet.
[b]supplied 5000 IU vitamin A; 700 IU vitamin D₃; 25 mg vitamin E; 2.5 mg vitamin K₃; 1.5 mg vitamin B₁; 5 mg vitamin B₂; 0.02 mg vitamin B₁₂; 7.5 mg calcium pantothenate; 20 mg niacin; 0.5 mg folic acid; 0.04 mg biotin per kg of diet

measurement of intramuscular fat (IMF) content, enzyme activities, and messenger RNA (mRNA) analysis, and additional longissimus samples were held at 4 °C for meat quality measurements. Fresh samples of backfat adipose tissue (1 cm^3) were fixed in 4 % paraformaldehyde in PBS (pH 7.3) for histology. Liver, pituitary, and hypothalamus tissue samples also were collected immediately and held, as described above, for mRNA extraction.

Measurement of hormones and biochemical variables in plasma

The plasma concentrations of high-density lipoprotein (HDL), low-density lipoprotein (LDL), free fatty acid (FFA), cholesterol, and triglyceride (TG) were determined using an automatic analyzer (cx5, Beckman Coulter INC, Brea, CA), and the activity of lipase was determined using an ELISA kit (Luyu Bioengineering, Shanghai, China). The concentrations of cAMP, GH, IGF-I, IGFBP3, T3, T4, leptin, AD, and insulin were measured using ELISA kits (GBD Co, Ltd, USA).

Meat quality measurements

The pH of muscle samples was measured at 45 min, 24 h, and 48 h postmortem using a pH meter (HI 8242C, Beijing Hanna Instruments Science & Technology, Beijing, China). Drip loss was measured, as described by Ma et al. [17]. Meat color CIE LAB values (L*, relative lightness; a*, relative redness; b*, relative yellowness) were determined on the transverse surface of the meat sample after it was cut and exposed to air for 45 min with a colorimeter (CR-410, Minolta, Suita-shi, Osaka, Japan); Shear force was measured using an Instron Universal Mechanical Machine (Instron model 4411; Instron, Canton, MA), as described by Ma et al. [17].

Measurement of intramuscular fat content

The muscle samples were lyophilized and grounded to powders. The IMF content was measured by petroleum ether (30 to 60 °C boiling point) extraction using the Soxtec 2055 fat extraction system (Foss Tecator AB, Sweden), as described by Ma et al. [17].

Diameter and the density of adipocytes

Fixed tissues were embedded in paraffin, sectioned at 5 - micrometer (mm), dewaxed, and then stained with hematoxylin and eosin (Beijing Biosynthesis Biotechnology Co, Ltd, Beijing, China). The sections (ten sections per sample) were viewed at ×10 magnification using a Motic BA400 microscope, and the diameter and density of the adipocytes were determined with Motic image software (Motic-Optic Industrial Group Co. Ltd, Xiamen, China).

Gene microarray analysis

Total RNA was isolated from backfat tissue from experiment 1 using TRIzol reagent (Invitrogen, Carlsbad, CA) according to the manufacturer's instructions. The quality and quantity of RNA were assessed by OD$_{260}$/OD$_{280}$. Five micrograms of total RNA was converted to double-stranded complementary DNA (cDNA) using the RT-kit (QIAGEN, Shanghai, China) with an oligo (dT) primer containing a T7 RNA polymerase promoter. Biotin-labeled complementary RNA (cRNA) was synthesized from purified double-stranded cDNA using a Bio-Array high-yield RNA transcript labeling kit (QIAGEN). Approximately 20 mg cRNA was fragmented to 50–300 bases and hybridized to Porcine Oligo Microarray chips (Agilent, Santa Clara, CA). A total of six chips were used here: three replicates for controls and pigs receiving db-cAMP (mRNA was pooled for the three pigs each replicate). The hybridized arrays were washed, stained, and scanned following the Porcine Oligo Microarray GeneChip Expression Analysis manual.

Real-time quantitative PCR of selected genes in backfat, liver, pituitary, and hypothalamus tissue

Total RNA was isolated (as above) from hypothalamus, pituitary, liver, and backfat tissue and stored at −80 °C. cDNA was produced using a commercial kit containing Reverse Transcriptase XL (AMV) and RNAsin (Invitrogen). Real-time PCR was performed using an ABI 7500 Mastercycler (Applied Biosystems, Foster City, CA) with qPCR Mix (TaKaRa, BIOINC, Japan). The gene (ADCYAP1, GHRH, CRH, POMC, PC1, PC2) expression levels were determined in hypothalamus tissue; the gene (GHRHR, GH, CRHR, POMC, TRHR, TSH) expression levels were determined in pituitary tissue; the gene (GHR, IGF-1) expression levels were determined in liver tissue. The selected genes (SAL1, STAR, CYP2A19, STAT1, SYK, CCL2, AIF1, ITGB2, CCR1 and CXCL2) of backfat were chosen from the results of the chip analysis results and beta-actin (reference transcript gene) was designed from the GenBank sequences.

Statistical analysis

Values were expressed as means ± SEM. Data were analyzed by t tests (Statistical Analysis Software version 8.1; SAS Institute, Inc, Cary, NC). Base on this, the effects of db-cAMP in experiments 1 and 2 were reanalyzed using two-way ANOVA followed by an appropriate post hoc t test. P values <0.05 were considered to be significant, and P values <0.01 were considered to be extremely significant.

Gene chip expression data analysis was performed using PCA project in the SAS system online. False discovery rate (FDR) correction was applied using the step-up method. Probe sets that met a FDR value of ≤0.05 and average fold change (FC) of at least 2 in either direction were selected for further study. The GenMAPP-CS software package (http://www.genmapp.org) was used for gene ontology (GO) and pathway analysis.

Results

Effect of dietary db-cAMP on growth performance and carcass characteristics

Dietary supplementation with 15 mg/kg db-cAMP did not affect ($P > 0.05$) final body weight, ADG, ADFI, or F:G ratio of the pigs in either experiments (Table 2). There were no significant effects of treatment on dressing percentage, longissimus muscle area, or lean percentage of the pigs in either experiment (Table 2). Dietary db-cAMP decreased the fat percentage of the pigs by 16.1 % in experiment 1 (135-day) and 12.1 % in experiment 2 (170-day) ($P < 0.05$), it also deceased the average backfat thickness by 22.4 % in experiment 1 and by 17.8 % in experiment 2 ($P < 0.05$), and the differences were greater in experiment 1 than that in experiment 2 ($P < 0.05$).

Effect of db-cAMP on meat quality of finishing pigs

There were no differences on meat quality traits (e.g., pH value, drip loss, shear force, and meat color) between the control and db-cAMP-supplemented pigs in either experiment except for the decreased a* value of the meat in experiment 1 (Table 2).

Effect of db-cAMP on biochemical indices in serum

Dietary supplementation with db-cAMP did not affect the plasma concentrations of cholesterol, TG, FFA, HDL, or LDL and the activity of lipase in either experiment. Dietary supplementation with db-cAMP increased the plasma concentrations of GH, IGF-I, T3, T4, and cAMP in experiment 1 and strikingly decreased the plasma concentration of leptin in experiment 2 (Table 3).

Effect of db-cAMP on adipose tissue histology

Figure 1 showed that dietary supplementation with 15 mg/kg db-cAMP increased the number of adipocytes per field and decreased the average diameter ($P < 0.05$) of backfat cell by 4.0 % in experiment 1 and by 7.0 % in experiment 2.

Table 2 Effects of db-cAMP on growth performance, carcass traits and meat quality in finishing pigs

Variable		Experiment 1		Experiment 2	
		Controls	db cAMP	Controls	db cAMP
Final weight (kg)		72.24±2.46	73.64±1.77	105.93±2.06	105.11±1.72
Average daily feed intake (kg)		2.32±0.15	2.25±0.17	2.85±0.08	2.72±0.10
Average daily gain (kg)		0.73±0.05	0.74±0.04	0.79±0.03	0.76±0.04
F/G		3.35±0.03	3.04±0.14	3.69±0.16	3.60±0.12
Dressing percentage (%)		73.80±1.25	73.40±0.56	78.22±0.87	77.84±0.76
Longissimus muscle area (cm²)		34.10±2.82	35.40±1.12	55.45±3.59	61.35±4.64
Lean percentage (%)		62.02±1.51	64.73±0.58	61.75±0.75	63.80±0.85
Fat percentage (%)#		19.55±1.06	16.41±0.32*	23.34±1.14	20.52±1.19*
Backfat thickness (cm)					
First rib#		3.70±0.19	2.89±0.32*	3.45±0.26	2.84±0.33
Tenth rib		1.67±0.11	1.33±0.16	1.89±0.21	1.56±0.33
Last rib		1.59±0.15	1.20±0.12	1.61±0.16	1.30±0.16
Average backfat thickness#		2.32±0.15	1.80±0.10**	2.31±0.09	1.90±0.08**
Drop loss (%) (24 h)		2.42±0.10	2.60±0.09	2.45±0.19	2.37±0.13
Intramuscular fat (%)		2.01±0.34	2.12±0.49	2.04±0.55	2.36±0.97
Shear force (48 h)		38.16±2.8	34.26±2.0	43.42±2.0	35.56±1.9
pH	45 min	6.38±0.13	6.41±0.07	6.28±0.14	6.52±0.05
	24 h	5.31±0.04	5.43±0.04	5.23±0.02	5.39±0.03
L*	45 min	50.64±1.0	49.65±0.6	46.56±0.4	45.40±1.0
	24 h	56.23±2.0	54.43±0.6	54.51±0.7	54.08±0.9
a*	45 min	16.83±0.6	14.94±0.3*	14.08±0.6	15.08±0.4
	24 h	17.19±0.6	15.46±0.5*	16.48±0.5	17.12±0.5
b*	45 min	3.89±0.2	3.64±0.4	3.28±0.3	2.94±0.1
	24 h	7.02±0.4	6.33±0.3	8.04±0.6	8.21±1.0

Within stages, means with * differ ($P < 0.05$) and those with ** differ ($P < 0.01$)
Within the same line, # means the effects of dbcAMP in experiment 1 is differ from experiment 2

Table 3 Effects of db-cAMP on serum biochemical indices and hormones in finishing pigs

Variable	Experiment 1		Experiment 2	
	controls	db cAMP	controls	db cAMP
Cholesterol (mmol/L)	2.45±0.08	2.34±0.11	1.96±0.11	2.08±0.06
TG (mmol/L)	0.36±0.04	0.38±0.04	0.28±0.02	0.29±0.03
Lipase (U/L)	48.3±6.6	62.1±13.5	42.7±3.6	69.9±15.2
FFA (□mol/L)	142.7±18.2	253.8±25.2	203.1±34.9	316.1±90.1
HDL (mmol/L)	0.54±0.08	0.58±0.06	0.71±0.05	0.77±0.03
LDL (mmol/L)	1.52±0.09	1.48±0.06	1.30±0.08	1.36±0.06
GH (ng/mL)	8.79±0.34	11.92±0.67*	8.87±0.24	9.26±0.65
IGF-1 (ng/mL)	337±23.5	431±24.2*	333±46.5	337±44.8
IGFBP3 (ng/mL)	63.8±5.7	86.6±10.0	67.6±12.4	68.4±13.2
T3 (ng/mL)	8.46±1.19	16.27±4.15*	11.35±1.17	11.37±1.65
T4 (ng/mL)	2.81±0.09	4.13±0.52*	3.41±0.19	3.42±0.35
Leptin (ng/mL)	1.44±0.44	0.99±0.23	7.15±1.45	2.10±0.22*
AD (ng/mL)	17.31±1.59	23.53±3.48	12.65±1.33	13.83±2.09
Insulin (ng/mL)	1.98±0.03	1.81±0.05	2.01±0.03	2.01±0.04
cAMP (pmol/mL)	73.69±3.69	127.36±28.8*	85.41±9.49	87.98±3.22

Within stages, means with * differ ($P < 0.05$)

TG, triglyceride; FFA, Free fatty acid; HDL, High-density lipoprotein; LDL, Low-density lipoprotein; IGFBP3, Insulin-like growth factor binding protein 3; T3, Triiodothyronine; T4, Thyroxine; AD, Adrenaline

Effect of db-cAMP on gene expression in hypothalamus, pituitary gland, and liver of finishing pigs

Changes in relative transcript abundance of genes of particular interest in the hypothalamus, pituitary, and liver are presented in Table 4. Treatments with db-cAMP increased the relative abundance of *ADCYAP1*, *GHRH*, *CRH*, *POMC*, and *PC1* (all $P < 0.05$) in the hypothalamus in experiment 1. Similar increases also occurred in pituitary abundance of *GHRHR* ($P < 0.05$), *GH* ($P < 0.01$), and *POMC* ($P < 0.05$) and hepatic expression of *GHR* and *IGF-1* ($P < 0.01$) in experiment 1. At the completion of experiment 2, db-cAMP treatment increased the relative abundance of *GHRH* ($P < 0.05$), *CRH* ($P < 0.05$), *POMC* ($P < 0.01$), and *PC1* ($P < 0.05$) in hypothalamus, *GH* ($P < 0.05$) and *POMC* ($P < 0.05$) in the pituitary gland, and hepatic expression of *IGF-1* ($P < 0.05$). The effect of db-cAMP on these gene expression was greater in experiment 1 than those in experiment 2 ($P < 0.05$), and db-cAMP increased the gene expressions of *GHRH*, *CRH*, *PC1*, *PC2*, *GHRHR*, *GH*, *POMC*, *GHR* and IGF-I by 173, 63, 142, 57, 32, 140, 131, 93, and 128 % in experiment 1 and 89, 45, 55, 15, 0, 115,95, 8, and 93 % in experiment 2.

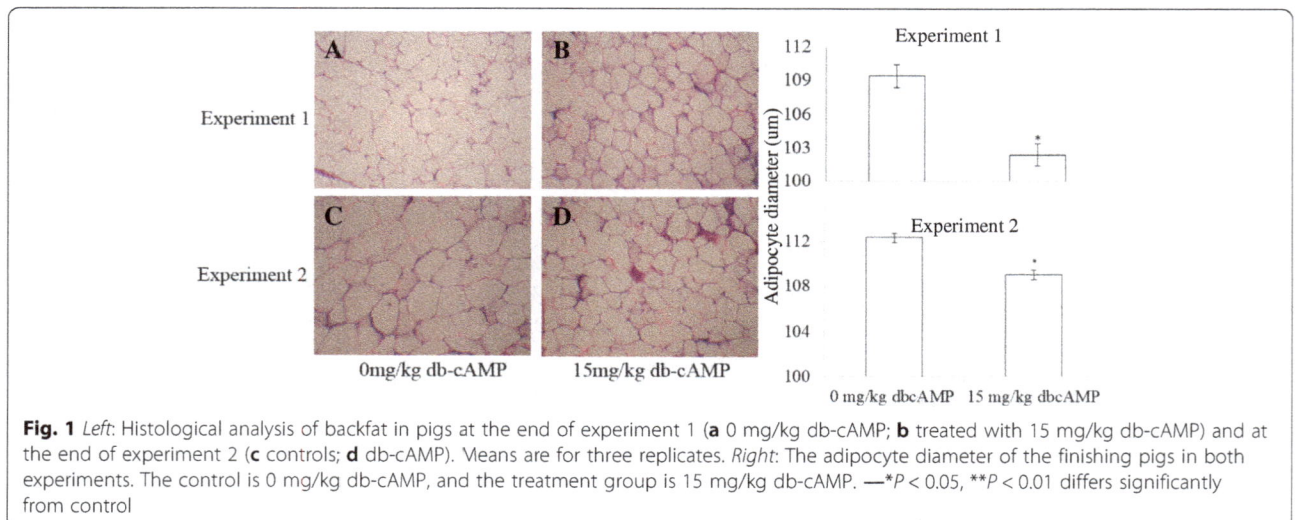

Fig. 1 *Left*: Histological analysis of backfat in pigs at the end of experiment 1 (**a** 0 mg/kg db-cAMP; **b** treated with 15 mg/kg db-cAMP) and at the end of experiment 2 (**c** controls; **d** db-cAMP). Means are for three replicates. *Right*: The adipocyte diameter of the finishing pigs in both experiments. The control is 0 mg/kg db-cAMP, and the treatment group is 15 mg/kg db-cAMP. —*$P < 0.05$, **$P < 0.01$ differs significantly from control

Table 4 Effects of db-cAMP on relative gene expression in the hypothalamus, pituitary gland and liver of finishing pigs

Variable	Experiment 1		Experiment 2	
	controls	db cAMP	controls	db cAMP
Hypothalamus				
ADCYAP1	0.56±0.02	0.78±0.02*	0.41±0.02	0.59±0.02
GHRH#	0.51±0.04	1.39±0.05**	0.38±0.05	0.72±0.08*
CRH#	0.94±0.03	1.53±0.06*	0.66±0.02	0.97±0.05*
POMC	0.81±0.01	1.00±0.01*	0.46±0.03	1.81±0.01**
PC1#	0.33±0.02	0.80±0.05*	0.64±0.04	0.99±0.01*
PC2#	0.35±0.02	0.55±0.03	0.71±0.02	0.82±0.01
Pituitary gland				
GHRHR#	0.72±0.01	0.95±0.01*	0.45±0.01	0.46±0.01
GH#	0.50±0.02	1.20±0.01**	0.39±0.01	0.84±0.03*
CRHR	0.59±0.03	0.62±0.03	0.59±0.01	0.75±0.08
POMC#	0.49±0.02	1.13±0.01*	0.42±0.01	0.82±0.01*
TRHR	0.51±0.01	0.58±0.03	0.39±0.02	0.53±0.01
TSH	1.44±0.04	1.49±0.02	0.66±0.04	0.88±0.03
Liver				
GHR#	0.55±0.01	1.06±0.03**	0.86±0.01	0.93±0.05
IGF-1#	0.50±0.01	1.14±0.01**	0.57±0.01	1.10±0.02*

Within stages, means with * differ ($P < 0.05$) and those with ** differ ($P < 0.01$).
Within the same line, # means the effects of dbcAMP in experiment 1 is differ from experiment 2.

Microarray analysis of backfat

To better understand the mechanism of the effect of dietary db-cAMP on fat deposition of the pigs, the backfat samples of experiment 1 were examined by microarrays and SAS analysis with thresholds for low probability values (FDR) set at $P < 0.05$ and log-fold change >1. Principal component analysis showed that differences between the control and treated pigs had high similarity, especially within the three control replicates.

Compared with the controls, the expression of 739 gene sets in treated animals changed significantly ($P < 0.05$, fold change >2, or <0.5); 248 gene sets were up-regulated (red), and 491 gene sets were down-regulated (green). Of the 739, only 84 gene sets have detailed comments and can be found in public databases for pigs; 14 were up-regulated and 70 down-regulated (Table 5). The heatmap plot (Fig. 2) showed that most of these genes (83 %) were down-regulated in pigs supplemented with db-cAMP compared with the controls.

Gene ontology analysis (SAS) showed that, compared with the controls, differentially expressed genes in db-cAMP supplemented pigs were significantly enriched in the categories listed in Table 6. The highest enrichment occurred in cell activation and immune functions, including leukocyte functions. Pathway analysis of the 84 differentially expressed genes in pigs supplemented with db-cAMP exposed the top five significant pathway maps involving 30 genes, and all of these were down-regulated (Fig. 3). The pathways, chemokine signaling, cell adhesion molecules (CAMs), Toll-like receptor signaling, cytokine-cytokine receptor interaction, antigen processing and presentation, and type I diabetes mellitus are consistent with the dietary supplementation causing a significant change in immune or inflammatory status of the adipose tissue.

Verification test

A selection of ten genes with relatively large change and related to fat metabolism or cell signaling were chosen to verify that their relative transcript abundance determined by the gene chips could be confirmed using real-time, quantitative PCR. For nine genes (Fig. 4), there was high correlation between the results of the mRNA array and qPCR methods (the average R^2 89 %).

Discussion

Consistent with others' findings [39], the present dietary supplementation with 15 mg/kg db-cAMP significantly decreased the backfat thickness and fat percentage of finishing pigs in both experiments while it did not affect growth performance or meat quality in either experiment, but Tian [36] found that db-cAMP stimulated the growth performance of pigs. The present research also showed that db-cAMP decreased the backfat thickness and backfat percentage more marked in the earlier

Table 5 The differentially expressed genes in adipocytes of finishing pigs treated with db-cAMP

Gene ID	Gene name	Gene description	P value	Fold change
Up-regulated				
396739	SAL1	salivary lipocalin	0.0025	22.14
407247	LHCGR	luteinizing hormone/choriogonadotropin receptor	0.044	5.18
641359	SULT2A1	sulfotransferase family, cytosolic, 2A, dehydro- epiandrosterone (DHEA)-preferring, member 1	0.0412	4.37
396597	STAR	steroidogenic acute regulatory protein	0.0043	4.14
403149	CYP2A19	cytochrome P450 2A19	0.0096	3.40
397290	HOXD10A	homeobox protein A10	0.0209	2.87
100124377	SBAB-707F1.10	solute carrier family 44, member 4	0.0353	2.58
397670	RH	Rh protein	0.0444	2.56
733668	DIRAS3	DIRAS family, GTP-binding RAS-like 3	0.0036	2.41
397324	ACACA	acetyl-Coenzyme A carboxylase alpha	0.0252	2.40
396861	LCN1	lipocalin 1 (tear prealbumin)	0.0062	2.29
100048933	ZFAND5	zinc finger, AN1-type domain 5	0.0113	2.25
100216478	TEF1	transcriptional enhancer factor 1	0.0200	2.19
414420	RPS28	ribosomal protein S28	0.0228	2.10
Down-regulated				
100157574	LOC100157574	similar to family with sequence similarity 49, member B	0.0022	0.50
100156398	LOC100156398	mini-chromosome maintenance complex component 4	0.0333	0.50
100154512	LOC100154512	similar to tripartite motif-containing 38	0.046	0.49
397330	XPO1	exportin 1 (CRM1 homolog, yeast)	0.0159	0.49
396599	MCSF ALPHA	macrophage colony stimulating factor alpha	0.0219	0.49
733579	LOC733579	tripartite motif protein TRIM5	0.0241	0.49
396655	STAT1	signal transducer and activator of transcription 1	0.0379	0.49
397177	DUOX1	dual oxidase 1	0.0234	0.48
100157208	LOC100157208	similar to Tectonic-3	0.0314	0.48
397222	MEOX2	mesenchyme homeobox 2	0.0095	0.48
100125540	SYK	spleen tyrosine kinase	0.0183	0.48
397108	GP91-PHOX	NADPH oxidase heavy chain subunit	0.0339	0.48
100154251	LOC100154251	similar to pleckstrin 2	0.0409	0.47
100048944	CPEB1	cytoplasmic polyadenylation element binding protein 1	0.0375	0.47
100158101	LOC100158101	similar to Rho GTPase-activating protein 30	0.0053	0.47
100048955	C5AR1	complement component 5a receptor 1	0.0121	0.47
100037274	TAF4B	TAF4b RNA polymerase II, TATA box binding protein (TBP)-associated factor, 105 kDa	0.0089	0.46
397041	LGALS4	lectin, galactoside-binding, soluble, 4	0.0439	0.46
100049698	SNCAIP	synuclein, alpha interacting protein	0.0078	0.45
595128	OAS2	2'-5'-oligoadenylate synthetase 2, 69/71 kDa	0.0401	0.453
397422	CCL2	chemokine (C-C motif) ligand 2	0.0181	0.45
387287	HCRTR1	hypocretin (orexin) receptor 1	0.0387	0.45
100124526	CD1D	CD1d molecule	0.0189	0.45
397271	AIF1	allograft inflammatory factor 1	0.0132	0.44
396935	PCCB	propionyl Coenzyme A carboxylase, beta polypeptide	0.0326	0.44
733649	TAP1	transporter 1, ATP-binding cassette, sub-family B (MDR/TAP)	0.0419	0.44
100156191	LOC100156191	zygote arrest 1-like protein	0.0402	0.44

Table 5 The differentially expressed genes in adipocytes of finishing pigs treated with db-cAMP *(Continued)*

414912	PU.1	transcription factor PU.1	0.0044	0.43
100157355	LOC100157355	similar to spindle and KT associated 1	0.0325	0.43
404704	CD4	CD4 molecule	0.0029	0.43
100126851	SERPINB9	serpin peptidase inhibitor, clade B (ovalbumin), member 9	0.0464	0.42
396723	DDX58	DEAD (Asp-Glu-Ala-Asp) box polypeptide 58	0.0049	0.42
396943	ITGB2	integrin, beta 2 (complement component 3 receptor 3 and 4 subunit)	0.0088	0.41
397141	NPL	N-acetylneuraminate pyruvate lyase	0.0157	0.40
100037296	TLR7	toll-like receptor 7	0.0053	0.40
100048946	RNASEL	Ribonuclease-L(2',5'-oligoisoadenylate-synthetase- dependent)	0.0105	0.40
100048958	GNA14	guanine nucleotide binding protein (G protein), alpha 14	0.0486	0.40
397441	CD86	CD86 molecule	0.0208	0.40
399500	IL6	interleukin 6 (interferon, beta 2)	0.0176	0.39
397590	PGHS-2	prostaglandin G/H synthase-2	0.024	0.38
100049665	KRT2	keratin 2	0.019	0.38
445460	C1QC	complement component 1, q subcomponent, C chain	0.0045	0.38
100156254	LOC100156254	similar to Plastin-2 (L-plastin) (Lymphocyte cytosolic protein 1) (LCP-1) (LC64P)	0.0435	0.38
100155269	LOC100155269	similar to lymphocyte antigen 9	0.0131	0.37
396900	AMCF-II	alveolar macrophage-derived chemotactic factor-II	0.0494	0.37
404772	GEM	GTP binding protein overexpressed in skeletal muscle	0.0291	0.36
397414	UF	uteroferrin	0.0066	0.36
100153090	LOC100153090	similar to Cathepsin S	0.0411	0.36
414373	CCR3	chemokine (C-C motif) receptor 3	0.0179	0.3
100152784	LOC100152784	Vascular non-inflammatory molecule 3 precursor (Vanin-3)	0.0392	0.35
399541	TLR4	toll-like receptor 4	0.0474	0.35
606745	LOC606745	A2b adenosine receptor	0.0159	0.35
100049673	HPS3	Hermansky-Pudlak syndrome 3	0.038	0.35
396624	OX40L	OX40L protein	0.0323	0.35
414374	CCR1	chemokine (C-C motif) receptor 1	0.0196	0.34
100152550	LOC100152550	similar to EF-hand domain (C-terminal) containing 1	0.038	0.34
503658	ENPP2	ectonucleotide pyrophosphatase/phosphodiesterase 2	0.0481	0.33
397079	CECR1	cat eye syndrome chromosome region, candidate 1	0.0057	0.33
396880	IL8	interleukin 8	0.0091	0.32
396985	PLAU	plasminogen activator	0.0474	0.32
100154994	LOC100154994	similar to serine proteinase inhibitor, clade B, member 10	0.0192	0.31
574057	PDCD1LG2	programmed cell death 1 ligand 2	0.0178	0.30
396726	FASLG	Fas ligand (TNF superfamily, member 6)	0.0261	0.30
414904	CXCL2	chemokine (C-X-C motif) ligand 2	0.0093	0.30
100156373	LOC100156373	similar to villin 1	0.0067	0.28
397373	MYO7A	myosin VIIA	0.0473	0.27
397102	AMBN	ameloblastin	0.0329	0.19
100049669	GPNMB	glycoprotein (transmembrane) nmb	0.0447	0.18
396662	CD2	CD2 molecule	0.0212	0.16
100135044	SBAB-591C4.5	MHC class II, DQ alpha	0.0027	0.09

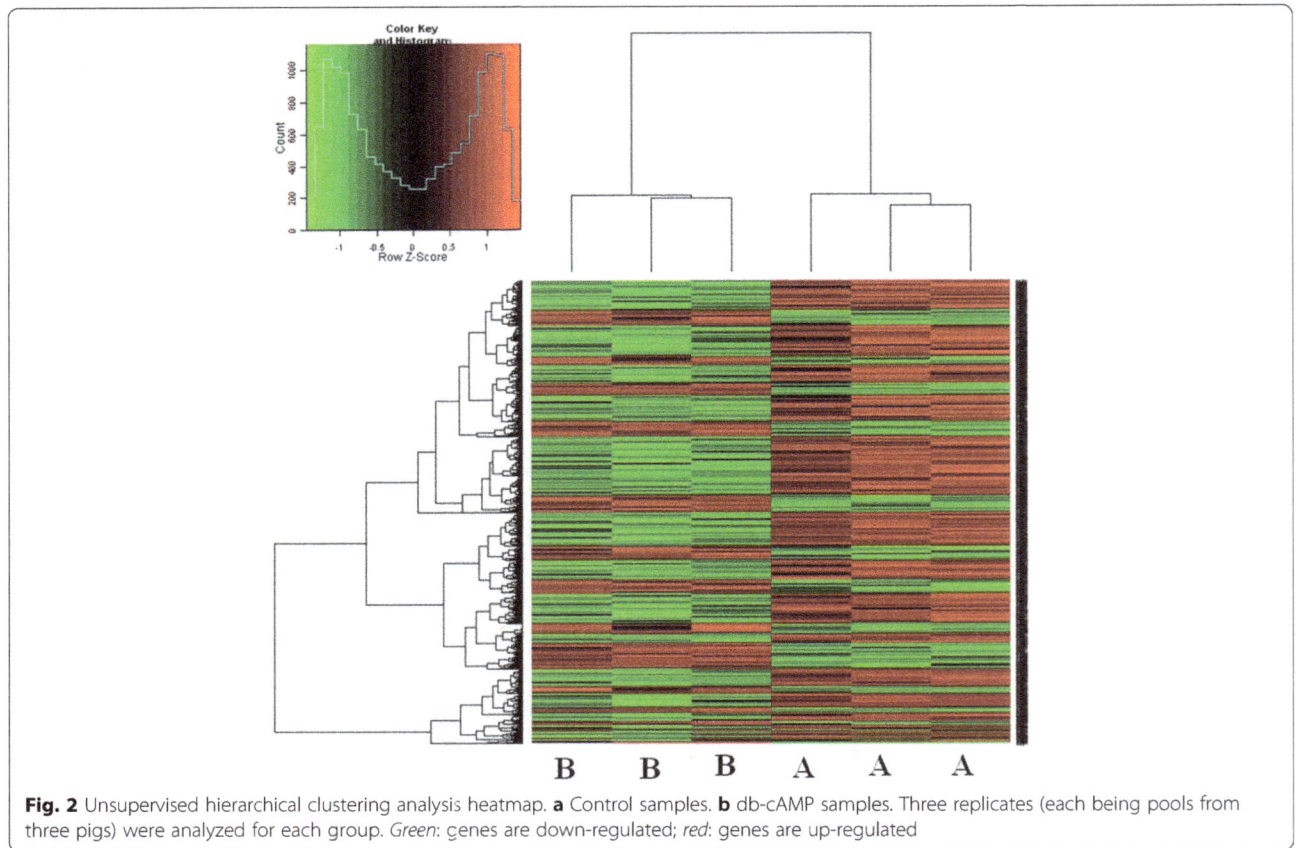

Fig. 2 Unsupervised hierarchical clustering analysis heatmap. **a** Control samples. **b** db-cAMP samples. Three replicates (each being pools from three pigs) were analyzed for each group. *Green*: genes are down-regulated; *red*: genes are up-regulated

stages than the later stages of finishing pigs, which implied that supplementation of db-cAMP in the earlier phase is better than the later phase of finishing pigs. This additive also was found to improve carcass composition and increase longissimus area and lean percentages in other experiment [39]. In our experiment, the longissimus area had a trend to increase after treated with db-cAMP. The changes in adipocyte volume can be used to estimate fat deposition in pigs [33] and adult rats [24]. The result of our experiment verified the previous

Table 6 Significant GO of differentially expressed genes

GO ID	Annotation	Number Changed/number measured (%)	Enrichment test p-value	Q value
GO:0001775	cell activation	15/150 (10)	0.0001	0.0202
GO:0050900	leukocyte migration	7/42 (16.67)	0.0005	0.0501
GO:0045321	leukocyte activation	12/123 (9.76)	0.0005	0.0501
GO:0042330	Taxis	9/76 (11.84)	0.0007	0.0569
GO:0002376	immune system process	24/410 (5.85)	0.0010	0.0681
GO:0001816	cytokine production	8/90 (8.89)	0.0072	0.3915
GO:0048583	regulation of response to stimulus	13/206 (6.31)	0.0101	0.4143
GO:0045058	T cell selection	3/16 (18.75)	0.0168	0.4460
GO:0009605	response to external stimulus	22/456 (4.82)	0.0168	0.4460
GO:0002682	regulation of immune system process	11/173 (6.36)	0.0170	0.4460
GO:0030029	actin filament-based process	10/154 (6.49)	0.0200	0.4460
GO:0006955	immune response	15/277 (5.42)	0.0205	0.4460
GO:0002520	immune system development	10/161 (6.21)	0.0260	0.5319
GO:0043900	regulation of multi-organism process	2/10 (20)	0.0463	0.7559

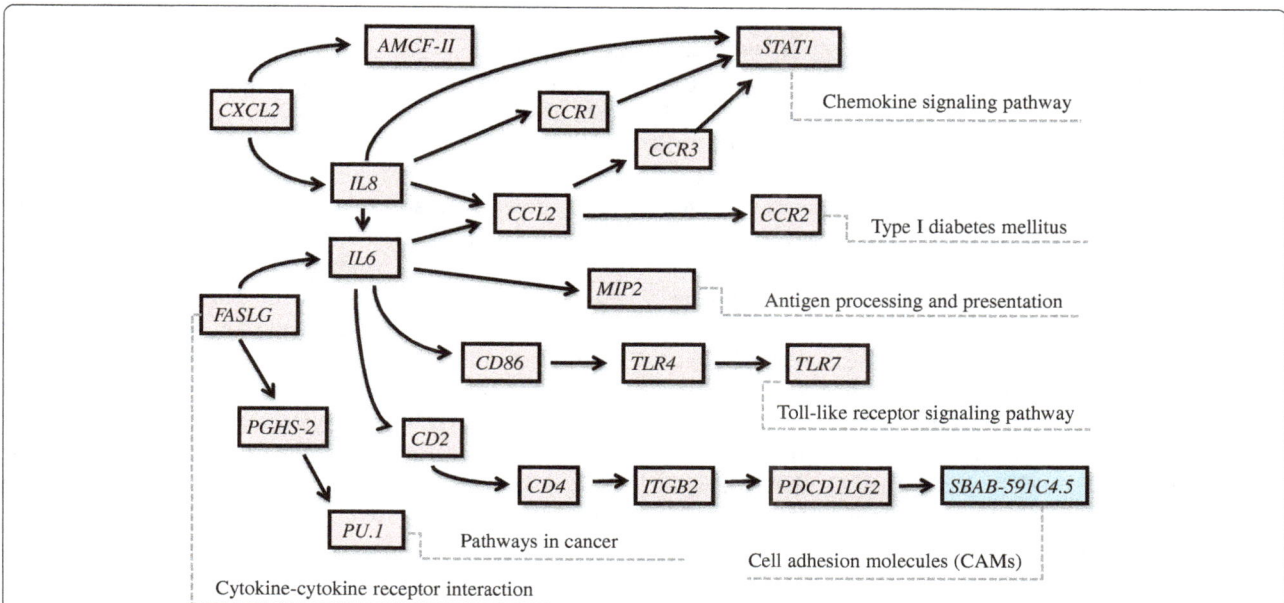

Fig. 3 Pathway analysis of the differently expressed genes involved in several changed pathways of the db-cAMP treatment group compared with the control group. *Green*: genes are down-regulated; *red*: genes are up-regulated

found that dietary db-cAMP decreased the diameter of adipocytes [38] in two different stages of finishing pigs, which may be caused by inhibiting the proliferation of preadipocytes and their differentiation [21], but the mechanism of db-cAMP inhibiting the proliferation and differentiation of preadipocytes is not illuminated yet. Db-cAMP increasing the activities of lipolytic enzymes [4] and inhibiting lipogenesis [21] was another reason for the backfat thickness decreased. The present study found that db-cAMP strikingly increased the plasma concentrations of cAMP at the earlier phase of finishing

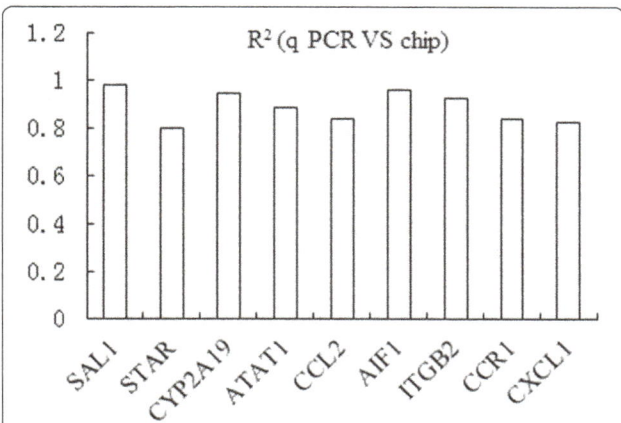

Fig. 4 The correlation coefficient of selected genes expressing level by RT-qPCR and gene chip data. *Vertical axis*: the value of correlation coefficient of the gene expression level by RT-qPCR and gene chip data; *horizontal axis*: detected genes

pigs and decreased the plasma concentrations of leptin at the later phase of finishing pigs, which verified the finding of Maeda and Horiuchi [19].

Dietary db-cAMP clearly influenced fat metabolism related to hormone and genes in the hypothalamus and pituitary, most notably in the earlier phase of finishing pigs; this is our novel founding. Both GH and its downstream peptide IGF-I and T3 and T4 were at higher concentrations in db-cAMP-treated pigs. Underlying these changes, there were increases in several gene expression level in the hypothalamus, pituitary, and liver in supplemented pigs. These included hypothalamic expression of *ADCYAP1* which activates adenylyl cyclase to increase endogenous cAMP and stimulates secretion of *GHRH* and *CRH* [3, 20], *GHRH*, *CRH*, *POMC*, and *PC1* genes. Supplementation with db-cAMP increased pituitary expression of *GHRHR* and *GH* and hepatic expression of *GHR* and *IGF-1*, all of which indicated enhanced activity of the GHRH-GH-IGF-1 axis. Some of these responses were also evident, though of less magnitude, in the second stage of finishing (day 170), consistent with higher circulating concentrations of GH and IGF-1 in the supplemented pigs. In experiment 1, supplemented pigs had higher plasma concentrations of T3 and T4 though no changes in pituitary expression of *TRHR* or *TSH*. The thyroid hormones promote and, in cooperation with GH and IGF-1, stimulate lipolysis [8, 37]. The findings described here help explain that db-cAMP increased the plasma contents of GH, IGF-1, T3, and T4 [6, 21, 39]. Dietary supplementation with db-cAMP also influenced the POMC axis with increasing the expression of *POMC* both in hypothalamus and pituitary and *CRH*, *PC1*, and *PC2* in hypothalamus. This system is implicated in the regulation of lipolysis and interactions between CRH and POMC [2, 9, 28], which also was affected by the dietary energy level and energy intake [22] and hydrolyzed by PC1 and PC2 [14, 34]. The changes detected here suggest some involvement of the POMC system in the effects of db-cAMP on lipid metabolism and fat accretion, and the possible mechanisms need to be further researched.

Db-cAMP decreasing the backfat thickness and backfat percentage was verified by the 2 experiments using different phases of finishing pigs in this present study, and we found new mechanism of db-cAMP regulating fat metabolism by mRNA array analysis that was db-cAMP affected the immune/inflammatory reaction. As the backfat thickness was obviously reduced by dietary db-cAMP in the earlier phase of the finishing pigs, gene expression in this tissue also was examined to expose likely underlying mechanisms. Go analysis result showed that db-cAMP inhibited the proliferation and differentiation of fat cells and reduces the deposition of adipose tissue through inhibiting adipose tissue cell activation, cell tropism, leukocyte activation, migration, and the immune system activation of the fattening pig. A relatively low proportion (11 %) of the differentially expressed gene sets was adequately documented, and of these, the bulk (83 %) was down-regulated in db-cAMP-treated pigs. It was of interest that the most striking changes occurred, not in genes obviously related to lipid metabolism but in cohorts associated with immune/inflammatory functions related to insulin sensitive or lipolysis. There is increasing recognition that inflammatory reactions in adipose tissue contribute to adiposity and appear to be linked to the metabolic syndrome and type I diabetes. The differentially expressed genes identified here were most obviously associated with pathways including chemokine signaling, CAMs, antigen processing and presentation, Toll-like receptor signaling, cancer, cytokine-cytokine receptor interaction, and type I diabetes mellitus. The chemokine member *CCL2* was highly expressed in adipose tissue and contributed to the cells becoming insulin resistant [10, 26] while *CXCL2* (or *MIP-2*), encoding macrophage inflammatory protein 2-alpha (MIP2-alpha), was the main marker of inflammatory reaction in metabolic syndrome [16, 35]. Another cytokine IL-8 [18] was highly expressed in hypertrophied adipocytes [1], and its inhibition decreased the likelihood of obesity and type 2 diabetes [15]. Cytokine receptors such as *CCR1*, *CCR2*, *CCR3*, and *CCR5* also related to insulin sensitivity [12], in turn closely connected with the size of adipocytes [32]. These genes also were down-regulated and stimulated lipolysis [23]. Although in the

present experiment db-cAMP did not decrease the concentration of plasma insulin, it could decrease the insulin sensitivity and stimulate the lipolysis, which reasons need further research. The CAMs pathway included a number of differentially expressed genes involved in inflammatory infiltration, reactions, and responses [25]. Their down-regulation in pigs treated with db-cAMP suggests diminished inflammatory sensitivity, perhaps resulting in reduced fat accretion. This interpretation was further supported by the diminished expression of several genes involved in Toll-like receptor signaling pathways critically involved in mediating inflammatory responses including in adipocytes, some of which were readily influenced by high-energy diets [27] and contributed to other pro-inflammatory factors secretion and insulin resistance [13]. The differential expression of these genes in backfat exposed by microarray analysis was, for the most part, convincingly supported by quantitative PCR measurements so they appear to be legitimate.

Conclusions

The results obtained from these analyses indicated that dietary supplementation of finishing pigs with db-cAMP resulted in significantly reduced accumulation of subcutaneous fat without changing growth performance or carcass characteristics, apparently stemmed from suppression of the inflammatory system within the adipose tissue related to insulin sensitive or lipolysis. There were additional systemic effects of treatment detected within major endocrine GHRH-GH-IGF-1 axis and POMC system, which are known to be involved in growth and energy metabolism. Any reduction in excessive fat deposition in finishing animals has economic and food quality consequences, so improved understanding of the underlying mechanisms allows exploring new strategies for manipulating fat accretion. This study has contributed to explaining how dietary supplemental db-cAMP provides a potential approach to achieving a more desirable animal product. In addition, this study illustrated that db-cAMP regulated fat deposition through improving the immune system, which is of potential value to dissect molecular pathways influencing fat deposition by db-cAMP. It would be benefit for health of human clinically used for weight loss.

Abbreviations

AD: adrenaline; ADCYAP1: adenylate cyclase activating polypeptide; *CRH*: corticotropin releasing hormone; *CRHR*: corticotropin releasing hormone receptor; db-cAMP: dibutyryl-cAMP; GH: growth hormone; GHR: growth hormone receptor; GHRH: growth hormone releasing hormone; GHRHR: growth hormone releasing hormone receptor; IGF-1: insulin-like growth factor-1; IGFBP3: insulin-like growth factor binding protein 3; PC: prohormone convertase; POMC: pro-opiomelanocortin; T3: triiodothyronine; T4: thyroxine; TRHR: thyrotropin-releasing hormone receptor; TSH: thyroid stimulating hormone.

Acknowledgements

This work was supported by grants from the earmarked fund for Modern Agro-industry Technology Research System (CARS-36), the National '973' Project of China (2012CB124706-5, 2012CB124706-4), and Guangdong innovation competence and building project (2012B060600005). We thank W. Bruce Currie (Emeritus Professor, Cornell University) for helping us in editing the manuscript.

Authors' contributions

XM carried out the mRNA array experiment, participated in analyzing the data, and drafted the manuscript. WF carried out the animal experiment. ZJ designed the experiment and supplied the fund. LW participated in the design of the study and performed the statistical analysis. XY participated in the lab experiment. KG helped to do the experiment and draft the manuscript. All authors read and approved the final manuscript.

Competing interests

The authors declare that they have no competing interests.

Author details

[1]Institute of Animal Science, Guangdong Academy of Agricultural Sciences, 510640 Guangzhou, China. [2]The Key Laboratory of Animal Nutrition and Feed Science (South China) of Ministry of Agriculture, 510640 Guangzhou, China. [3]State Key Laboratory of Livestock and Poultry Breeding, 510640 Guangzhou, China. [4]Guangdong Public Laboratory of Animal Breeding and Nutrition, 510640 Guangzhou, China. [5]Guangdong Key Laboratory of Animal Breeding and Nutrition, 510640 Guangzhou, China.

References

1. Boisvert WA. Modulation of atherogenesis by chemokines. Trends Cardiovasc Med. 2004;14:161–5.
2. Breen TL, Conwell IM, Wardlaw SL. Effects of fasting, leptin, and insulin on AGRP and POMC peptide release in the hypothalamus. Brain Res. 2005;1032:141–8.
3. Canny BJ, Rawlings SR, Leong DA. Pituitary adenylate cyclase activating polypeptide specifically increase cytosolic calcium ion concentration in rat gonadotropes and somatotropes. Endocrinology. 1992;130:211–5.
4. Carmen GY, Víctor SM. Signaling mechanisms regulating lipolysis. Cell Signal. 2006;18:401–8.
5. Chaves VE, Júnior FM, Bertolini GL. The metabolic effects of growth hormone in adipose tissue. Endocrine. 2013;44:293–302.
6. Cheng ML, Zhang X, Gao SS, Liu W, Yan DL. Regulation of dbcAMP on endocrine metabolism of pigs. Chin J Anim HusVet. 2005;32:3–5. Chinese Journal.
7. Egan JJ, Greenberg AS, Chang MK. Mechanism of hormone-stimulated lipolysis in adipocytes: translocation of hormone-sensitive lipase to the lipid storage droplet. Proc Natl Acad Sci. 1992;89:8537–41.
8. Ezzat S, Laks D, Oster J, Melmed S. Growth hormone regulation in primary fetal and neonatal rat pituitary cell culture: the role of thyroid hormone. Endocrinology. 1991;128:937–43.
9. Gagner JP, Drouin J. Tissue-specific regulation of pituitary proopiomelanocortin gene transcription by corticotropin-releasing hormone, 3′,5′-cyclic adenosine monophosphate, and glucocorticoids. Mol Endocrinol. 1987;1:677–52.
10. Gerhardt CC, Romero IA, Cancello R, Camoin L, Strosberg AD. Chemokines control fat accumulation and leptin secretion by cultured human adipocytes. Mol Cell Endocrinol. 2001;175:81–92.
11. Hernandez A, Garcia-Jimenez C, Santisteban P, Obregon MJ. Regulation of malic- enzyme-gene expression by cAMP and retinoic acid in differentiating brown adipocytes. Eur J Biochem. 1993;215:285–90.
12. Huber J, Kiefer FW, Zeyda M, Ludvik B, Silberhumer GR, Prager G, et al. CC chemokine and CC chemokine receptor profiles in visceral and subcutaneous adipose tissue are altered in human obesity. J Clin Endocrinol Metab. 2008;93:3215–21.
13. Hwa Cho H, Bae YC, Jung JS. Role of toll-like receptors on human adipose-derived stromal cells. Stem Cells. 2006;24:2744–52.
14. Karsi A, Waldbieser GC, Small BC, Wolters WR. Genomic structure of the proopiomelanocortin gene and expression during acute low-water stress in channel catfish. Gen Comp Endocrinol. 2005;143:104–12.
15. Kobashi C, Asamizu S, Ishiki M, Iwata M, Usui I, Yamazaki K, et al. Inhibitory effect of IL-8 on insulin action in human adipocytes via MAP kinase pathway. J Inflamm (Lond). 2009;6:25.
16. Leinonen E, Hurt-Camejo E, Wiklund O, Hultén LM, Hiukka A, Taskinen MR. Insulin resistance and adiposity correlate with acute-phase reaction and soluble cell adhesion molecules in type 2 diabetes. Atherosclerosis. 2003;166:387–94.
17. Ma XY, Lin YC, Jiang ZY, Zheng CT, Zhou GL. Dietary arginine supplementation enhances antioxidative capacity and improves meat quality of finishing pigs. Amino Acids. 2010;38:95–102.
18. Mackay CR. Chemokines: immunology's high impact factors. Nat Immunol. 2001;2:95–101.
19. Maeda T, Horiuchi N. Simvastatin suppresses leptin expression in 3 T3-L1 adipocytes via activation of the cyclic AMP-PKA pathway induced by inhibition of protein prenylation. J Biochem. 2009;145:771–81.
20. Mei YA, Vaudry D, Basille M, Castel H, Fournier A, Vaudry H, et al. PACAP inhibits delayed rectifier potassium current via a cAMP/PKA transduction pathway: evidence for the involvement of I k in the anti-apoptotic action of PACAP. Eur J Neurosci. 2004;19:1446–58.
21. Mills SE, Liu CY. Sensitivity of lipolysis and lipogenesis to dibutyryl-cAMP and beta-adrenergic agonists in swine adipocytes in vitro. J Anim Sci. 1990;68:1017–23.
22. Mizuno TM, Kleopoulos SP, Bergen HT, Roberts JL, Priest CA, Mobbs CV. Hypothalamic pro-opiomelanocortin mRNA is reduced by fasting in ob/ob and db/db mice, but is stimulated by leptin. Diabetes. 1998;47:294–7.
23. Mokry FB, Higa RH, de Alvarenga Mudadu M, Oliveira de Lima A, Meirelles SL, Barbosa da Silva MV, et al. Genome-wide association study for backfat thickness in Canchim beef cattle using Random Forest approach. BMC Genet. 2013;14:47.
24. Nall JL, Wu G, Kim KH, Choi CW, Smith SB. Dietary supplementation of L-arginine and conjugated linoleic acid reduces retroperitoneal fat mass and increases lean body mass in rats. J Nutr. 2009;139:1279–85.
25. Nicholas JG. Cell adhesion molecules in context: CAM function depends on the neighborhood. Cell Adh Migr. 2011;5:48–51.
26. Permana PA, Menge C, Reaven PD. Macrophage-secreted factors induce adipocyte inflammation and insulin resistance. Biochem Biophys Res Commun. 2006;341:507–14.
27. Pietsch J, Batra A, Stroh T, Fedke I, Glauben R, Okur B, et al. Toll-like receptor expression and response to specific stimulation in adipocytes and preadipocytes: on the role of fat in inflammation. Ann N Y Acad Sci. 2006; 1072:407–9.
28. Poplawski MM, Boyadjieva N, Sarkar DK. Vasoactive intestinal peptide and corticotropin releasing hormone increase beta-endorphin release and propinomelanocortin messenger RNA levels in primary cultures of hypothalamic cells: effects of acute and chronic ethanol treatment. Alcohol Clin Exp Res. 2005;29:648–55.
29. Science and Technology Ministry of China. The guiding suggestion about treating experimental animals amicably. Document no. 2006; 398. (Chinese Version)
30. Schofield JG. Role of cyclic 3′,5′-adenosine monophosphate in relation of hormone in vitro. Nature. 1967;215:1382–3.
31. Schmidt M, Evellin S, Weernink PA, von Dorp F, Rehmann H, Lomasney JW, et al. A new phospholipase-C-calcium signaling pathway mediated by cyclic AMP and a Rap GTPase. Nat Cell Biol. 2001;3:1020–4.
32. Salans LB, Dougherty JW. The effect of insulin upon glucose metabolism by adipose cells of different size. J Clin Invest. 1971;50:1399–410.
33. Steffen DG, Chai EY, Brown LJ, Mersmann HJ. Effects of diet on swine glyceride lipid metabolism. J Nutr. 1978;108:911–8.
34. Tanaka S. Comparative aspects of intracellular proteolytic processing of peptide hormone precursors: studies of proopiomelanocortin processing. Zoolog Sci. 2003;20:1183–98.
35. Tataranni PA, Ortega E. A burning question: does an adipokine-induced activation of the immune system mediate the effect of overnutrition on type 2 diabetes? Diabetes. 2005;54:917–27.
36. Tian YB. Effect of dbcAMP on growth performance and meat quality of pigs. Guangxi Sci. 2003;10:305–8. Chinese Journal.
37. Valcavi R, Zini M, Portioli I. Thyroid hormone and growth hormone secretion (review). J Endocrinol Invest. 1992;15:313–30.

15

Brain xanthophyll content and exploratory gene expression analysis: subspecies differences in rhesus macaque

Emily S. Mohn[1], John W. Erdman Jr.[2], Martha Neuringer[3], Matthew J. Kuchan[4] and Elizabeth J. Johnson[1,5*]

Abstract

Background: The dietary xanthophylls, lutein and zeaxanthin, accumulate in primate retina and brain, and emerging evidence indicates neural lutein content may be beneficial for cognition. Neural xanthophyll content in primates varies greatly among individuals, and genetic factors are likely to be significant contributors. Subspecies of rhesus macaques originating from different geographic locations are known to differ genetically, but the effect of origin on gene expression and carotenoid status has not been determined. The study objective was to determine whether xanthophyll status and expression of carotenoid-related genes, as well as genes with known variants between subspecies, differ between the brains of adult rhesus monkeys of Indian and Chinese origin.

Methods: Samples of prefrontal cortex, cerebellum, and striatum were collected from adult monkeys ($n = 9$) fed a standard stock diet containing carotenoids. Serum and brain carotenoids were determined using reverse-phase high-performance liquid chromatography. For each brain region, RNA sequencing and real-time quantitative polymerase chain reaction were used to determine differentially expressed genes between the subspecies.

Results: Indian-origin monkeys had higher xanthophyll levels in brain tissue compared to Chinese-origin monkeys despite consuming similar amounts of dietary carotenoids. In a region-specific manner, four genes related to carotenoid and fatty acid metabolism (BCO2, RPE65, ELOVL4, FADS2) and four genes involved in the immune response (CD4, CD74, CXCL12 LTBR) were differentially expressed between Indian- and Chinese-origin monkeys. Expression of all four genes involved in carotenoid and fatty acid metabolism were correlated with brain xanthophyll concentration in a region-specific manner.

Conclusions: These results indicate that origin is related to differences in both gene expression and xanthophyll content in the brain. Findings from this study may have important implications regarding genetic diversity, lutein status, and cognition in primates.

Keywords: Lutein, Zeaxanthin, Rhesus monkey, Subspecies, Brain, RNA-sequencing

Background

Lutein is a xanthophyll carotenoid found in a variety of colorful fruits and vegetables, as well as in dark leafy greens and eggs [1]. Animals cannot synthesize lutein, and therefore its presence in the body is a result of dietary consumption [2]. Lutein and its isomer zeaxanthin

accumulate in the macula of the primate retina to form macular pigment (MP). In the macula, lutein and zeaxanthin function to protect the eye from oxidative damage both by filtering harmful blue light and by their antioxidant activity [3, 4]. More recently it has been discovered that lutein, and in smaller amounts, zeaxanthin, also preferentially accumulate in the primate brain [5–7]. Current evidence indicates that lutein may have an important role in maintaining and improving brain function and cognition, with studies showing that MP optical density (MPOD) [8–11], as well as serum and brain lutein concentrations, are associated with better cognition in humans [6].

* Correspondence: Elizabeth.Johnson@tufts.edu
[1]Jean Mayer United States Department of Agriculture Human Nutrition Research Center on Aging, Tufts University, Boston, MA, USA
[5]Antioxidants Research Laboratory, 711 Washington Street, Boston, MA 02111, USA
Full list of author information is available at the end of the article

It is well established that there is a high amount of inter-individual variability in serum carotenoid levels [12, 13]. A major contributing factor is the large variability in intestinal absorption of carotenoids [14]. Additionally, MP response to dietary and supplemental lutein/zeaxanthin is highly variable [15–17]. Genomic studies have identified a number of single nucleotide polymorphisms (SNPs) in genes involved in carotenoid uptake, transport, and metabolism that are related to MPOD and risk for age-related macular degeneration (AMD) [18, 19]. While a number of studies have documented significant variability in efficiency of uptake and storage of lutein and zeaxanthin in the eye, it is not clear whether the same variability is observed in the brain. However, it is likely that these tissues share similar mechanisms for xanthophyll uptake and deposition given that lutein is selectively taken up into this tissue just as it is in the retina [6, 7]. Evidence to support this hypothesis has been shown in both human and non-human primates where MP was significantly correlated with lutein concentrations in the brain [20, 21].

Like humans, but unlike other animal models, rhesus macaques (*Macaca mulatta*) have been shown to absorb and preferentially store xanthophylls in the eye and brain [20, 22], making them an ideal model for studying factors influencing the accumulation of lutein and zeaxanthin into neural tissue. Another advantage of using these non-human primates is that rhesus monkeys of different geographical origin (Indian and Chinese) have been shown to be genetically different, with a number of SNPs distinguishing the two subspecies from one another [23]. Therefore, utilizing both subspecies of monkeys in carotenoid research provides a unique opportunity for studying the nutrigenomics of xanthophyll absorption, deposition, and storage/metabolism in neural tissue. However, to date, no studies have investigated whether accumulation of xanthophylls in neural tissue differs between rhesus monkeys of Indian and Chinese origin when provided very similar carotenoid-containing foods. Additionally, no studies have determined the relationship between rhesus monkey origin and expression of genes related to xanthophyll metabolism and function.

The objective of this study was twofold: (1) to determine whether xanthophyll status in serum and brain differs between rhesus monkeys of different subspecies and (2) to investigate whether the brains of rhesus monkeys of Indian and Chinese origin differs in the expression of genes involved in carotenoid uptake, transport, and metabolism as well as genes with known variants between subspecies. Brain regions of interest included the prefrontal cortex (PFC), cerebellum (CER), and striatum (STR), since these regions play important but distinct roles in cognitive function [24–26].

Methods

Study animals and diet

Post-mortem brain samples from nine rhesus monkeys (*M. mulatta*) ranging from 7 to 16 years of age were obtained from the Tissue Distribution Program at the Oregon National Primate Research Center (ONPRC) at Oregon Health and Science University. All animals were fed a standard monkey stock diet (LabDiet #5037, St. Louis, MO) that was determined by reverse-phase high-performance liquid chromatography (HPLC) [27] to contain ~16 μmol/kg of lutein, ~6 μmol/kg of zeaxanthin, ~5 μmol/kg β-carotene, ~1 μmol/kg α-carotene, and ~0.1 μmol/kg cryptoxanthin, plus a variety of supplemental fruits and vegetables two times/week (seasonal: bananas, apples, oranges, spinach, cucumber, carrots). All Indian-origin monkeys were born at the ONPRC, while monkeys of Chinese origin were obtained as young adults and lived for 3 years at the ONPRC prior to termination. After termination, PFC, CER, and STR were dissected, frozen at −0 °C and shipped on dry ice overnight to Tufts University for analysis. Tissues were kept frozen at −80 °C until analysis.

Carotenoid extraction from brain regions and serum

Extraction of carotenoids from brain regions was adapted from previous methods [28] and has been described in detail [20]. Seven of the nine monkeys had serum collected at termination that was available for carotenoid analysis. Carotenoids were extracted from serum as previously described [29]. HPLC was used to separate and quantify carotenoids [29]. For serum, total lutein (sum of *cis* and *trans* isomers) was used for the data analysis. In the brain, only the *trans* isomer of lutein was detected. For the other carotenoids, including zeaxanthin, only the *trans* isomers were detected in serum and brain. Carotenoid data (both serum and brain) are expressed as mean ± standard error of mean.

Total RNA extraction from rhesus monkey brain for RNA sequencing and RT-PCR

From the nine monkeys, three from each subspecies were selected for RNA sequencing (RNA-seq) analysis that were matched for age (13 ± 4 years and 11 ± 1 year for Indian- and Chinese-origin monkeys, respectively) and sex (two females and one male in each group). Total RNA was isolated from PFC, CER, and STR using the RNeasy lipid tissue mini kit (Qiagen) per manufacturer's instructions. RNA purity and concentrations were determined using a NanoDrop ND-1000 (Thermo Fisher Scientific). All RNA samples had a 260/280 ratio greater than 2.05. One to 2 μg RNA was aliquoted for RNA-seq analysis. RNA integrity was determined to be satisfactory for sequencing using an AATI (Advanced Analytical Technologies, Inc) Fragment Analyzer. One microgram

RNA was aliquoted for real-time quantitative polymerase chain reaction (RT-PCR).

Library preparation, next-generation RNA sequencing, and processing of reads

RNA-seq was performed in order to explore differences in gene expression profiles in the brains of rhesus monkeys of different origin. RNA-seq uses next-generation sequencing to characterize genome-wide RNA sequences and determine their abundance in a given sample with extremely high resolution. Due to its high sensitivity and broad scope, RNA-seq is quickly becoming the preferred method over microarrays for differential gene expression studies [30].

For library preparation, the TruSeq RNA library preparation kit (Illumina, Inc) was used according to the manufacturer's protocol. Single-end 50-bp sequencing was performed on the HiSeq 2500, High Output v4 (eight lanes flow cell) system. For this analysis six samples were sequenced per lane (total of three lanes used, one for each brain region). Quality control of the resulting reads was performed using the FastQC tool on the Tufts Galaxy server. Additional file 1: Table S1 shows the average number of reads and the mean quality score (PHRED format) for Indian- and Chinese-origin groups for each brain region.

Mapping of RNA-seq reads using TopHat

Sequence reads were aligned to the Ensembl rhesus monkey reference genome (mmul1) using TopHat for Illumina (version 1.5.0) on the Tufts University Galaxy server. TopHat aligns reads to mammalian-sized genomes using the high-throughput short read aligner Bowtie and then analyzes the mapping results to identify splice junctions between exons [31]. Default settings for TopHat were used.

Differential expression testing using Cuffdiff

Using the resulting BAM files (.bam) containing mapped reads from TopHat and a reference *M. mulatta* iGenome GTF annotation file, transcripts were assembled and normalized to fragments per kilobase of exon per million fragments (FPKM) expression units to estimate the relative abundance of transcripts. Differential expression of FPKM estimates was determined using Cuffdiff [32]. Differential gene expression is expressed as fold change between Indian- and Chinese-origin monkeys. Differences in gene expression between monkeys of different origin were determined using two-tailed Student's *t* tests. Resulting *p* values were adjusted for multiple testing using the Benjamini-Hochberg (false discovery rate) correction (*q* value).

Validation using RT-PCR

Genes with statistically significant ($P < 0.05$) fold changes ranging from 1.25 to 3.69 (for upregulated genes) and −1.52 to −2.44 (for downregulated genes) between Indian and Chinese-origin monkeys were selected for differential expression analysis using real-time quantitative polymerase chain reaction. Complementary DNA (cDNA) was generated from total RNA (1 µg) and RT-PCR was performed using SYBR Green (Applied Biosystems 7300, Carlsbad, CA). Relative expression was calculated using the $2^{-\Delta\Delta CT}$ method. After testing three different reference genes (actin gamma 1 (*ACTG1*), ribosomal protein L13a (*RPL13a*), and alpha-1,2-mannosyltransferase (*ALG9*)), *ACTG1* was determined to have the lowest variability between monkeys of different origins and among different brain regions. Therefore, it was chosen as the endogenous control for this study. Primer sequences are listed in Additional file 1: Table S2. The data is expressed as the relative RNA expression of Chinese- to Indian-origin monkeys.

Statistical analysis

Two-tailed student's *t* test was performed to determine differences in each carotenoid and in gene expression between monkeys of different origins. Pearson's correlation analysis was performed to determine the association between brain xanthophyll concentration and gene expression. Given the exploratory nature of this pilot study, significance was set at the 0.1 level.

Results

Carotenoid profile in serum

Mean carotenoid profiles in serum of all Indian- and Chinese-origin monkeys for which samples were available (*n* = 7; three Indian-origin, four Chinese-origin) are shown in Fig. 1a. Lutein was the major carotenoid detected in serum for both Indian- (318 ± 127 nmol/L) and Chinese-origin (94.3 ± 26.5 nmol/L) rhesus monkeys. Other carotenoids detected in both subspecies included zeaxanthin (70.2 ± 28.7 nmol/L and 18.6 ± 5.0 nmol/L, Indian and Chinese, respectively) and β-carotene (35.7 ± 15.5 nmol/L and 11.90 ± 2.86 nmol/L, Indian and Chinese respectively). Cryptoxanthin and α-carotene were only detected in one monkey, which was of Indian origin. Between subspecies, lutein and zeaxanthin concentrations were greater in monkeys of Indian origin compared to Chinese origin (*p* = 0.09). β-carotene concentrations also tended to be higher in monkeys of Indian origin, but this was not statistically significant (*p* = 0.14).

Serum carotenoid profiles in the subset of monkeys selected for brain gene expression analysis are shown in Fig. 1b (*n* = 4, two Indian-origin, two Chinese-origin). The average lutein concentration in the Indian-origin

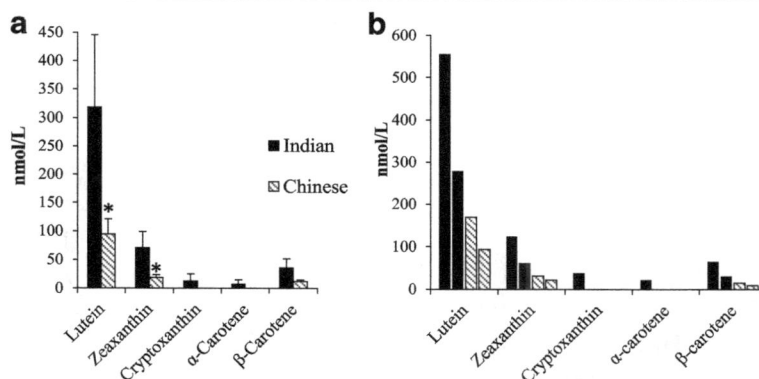

Fig. 1 Mean (±SEM) carotenoid content in serum of rhesus macaque of different origin in **a** ($n = 4$ Chinese, $n = 3$ Indian) and **b** subset used for gene expression analysis ($n = 2$ for each origin). Lutein (cis+trans) and zeaxanthin (trans, no cis present) concentrations (nmol/L) were greater in monkeys of Indian origin vs. Chinese (Fig. 1a. *$p < 0.09$, Student's t test)

monkeys was 417 nmol/L, over three times greater than the average concentration of the Chinese-origin monkeys (132 nmol/L). For zeaxanthin, the average concentration in Indian-origin monkeys was 92.6 nmol/L while the concentration in Chinese monkeys was 26.4 nmol/L. Serum β-carotene concentration was four times higher in Indian-(47.7 nmol/L) versus Chinese-origin monkeys (11.9 nmol/L).

Lutein and zeaxanthin concentration in the brain

Lutein and zeaxanthin concentrations in PFC, CER, and STR of all Indian-($n = 4$) and Chinese-origin ($n = 5$) monkeys are shown in Fig. 2a and c, respectively. Rhesus monkeys had the same distribution pattern of lutein and zeaxanthin among the three regions regardless of origin. Namely, xanthophyll levels tended to be the highest in STR, followed by PFC and the lowest in CER (Indian origin $p = 0.1$; Chinese origin $p < 0.05$). In PFC and CER, lutein concentrations were greater in monkeys of Indian origin compared to those of Chinese origin (Fig. 2a, $p = 0.08$ for both). Similarly, zeaxanthin concentrations were higher in the PFC and CER of these animals compared to Chinese (Fig. 2c, $p < 0.05$ for both). Lutein and zeaxanthin concentrations also tended to be higher in the STR of Indian-origin monkeys compared to Chinese origin; however, this was not statistically significant ($p = 0.14$ and $p = 0.16$, respectively).

Lutein and zeaxanthin concentrations in PFC, CER, and STR of Indian- and Chinese-origin monkeys selected for gene expression analysis ($n = 3$ per group) are shown in Fig. 2b and d, respectively. Both lutein and zeaxanthin concentrations were significantly higher in PFC and CER of Indian-origin monkeys compared to Chinese-origin ($p < 0.05$ for all comparisons). Individual xanthophyll concentrations for this subset of rhesus monkeys are shown in Additional file 2: Figures S1, S2, and S3.

Differences in gene expression between monkeys of Indian and Chinese origin using RNA-Seq

Given that xanthophyll concentrations differ in the brain between Indian- and Chinese-origin rhesus monkeys, we elected to focus this analysis on genes that are known to be related to carotenoid uptake/transport (NPC1L1, ABCG5, ABCA1, SCARB1, LIPC), carotenoid binding in neural tissue (GSTP1, STARD3) and carotenoid metabolism (BCO1, BCO2), as well as genes involved in long-chain omega-3 polyunsaturated fatty acid (PUFA) metabolism and synthesis (ELOVL2/4/5 and FADS1/2), which have been shown to be related to xanthophyll uptake and accumulation in neural tissue [18, 19] and genes related to maculopathies and low macular xanthophyll status (RPE65, ALDH3A2) (Table 1). In the PFC, BCO2 (1.64 fold change, $p < 0.01$) and ELOVL4 (1.25 fold change, $p < 0.05$) have higher expression in monkeys of Chinese origin compared to Indian origin. Similarly, in the striatum, BCO2 expression was higher in Chinese-origin monkeys compared to Indian (1.69 fold change, $p = 0.01$). In this region, expression of the fatty acid desaturase genes FADS1 (1.55 fold change, $p = 0.01$) and FADS2 (1.32 fold change, $p = 0.05$), as well as the cholesterol transporter, ABCA1 (1.43 fold change, $p = 0.06$), and receptor, SCARB1 (1.20 fold change, $p = 0.09$), were also higher in Chinese monkeys compared to Indian. In the CER, only RPE65 had a significant fold change, with lower expression (−2.44 fold change, $p = 0.03$) in monkeys of Chinese origin compared to Indian origin. However, all gene expression differences lost statistical significance when adjusted for multiple comparisons ($q > 0.1$).

A number of known single nucleotide polymorphisms (SNPs) have previously been identified between rhesus monkeys of Indian and Chinese origin [23]. However, whether there are also differences in expression of these genes between the different

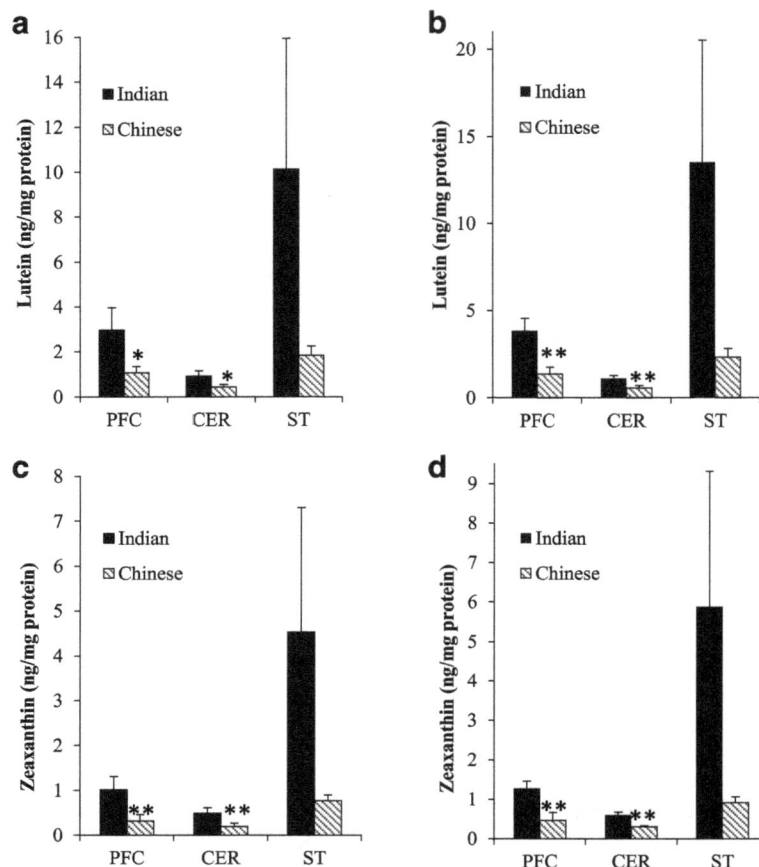

Fig. 2 Mean xanthophyll concentrations (ng/mg protein) ±SEM in prefrontal cortex (PFC), cerebellum (CER), and striatum (STR) of rhesus macaques of different origin. Lutein concentrations were greater in monkeys of Indian origin compared to Chinese in PFC and CER in **a** all monkeys analyzed (*$p < 0.1$, Student's t test, $n = 5$ Indian, $n = 4$ Chinese) and **b** in subset of monkeys selected for gene expression analysis (**$p < 0.05$, Student's t test, $n = 3$ per group). Zeaxanthin concentrations were greater in monkeys of Indian origin compared to Chinese in PFC and CER in **c** all monkeys analyzed ($n = 9$) and **d** in subset of monkeys selected for gene expression analysis ($n = 6$), **$P < 0.05$ for both, Student's t test

subspecies has not yet been determined. Therefore, we also elected to look at differences in expression of these genes (Table 2). Of the 27 genes analyzed, 9 were differentially expressed in at least one brain region. In all three regions, *CD74* and *CD4*, genes that encode proteins important for antigen presentation and immune function, were differentially expressed ($p \leq 0.0001$), with expression levels higher in Chinese monkeys compared to Indian. In STR, *CXCL12*, a gene encoding a chemokine, expression was also significantly higher in Chinese-origin monkeys (3.22 fold change, $p < 0.001$). Fold change expression of these three genes in PFC and STR remained statistically significant after adjusting for multiple comparisons ($q < 0.01$).

Expression of *CCR1*, gene encoding a chemokine receptor, was also greater in the PFC (1.94 fold change, $p = 0.02$) and STR (1.57 fold change, $p = 0.07$) of Chinese-origin monkeys compared to Indian-origin

animals. Another gene related to inflammation, and a member of the tumor necrosis factor (TNF) family, *LTBR*, was differentially expressed in PFC, with expression being lower in monkeys of Chinese origin. However, differences in expression of both these genes lost significance after adjusting for multiple comparisons ($q > 0.1$). Three genes related to neurotransmission (*SNCA*, *NOS1*, *NPY*) were differentially expressed. Specifically, *SNCA*, which encodes a protein (alpha-synuclein) that regulates presynaptic transmission, was observed to have higher expression in monkeys of Chinese origin in both PFC (1.21 fold change, $p = 0.1$) and STR (1.41 fold change, $p = 0.04$). *NOS1* expression was higher in Chinese-origin monkeys compared to Indian (1.57 fold change, $p = 0.05$) while *NPY* expression was significantly lower in Chinese monkeys (–10.0 fold change, $p = 0.05$). Again, differences in expression lost significance after adjusting for multiple comparisons ($q > 0.1$).

Table 1 Relative expression of genes (fold change, Chinese vs. Indian) involved in xanthophyll uptake and metabolism in prefrontal cortex (PFC), cerebellum (CER), and striatum (STR) of Indian and Chinese-origin rhesus monkeys ($n = 3$ per group)

	Fold change-PFC	p value	Fold change-CER	p value	Fold change-STR	p value
BCO1	−1.15	0.77	2.75	0.99	1.84	0.37
BCO2	*1.64*	*0.006*	1.58	0.13	*1.69*	*0.01*
NPC1L1	1.54	0.34	−1.06	0.91	1.26	0.60
ABCG5	−1.37	0.99	1.17	0.68	1.06	0.91
ABCA1	1.05	0.84	−1.01	0.99	*1.43*	*0.06*
SCARB1	1.18	0.12	1.10	0.43	*1.20*	*0.09*
GSTP1	1.07	0.52	−1.09	0.59	1.15	0.38
STARD3	1.09	0.99	1.07	0.99	1.31	0.99
LIPC	−1.61	0.25	1.38	0.99	−1.37	0.46
ELOVL2	−1.02	0.87	1.06	0.71	1.08	0.67
ELOVL4	*1.25*	*0.04*	1.06	0.66	1.11	0.50
ELOVL5	1.14	0.49	−1.05	0.81	1.24	0.29
FADS1	1.17	0.15	1.20	0.20	*1.55*	*0.01*
FADS2	1.16	0.12	−1.04	0.75	*1.32*	*0.05*
RPE65	−1.28	0.44	*−2.44*	*0.03*	−1.37	0.26
ALDH3A2	−1.11	0.26	−1.05	0.61	1.02	0.89

Fold change calculated by dividing fragments per kilobase of transcript per million mapped reads (FPKM) Chinese origin by FPKM Indian origin. Genes in italics showed a significant difference in expression in at least one brain region. Genes in bold were selected for RT-PCR analysis

Differences in gene expression between monkeys of Indian and Chinese origin using RT-PCR

Although no carotenoid-related genes had significant q values between monkeys of different origin, we elected to perform differential gene expression analysis using RT-PCR for genes with expression difference p values ≤ 0.05 (*BCO2*, *ELOVL4*, *FADS1*, *FADS2*, *RPE65*). Similarly, for genes with known variants between rhesus monkeys of Indian and Chinese origin, we performed differential gene expression analysis not only on genes with a significant q value (*CXCL12*, *CD74*, *CD4*), but also genes with expression differences $p < 0.05$ (*LTBR*, *CCR1*, *SNCA*).

Results from RT-PCR analysis are shown in Fig. 3a–c. In the PFC, *RPE65* expression was significantly lower in monkeys of Chinese origin compared to those of Indian origin ($p < 0.01$). Regarding genes with known variants between subspecies, *CD74*, *CD4*, and *LTBR* were differentially expressed. Specifically, *CD74* and *CD4* expression was higher in Chinese-origin monkeys compared to Indian origin ($p < 0.1$). Conversely, *LTBR* expression was significantly lower in these monkeys compared to those of Indian origin ($p < 0.01$). In the CER, expression of *RPE65* was also lower in Chinese-origin monkeys compared to Indian ($p < 0.05$). Additionally, *FADS2* expression was higher in Chinese-origin monkeys ($p < 0.1$). Higher expression of *CD4* ($p < 0.1$) and *CXCL12* ($p = 0.06$) was also observed in monkeys of Chinese origin. In the STR, 5 of the 12 genes were differentially expressed. Differentially expressed genes related to carotenoid

uptake, transport, and metabolism included *BCO2* ($p < 0.01$), *ELOVL4* ($p < 0.01$), and *FADS1* ($p < 0.1$), all of which had higher expression in monkeys of Chinese origin. Differential expression of genes with known variants between Indian and Chinese origin included *CD4* ($p < 0.1$) and *LTBR* ($p < 0.01$), the former of which had higher expression and the latter, lower expression, in monkeys of Chinese origin compared to Indian origin. In Fig. 3, superscripts next to gene names indicate consistency in results between RNA-seq and RT-PCR analysis within each brain region.

In order to examine the cross-sectional relationship between brain xanthophyll content and expression of genes involved in carotenoid and fatty acid metabolism, correlation analyses was performed for each brain region (Table 3). Results from this analysis indicate positive associations between xanthophyll concentration and *RPE65* expression in PFC and CER ($p < 0.05$). In STR, xanthophyll concentration was inversely associated with *BCO2* expression ($p < 0.05$) and *ELOVL4* ($p < 0.1$). Additionally, *FADS1* and *FADS2* were negatively associated with xanthophyll content in STR and CER, respectively ($p < 0.1$).

Discussion

Xanthophyll status differs between rhesus monkeys of different origin

Indian-origin monkeys were found to have higher xanthophyll content in serum, with a combined 3.5 times greater concentration of xanthophylls, compared to

Table 2 Relative expression of genes (fold change, Chinese vs. Indian) with known variants between rhesus monkeys of different origin in the prefrontal cortex (PFC), cerebellum (CER), and striatum (STR) ($n = 3$ per group)

	Fold change-PFC	p value	Fold change-CER	p value	Fold change-STR	p value
CCL5	1.07	0.98	1.01	0.99	1.15	0.94
CXCL12	1.45	0.19	1.18	0.61	*3.22*	*0.00058*
XCL1	1.43	0.42	0.89	0.77	3.57	0.11
CCR4	1.50	0.67	1.27	0.72	1.19	0.79
CCR1	*1.94*	*0.02*	1.46	0.21	*1.57*	*0.07*
IL2RA	2.04	0.50	1.89	0.58	1.00	0.98
CD74	*2.11*	*0.0001*	*1.44*	*0.09*	2.52	0.0000043
CD4	*3.69*	*0.0000001*	*1.66*	*0.008*	3.59	0.0000006
CD44	−1.08	0.81	−1.12	0.31	1.27	0.38
TLR5	1.06	0.83	−1.20	0.63	1.02	0.94
LTBR	*−1.52*	*0.02*	−1.28	0.22	−1.06	0.80
FAS	1.27	0.58	1.24	0.57	−1.39	0.43
MAOA	1.06	0.72	1.03	0.89	1.04	0.86
BCHE	1.13	0.15	1.43	0.12	−1.01	0.99
NOS1	1.06	0.82	1.24	0.25	*1.57*	*0.05*
NPY	1.00	0.99	*−10.0*	*0.05*	1.18	0.36
PYY	1.08	0.92	1.92	0.65	3.04	0.41
SLC5A7	1.56	0.19	1.67	0.19	1.01	0.95
SLC6A4	1.67	0.67	−3.23	0.27	−1.75	0.69
SNCA	*1.21*	*0.10*	1.08	0.63	*1.41*	*0.04*
INHBB	−1.11	0.68	−1.08	0.82	1.13	0.68
SIRT1	1.13	0.51	1.08	0.64	1.23	0.34
HTATSF1	1.10	0.35	1.03	0.82	1.13	0.41
STAR	−1.52	0.18	−1.30	0.49	−1.04	0.91
ADRBK2	1.21	0.19	1.11	0.49	*1.52*	*0.08*
ITGA4	−1.10	0.74	1.01	0.99	1.80	0.32
SASH1	1.13	0.35	1.21	0.31	1.30	0.12

Fold change calculated by dividing fragments per kilobase of transcript per million mapped reads (FPKM) Chinese origin by FPKM Indian origin. Genes in italics showed a significant difference in expression in at last one brain region. Genes bold were selected for RT-PCR analysis

monkeys of Chinese origin, despite eating the same stock diet. Although we cannot rule out a contribution of modest differences in preference for seasonal fruits and vegetables, it is much more likely that these differences are due to differing efficiencies in their ability to absorb, transport, and metabolize lutein and zeaxanthin.

Indian-origin monkeys were also observed to have higher xanthophyll concentrations in each brain region compared to Chinese-origin monkeys. However, variability within each group was high, particularly for the ST of Indian-origin monkeys. Therefore, origin does not account for all of the variability observed with neural lutein content among primates. In addition, monkeys of both subspecies tended to have lower levels of lutein in CER compared with PFC and ST, two regions more closely linked to cognitive function. Specifically, lutein is known to be related to improved working memory,

executive function, and language in humans, all of which involve function of the PFC and STR [6, 33].

Expression of carotenoid-related genes in rhesus monkey brain

As determined by PCR, differential gene expression analysis indicated region-specific differences in expression of four carotenoid metabolism genes in Chinese- versus Indian-origin monkeys. The CER had the fewest number of differentially expressed carotenoid-related genes, only *RPE65* and *FADS2*, which is consistent with this region having the smallest difference in xanthophyll concentrations (~2 times higher in Indian vs. Chinese) compared to the other regions (~3 times in PFC, ~5.5 in STR), which had a combined four differentially expressed genes (*BCO2, RPE65, ELOVL4, FADS1*). Our findings also

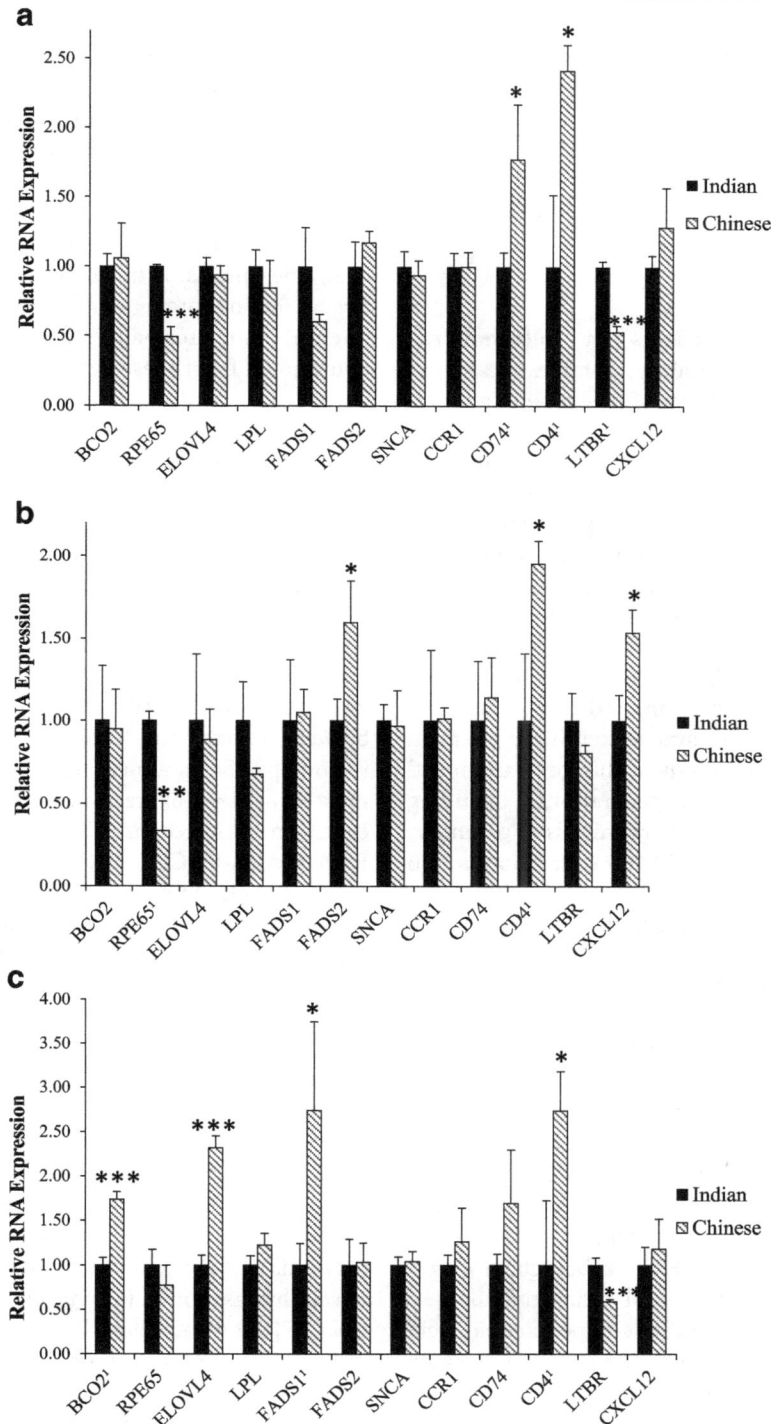

Fig. 3 Relative Expression (±SEM) of genes selected for RT-PCR analysis in. **a** Prefrontal Cortex. **b** Cerebellum. **c** Striatum of Indian and Chinese-origin rhesus monkeys (*n* = 3 per origin). ***p < 0.01, **p < 0.05, *p < 0.1. [1]*Superscript* next to gene name indicates significant *p* value also observed in RNA-seq analysis for the same brain region

indicate that brain xanthophyll concentration is directly associated with expression of these genes in a region-specific manner.

The *BCO2* gene encodes a mitochondrial enzyme responsible for the degradation of carotenoids. Evidence indicates that this enzyme is induced to prevent

Table 3 Cross-sectional relationship between xanthophyll concentration (ng/mg protein) and gene expression (fold change) in rhesus monkeys of different origin in prefrontal cortex (PFC), cerebellum (CER), and striatum (STR) ($n = 6$)

	BCO2	RPE65	ELOVL4	FADS1	FADS2
Prefrontal cortex	–	0.84**	0.65	0.58	–0.67
Cerebellum	–	0.83**	–	–	–0.68*
Striatum	–0.86**	–	–0.68*	–0.77*	–

*$P \leq 0.1$
**$P < 0.05$

over-accumulation of carotenoids in mitochondria, which can lead to mitochondrial dysfunction and oxidative stress [34]. Higher expression of this gene in animals of Chinese origin versus Indian origin and an inverse correlation between xanthophyll concentration and BCO2 expression in STR suggest that differences in neural xanthophyll content between origins may be due, in part, to differences in metabolism/degradation. The RPE65 gene also encodes a carotenoid oxygenase, which has a well-established function in the retina as a critical participant in the visual cycle where it produces 11-cis-retinol [35]. This gene has been linked to macular pigment response to supplementation, and thus, it appears to be related to retinal lutein and zeaxanthin content in some capacity [17, 18]. Mutations in this gene are linked with blindness and retinal degenerations, including Leber congenital amaurosis and retinitis pigmentosa [36]. Our findings indicate that RPE65 expression is also related to lutein and zeaxanthin content in the brain. However, it is not clear what function this enzyme possesses in brain tissue. Therefore, it is difficult to speculate on the relationship between brain xanthophyll content and RPE65 expression at this time.

FADS1 and FADS2 encode the enzymes delta-5 desaturase and delta-6 desaturase, respectively. They are the rate-limiting enzymes and main determinants for the synthesis of long-chain polyunsaturated fatty acids (PUFA), including eicosapentaenoic acid (EPA) and docosahexaenoic acid (DHA), from their precursors [37]. ELOVL4 mediates fatty acid elongation, in particular, the synthesis of very-long-chain PUFAs (carbon chain length 24–36), which are present in neural retina membranes. Circulating levels of EPA and docosapentaenoic acid (DPA) [38] and SNPs in all three genes are associated with MPOD [18]. Furthermore, ELOVL4 mutations underlie autosomal-dominant Stargardt disease, a form of early-onset macular degeneration [39]. Given that lutein and zeaxanthin are likely taken up into the brain through similar mechanisms as in the eye, there may be a similar relationship in both tissues between long-chain PUFAs (particularly EPA and DHA) and xanthophyll concentrations (or vice versa). This evidence is also consistent with previous findings that brain concentrations

of lutein and DHA may interact with one another to influence cognitive function in humans [40, 41]. One potential explanation for the inverse associations between xanthophyll concentration and expression of ELOVL4, FADS1, and FADS2 may be a compensatory mechanism. That is, lower xanthophyll levels in the brain may trigger upregulation of enzyme expression to maintain functions common to xanthophylls and long-chain PUFAs, such as membrane fluidity or anti-inflammatory actions. However, the mechanisms underlying the relationship between brain lutein and PUFA composition remain unclear, and cause-and-effect relationships cannot be determined from these data.

Brain expression of genes with SNPs between Indian- and Chinese-origin rhesus monkeys

Given the well-established genetic divergence between Indian- and Chinese-origin monkeys, we sought to determine whether genes with known SNPs between subspecies also differed in their expression levels in brain tissue. Our findings indicate that among the 27 identified genes with SNPs, three genes related to immune function (CD4, CD74, LTBR) and one related to chemokine expression (CXCL12) were differentially expressed between Indian- and Chinese-origin monkeys in a brain region-specific manner. CD4 expression showed the most consistent expression differences, differing significantly in all three brain regions as evaluated by both RNA-seq and PCR. Higher expression of CD4, CD74, CXCL12, and lower expression of LTBR in Chinese-origin monkeys is consistent with what is known regarding simian immune-deficiency virus (SIV) infection and progression susceptibility in the two subspecies. Specifically, Chinese-origin monkeys are more resistant to SIV with slower disease progression than their Indian-origin counterparts [42–45]. Our findings support evidence that Chinese-origin monkeys may have stronger immune responses, particularly in the face of SIV infection.

Studies in diverse animal models (mice, dogs, cats, and birds) show enhanced immune responses with lutein supplementation [46]. With regard to HIV specifically, limited data indicates that circulating concentrations of lutein and zeaxanthin are lower in individuals with HIV versus controls [47]. However, all of these studies focused on systemic immune function, with no current evidence to date on the relationship between lutein and immunity in the brain. Research on age-related macular degeneration (AMD) in humans has provided evidence that the alternative complement pathway underlies the pathogenesis of AMD, and this pathway can be suppressed by the xanthophylls [46, 48]. Given that Chinese-origin monkeys may have more efficient immune systems than monkeys of Indian origin, it is possible they require, and therefore accumulate, less lutein and zeaxanthin for normal function in brain tissue.

Conclusions

To our knowledge, this is the first study to explore the effect of genetic divergence (i.e., monkey subspecies based on geographic origin) on lutein concentrations and gene expression profiles in the primate brain. Findings from this study indicate that rhesus monkeys of Indian and Chinese origin differ in serum and brain lutein and zeaxanthin status despite eating the same standard stock diet during their adult life. Furthermore, neural xanthophyll content may be related to expression of genes involved in carotenoid and fatty acid metabolism in the brain. However, given that this is an exploratory pilot study, these results must be replicated with a larger sample size to confirm this relationship. Future studies determining whether these differences in gene expression actually translate to changes in protein expression should also be performed. Additionally, given that *RPE65* was consistently differentially expressed in the brains of monkeys of Chinese and Indian origin, functional studies determining the specific role of this protein in the brain are warranted in order to determine its relationship to the brain concentrations of lutein and zeaxanthin.

The first limitation of this cross-sectional, correlational study is that the results do not provide information on the causal effect of differences in gene expression due to origin on neural lutein and zeaxanthin status, or vice versa. Another limitation is that, unlike the Indian-origin monkeys, Chinese-origin monkeys were imported to the ONPRC as adults. Therefore, we cannot account for earlier long-term epigenetic (e.g., environmental and dietary) factors that may have influenced gene expression in these animals as adults. However, animals lived in the same environment and consumed the same diet for at least 3 years before termination, thus limiting the number of variables for a significant amount of time leading up to blood and tissue collection. A major strength of this study is that these results provide valuable knowledge regarding factors related to variability in carotenoid status, and in particular, lutein and zeaxanthin levels, among genetically diverse rhesus monkeys. This information should be considered when designing and implementing studies on carotenoids in rhesus macaques. Furthermore, numerous studies have linked neural xanthophyll concentrations, particularly lutein, to cognitive performance in humans [6, 8–11]. Therefore, our findings have important implications regarding the influence of genetics on the role of lutein (and zeaxanthin) in cognition in primates. However, future studies must be conducted to evaluate the association between differences in carotenoid-related gene expression profiles and carotenoid-related function in brain tissue in order to determine the functional impact of differences in brain xanthophyll status due to genetics on brain health, function, and overall cognition.

Acknowledgements
Authors would like to acknowledge Emily E. Johnson and the ONPRC Veterinary Pathology Service for assistance with tissue collection, the Tufts University Genomics Core Facility (TUCF) for performing the cDNA library preparation and RNA sequencing for all samples, and Dr. Albert Tai of the TUCF for providing guidance on cleaning, mapping, and analyzing the raw sequencing data in Galaxy.

Funding
This work was supported by a grant from Abbott Nutrition through the Center for Nutrition, Learning, and Memory at the University of Illinois and USDA (58-1950-0-014) and NIH grant P51OD011092.

Authors' contributions
All authors contributed to the conception and design of the study. MN performed brain dissections. ESM performed carotenoid analyses, RNA isolations, and RT-PCR experiments, analyzed all the data, and wrote the paper. All authors read and approved the manuscript.

Competing interests
MJK is an employee of Abbott Nutrition. ESM, JWE Jr, MN, and EJJ report no conflicts of interest.

Author details
[1]Jean Mayer United States Department of Agriculture Human Nutrition Research Center on Aging, Tufts University, Boston, MA, USA. [2]Department of Food Science and Human Nutrition, University of Illinois at Urbana-Champaign, Urbana, IL, USA. [3]Division of Neuroscience, Oregon National Primate Research Center, Oregon Health and Science University, Beaverton, Oregon, USA. [4]Abbott Nutrition, Columbus, Ohio, USA. [5]Antioxidants Research Laboratory, 711 Washington Street, Boston, MA 02111, USA.

References
1. Abdel-Aal E-SM, Akhtar H, Zaheer K, Ali R. Dietary sources of lutein and zeaxanthin carotenoids and their role in eye health. Nutrients. 2013;5:1169–85.
2. Rao AV, Rao LG. Carotenoids and human health. Pharmacol Res. 2007;55:207–16.
3. Krinsky NI, Landrum JT, Bone RA. Biologic mechanisms of the protective role of lutein and zeaxanthin in the eye. Annu Rev Nutr. 2003;23:171–201.
4. Ozawa Y, Sasaki M, Takahashi N, Kamoshita M, Miyake S, Tsubota K. Neuroprotective effects of lutein in the retina. Curr Pharm Des. 2012;18:51–6.
5. Craft NE, Haitema TB, Garnett KM, Fitch KA, Dorey CK. Carotenoid, tocopherol, and retinol concentrations in elderly human brain. J Nutr Health Aging. 2004;8:156–62.
6. Johnson EJ, Vishwanathan R, Johnson MA, Hausman DB, Davey A, Scott TM, et al. Relationship between serum and brain carotenoids, α-tocopherol, and retinol concentrations and cognitive performance in the oldest old from the Georgia Centenarian Study. J Aging Res. 2013;2013:951786.
7. Vishwanathan R, Kuchan MJ, Sen S, Johnson EJ. Lutein and preterm infants with decreased concentrations of brain carotenoids. J Pediatr Gastroenterol Nutr. 2014;59:659–65.
8. Feeney J, Finucane C, Savva GM, Cronin H, Beatty S, Nolan JM, et al. Low macular pigment optical density is associated with lower cognitive performance in a large, population-based sample of older adults. Neurobiol Aging. 2013;34:2449–56.
9. Kelly D, Coen RF, Akuffo KO, Beatty S, Dennison J, Moran R, et al. Cognitive function and its relationship with macular pigment optical density and serum concentrations of its constituent carotenoids. J Alzheimers Dis JAD. 2015;48:261–77.
10. Renzi LM, Dengler MJ, Puente A, Miller LS, Hammond BR. Relationships between macular pigment optical density and cognitive function in unimpaired and mildly cognitively impaired older adults. Neurobiol Aging. 2014;35:1695–9.
11. Vishwanathan R, Iannaccone A, Scott TM, Kritchevsky SB, Jennings BJ, Carboni G, et al. Macular pigment optical density is related to cognitive function in older people. Age Ageing. 2014;43(2):271–5.

12. Borel P. Genetic variations involved in interindividual variability in carotenoid status. Mol Nutr Food Res. 2012;56:228–40.

13. Borel P, Desmarchelier C, Nowicki M, Bott R, Morange S, Lesavre N. Interindividual variability of lutein bioavailability in healthy men: characterization, genetic variants involved, and relation with fasting plasma lutein concentration. Am J Clin Nutr. 2014;100:168–75.

14. Johnson E. Human Studies on Bioavailability and Serum Response of Carotenoids. In: Handbook of Antioxidants [Internet]. CRC Press; 2001 [cited 2016 Jul 8]. Available from: http://www.crcnetbase.com/doi/abs/10.1201/9780203904046.ch14.

15. Hammond BR, Johnson EJ, Russell RM, Krinsky NI, Yeum KJ, Edwards RB, et al. Dietary modification of human macular pigment density. Invest Ophthalmol Vis Sci. 1997;38:1795–801.

16. Johnson EJ, Hammond BR, Yeum K-J, Qin J, Wang XD, Castaneda C, et al. Relation among serum and tissue concentrations of lutein and zeaxanthin and macular pigment density. Am J Clin Nutr. 2000;71:1555–62.

17. Yonova-Doing E, Hysi PG, Venturini C, Williams KM, Nag A, Beatty S, et al. Candidate gene study of macular response to supplemental lutein and zeaxanthin. Exp Eye Res. 2013;115:172–7.

18. Meyers KJ, Johnson EJ, Bernstein PS, Iyengar SK, Engelman CD, Karki CK, et al. Genetic determinants of macular pigments in women of the carotenoids in Age-Related Eye Disease Study. Invest Ophthalmol Vis Sci. 2013;54:2333–45.

19. Meyers KJ, Mares JA, Igo RP, Truitt B, Liu Z, Millen AE, et al. Genetic evidence for role of carotenoids in age-related macular degeneration in the Carotenoids in Age-Related Eye Disease Study (CAREDS). Invest Ophthalmol Vis Sci. 2014;55:587–99.

20. Vishwanathan R, Neuringer M, Snodderly DM, Schalch W, Johnson EJ. Macular lutein and zeaxanthin are related to brain lutein and zeaxanthin in primates. Nutr Neurosci. 2013;16:21–9.

21. Vishwanathan R, Schalch W, Johnson EJ. Macular pigment carotenoids in the retina and occipital cortex are related in humans. Nutr Neurosci. 2015;19:95–101.

22. Neuringer M, Sandstrom MM, Johnson EJ, Snodderly DM. Nutritional manipulation of primate retinas, I: effects of lutein or zeaxanthin supplements on serum and macular pigment in xanthophyll-free rhesus monkeys. Invest Ophthalmol Vis Sci. 2004;45:3234–43.

23. Ferguson B, Street SL, Wright H, Pearson C, Jia Y, Thompson SL, et al. Single nucleotide polymorphisms (SNPs) distinguish Indian-origin and Chinese-origin rhesus macaques (Macaca mulatta). BMC Genomics. 2007;8:43.

24. O'Callaghan C, Bertoux M, Hornberger M. Beyond and below the cortex: the contribution of striatal dysfunction to cognition and behaviour in neurodegeneration. J Neurol Neurosurg Psychiatry. 2014;85:371–8.

25. Peters A, Morrison JH, Jones EG. Cerebral Cortex: Neurodegenerative and age-related changes in structure and function of the cerebral cortex. New York: Kluwer Academic/Plenum Publishers; 1999.

26. Strick PL, Dum RP, Fiez JA. Cerebellum and nonmotor function. Annu Rev Neurosci. 2009;32:413–34.

27. Muzhingi T, Yeum K-J, Russell RM, Johnson EJ, Qin J, Tang G. Determination of carotenoids in yellow maize, the effects of saponification and food preparations. Int J Vitam Nutr Res Int Z Für Vitam- Ernährungsforschung J Int Vitaminol Nutr. 2008;78:112–20.

28. Park J, Hwang H, Kim M, Lee-Kim Y. Effects of dietary fatty acids and vitamin E supplementation on antioxidant vitamin status of the second generation rat brain sections. Korean J Nutr. 2001;34:754–61.

29. Johnson EJ, Neuringer M, Russell RM, Schalch W, Snodderly DM. Nutritional manipulation of primate retinas, III: Effects of lutein or zeaxanthin supplementation on adipose tissue and retina of xanthophyll-free monkeys. Invest Ophthalmol Vis Sci. 2005;46:692–702.

30. Finotello F, Camillo BD. Measuring differential gene expression with RNA-seq: challenges and strategies for data analysis. Brief Funct Genomics. 2014;14(2):130–42.

31. Trapnell C, Pachter L, Salzberg SL. TopHat: discovering splice junctions with RNA-Seq. Bioinformatics. 2009;25:1105–11.

32. Trapnell C, Williams BA, Pertea G, Mortazavi A, Kwan G, van Baren MJ, et al. Transcript assembly and abundance estimation from RNA-Seq reveals thousands of new transcripts and switching among isoforms. Nat Biotechnol. 2010;28:511–5.

33. Johnson E, Vishwanathan R, Mohn E, Haddock J, Rasmussen H, Scott T. Avocado consumption increases neural lutein and improves cognitive function. FASEB J. 2015;29(1 Supplement):32.8.

34. Amengual J, Lobo GP, Golczak M, Li HNM, Klimova T, Hoppel CL, et al. A mitochondrial enzyme degrades carotenoids and protects against oxidative stress. FASEB J Off Publ Fed Am Soc Exp Biol. 2011;25:948–59.

35. Lobo GP, Amengual J, Palczewski G, Babino D, von Lintig J. Mammalian carotenoid-oxygenases: key players for carotenoid function and homeostasis. Biochim Biophys Acta. 2012;1821:78–87.

36. Cideciyan AV. Leber congenital amaurosis due to RPE65 mutations and its treatment with gene therapy. Prog Retin Eye Res. 2010;29:398–427.

37. Tosi F, Sartori F, Guarini P, Olivieri O, Martinelli N. Delta-5 and delta-6 desaturases: crucial enzymes in polyunsaturated fatty acid-related pathways with pleiotropic influences in health and disease. Adv Exp Med Biol. 2014;824:61–81.

38. Delyfer M-N, Buaud B, Korobelnik J-F, Rougier M-B, Schalch W, Etheve S, et al. Association of macular pigment density with plasma ω-3 fatty acids: the PIMAVOSA study. Invest Ophthalmol Vis Sci. 2012;53:1204–10.

39. Bernstein PS, Tammur J, Singh N, Hutchinson A, Dixon M, Pappas CM, et al. Diverse macular dystrophy phenotype caused by a novel complex mutation in the ELOVL4 gene. Invest Ophthalmol Vis Sci. 2001;42:3331–6.

40. Johnson EJ, McDonald K, Caldarella SM, Chung H-Y, Troen AM, Snodderly DM. Cognitive findings of an exploratory trial of docosahexaenoic acid and lutein supplementation in older women. Nutr Neurosci. 2008;11:75–83.

41. Mohn E, Vishwanathan R, Schalch W, Lichtenstein AH, Matthan NR, Poon LW, et al. The relationship of Lutein and DHA in Age-Related Cognitive Function. Boston: Poster Presentation presented at: Experimental Biology Conference; 2013.

42. Ling B, Veazey RS, Luckay A, Penedo C, Xu K, Lifson JD, et al. SIV(mac) pathogenesis in rhesus macaques of Chinese and Indian origin compared with primary HIV infections in humans. AIDS Lond Engl. 2002;16:1489–96.

43. Marshall WL, Brinkman BM, Ambrose CM, Pesavento PA, Uglialoro AM, Teng E, et al. Signaling through the lymphotoxin-beta receptor stimulates HIV-1 replication alone and in cooperation with soluble or membrane-bound TNF-alpha. J Immunol Baltim Md 1950. 1999;162:6016–23.

44. Monceaux V, Viollet L, Petit F, Cumont MC, Kaufmann GR, Aubertin AM, et al. CD4+ CCR5+ T-cell dynamics during simian immunodeficiency virus infection of Chinese rhesus macaques. J Virol. 2007;81:13865–75.

45. Trichel AM, Rajakumar PA, Murphey-Corb M. Species-specific variation in SIV disease progression between Chinese and Indian subspecies of rhesus macaque. J Med Primatol. 2002;31:171–8.

46. Kijlstra A, Tian Y, Kelly ER, Berendschot TTJM. Lutein: more than just a filter for blue light. Prog Retin Eye Res. 2012;31:303–15.

47. Lacey CJ, Murphy ME, Sanderson MJ, Monteiro EF, Vail A, Schorah CJ. Antioxidant-micronutrients and HIV infection. Int J STD AIDS. 1996;7:485–9.

48. Erdman JW, Smith JW, Kuchan MJ, Mohn ES, Johnson EJ, Rubakhin SS, et al. Lutein and brain function. Foods Basel Switz. 2015;4:547–64.

16

Metallothioneins 1 and 2, but not 3, are regulated by nutritional status in rat white adipose tissue

Sylwia Szrok[1], Ewa Stelmanska[1], Jacek Turyn[1], Aleksandra Bielicka-Gieldon[2], Tomasz Sledzinski[3] and Julian Swierczynski[1*]

Abstract

Background: Cumulating evidence underlines the role of adipose tissue metallothionein (MT) in the development of obesity and type 2 diabetes. Fasting/refeeding was shown to affect MT gene expression in the rodent liver. The influence of nutritional status on MT gene expression in white adipose tissue (WAT) is inconclusive. The aim of this study was to verify if fasting and fasting/refeeding may influence expression of MT genes in WAT of rats.

Results: Fasting resulted in a significant increase in MT1 and MT2 gene expressions in retroperitoneal, epididymal, and inguinal WAT of rats, and this effect was reversed by refeeding. Altered expressions of MT1 and MT2 genes in all main fat depots were reflected by changes in serum MT1 and MT2 levels. MT1 and MT2 messenger RNA (mRNA) levels in WAT correlated inversely with serum insulin concentration. Changes in MT1 and MT2 mRNA levels were apparently not related to total zinc concentrations and MTF1 and Zn transporter mRNA levels in WAT. Fasting or fasting/refeeding exerted no effect on the expression of MT3 gene in WAT. Addition of insulin to isolated adipocytes resulted in a significant decrease in MT1 and MT2 gene expressions. In contrast, forskolin or dibutyryl-cAMP (dB-cAMP) enhanced the expressions of MT1 and MT2 genes in isolated adipocytes. Insulin partially reversed the effect of dB-cAMP on MT1 and MT2 gene expressions.

Conclusions: This study showed that the expressions of MT1 and MT2 genes in WAT are regulated by nutritional status, and the regulation may be independent of total zinc concentration.

Keywords: Metallothioneins, Insulin, cAMP, Fasting, WAT

Background

Metallothioneins (MTs) constitute the family of cysteine- and metal-rich, low molecular mass (61 to 68 amino acid) single-chain proteins [41, 47]. Four MT isoforms, MT1, MT2, MT3, and MT4, were found in mammals [47]. MT1 and MT2 are predominant isoforms expressed in many animal tissues. MT1 and MT2 expression is induced by several factors including metals, some drugs, glucocorticosteroids, oxidative stress, and inflammatory mediators [47]. MT3 (also referred to as growth inhibitory factor (GIF)) and MT4 genes are expressed in the brain (predominantly in Zn-containing neurons of the hippocampus, pineal gland, and retina) and stratified squamous epithelial cells [1, 14, 47]. Expression of MT3 was also

found in some peripheral organs of rats [20]. Although MT3 and MT4 are often referred to as non-inducible proteins [47], some data imply that also MT3 may be, at least in part, an inducible protein, and its expression is modulated by metal concentrations [14]. While all MT isoforms show similar metal binding capacities, they likely have different biological functions. Available evidence suggests that MT1 and MT2 may be involved in (a) protection against heavy metal- and reactive oxygen species-induced toxicity [36], (b) Zn and Cu homeostasis, as they sequester and/or dispense Zn and Cu [40], and (c) acute phase response [4]. Noticeably, however, mice with disrupted MT1 and MT2 genes were viable and developed normally under standard conditions, despite greater susceptibility to cadmium toxicity [31]. Moreover, it has been suggested that the increased level of MT1 in mice might have an important role in reducing morbidity in old animals [29]. Recent studies imply that both MT1 and MT2 may

* Correspondence: juls@gumed.edu.pl
[1]Department of Biochemistry, Medical University of Gdansk, Debinki 1, 80-211 Gdansk, Poland
Full list of author information is available at the end of the article

influence mammal longevity [21]. Moreover, MTs were postulated to play a role in the prevention of cardiomyopathy [5, 6] and intermittent hypoxia-induced renal injury [50]. Relatively little is known about the biological functions of MT3 and MT4. MT3 knockout mice developed normally under standard conditions but were more susceptible to kanic acid-induced seizures and showed a greater degree of resultant hippocampal neuronal injury [15]. The potential role of MT3 in the progression of neurodegenerative diseases still raises some controversies; while according to some authors MT3 acts as a protective factor against neurodegenerative diseases, others showed that it may stimulate progression thereof [1, 14, 19, 22]. The evidence from in vivo studies suggests that ectopic expression of MT3 encoding gene stimulates pancreatic acinar necrosis; however, the molecular basis for this toxic effect is unknown [34]. MT4 is likely involved in the regulation of Zn metabolism during the differentiation of epithelial cells [33].

The list of tissues/organs that express MTs encoding genes includes also brown and white adipose tissue [3, 43, 45]. Some evidence from animal studies implies that MT1 and MT2 may be involved in the regulation of energy balance [2]. Furthermore, these MTs may play a role in the prevention of high-fat diet-induced obesity [37]. Moreover, human studies documented enhanced expression of MT2a encoding gene in adipose tissue from an obese subject [7, 11] and patients with type 2 diabetes [16]. This implies that the upregulation of MT gene expression in human adipose tissue may exert a detrimental effect promoting obesity or be a consequence of obesity. In view of data mentioned above, further studies are needed to establish whether MTs really play a role in the etiopathogenesis of obesity and type 2 diabetes. Both these conditions are strongly influenced by the amount of consumed food [18] and intracellular zinc homeostasis [38, 42, 46, 48]. Among other factors, intracellular zinc homeostasis is regulated by MTs [8, 26, 30]. It has been shown that overexpression of MTs quickly diminishes intracellular zinc concentration in cell culture [28]. Thus, it is likely that overexpression of genes coding MT in vivo could decrease zinc concentration in adipocytes, and subsequently biosynthesis of zinc finger proteins, which are the important transcription factors regulating adipogenesis, obesity, and related diseases [48].

Higashimoto et al. [17] and Kondoh et al. [25] found that the liver content of MTs in fasted mice increases significantly, perhaps due to starvation-stimulated synthesis of MTs. In contrast, fasting and refeeding exert no effect on MT1 gene expression in epididymal white adipose tissue of mice [43, 45]. Surprisingly, a significant increase in MT gene expression was observed in a primary culture of rat adipocytes incubated with cAMP or insulin [44]. The abovementioned discrepancies

between the results of in vivo (especially, no effect of fasting and fasting/refeeding on MT gene expression in white adipose tissue (WAT)) and in vitro studies (stimulatory effect of cAMP and insulin on MTs genes in primary adipocyte culture) require further clarification.

The aim of this study was to analyze factors that potentially may regulate expression of genes coding MTs in rat WAT. We concentrated especially on the effects of fasting and fasting/refeeding on MT gene expression in main fat depots of rats, as well as an effect of insulin and cAMP on MT messenger RNA (mRNA) levels in isolated adipocytes.

Methods

Animals and treatment, tissue and blood collection

The experiment included 10-week-old male Wistar rats. The animals were housed at 22 °C in individual wire-mesh cages, under a 12:12 h light to dark cycle with lights on at 7:00 a.m. The rats were randomly assigned to seven groups (10 animals each): (a) control (ad libitum-fed animals with free access to food and tap water); (b) fasted for 24, 48, or 72 h, and (c) fasted for 48 h and then refed ad libitum for 12, 24, or 48 h.

The rats were killed by decapitation (between 8:00 and 10:00 a.m.). White adipose tissue: retroperitoneal, epididymal, and inguinal, as well as liver and esophagus, were harvested, weighed, and frozen in liquid nitrogen immediately upon collection and stored at –80 °C until analysis. Blood samples were obtained from the cervical artery. After 1 h, the blood cells were removed by centrifugation at $1500 \times g$ for 10 min. Obtained serum samples were stored at –80 °C until analysis.

All institutional and national guidelines for the care and use of laboratory animals were followed.

The study was approved by the Local Ethics Committee for Experimental Animals in Gdansk, Poland (14/2012).

Isolation and primary culture of rat adipocytes

Adipocytes from epididymal WAT of 10-week-old male rats were isolated by collagenase digestion as described by [35]. The tissue was placed in polypropylene tubes with Krebs-Ringer buffer (37 °C) containing 1 % bovine serum albumin suitable for cell culture (Sigma-Aldrich, USA), 5.5-mM glucose, 20-mM HEPES (pH 7.6), and 1-mg/ml collagenase (type II; Sigma-Aldrich, USA). The tissue was finely cut with scissors and incubated at 37 °C for 1 h with continuous shaking. After the incubation, the tissue was filtered using 180-µm nylon filters. Adipocytes were washed three times with Krebs-Ringer buffer. The adipocytes isolated from each rat were divided into equal portions and transferred onto incubation plate (Corning, USA) with 2-ml Dulbecco's modified Eagle's medium (DMEM) (Sigma-Aldrich, USA) with 5.5-mM glucose supplemented with 1 % bovine serum albumin. The adipocytes were incubated at 37 °C (under 5 % CO_2 plus 95 % O_2) for 24 h: (a) without addition (control) or (b) in the presence of insulin (10 µg/ml), (c) forskolin (12 µM) (Sigma-Aldrich, USA), (d) 0.2-mM dibutyryl-cAMP (dB-cAMP) (Sigma-Aldrich, USA), and (e) insulin (10 µg/ml) plus dB-cAMP (0.2 mM).

RNA isolation

Total RNA (from rat adipose tissue and liver, as well as from isolated adipocytes) was extracted using the Purezol reagent (Bio-Rad, USA) according to the manufacturer's protocol. Concentration of the RNA was determined on the basis of absorbance at 260 nm. All samples had 260/280 nm absorbance ratio of approximately 2.0.

Reverse transcription

First-strand complementary DNA (cDNA) was synthesized from 4 µg of total RNA (RevertAidTM First Strand cDNA Synthesis Kit; Thermo Scientific, USA). Prior to amplification of cDNA, each RNA sample was treated with RNase-free DNase I (Thermo Scientific, USA) at 37 °C for 30 min.

Real-time PCR

Real-time PCR amplification was performed in a 20-µl volume using iQ SYBR Green Supermix (Bio-Rad, USA). Each reaction mix contained cDNA and 0.3 µM of each primer. Primers were designed using Primer-BLAST software (NCBI, USA) and synthesized at Genomed (Poland). Forward and reverse primer sequences are presented in supplementary material (Additional file 1: Table S1). The samples were incubated at 95 °C for 5 min to obtain an initial denaturation and polymerase activation, followed by 35 PCR cycles of amplification (92 °C for 20 s, 57 °C for 20 s, and 72 °C for 40 s). Control reactions, with omission of the RT step or with no template cDNA added, were performed for each assay. All the samples were run in triplicate. To adjust for variations in the amount of added RNA and efficiency of the reverse transcription, β-actin, cyclophilin, and TBP mRNAs were quantified in corresponding samples of WAT and liver, and the results were normalized to these values. Since the results regarding MT mRNA levels in WAT and liver obtained with β-actin, cyclophilin, and TBP were essentially similar, we presented the relative gene expression only as precisely corresponding mRNA/β-actin mRNA in the "Results" section. Relative quantities of the transcripts were calculated using the $2^{-\Delta\Delta CT}$ formula [27]. The results are expressed in arbitrary units, with one unit corresponding to mean mRNA level for the control group. Amplification

of specific transcripts was further confirmed by obtaining melting curve profiles and subjecting the amplification products to 1 % agarose gel electrophoresis.

Western blots

Western blots were performed as recently described [39]. Briefly, frozen liver or adipose tissue were homogenized in 20-mM Tris-HCl buffer (pH 7.8) containing 0.2 % Triton X-100 and protease inhibitor cocktail (Sigma-Aldrich, USA) and centrifuged (30 000×g for 20 min). Aliquots of the supernatants containing 20-µg protein (estimated by Lowry's method) and the molecular mass protein markers were separated by 10 % SDS-PAGE and electroblotted to Immun-Blot PVDF Membrane (Bio-RAD, USA). The membranes were blocked with 5 % albumin in phosphate buffered saline (PBS) with 0.05 % Tween 20 (Sigma-Aldrich, USA). Subsequently, the membranes were incubated with antibodies diluted in blocking buffer. Monoclonal mouse antibodies against both MT1 and MT2 (MT1/2) (UC1MT) were purchased from Abcam (GB). Anti-actin (A5060), as well as HRP-conjugated secondary anti-rabbit (A0545) and anti-mouse antibodies (A9044), was obtained from Sigma-Aldrich (USA). The bands were visualized using ChemiDoc XRS (Bio-Rad, USA) and compared with respective molecular mass protein markers (SM26634) obtained from Thermo Scientific (USA), visualized on the membrane after electroblotting.

Serum samples were diluted with 20-mM Tris-HCl buffer (pH 7.8), and aliquots of the diluted solution containing 20-µg serum protein (protein estimated by Lowry's method) were separated by 10 % SDS-PAGE and electroblotted to Immun-Blot PVDF Membrane (Bio-RAD, USA). Further steps of western blots were performed as described above for liver or adipose tissue samples.

Serum insulin concentration assay

Serum insulin concentrations were determined by enzyme-linked immunosorbent assay (ELISA) (RAI008R; Biovendor, Czech Republic).

Determination of total zinc levels in adipose tissues

The total amount of Zn in adipose tissues was determined by flame atomic absorption spectrometry (spectrometer AAnalyst 400 Perkin Elmer) after dry ashing at 450 °C. Approximately 0.3 g of epididymal adipose tissue was combusted with gradual increase of temperature (50 °C/h). The obtained ash was treated with 5 ml of hydrochloric acid (6 M), and then, the acid solution was evaporated to dryness. The obtained residue was dissolved in 5 ml of nitric acid (0.1 M) and used for zinc determination at 213.9 nm. All analyses were done in triplicate. The accuracy and precision of the used method was assured by simultaneous analysis of certified reference material M-3 HerTis (Herring Tissue).

Statistics

Statistical significance of intergroup differences was verified on the basis of one-way analysis of variance (ANOVA) with Tukey's post hoc test. If data were not normally distributed, they were verified by non-parametric Kruskal–Wallis test. Pearson's correlation coefficient was calculated to assess the correlation between body weight or adipose tissue mass and relative MT mRNA level. All results are presented as means ± standard deviations (SD). The differences were considered significant at $p < 0.05$. Sigma Stat software was used for all statistical analyses.

Results

Using real-time PCR, we detected MT1, MT2, and MT3 mRNA in epididymal, retroperitoneal, and inguinal white adipose tissue (Fig. 1). MT4 mRNA was not found in any of the main fat depots (Fig. 1). The esophagus served as a positive control for MT4 mRNA (Fig. 1). As expected, in the liver, no MT3 mRNA was found (Fig. 1). After a 24-h fast, a significant increase in MT1 (Fig. 2a) and MT2 (Fig. 2b) mRNA levels was observed in epididymal, retroperitoneal, and inguinal WAT. After a 48-h fast, MT1 and MT2 mRNA levels in epididymal and retroperitoneal WAT were several-fold higher than in the controls (Fig. 2a, b). Fasting exerted less prominent effects on MT1 and MT2 mRNA levels in inguinal WAT (Fig. 2a, b), what points to likely differences in fasting

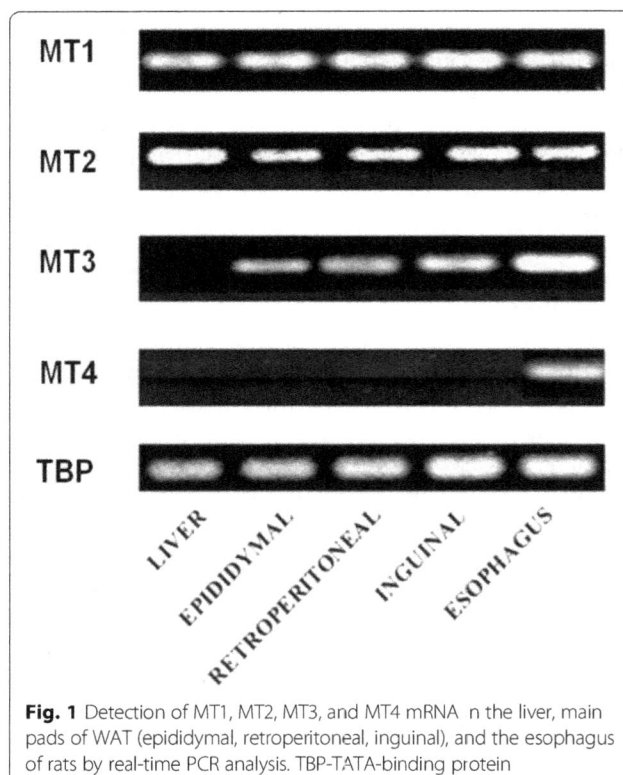

Fig. 1 Detection of MT1, MT2, MT3, and MT4 mRNA in the liver, main pads of WAT (epididymal, retroperitoneal, inguinal), and the esophagus of rats by real-time PCR analysis. TBP-TATA-binding protein

response of various WAT depots. The effects of a 72-h fast on MT1 and MT2 mRNA levels in WAT were comparable to those observed after 48 h (Fig. 2a, b). Fasting exerted no significant effects on MT3 mRNA levels in any of the main fat depots (Fig. 2c). An increase in MT1 and MT2 mRNA levels was observed for liver MTs (Fig. 3). The differences in MT1 and MT2 mRNA levels in the WAT and liver of control and fasted rats were reflected by their WAT, liver, and serum MT1 and MT2 protein levels determined by western blot analysis (Fig. 4). When the rats were fed ad libitum after a 48-h fast, their MT1 mRNA levels in retroperitoneal, epididymal, and inguinal WAT were normalized within 12 h (Fig. 5a). Similar effects were also observed for MT2 mRNA levels in retroperitoneal, epididymal, inguinal WAT (Additional file 2: Table S2) and liver MT1 and MT2 (Fig. 5b, c, respectively). Fasting/refeeding exerted no effects on MT3 mRNA levels in any of the main WAT depots (Additional file 2: Table S2). The differences in MT1 and MT2 mRNA levels in the WAT and liver of fasted and refed rats were consistent with the differences in their WAT and liver MT1 and MT2 protein levels determined by western blot analysis (Fig. 5d). Changes in MT1 and MT2 mRNA as well as protein levels apparently were not related to the epididymal WAT total zinc concentrations expressed as μg/mg protein (Fig. 5e) or as μg/g tissue (Additional file 3: Table S3). Moreover, in contrast to MT1 and MT2 mRNA and proteins, ZnT1 mRNA (Fig. 5f) and MTF1 mRNA (Fig. 5g) levels were not affected by fasting or fasting/refeeding. It should be mentioned that others examined Zn transporter mRNAs like ZnT6, ZnT9, ZIP6, ZIP8, and ZIP14 were also not affected by fasting or fasting/refeeding (Additional file 4: Table S4). Thus, the data presented on Fig. 5 suggest that the changes induced by fasting or fasting/refeeding in MT1 and MT2 mRNA levels may be independent of zinc. Body and fat mass (sum of retroperitoneal + epididymal + inguinal WAT) for control (not treated), fasted, and fasted/refed rats are presented in Table 1. Based on data presented in Fig. 2 and Table 1, correlation coefficient between body mass and MT mRNA levels as well between fat mass and MT mRNA levels was calculated. As indicated in Table 2, there was a negative correlation between MT1 mRNA level and body mass or fat mass. Essentially similar correlation for MT2 mRNA was found. As expected, no correlation was revealed in the case of MT3 (Table 2).

To obtain more information about potential factor(s) that may contribute to food intake-related changes in MT1 and MT2 gene expressions, we determined serum concentrations of insulin in control, fasted, and refed rats. As shown in Fig. 6, fasting was associated with a significant decrease in serum insulin, whereas refeeding resulted in an increase of this parameter. An inverse association between serum insulin and MT1 and MT2

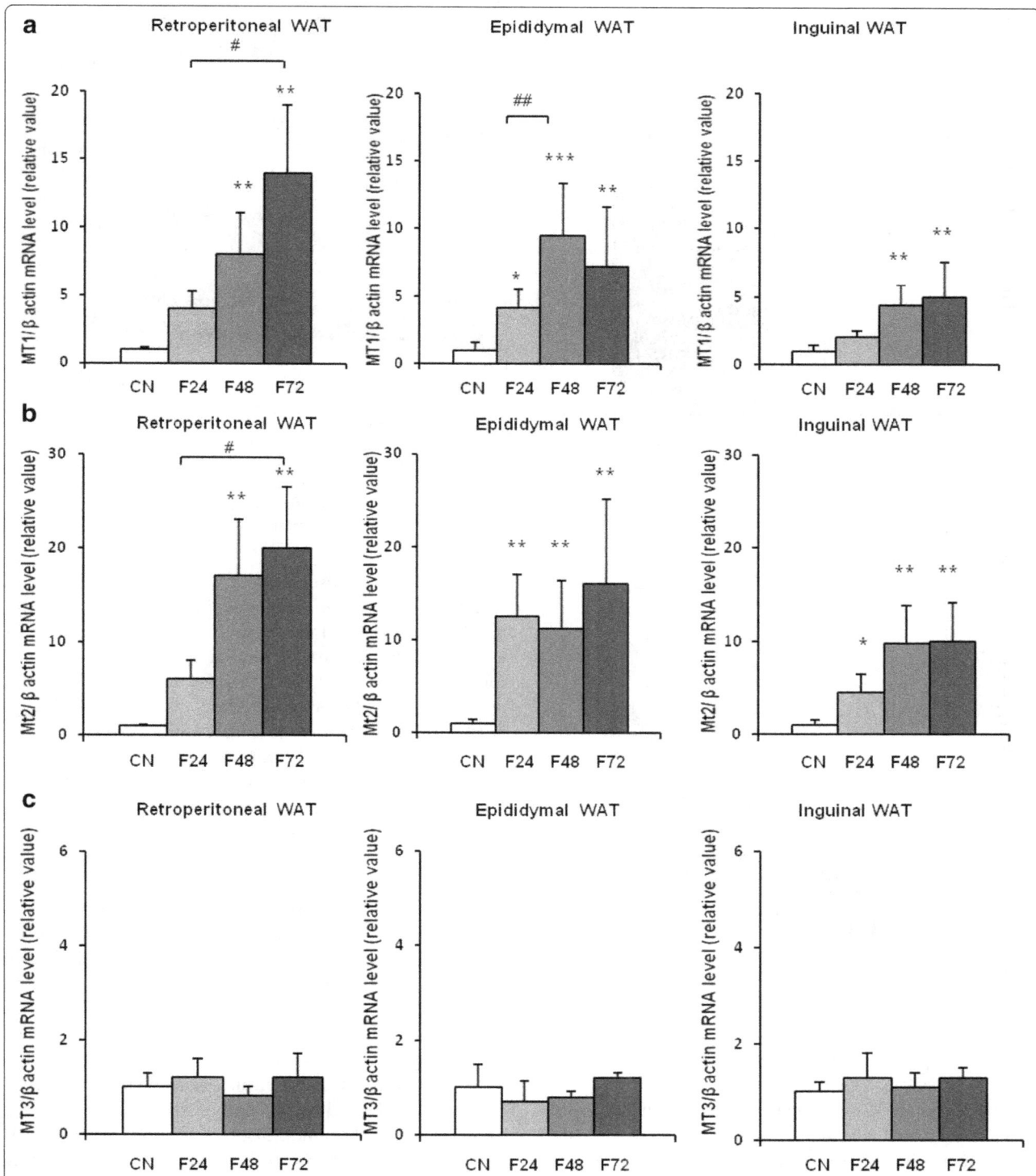

Fig. 2 The influence of fasting on MT mRNA level in WAT of rats. MT1 (**a**), MT2 (**b**), and MT3 (**c**) mRNA levels relative to β-actin mRNA levels in retroperitoneal, epididymal, and inguinal WAT of rats fed ad libitum (CN) and fasted rats: 24 h (F24), 48 h (F48), and 72 h (F72) are shown on the graphs (mean ± S.D., $n = 10$) *$p < 0.05$, **$p < 0.01$, ***$p < 0.001$. Note that MT3 mRNA levels in retroperitoneal, epididymal, and inguinal of control rats were significantly lower than MT1 and MT2

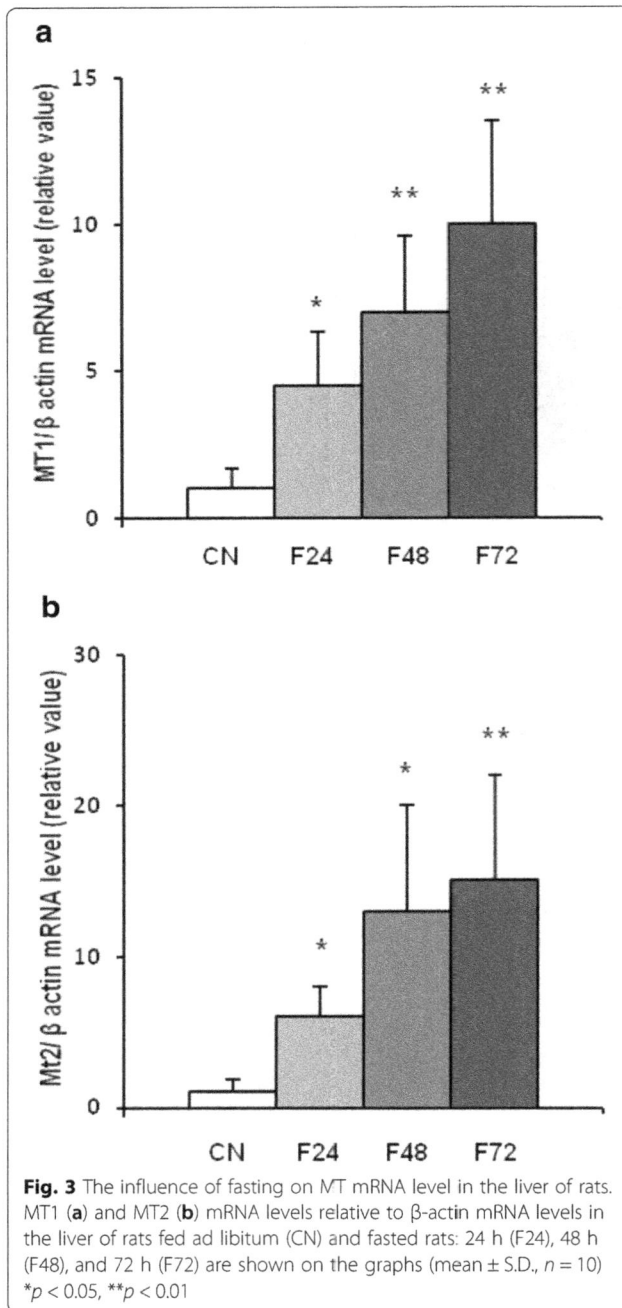

Fig. 3 The influence of fasting on MT mRNA level in the liver of rats. MT1 (**a**) and MT2 (**b**) mRNA levels relative to β-actin mRNA levels in the liver of rats fed ad libitum (CN) and fasted rats: 24 h (F24), 48 h (F48), and 72 h (F72) are shown on the graphs (mean ± S.D., n = 10) *p < 0.05, **p < 0.01

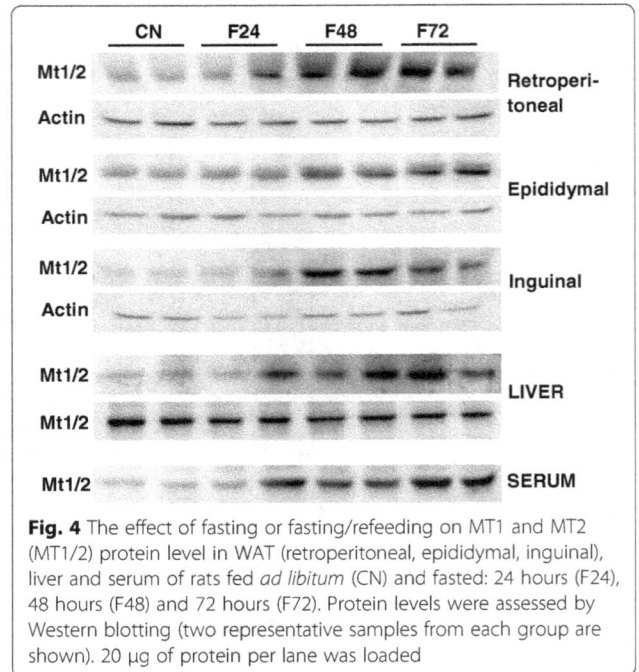

Fig. 4 The effect of fasting or fasting/refeeding on MT1 and MT2 (MT1/2) protein level in WAT (retroperitoneal, epididymal, inguinal), liver and serum of rats fed ad libitum (CN) and fasted: 24 hours (F24), 48 hours (F48) and 72 hours (F72). Protein levels were assessed by Western blotting (two representative samples from each group are shown). 20 µg of protein per lane was loaded

mRNA levels in WAT suggests that insulin may influence, at least partially the expressions of MT1 and MT2 encoding genes. To verify this hypothesis, we studied the effects of insulin on MT1 and MT2 levels in isolated adipocytes from epididymal WAT. As shown in Fig. 7, exposure of adipocytes to insulin (which theoretically should mimic a fed state) was reflected by a significant decrease in MT1 mRNA level. When dB-cAMP was added to the primary culture (which theoretically should mimic a fasted state), a significant increase in MT1 mRNA level was observed (Fig. 7a). Further, addition of insulin to adipocytes incubated in the presence of dB-cAMP was reflected by a significant decrease in MT1 mRNA levels. Essentially, similar results were obtained for MT2 mRNA level (Fig. 7a). Incubation with insulin or/and dB-cAMP exerted no effects on MT3 mRNA level in the primary culture of isolated adipocytes (Fig. 7a). Moreover, MT1 and MT2 mRNA in isolated rat adipocytes was also upregulated by forskolin (Fig. 7b), a compound increasing the intracellular cAMP. No significant effect of forskolin on MT3 mRNA level was found (Fig. 7b).

Discussion

Our present study showed that (a) MT1, MT2, and MT3 isoforms, but not MT4, are expressed in all main fat depots (retroperitoneal, epididymal, and inguinal) of rats, (b) MT1 and MT2 encoding genes are overexpressed in all main fat depots of fasted rats, (c) refeeding of fasted rats leads to a decrease in the expressions of MT1 and MT2 encoding genes in WAT, and (d) expression of MT3 encoding gene in retroperitoneal, epididymal, and inguinal WAT is not affected by fasting/refeeding. The magnitude of induction of MT1 and MT2 mRNA (and protein) levels is dependent on adipose tissue localization, since fasting exerted less prominent effects on MT1 and MT2 mRNA levels in inguinal (subcutaneous) than in epididymal and retroperitoneal WAT (Fig. 2a, b). The differences between MT levels in omental and subcutaneous human adipose tissue were also reported by Kim et al. [23]. Furthermore, our data imply that the effects of fasting on MT1 and MT2 mRNA levels in WAT are generally similar to those

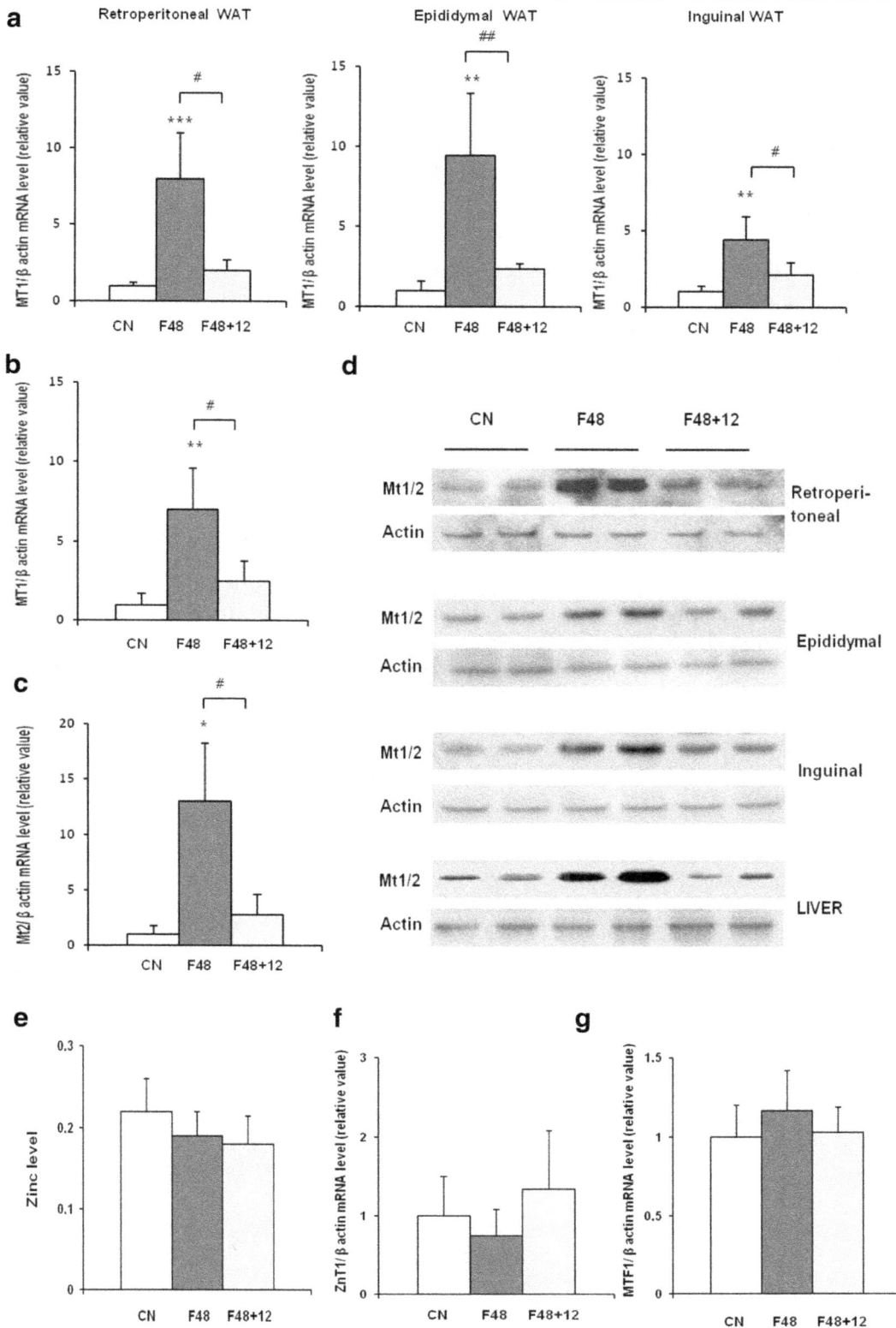

Fig. 5 (See legend on next page.)

(See figure on previous page.)
Fig. 5 The influence of fasting or fasting/refeeding on MT1 mRNA level in WAT (**a**), liver (**b**, **c**), MT1 and MT2 (MT1/2) protein level in WAT and liver of rats (**d**), zinc level (µg/mg protein) in epididymal WAT (**e**), ZnT1 mRNA level in epididymal WAT (**f**), and MTF1 mRNA level in epididymal WAT(**g**). MT1 mRNA levels relative to β-actin expression in WAT (retroperitoneal, epididymal, and inguinal) and liver of rats fed ad libitum (CN), fasted 48 h (F48), and fasted 48 h and refed 12 h (F48 + 12) are shown on the graphs (mean ± S.D., $n = 10$) *$p < 0.05$, **$p < 0.01$, ***$p < 0.001$; MT1 and MT2 protein level in WAT and liver of rats fed ad libitum (CN), fasted 48 h (F48), and fasted 48 h and refed 12 h (F48 + 12) protein levels were assessed by western blotting (two representative samples from each group are shown, 20 µg of protein per lane was loaded); ZnT1 and MTF1 mRNA levels relative to β-actin mRNA levels in WAT (epididymal) of rats fed ad libitum (CN), fasted 48 h (F48), and fasted 48 h and refed 12 h (F48 + 12) are shown on the graphs (mean ± S.D., $n = 10$)

observed in the liver (Figs. 2 and 3). Thus, the effect of fasting on the liver content of MTs presented here confirms the results reported previously by Higashimoto et al. [17] and Kondoh et al. [25] in mice.

Our findings differ considerably from those reported previously by Trayhurn et al. [44] according to whom MT1 mRNA levels in epididymal WAT of fasted and fasted/refed mice were similar to the controls. In contrast, our fasted rats presented significantly higher MT1 and MT2 mRNA levels than the control animals. Moreover, we showed that the effects of fasting on MT mRNA levels are time-dependent, reaching its peak after a 48-h fast. Thus, one possible explanation for the discrepancy between the data published by Trayhurn et al. [43] and the results of our study (beside different animal model used) may be a duration of fasting. In Trayhurn et al.'s [43] experiment, mice were fasted for up to 16 h. As shown in Fig. 2, the level of MT1 mRNA (as well as MT2 RNA) in epididymal WAT increased approximately twofold after 24-h fast and several fold after 48 and 72 h fast compare to the control.

The effects of fasting on the expressions of MT1 and MT2 encoding genes in the liver and WAT (as well as on the serum concentrations of MT1 and MT2), measured at both mRNA and protein level, were completely reversed after a 12-h refeeding ad libitum. This implies that the expressions of MT1 and MT2 encoding genes in all main fat depots of rats are highly sensitive to nutritional status. Consequently, the levels of MT1 and MT2 in WAT and blood slightly fluctuate throughout the day in response to food intake.

Interestingly, the results presented here indicate that the expression of genes encoding MT1 and MT2 regulated by fasting and fasting/refeeding could be independent of total zinc content in WAT. Induction of gene encoding MT1 expression in rat brown adipose tissue [32] and mouse liver [13] independent of zinc has been also reported previously. However, regarding the fact that intracellular zinc homeostasis is regulated by MTs [8, 26, 30], overexpression of genes coding MTs in fasted rats and subsequently the increase in MTs levels could decrease free zinc ion (but not total zinc levels) concentration in adipocytes necessary for zinc finger protein biosynthesis. This may affect zinc finger protein biosynthesis and subsequently, adipose tissue function [48]. It is well documented that the zinc finger proteins regulate adipogenesis and lipid metabolism in adipose tissue [48]. Thus, one may suppose that increased MT1 and MT2 levels may lead to decrease in intracellular zinc finger protein levels and subsequently to inhibition of adipogenesis and lipid accumulation in adipose tissue. Diminished levels of intracellular MTs may lead to the increase of zinc finger protein levels and subsequently to the activation of adipogenesis and increase in lipid accumulation in adipose tissue, which in turn may lead to obesity.

Table 1 The body and WAT (retroperitoneal, epididymal, inguinal) mass of control, fasted, fasted and refed rats

Group	Body weight (g)	Adipose tissue mass (g)
Control (ad libitum)	261 ± 10	6.4 ± 1.1
Fasted 24 h	227 ± 9***	5.4 ± 1.1*
Fasted 48 h	216 ± 9***	4.9 ± 1.0*
Fasted 72 h	205 ± 8*** ##	4.1 ± 0.9* #
Fasted 48 h + ad libitum	242 ± 9* ##	4.7 ± 1.4**

The body mass and adipose tissue of rats maintained on fasting and fasting and refeeding (mean ± S.D., $n = 10$). *$p < 0.05$, **$p < 0.01$, ***$p < 0.001$ compared to the control group, #$p < 0.05$, ##$p < 0.01$ compared to 24-h fasted group

Table 2 Correlation coefficients between body weight and MT mRNA level in retroperitoneal, epididymal, or inguinal WAT and the sum of adipose tissue mass and MT mRNA relative level in retroperitoneal, epididymal, or inguinal WAT

WAT	mRNA	Body weight		Adipose tissue mass	
		R	p	R	p
Retroperitoneal	MT1	−0.60	<0.001	−0.63	<0.001
	MT2	−0.54	<0.01	−0.52	<0.01
	MT3	0.12	ns	0.02	ns
Epididymal	MT1	−0.66	<0.001	−0.48	<0.01
	MT2	−0.52	<0.01	−0.43	<0.02
	MT3	−0.12	ns	−0.05	ns
Inguinal	MT1	−0.82	<0.001	−0.66	<0.001
	MT2	−0.83	<0.001	−0.54	<0.01
	MT3	0.18	ns	0.12	ns

R correlation coefficients; ns non-significant

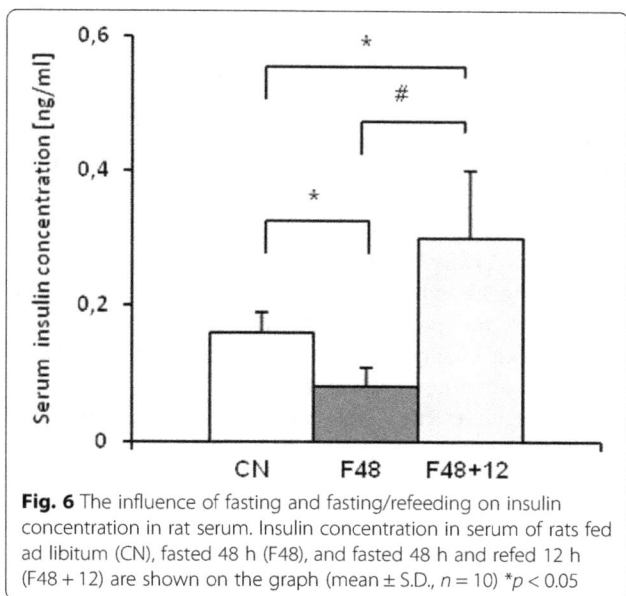

Fig. 6 The influence of fasting and fasting/refeeding on insulin concentration in rat serum. Insulin concentration in serum of rats fed ad libitum (CN), fasted 48 h (F48), and fasted 48 h and refed 12 h (F48 + 12) are shown on the graph (mean ± S.D., n = 10) *p < 0.05

Accordingly, the data reported previously indicate that MTs (1 and 2) null mice are obese [2, 37].

It should be noted that besides MTs, intracellular zinc homeostasis may be regulated by zinc transporters, SLC30A (also named ZnT) and SLC39A (also named ZIP) [42]. However, the results presented in this paper indicate no association between MTs and Zn transporter mRNA levels.

Moreover, we showed that a 24-h incubation with dB-cAMP (or forskolin) results in increase, whereas a 24-h exposure to insulin leads to decrease in MT1 and MT2 mRNA levels in isolated adipocytes (Fig. 7). Thus, the effect of cAMP on MT gene expression in isolated rat adipocytes is similar to that reported by Trayhurn [44]. However, in contrast to our results, Trayhurn et al. [44] found increase in MT gene expressions in rat adipocytes incubated with insulin. Based on the data indicating that insulin leads to decrease of cAMP concentrations in adipocytes [12], the data reported by Trayhurn et al. [44] are difficult to explain. Moreover, our results are in line

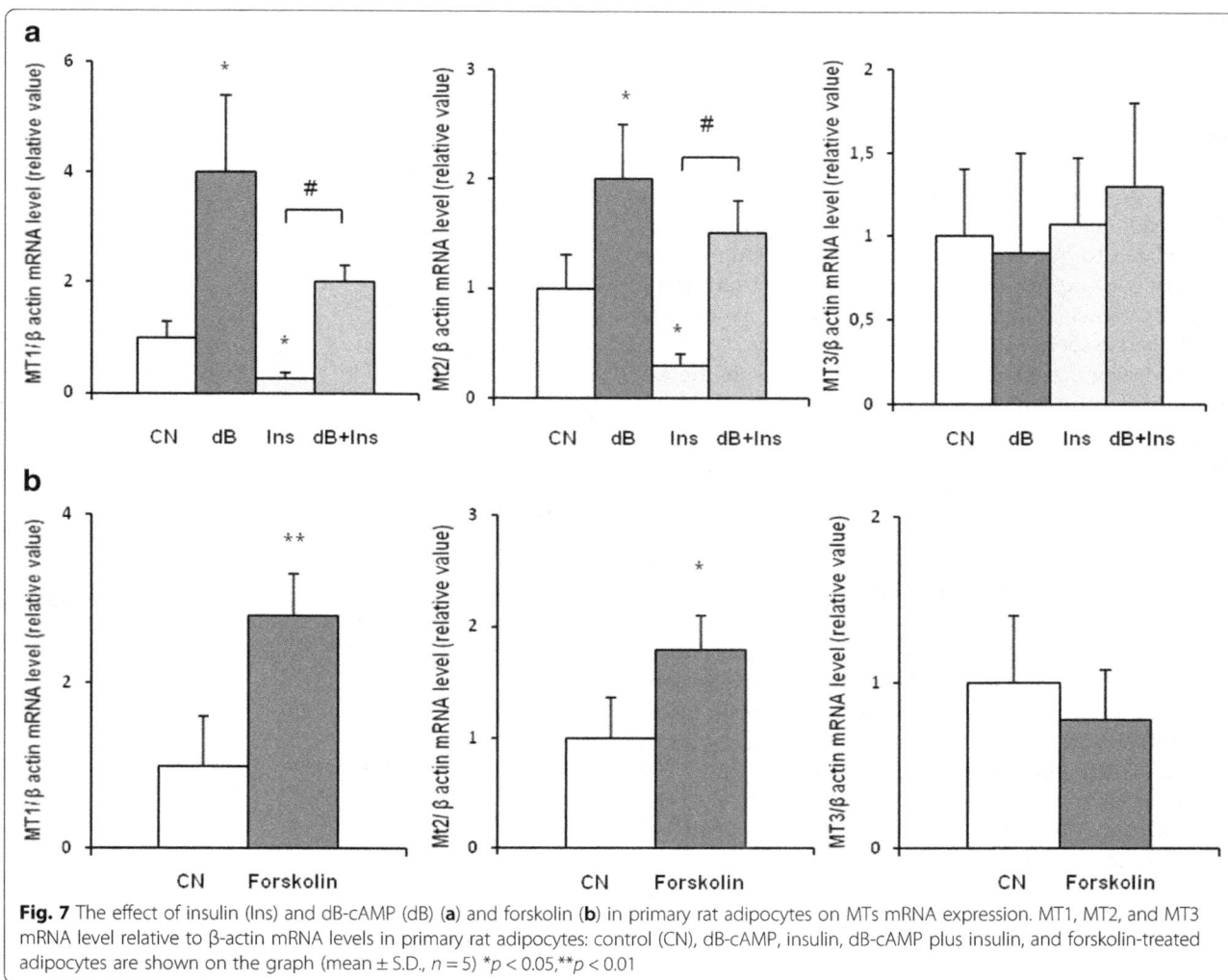

Fig. 7 The effect of insulin (Ins) and dB-cAMP (dB) (**a**) and forskolin (**b**) in primary rat adipocytes on MTs mRNA expression. MT1, MT2, and MT3 mRNA level relative to β-actin mRNA levels in primary rat adipocytes: control (CN), dB-cAMP, insulin, dB-cAMP plus insulin, and forskolin-treated adipocytes are shown on the graph (mean ± S.D., n = 5) *p < 0.05,**p < 0.01

with data reported by Costarelli et al. [9], who found inverse relationship between human plasma insulin and MT concentrations.

Taken together, the results of our study imply that nutritional status plays a key role in the regulation of MT1 and MT2 encoding genes in WAT. Inverse relationship between serum insulin concentration and MTs (1 and 2) mRNA levels in WAT (Figs. 5a and 6) as well as the decrease in MT1 and MT2 mRNA levels by insulin in isolated adipocytes (Fig. 7) suggests that the effect of nutritional status on MT1 and MT2 is mediated by insulin. Previous studies showed that MT promoter has the sequence for AP-2 (activating protein-2), a transcription factor via which cAMP upregulates mRNA level in the liver [10]. Insulin is likely to suppress MT1 and MT2 encoding genes upon binding to adipocyte insulin receptors and their activation; this results in the phosphorylation of insulin receptor substrates, activation of the phosphatidylinositol kinase 3 (PI3K)-kinase B/Akt (PKB/Akt)-phosphodiesterase 3B pathway, and degradation of cAMP in adipocytes [12]. These events lead to a decrease in the intracellular concentrations of cAMP and resultant decrease in MT1 and MT2 mRNA levels. Consequently, both lack of insulin and insulin insensitivity may upregulate MT1 and MT2 encoding genes in WAT of rats. However, it is not excluded that insulin stimulated glucose influx into adipocytes could be responsible for the inhibition of gene expression encoding MT1 and MT2 in WAT. Although our experimental data cannot be directly extrapolated to humans, the previously reported increase in MT2a gene expression in the adipose tissue from type 2 diabetic patients [16] and obese subject [7, 11] might be at least in part associated with insulin insensitivity.

Considering that glucocorticosteroids stimulate the expression of gene encoding MT1 and MT2 in the liver [24], one can suppose that fasting-induced increase in these steroid levels [49] may also at least in part contribute to the observed upregulation of MTs (1 and 2) in WAT and liver in vivo.

According to Trayhurn et al. [43], MT is a secretory protein synthesized in WAT (though the primary structure of MT is inconsistent with that of the classic secretory protein), and as such, may exert systemic biological effects. Our presented findings imply that enhanced expressions of MT1 and MT2 genes in WAT and liver (observed at both mRNA and protein levels) correlate strongly with an increase in the serum concentrations of MT1 and MT2 (Fig. 4). Therefore, liver and WAT might contribute to elevated serum MT levels. Consequently, the results of our study seem to support the hypothesis that MTs are secretory products of WAT, as proposed by Trayhurn et al. [43]. However, it is not excluded that some amount of MTs are released from blood cells during the preparation of serum.

Conclusions

In conclusion, our findings imply that the genes encoding MT1 and MT2, but not MT3, in retroperitoneal, epididymal, and inguinal WAT of rats are regulated by nutritional status and that insulin plays an important role in this process. Changes in MT1 and MT2 mRNA levels were not related to (a) total zinc concentrations, (b) MTF1 mRNA level, and (c) Zn transporters mRNA levels in WAT. This suggests that the regulation of MT1 and MT2 gene expression by fasting and fasting/refeeding may be independent of total zinc concentrations. It is likely that changes in WAT MT1 and MT2 levels induced by nutritional status could be an important system to regulate intracellular distribution, but not total concentrations of zinc.

Abbreviations

cAMP, cyclic adenosine monophosphate; Cu, copper; dB-cAMP, dibutyryl cyclic adenosine monophosphate; DMEM, Dulbecco's Modified Eagle's Medium; HEPES, N-(2-Hydroxyethyl)piperazine-N'-(2-ethanesulfonic acid); MT, metallothionein; MTF1, metal-responsive transcription factor; PCR, polymerase chain reaction; RNA, ribonucleic acid; SD, standard deviations; TBP, TATA-box binding protein; WAT, white adipose tissue; Zn, zinc

Acknowledgements

The authors would like to thank Mrs Elzbieta Goyke for her technical assistance.

Funding

The research was funded by the Ministry of Science and Higher Education (Poland) for the Medical University of Gdansk: grant no. MN-01-0043/08, MN- 01-01253/08/256; ST-41 and ST-40. Publication of this manuscript was supported by the Ministry of Science and Higher Education of the Republic of Poland, from the quality-promoting subsidy, under the Leading National Research Centre (KNOW) program for the years 2012–2017.

Authors' contributions

SSz carried out the molecular genetic and western blot studies, adipocyte isolation, animal procedures, and statistical analysis and helped to draft the manuscript. ES participated in the immunoassay. JT designed all the oligonucleotides and participated in the animal procedures. ABG determined the zinc concentration. TS helped in the adipocyte isolation and statistical analysis. JS conceived the study, participated in its design and coordination, and drafted the manuscript. All authors read and approved the final manuscript.

Competing interests

The authors declare that they have no competing interests.

Author details

Department of Biochemistry, Medical University of Gdansk, Debinki 1, 80-211 Gdansk, Poland. [2]Department of Environmental Technology, University of Gdansk, Wita Stwosza 63, 80-952 Gdansk, Poland. [3]Department of Pharmaceutical Biochemistry, Medical University of Gdansk, Debinki 1, 80-211 Gdansk, Poland.

References

1. Aschner M. The functional significance of brain metallothioneins. FASEB J. 1996;10:1129–36.
2. Beattie JH, Wood AM, Newman AM, Bremner I, Choo KH, Michalska AE, et al. Obesity and hyperleptinemia in metallothionein (-I and -II) null mice. Proc Natl Acad Sci USA. 1998;95:358–63.
3. Beattie JH, Wood AM, Trayhurn P, Jasani B, Vincent A, McCormack G, et al. Metallothionein is expressed in adipocytes of brown fat and is induced by catecholamines and zinc. Am J Physiol Regul Integr Comp Physiol. 2000;278: R1082–9.
4. Bremner I, Beattie JH. Metallothionein and the trace minerals. Annu Rev Nutr. 1990;10:63–83.
5. Cai L. Suppression of nitrative damage by metallothionein in diabetic heart contributes to the prevention of cardiomyopathy. Free Radic Biol Med. 2006;41:851–61.
6. Cai L. Diabetic cardiomyopathy and its prevention by metallothionein: experimental evidence, possible mechanisms and clinical implications. Curr Med Chem. 2007;14:2193–203.
7. Cancello R, Zulian A, Gentilini D, Mencarelli M, Della BA, Maffei M, et al. Permanence of molecular features of obesity in subcutaneous adipose tissue of ex-obese subjects. Int J Obes. 2013;37:867–73.
8. Colvin R, Holmes WR, Fontaine CP, Maret W. Cytosolic zinc buffering and muffling: their role in intracellular zinc homeostasis. Metallomics. 2010;2: 306–17.
9. Costarelli L, Muti E, Malavolta M, Cipriano C, Giacconi R, Tesei S, et al. Distinctive modulation of inflammatory and metabolic parameters in relation to zinc nutritional status in adult overweight/obese subjects. J Nutr Biochem. 2010;21:432–7.
10. Davis SR, Cousins RJ. Metallothionein expression in animals: a physiological perspective on function. J Nutr. 2000;130:1085–8.
11. Do MS, Nam SY, Hong SE, Kim KW, Duncan JS, Beattie JH, et al. Metallothionein gene expression in human adipose tissue from lean and obese subjects. Horm Metab Res. 2002;34:348–51.
12. Duncan RE, Ahmadian M, Jaworski K, Sarkadi-Nagy E, Sul HS. Regulation of lipolysis in adipocytes. Annu Rev Nutr. 2007;27:79–101.
13. Durnam DM, Hoffman JS, Quaife CJ, Benditt EP, Chen HY, Brinster RL, et al. Induction of mouse metallothionein-I mRNA by bacterial endotoxin is independent of metals and glucocorticoid hormones. Proc Natl Acad Sci USA. 1984;81:1053–6.
14. Ebadi M, Iversen PL, Hao R, Cerutis DR, Rojas P, Happe HK, et al. Expression and regulation of brain metallothionein. Neurochem Int. 1995;27:1–22.
15. Erickson JC, Hollopeter G, Thomas SA, Froelick GJ, Palmiter RD. Disruption of the metallothionein-III gene in mice: analysis of brain zinc, behavior, and neuron vulnerability to metals, aging, and seizures. J Neurosci. 1997;17: 1271–81.
16. Haynes V, Connor T, Tchernof A, Vidal H, Dubois S. Metallothionein 2a gene expression is increased in subcutaneous adipose tissue of type 2 diabetic patients. Mol Genet Metab. 2013;108:90–4.
17. Higashimoto M, Sano M, Kondoh M, Sato M. Different responses of metallothionein and leptin induced in the mouse by fasting stress. Biol Trace Elem Res. 2002;89:75–84.
18. Hotamisligil GS. Inflammation and metabolic disorders. Nature. 2006;444: 860–7.
19. Hozumi I, Asanuma M, Yamada Y, Uchida Y. Metallothioneins and neurodegenerative diseases. J Health Science. 2004;50:323–31.
20. Hozumi I, Suzuki JS, Kanazawa H, Hara A, Saio M, Inuzuka T, et al. Metallothionein-3 is expressed in the brain and various peripheral organs of the rat. Neurosci Lett. 2008;438:54–8.
21. Kadota Y, Aki Y, Toriuchi Y, Mizuno Y, Kawakami T, Sato M, et al. Deficiency of metallothionein-1 and -2 genes shortens the lifespan of the 129/Sv mouse strain. Exp Gerontol. 2015;66:21–4.
22. Kawashima T, Doh-ura K, Torisu M, Uchida Y, Furuta A, Iwaki T. Differential expression of metallothioneins in human prion diseases. Dement Geriatr Cogn Disord. 2000;11:251–62.
23. Kim JR, Ryu HH, Chung HJ, Lee JH, Kim SW, Kwun WH, et al. Association of anti-obesity activity of N-acetylcysteine with metallothionein-II down-regulation. Exp Mol Med. 2006;38:162–72.
24. Klaassen CD, Lehman-McKeeman LD. Regulation of the isoforms of metallothionein. Biol Trace Elem Res. 1989;21:119–29.
25. Kondoh M, Kamada K, Kuronaga M, Higashimoto M, Takiguchi M, Watanabe Y, et al. Antioxidant property of metallothionein in fasted mice. Toxicol Lett. 2003;143:301–6.
26. Krezel A, Maret W. Zinc-buffering capacity of a eukaryotic cell at physiological pZn. J Biol Inorg Chem. 2006;11:1049–62.
27. Livak KJ, Schmittgen TD. Analysis of relative gene expression data using real-time quantitative PCR and the 2(-Delta Delta C(T)) Method. Methods. 2001;25:402–8.
28. Malaiyandi LM, Dineley KE, Reynolds IJ. Divergent consequences arise from metallothionein overexpression in astrocytes: zinc buffering and oxidant-induced zinc release. Glia. 2004;45:346–53.
29. Malavolta M, Basso A, Piacenza F, Giacconi R, Costarelli L, Pierpaoli S, et al. Survival study of metallothionein-1 transgenic mice and respective controls (C57BL/6J): influence of a zinc-enriched environment. Rejuvenation Res. 2012;15:140–3.
30. Maret W. Molecular aspects of human cellular zinc homeostasis: redox control of zinc potentials and zinc signals. Biometals. 2009;22:149–57.
31. Michalska AE, Choo KH. Targeting and germ-line transmission of a null mutation at the metallothionein I and II loci in mouse. Proc Natl Acad Sci USA. 1993;90:8088–92.
32. Peresleni T, Noiri E, Bahou WF, Goligorsky MS. Antisense oligodeoxynucleotides to inducible NO synthase rescue epithelial cells from oxidative stress injury. Am J Physiol. 1996;270:F971–7.
33. Quaife CJ, Findley SD, Erickson JC, Froelick GJ, Kelly EJ, Zambrowicz BP, et al. Induction of a new metallothionein isoform (MT-IV) occurs during differentiation of stratified squamous epithelia. Biochemistry. 1994;33:7250–9.
34. Quaife CJ, Kelly EJ, Masters BA, Brinster RL, Palmiter RD. Ectopic expression of metallothionein-III causes pancreatic acinar cell necrosis in transgenic mice. Toxicol Appl Pharmacol. 1998;148:148–57.
35. Rodbell M. Metabolism of isolated fat cells. Effects of hormones on glucose metabolism and lipolysis. J Biol Chem. 1964;239:375–80.
36. Sato M, Kondoh M. Recent studies on metallothionein: protection against toxicity of heavy metals and oxygen free radicals. Tohoku J Exp Med. 2002; 196:9–22.
37. Sato M, Kawakami T, Kondoh M, Takiguchi M, Kadota Y, Himeno S, et al. Development of high-fat-diet-induced obesity in female metallothionein-null mice. FASEB J. 2010;24:2375–84.
38. Smidt K, Pedersen S, Brock B, Schmitz O, Fisker S, Bendix J, et al. Zinc-transporter genes in human visceral and subcutaneous adipocytes: lean versus obese. Mol Cell Endocrinol. 2007;264:68–73.
39. Stelmanska E, Szrok S, Swierczynski J. Progesterone-induced down-regulation of hormone sensitive lipase (Lipe) and up-regulation of G0/G1 switch 2 (G0s2) genes expression in inguinal adipose tissue of female rats is reflected by diminished rate of lipolysis. J Steroid Biochem Mol Biol. 2015; 147:31–9.
40. Suzuki KT, Someya A, Komada Y, Ogra Y. Roles of metallothionein in copper homeostasis: responses to Cu-deficient diets in mice. J Inorg Biochem. 2002;88:173–82.
41. Swindell WR. Metallothionein and the biology of aging. Ageing Res Rev. 2011;10:132–45.
42. Tepaamorndech S, Kirschke CP, Pedersen TL, Keyes WR, Newman JW, Huang L. Zinc transporter 7 deficiency affects lipid synthesis in adipocytes by inhibiting insulin-dependent Akt activation and glucose uptake. FEBS J. 2016;283:378–94.
43. Trayhurn P, Duncan JS, Wood AM, Beattie JH. Metallothionein gene expression and secretion in white adipose tissue. Am J Physiol Regul Integr Comp Physiol. 2000a;279:R2329–35.
44. Trayhurn P, Duncan JS, Wood AM, Beattie JH. Regulation of metallothionein gene expression and secretion in rat adipocytes differentiated from preadipocytes in primary culture. Horm Metab Res. 2000b;32:542–7.
45. Trayhurn P, Beattie JH. Physiological role of adipose tissue: white adipose tissue as an endocrine and secretory organ. Proc Nutr Soc. 2001;60:329–39.
46. Tsave O, Halevas E, Yavropoulou MP, Kosmidis PA, Yovos JG, Hatzidimitriou A, et al. Structure-specific adipogenic capacity of novel, well-defined ternary Zn(II)-Schiff base materials. Biomolecular correlations in zinc-induced differentiation of 3T3-L1 pre-adipocytes to adipocytes. J Inorg Biochem. 2015;152:123–37.
47. Vasak M, Meloni G. Chemistry and biology of mammalian metallothioneins. J Biol Inorg Chem. 2011;16:1067–78.
48. Wei S, Zhang L, Zhou X, Du M, Jiang Z, Hausman GJ, et al. Emerging roles of zinc finger proteins in regulating adipogenesis. Cell Mol Life Sci. 2013;70: 4569–84.

17

Dietary and genetic risk scores and incidence of type 2 diabetes

Ulrika Ericson[1,2]*, George Hindy[1], Isabel Drake[1], Christina-Alexandra Schulz[1], Louise Brunkwall[1], Sophie Hellstrand[1], Peter Almgren[1] and Marju Orho-Melander[1]

Abstract

Background: Both lifestyle and genetic predisposition determine the development of type 2 diabetes (T2D), and studies have indicated interactions between specific dietary components and individual genetic variants. However, it is unclear whether the importance of overall dietary habits, including T2D-related food intakes, differs depending on genetic predisposition to T2D. We examined interaction between a genetic risk score for T2D, constructed from 48 single nucleotide polymorphisms identified in genome-wide association studies, and a diet risk score of four foods consistently associated with T2D in epidemiological studies (processed meat, sugar-sweetened beverages, whole grain and coffee). In total, 25,069 individuals aged 45–74 years with genotype information and without prevalent diabetes from the Malmö Diet and Cancer cohort (1991–1996) were included. Diet data were collected with a modified diet history method.

Results: During 17-year follow-up, 3588 incident T2D cases were identified. Both the diet risk score (HR in the highest risk category 1.40; 95% CI 1.26, 1.58; P trend $= 6 \times 10^{-10}$) and the genetic risk score (HR in the highest tertile of the genetic risk score 1.67; 95% CI 1.54, 1.81; P trend $= 7 \times 10^{-35}$) were associated with increased incidence of T2D. No significant interaction between the genetic risk score and the diet risk score ($P = 0.83$) or its food components was observed. The highest risk was seen among the 6% of the individuals with both high genetic and dietary risk scores (HR 2.49; 95% CI 2.06, 3.01).

Conclusions: The findings thus show that both genetic heredity and dietary habits previously associated with T2D add to the risk of T2D, but they seem to act in an independent fashion, with the consequence that all individuals, whether at high or low genetic risk, would benefit from favourable food choices.

Keywords: Diet, Food intake, Gene-environment interactions, Cohort study, Type 2 diabetes

Background

The prevalence of type 2 diabetes (T2D) is increasing worldwide, and it is of great concern to identify modifiable lifestyle factors including diet. However, both lifestyle and genetic predisposition determine the development of the disease [1], and some studies have indicated interactions between specific dietary components and individual genetic variants [2, 3]. Yet, few findings have been replicated, and it is unclear whether the importance of overall dietary habits, including T2D-related food intakes, differs depending on overall genetic predisposition to T2D.

Single nucleotide polymorphisms (SNPs) associated with T2D have been identified in genome-wide association studies (GWAS) [4, 5]. Moreover, high intakes of processed meat [6–8] and sugar-sweetened beverages (SSB) [9–11] have in meta-analyses of observational studies consistently been associated with increased risk of developing T2D, whereas high intakes of whole grain [12, 13] foods and coffee [14, 15] have been associated with decreased risk. Probable mechanisms behind these associations have been proposed [16–19]. Inverse associations with intakes of fruits and vegetables [20, 21], dairy products [22] (especially fermented dairy) [22–24]) and fatty fish [25] have also been observed, but these findings are less conclusive [23, 26, 27] or may be explained by intake of specific products within these food groups [20, 21, 23, 24, 28–30].

It has been indicated that associations between western dietary patterns and T2D may differ between individuals depending on genetic susceptibility, but dietary habits assessed by a Mediterranean diet score were not found to interact with a genetic risk score (GRS) for T2D in the

---

* Correspondence: Ulrika.Ericson@med.lu.se
[1]Diabetes and Cardiovascular Disease, Genetic Epidemiology, Department of Clinical Sciences, Malmö, Lund University, Malmö, Sweden
[2]Clinical Research Centre, Building 60, floor 13, SUS in Malmö, entrance 72, Jan Waldenströms gata 35, SE-205 02 Malmö, Sweden

EPIC InterAct study [31]. However, we are not aware of any previous study examining whether a diet risk score (DRS), based on specific food intakes previously found to associate with T2D, interacts with a GRS. Besides, a diet quality index, based on Swedish nutrition recommendations, that has been associated with cardiovascular disease could not be linked to incidence of T2D in the Malmö Diet and Cancer (MDC) Study [32], suggesting that the index components chosen to reflect overall diet quality may not capture food intakes of particular relevance in the development of T2D.

Our aim was to examine T2D incidence in the MDC study according to a DRS of the four foods and beverages most consistently reported to associate with T2D in epidemiological studies (processed meat, sugar-sweetened beverages, whole grain and coffee), and a GRS of 48 GWAS-identified T2D SNPs [5], as well as their interaction. We also examined interactions between the GRS and each of the diet components included in the DRS.

Methods

Study population and data collection
The MDC study is a population-based prospective cohort study in southern Sweden with baseline examinations in 1991–1996. Women born in 1923–1950 and men born in 1923–1945, living in the city of Malmö, were invited. Details of the cohort and the recruitment are described elsewhere [33]. The participants filled out questionnaires covering socio-economic and lifestyle and underwent a diet history assessment. Anthropometric measurements were conducted by nurses. Body composition was estimated with a bioelectrical impedance analyser. During the screening period, 28,098 participants (40% of the eligible persons) completed all baseline examinations. Of the non-participants, 49% did not reply to the invitation letter, 39% answered that they were not willing to take part, 7% died or moved before they had received an invitation and 5% failed to complete all baseline examinations.

We excluded 1230 participants, based on self-reported diabetes diagnosis, self-reported diabetes medication or information from medical registries (see below). We were then left with 26,868 individuals, of whom 25,430 individuals had available DNA, and out of those, 25,069 individuals were successfully genotyped for > 60% of the SNPs included in the GRS; these individuals constituted our study population. A random 50% subsample of those who participated in MDC study between 1991 and 1994 were invited to be involved in additional baseline examinations. All additional measurements were made at baseline with a median time lag of 7 months after the first visit. In total, 6103 individuals participated in the additional examinations (the MDC cardiovascular sub-cohort, MDCS-CC). Out of those, 4193 individuals were successfully genotyped for additional SNPs included in an extended GRS. The ethical committee at Lund University has approved the study (LU 51-90), and the participants have given their written informed consent.

GRS for T2D
Weighted GRSs for T2D was calculated in PLINK from 48 T2D SNPs identified in 37 GWAS and confirmed or identified in a meta-analysis by Morris et al. [5] (Additional file 1: Table S1). Out of 63 identified SNPs in Morris et al., 9 were excluded as they were in linkage disequilibrium with other SNPs that we included in the GRS (rs6795735, rs10440833, rs1920792, rs4430796, rs757110, rs1387153, rs13081389, rs12255372 and rs4760790), 2 were excluded due to sex-specific associations in GWAS (rs11063069 and rs8108269) [5], 1 due to imprinting (rs2334499) [34] and 3 due to deviation from HWE (rs757210, rs4607517 and rs2796441) in our study. If the individuals had missing values for any of the 48 SNPs, it was substituted in PLINK by the mean of the risk alleles for that SNP calculated from the other individuals. Genotypes at each locus were coded as 0, 1 and 2, according to the number of T2D-increasing risk alleles, and a weighted GRS was calculated in PLINK such that each risk allele was weighted by their previously published effect sizes [5]. The weighted GRS was divided into tertiles.

Extended GRS for T2D for secondary analyses in a subsample
An extended weighted GRS for T2D was calculated in PLINK from 68 T2D SNPs in a subsample of the MDC cohort (individuals with genotype information on 68 T2D SNPs and without prevalent diabetes from the MDC cardiovascular sub-cohort). The extended GRS included 20 of the additional SNPs identified after the meta-analysis by Morris et al. until Fuchsberger et al. [35] (Additional file 1: Table S9).

Genotyping
A MALDI-TOF mass spectrometer (Sequenom MassArray, Sequenom, San Diego, CA) was used to genotype DNA samples using Sequenom reagents and protocols. Proxy SNPs were identified using SNAP version 2.2.2 when commercial primers were not available. SNPs that failed Sequenom genotyping were genotyped individually using TaqMan or KASPar allelic discrimination on an ABI 7900HT (Applied Biosystems, Life Technologies, Carlsbad, CA). All included 48 SNPs had genotyping success rate above 93%, and 45 of the SNPs had a success rate above 95%. The concordance rate was > 99% for all 48 SNPs, including the three SNPs with success rates between 93 and 95%, in 5500 samples which were

additionally re-genotyped using Human Omni Express Exome Bead Chip Kit (Illumina, San Diego, CA, USA).

Dietary data

Dietary data was collected once during the baseline period. An interview-based, modified diet history method was used that combined (i) a 7-day menu book for recording of intakes from meals that vary from day to day (usually lunch and dinner meals) and cold beverages, (ii) a 168-item diet questionnaire for assessment of consumption frequencies and portion sizes of regularly eaten foods not covered by the menu book and (iii) a 45-min interview. The MDC method has previously been described in detail [36].

Diet analyses were adjusted for the variable "diet method version", because slightly altered coding routines of dietary data were introduced in September 1994 to shorten the interview time (from 60 to 45 min). This resulted in two slightly different method versions without major influence on the ranking of individuals [36]. The relative validity of the original MDC method was evaluated in the Malmö Food study 1984–1985, comparing the method with 18-day weighed food records [37, 38]. The Pearson correlation coefficients, adjusted for total energy, were in women and men respectively for fibre 0. 69/0.74, bread 0.58/0.50, cereals 0.73/0.74, meat 0.92/0. 84, fruits 0.77/0.60, vegetables 0.53/0.65, milk 0.84/0.83, cheese 0.59/0.47 and fish 0.70/0.35 [37, 38].

Food intakes were converted to nutrient intakes using the MDC nutrient database where information comes from the Swedish National Food Agency. Portions (instead of grams) were used in order to analyse the sum of whole grain products and the sum of fermented dairy products, because water contents and portion sizes differ. Standard portion sizes from the MDC study or from the National Food Agency were used [39]: fibre-rich soft bread (50 g/portion), fibre-rich crispbread (30 g/portion) , breakfast cereals (25 g/portion), yoghurt (200 g/portion) and cheese (20 g/portion).

Food variables were natural logarithm transformed to normalize the distribution. To handle log transformation of zero intakes, we added 0.01. Energy-adjusted variables were obtained by regressing the variables on non-alcohol energy intake. Tertiles were used as exposure categories. As more than 33% were zero-consumers of SSB, these individuals constituted the lowest intake category and the higher categories were defined as below or above the median among the consumers.

DRS for T2D

A DRS for T2D was constructed by classifying the individuals according to low, medium and high intakes of foods previously shown to consistently associate with incident T2D in meta-analyses of prospective cohort studies, as described in the introduction, i.e. processed meat (sausage and cured meat), SBB (beverages sweetened with energy containing sweeteners; mainly sucrose) , whole grains (fibre-rich breads and cereals) and coffee (total; very few consumed decaffeinated coffee). High points were assigned for intakes expected to associate with increased T2D risk based on the earlier studies. Unweighted diet risk levels were used, as different diet assessment methods and intake levels in published studies complicate extrapolation to absolute risk estimates. Thus, for processed meat and SSB, no points were assigned to those with low intake, 1 to those with medium intake and 2 points to those with high intake. For whole grains and coffee, no points were assigned to those with high intake, 1 to those with medium intake and 2 points to those with low intake. Finally, the points were summed up to the risk score that was divided into three groups: low DRS (0–2 points), medium DRS (3–5 points) and high DRS (6–8 points).

Extended DRS for T2D for secondary analyses

Although the most consistent associations with T2D have been observed for the food components we included in our DRS, some studies have also indicated that intake of other foods may be associated with risk of T2D. A recent meta-analysis suggested high intake of fruit to be protective [20], but the latest meta-analysis indicated no additional risk decrease at intakes above two servings per day [26]. Likewise, a non-linear association was seen for vegetable intake [26], although high intakes of specific types of vegetables, especially green leafy vegetables may be beneficial [20, 21, 28, 40]. Moreover, total intake of fruits and vegetables does not seem to associate with the risk of T2D [20, 26, 28, 40]. Dairy products have been suggested to be protective [22], especially fermented dairy products [23] such as yoghurt and cheese [22, 24], but it is unclear whether specific dairy foods or dairy components explain observed associations [23, 29, 30]. Lastly, findings regarding fatty fish are non-conclusive [25, 27].

For secondary analyses, extended scores were created that additionally included intakes (in tertiles) of fruit and vegetables, fermented dairy or high-fat fish. Thus, each extended score is included in total five foods or beverages. The extended scores summed up to low (0–3 points), medium (4–6 points) and high (7–10 points) DRS. Finally, we constructed an extended risk score simultaneously including intakes of the original components and all three additional components: low (0–4 points), medium (5–9 points) and high (10–14 points) DRS.

Ascertainment of T2D incidence

We identified 3588 incident cases of T2D during 433,888 person-years of follow-up via at least one of seven registries

(90% of cases) or at examinations during follow-up (10% of cases). The mean follow-up time was 17 ± 5.6 years (range 0–24). The subjects contributed person-time from date of enrolment to date of diabetes diagnosis, death, migration from Sweden or end of follow-up (December 2014), whichever occurred first. During follow-up, 0.5% had migrated from Sweden. If available, we used information on date of diagnosis from two registries prioritized in the following order: (i) the regional Diabetes 2000 registry of Scania [41] and (ii) the Swedish National Diabetes Registry [42]. These registries required a physician diagnosis according to established diagnosis criteria (fasting plasma glucose concentration ≥ 7.0 mmol/L or fasting whole blood concentration ≥ 6.1 mmol/L, measured at two occasions). Individuals with at least two HbA1c values above 6.0% with the Swedish Mono-S standardization system (corresponding to 6.9% in the US National Glycohemoglobin Standardization Program and 52 mmol/mol with the International Federation of Clinical Chemistry and Laboratory Medicine (IFCC) units) [43, 44] were categorized as diabetes cases in the Malmö HbA1c Registry. In addition, cases were identified via registries from the National Board of Health and Welfare: the Swedish National Inpatient Registry, the Swedish Hospital-based outpatient care, the Cause-of-death Registry and the Swedish Prescribed Drug Registry.

Other variables

Leisure time physical activity was based on reported minutes per week spent on 17 activities and activity-specific intensity factors. Smoking was defined as current, former and never. Alcohol consumption was defined as zero consumption (based on 7-day record and lifestyle questionnaire) and low (< 15 g/day, < 20 g/day), medium (15–30 g/day, 20–40 g/day) or high (> 30 g/day, > 40 g/day) in men and women respectively during the 7-day record. Highest level of education was defined as ≤ 8 years, 9–10 years, 11–13 years or university degree. Dietary change in the past (yes/no) was based on the question "Have you substantially changed your eating habits because of illness or other reasons?"

Statistical analysis

The SPSS statistical computer package (version 20.0; IBM Corporation, Armonk, NY, USA) was used for statistical analyses.

We examined baseline characteristics across categories of the GRS and DRS, and in cases and non-cases of T2D, with the general linear model for continuous variables (adjusted for age and sex) and with chi^2 test for categorical variables. Pearson correlation coefficients between energy-adjusted intakes of the foods in the DRS were computed.

We used Cox proportional hazards regression model to estimate hazard ratios (HRs) of diabetes incidence

associated with tertiles of the GRS and three groups of the DRS for T2D, as well as for each dietary intake included in the DRS (adjusted for energy intake using the residual method). Years of follow-up were used as underlying time variable. In order to assess the proportional hazards assumption, we used graphs and tested interactions between the underlying time variable and examined covariates. The assumption was considered to be satisfied for all covariates except age. The presented results are therefore from age-stratified cox models (per 1-year age interval).

The basic model included adjustments for sex (when applicable). Our presented full multivariate model additionally included adjustments for BMI and total energy intake as continuous variables and for the following categorical variables: diet assessment method version, season of diet data collection, leisure time physical activity, smoking, alcohol intake and education. Missing data were treated as separate categories. Additional models included adjustment for intakes of fruit and vegetables, fermented dairy and high-fat fish, when applicable, but gave similar findings. We also performed analyses excluding BMI from the full multivariate model, as BMI may mediate associations between diet and T2D, but the results were virtually unchanged. Finally, we included waist or body fat percent instead of BMI in the multivariate model. Tests for interaction between the GRS and diet were performed, both by introducing multiplicative factors of the tertiles [GRS tertile × diet tertile (treated as continuous variables)]. Tertiles were used in order to overcome problems with outliers and to minimize power issues due to small groups when ranking the individual according to both diet and genetics. However, to test a more sensitive model, we also examined interaction between continuous variables.

In sensitivity analysis, we excluded individuals with dietary change in the past (22% of the individuals). In a second sensitivity analysis, we excluded individuals with prevalent cardiovascular disease (coronary event or stroke) at baseline (3%). All statistical tests were two-sided, and statistical significance was assumed at $P < 0.05$.

Results

Baseline characteristics

The baseline levels of established risk factors for T2D, as well as potential confounders of dietary associations, differed between incident cases and non-cases of T2D (Additional file 1: Table S2). Individuals who developed diabetes during follow-up were older and had higher fasting levels of glucose and insulin, higher BMI, a more sedentary lifestyle, higher protein intake and lower fibre intake. In addition, among incident cases of T2D, there were more males, ever-smokers as well as individuals reporting dietary change in the past and fewer individuals with high level of education. Fasting blood glucose increased across the GRS tertiles (Table 1), and several risk factors for T2D and potential confounders differed across the DRS tertiles. The dietary factors included in the DRS did not differ across tertiles of the GRS. Moreover, correlations between the four factors included in the DRS were very weak (Additional file 1: Table S3).

The GRS and T2D

The GRS, designed based on previous GWAS findings, associated as expected with increased incidence of T2D (P for trend = 7×10^{-35}), with a HR for individuals in the highest tertile of the GRS of 1.67 (95% CI 1.54, 1.81), compared with individuals in the lowest tertile. Similar observations were made in both genders (Table 2).

The DRS and T2D

The DRS based on high intakes of processed meat and SSB, and on low intakes of whole grain and coffee, associated with increased incidence of T2D (P for trend = 6×10^{-10}), with 40% risk increase in the highest tertile (95% CI 26–56%). No major gender differences were seen (Table 2).

Components of the DRS and T2D

All components of the DRS showed significant associations with incident T2D; we observed increased incidences at high intakes of processed meat (HR in the highest tertile 1.11; 95% CI 1.03, 1.21; P for trend = 0.009) and SSB (HR in the highest tertile 1.13; 95% CI 1.05, 1.22; P for trend = 0.003) and decreased incidences at high intakes of whole grain (HR in the highest tertile 0.89; 95% CI 0.82, 0.96; P for trend = 0.004) and coffee (HR in the highest tertile 0.75; 95% CI 0.69, 0.81; P for trend = 1×10^{-11}) (Table 2). Similar tendencies were seen independently of gender, although the inverse association with coffee intake was significantly stronger in women (P for interaction with sex = 6×10^{-5}).

Interaction between the GRS and the DRS

We did not observe any interaction between the GRS and the DRS on incidence of T2D (P = 0.83). The magnitude of the association between the GRS and T2D was similar at low, medium and high diet risk (Table 3), and likewise associations with the DRS did not differ depending on the genetic risk for T2D (Table 4). In joint effect model with low GRS and low DRS as reference, the highest risk estimate was seen for individuals with both high (3rd tertile) GRS and high DRS (HR 2.49; 95% CI 2.06, 3.01) (Fig. 1, Additional file 1: Table S4).

Interaction between the GRS and components in the DRS

We did not observe any significant interactions between the components in the DRS and the GRS on incident T2D (Additional file 1: Table S5). Regarding whole grain intake and the GRS in gender-specific analyses, we observed some non-significant tendencies of interactions, although in opposite directions; in women, the magnitude of the inverse association between whole grain intake and T2D tended to decrease with higher genetic risk (P for interaction = 0.07), whereas it tended to increase with higher genetic risk in men (P for interaction = 0.07).

Secondary analyses with extended DRS for T2D

Extended DRSs, that additionally included intakes (in tertiles) of fruit and vegetables, fermented dairy or high-fat fish showed similar associations with T2D as the original DRS (Additional file 1: Table S6), and intakes of the additional food components in the extended scores did not show significant associations with T2D in gender-combined analyses, favouring our approach of not including these foods in the initial diet score. However, in women, fermented dairy intake was inversely associated with T2D (P for trend = 0.002) (P for interaction with sex = 0.02).

Furthermore, we did not observe any interactions between the GRS and the extended DRSs (Additional file 1: Table S7) (all P values for interactions ≥ 0.16) or their added food components (Additional file 1: Table S8), in gender-combined analyses. In women, our results suggested some possible, although unclear, modification by the GRS for the role of fruit and vegetable intake in T2D incidence (P for interaction = 0.04), and we found a non-significant tendency of stronger inverse association between fermented dairy and T2D among women with lower GRS (P for interaction = 0.07).

Secondary analyses in a subsample with extended GRS for T2D

In the subsample of the MDC study (n = 4193), with genetic data on 68 T2D associated SNPs, no statistical interaction was observed between the extended GRS and the DRS (P = 0.34) (Additional file 2: Figure S1). Higher DRS associated with an increased risk of T2D in the low (P for trend across DRS tertiles = 0.001), medium (P for trend = 0.003) and high tertile (P for trend = 0.04) of the extended GRS. Individuals with both high genetic susceptibility and unfavourable dietary habits had more than twice as high risk (HR 3.82; 95% CI 2.18, 6.71) of developing T2D compared to those with low genetic susceptibility and favourable dietary habits (reference HR = 1.00).

Table 1 Means (and standard deviations) or percentage distribution for baseline characteristics across tertiles of a weighted genetic risk score for type 2 diabetes and across categories of a diet risk score in 15,380 women and 9689 men from the Malmö Diet and Cancer Study

Tertile of genetic risk score

	n	All 1	All 2	All 3	P trend*	Women 1	Women 2	Women 3	P trend*	Men 1	Men 2	Men 3	P trend*
n		5699	15,188	4182		3767	9205	2408		1932	5983	1774	
Age (years)	25,069	58.3 (7.8)	58.2 (7.6)	58.2 (7.7)	0.32	57.3 (8.0)	57.3 (7.9)	57.3 (8.0)	0.86	59.5 (7.2)	59.0 (7.1)	59.1 (7.1)	0.04
BMI	25,035	25.7 (4.0)	25.7 (3.9)	25.6 (3.8)	0.12	25.3 (4.2)	25.4 (4.2)	25.3 4.0)	0.48	26.2 (3.5)	26.2 (3.4)	26.0 (3.4)	0.046
Fasting blood glucose (mmol/L)	4860	4.90 (0.6)	5.00 (0.7)	5.05 (0.8)	<0.001	4.78 (0.5)	4.88 (0.6)	4.94 (0.7)	<0.001	5.06 (0.6)	5.17 (0.8)	5.21 (1.0)	0.001
Fasting plasma insulin (mIU/L)	4819	7.8 (8.9)	7.7 (8.1)	7.7 (6.1)	0.89	7.3 (8.3)	7.0 (5.0)	7.2 (4.8)	0.75	8.5 (9.5)	8.7 (11.3)	8.6 (7.4)	0.93
HOMA-IR[†]	4571	1.60 (1.43)	1.59 (1.12)	1.61 (1.13)	0.76[†]	1.49 (1.54)	1.47 (1.04)	1.49 (0.96)	0.66[†]	1.76 (1.23)	1.77 (1.21)	1.80 (1.32)	0.29[†]
Alcohol intake (g/day)[‡]	23,551	11.6 (12.8)	11.5 (12.9)	11.3 (12.3)	0.11	8.5 (8.9)	8.3 (8.6)	8.3 (8.7)	0.21	16.4 (16.0)	16.4 (16.4)	15.9 (15.3)	0.26
Processed meat (g/day)	25,069	38 (30)	38 (30)	38 (30)	0.61	31 (23)	31 (23)	31 (23)	0.57	51 (35)	49 (36)	50 (36)	0.68
Sugar-sweetened beverages (g/day)	25,069	76 (145)	78 (150)	77 (145)	0.64	67 (125)	65 (121)	66 (127)	0.83	91 (171)	99 (187)	95 (170)	0.42
Whole grain (portions/day)	25,069	1.0 (1.0)	1.0 (1.0)	1.0 (1.0)	0.93	0.9 (0.9)	0.9 (0.9)	0.9 (0.9)	0.65	1.0 (1.2)	1.1 (1.2)	1.1 (1.2)	0.58
Coffee (g/day)	25,069	520 (390)	530 (400)	510 (400)	0.77	510 (380)	520 (390)	510 (390)	0.87	530 (400)	540 (420)	530 (410)	0.77
					P value				P value				P value
Smoking (ever) (%)	25,059	62.4	61.7	61.1	0.22	56.7	55.6	54.9	0.17	71.3	71.3	71.4	0.99
Leisure time physical activity, high (%)[§]	24,913	18.9	20.6	20.2	0.02	19.4	20.1	20.2	0.58	18.2	21.4	20.3	0.01
Education (>10 years) (%)	25,008	32.0	32.7	31.5	0.25	31.1	30.5	30.3	0.68	33.3	36.3	33.3	0.02

Diet risk score

	n	All Low	All Mid	All High	P trend*	Women Low	Women Mid	Women High	P trend*	Men Low	Men Mid	Men High	P trend*
n		5699	15,188	4182		3767	9205	2408		1932	5983	1774	
Age (years)	25,069	57.6 (7.4)	58.4 (7.7)	58.7 (8.0)	<0.001	56.6 (7.5)	57.4 (8.0)	57.8 (8.4)	<0.001	58.6 (6.8)	59.3 (7.1)	59.6 (7.2)	<0.001
BMI	25,035	25.4 (3.8)	25.6 (3.9)	26.0 (4.0)	<0.001	25.0 (3.9)	25.3 (4.2)	25.7 (4.2)	<0.001	26.1 (3.4)	26.1 (3.4)	26.6 (3.5)	<0.001
Fasting blood glucose (mmol/L)	4860	4.94 (0.7)	4.98 (0.7)	5.07 (0.9)	<0.001	4.82 (0.5)	4.89 (0.6)	4.92 (0.7)	0.005	5.13 (0.9)	5.12 (0.7)	5.28 (1.0)	0.03
Fasting plasma insulin (mIU/L)	4819	7.4 (7.3)	7.7 (8.0)	8.7 (7.6)	0.001	7.0 (8.1)	7.1 (5.4)	7.7 (4.8)	0.12	7.8 (5.4)	8.6 (10.6)	10.0 (9.8)	0.002
HOMA-IR[†]	4571	1.52 (1.49)	1.58 (1.07)	1.81 (1.35)	<0.001	1.46 (1.68)	1.46 (0.91)	1.66 (1.14)	<0.001	1.61 (1.04)	1.77 (1.23)	2.03 (1.54)	<0.001
Alcohol intake (g/day)[‡]	23,551	11.5 (12.0)	11.4 (12.6)	11.7 (13.8)	0.53	8.6 (8.5)	8.4 (8.7)	7.8 (8.9)	0.007	15.9 (15.7)	16.0 (15.7)	17.4 (16.8)	0.009
Processed meat (g/day)	25,069	22 (21)	40 (30)	55 (31)	<0.001	18 (16)	32 (23)	46 (24)	<0.001	28 (26)	51 (36)	69 (36)	<0.001
Sugar-sweetened beverages (g/day)	25,069	18 (70)	70 (140)	170 (200)	<0.001	12 (52)	66 (124)	150 (156)	<0.001	25 (91)	84 (161)	209 (235)	<0.001
Whole grain (portions/day)	25,069	1.6 (1.2)	0.9 (0.9)	0.4 (0.5)	<0.001	1.5 (0.9)	0.8 (0.8)	0.4 (0.4)	<0.001	1.9 (1.4)	1.0 (1.1)	0.4 (0.5)	<0.001

Table 1 Means (and standard deviations) or percentage distribution for baseline characteristics across tertiles of a weighted genetic risk score for type 2 diabetes and across categories of a diet risk score in 15,380 women and 9689 men from the Malmö Diet and Cancer Study (*Continued*)

Coffee (g/day)	25,069	700 (410)	510 (390)	310 (260)	<0.001	680 (400)	490 (370)	310 (270)	<0.001	735 (430)	530 (410)	320 (260)	<0.001
					P value				*P* value				*P* value
Smoking (ever) (%)	25,059	65.2	61.3	58.5	<0.001	60.7	55.0	50.6	<0.001	74.1	71.1	69.3	<0.004
Leisure time Physical Activity, high (%)§	24,913	22.3	19.3	18.9	<0.001	22.9	19.1	18.1	<0.001	21.2	19.5	19.8	0.30
Education (> 10 years) (%)	25,008	37.7	31.6	26.3	<0.001	35.7	30.4	23.6	<0.001	41.8	33.3	29.9	<0.001

*Adjusted for age and sex when applicable
†*P* value for ln transformed variables
‡Among those reporting that they consumed alcohol during the year before baseline examinations
§Highest quintile of leisure time physical activity

Table 2 Hazard ratios of incident type 2 diabetes according to a genetic risk score, and according to a diet risk score and its components, in 15,380 women and 9689 men from the Malmö Diet and Cancer Study

	All				Women				Men			
	Tertile*				Tertile*				Tertile*			
	1	2	3	P value for trend†	1	2	3	P value for trend†	1	2	3	P value for trend†
Cases/person-years	929/147393	1188/144429	1471/142031		478/92494	602/91511	764/91595		451/54897	586/52917	707/50436	
Genetic risk score	1.00	1.31 1.21, 1.43	1.67 1.54, 1.81	7×10^{-35}	1.00	1.28 1.13, 1.44	1.62 1.44, 1.81	1×10^{-16}	1.00	1.36 1.20, 1.53	1.72 1.53, 1.94	9×10^{-20}
Cases/person-years	673/102570	2194/262381	721/68902		350/69708	1154/164327	340/41567		323/32862	1040/98054	381/27336	
Diet risk score	1.00	1.19 1.09, 1.30	1.40 1.26, 1.56	6×10^{-10}	1.00	1.33 1.18, 1.50	1.45 1.26, 1.71	3×10^{-7}	1.00	1.07 0.95, 1.22	1.33 1.14, 1.55	0.0002
Processed meat	1.00	1.01 0.93, 1.10	1.11 1.03, 1.21	0.009	1.00	1.06 0.95, 1.19	1.12 1.01, 1.27	0.03	1.00	0.98 0.87, 1.11	1.11 0.98, 1.25	0.08
SSB	1.00	1.01 0.93, 1.10	1.13 1.05, 1.22	0.003	1.00	1.06 0.94, 1.20	1.12 1.01, 1.25	0.03	1.00	0.95 0.84, 1.07	1.14 1.01, 1.28	0.06
Whole grain	1.00	0.94 0.86, 1.01	0.89 0.82, 0.96	0.004	1.00	0.95 0.85, 1.05	0.90 0.80, 1.02	0.09	1.00	0.92 0.82, 1.03	0.87 0.77, 0.98	0.02
Coffee	1.00	0.87 0.81, 0.95	0.75 0.69, 0.81	1×10^{-11}	1.00	0.78 0.70, 0.87	0.63 0.56, 0.71	2×10^{-14}	1.00	0.97 0.87, 1.10	0.88 0.78, 0.99	0.04

*For the DRS the levels refer to low risk score (0–2 points), medium risk score (3–5 points) and high risk score (6–8 points) instead of tertiles
†Age-stratified model, adjusted for sex when applicable. Examination of dietary variables was also adjusted for diet method version, season, total energy intake, BMI, leisure time physical activity, alcohol intake, smoking and education

Table 3 Hazard ratios of incident type 2 diabetes according to a weighted genetic risk score in strata of a diet risk score based on intakes of processed meat, sugar-sweetened beverages (SSB), whole grain and coffee in 15,380 women and 9689 men from the Malmö Diet and Cancer Study

Diet risk score level/diet tertile	All Tertile of genetic risk score			P value for trend*	Women Tertile of genetic risk score			P value for trend*	Men Tertile of genetic risk score			P value for trend*
	1	2	3		1	2	3		1	2	3	
Diet risk score												
Low	1.00	1.38 1.13, 1.68	1.71 1.41, 2.08	4×10^{-8}	1.00	1.50 1.13, 1.99	1.75 1.34, 2.30	6×10^{-5}	1.00	1.25 0.94, 1.68	1.69 1.28, 2.22	2×10^{-4}
Medium	1.00	1.30 1.16, 1.45	1.66 1.49, 1.84	2×10^{-21}	1.00	1.22 1.05, 1.43	1.62 1.40, 1.87	4×10^{-11}	1.00	1.40 1.19, 1.64	1.71 1.47, 2.00	8×10^{-12}
High	1.00	1.32 1.09, 1.60	1.69 1.41, 2.03	1×10^{-8}	1.00	1.26 0.96, 1.67	1.50 1.16, 1.96	0.002	1.00	1.39 1.07, 1.83	1.85 1.44, 2.38	2×10^{-6}
$P_{interaction}$[†,‡]				0.83 (0.94)				0.40 (0.67)				0.60 (0.73)

*Age-stratified model, adjusted for sex when applicable
[†]Age-stratified model, adjusted for sex, diet method version, season, total energy intake, BMI, leisure time physical activity, alcohol intake, smoking and education
[‡]P for interaction treating tertiles as continuous variables and, in brackets, P for interaction between continuous variables of the GRS and the DRS

Statistical models with waist circumference and body fat percent

Replacing BMI with waist or body fat percent in our multivariate models did not substantially change our observations. However, no tendencies of interactions between whole-grain intake and the GRS remained in the gender-specific analyses, when waist or body fat percent replaced BMI.

Sensitivity analysis

After excluding individuals reporting dietary change in the past, our results remained virtually unchanged, indicating that unfavourable diet and genetic predisposition independently contribute to an increased risk of T2D. Excluding individuals with prevalent cardiovascular disease did not either change our findings (data not shown).

Discussion

A risk score, of food intakes consistently associated with risk of T2D (processed meat, SSB, whole grain and coffee), was in our population-based prospective study associated with increased incidence of T2D. The positive association was of similar magnitude independent of genetic predisposition to T2D, assessed using a GRS composed of 48 SNPs identified in GWAS for T2D (Fig. 2). Likewise, each food component of the DRS associated with incidence of T2D, independently of the GRS. The highest risk of T2D was seen in individuals with both high genetic and dietary risk scores. Adding foods less consistently associated with T2D, in scientific literature, to create an extended DRS did not importantly alter the findings regarding the original DRS, and lack of overall association between these foods and T2D in our study supports the initial approach of not including them in the DRS.

Table 4 Hazard ratios of incident type 2 diabetes according to a diet risk score based on intakes of processed meat, sugar-sweetened beverages (SSB), whole grain and coffee in strata of a weighted genetic risk score among 15,380 women and 9689 men from the Malmö Diet and Cancer Study

Diet risk score level/diet tertile	All Tertile of genetic risk score			Women Tertile of genetic risk score			Men Tertile of genetic risk score		
	1	2	3	1	2	3	1	2	3
Diet risk score									
Low	1.00	1.00	1.00	1.00	1.00	1.00	1.00	1.00	1.00
Medium	1.23 1.03, 1.46	1.17 1.01, 1.36	1.20 1.04, 1.37	1.48 1.16, 1.90	1.23 1.00, 1.51	1.32 1.09, 1.59	1.02 0.80, 1.31	1.12 0.89, 1.39	1.11 0.91, 1.36
High	1.42 1.15, 1.76	1.42 1.18, 1.71	1.40 1.18, 1.65	1.68 1.24, 2.27	1.45 1.11, 1.89	1.38 1.09, 1.76	1.21 0.90, 1.63	1.40 1.07, 1.83	1.40 1.10, 1.78
P_{trend}*	0.001	3×10^{-4}	8×10^{-5}	0.001	0.006	0.005	0.20	0.01	0.005
$P_{interaction}$*,[†]			0.83 (0.94)			0.40 (0.67)			0.60 (0.73)

*Age-stratified model, adjusted for sex, diet method version, season, total energy intake, BMI, leisure time physical activity, alcohol intake, smoking and education
[†]P for interaction treating tertiles as continuous variables and, in brackets, P for interaction between continuous variables of the GRS and the DRS

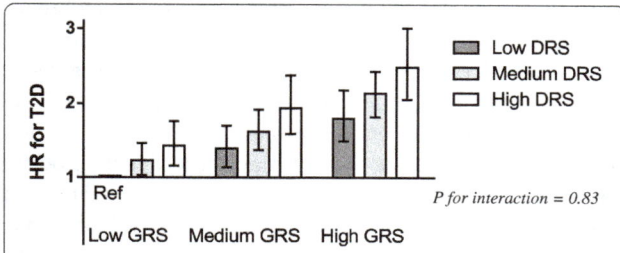

Figure 1 Hazard ratios of incident type 2 diabetes according to combinations of a genetic risk score and a dietary risk score for type 2 diabetes among individuals in the Malmö Diet and Cancer Study ($n = 25,069$). No statistical interaction was observed between the genetic and dietary risk scores ($P = 0.83$). Individuals with both high genetic susceptibility and unfavourable dietary habits had more than twice as high risk (HR 2.49; 95% CI 2.06, 3.01) of developing T2D compared to those with low genetic susceptibility and favourable dietary habits (reference HR = 1.00).

men, a higher score of a GRS, based on 10 T2D-associated SNPs, was found to accentuate the increased risk of T2D associated with a Western dietary pattern, characterized by meat, refined cereals, sweets and desserts [46]. Moreover, genetic variations in the *FTO* and *MC4R* genes have been reported to interact with a Mediterranean diet score on T2D [47], and a genetic variation in *ADRA2B* has been reported to interact with diet quality, based on fat and fibre intakes, on T2D [48]. Few results regarding interactions between GRSs and specific dietary components on T2D or related traits have been reported; no interaction was detected between a GRS of 15 SNPs and carbohydrates or fibre in the National Health and Nutrition Examination Survey [49], and meat intake was found to associate with fasting concentrations of glucose and insulin independently of a GRS in a meta-analysis of 14 cohorts [50]. Most indications of interactions between dietary factors and genetic variants have come off from investigations of single T2D SNPs and specific dietary factors [2, 3]. Regarding the components included in the DRS of our study and earlier reported interactions with T2D associated SNPs, fibre or whole-grain intakes have been found to interact with genetic variation in *TCF7L2*, by us and others, as well as with variation in *NOTCH2* and *ZBED3* [2, 51, 52]. In addition, interaction between coffee consumption and genetic variation in *CDCAL1* and *IGF2BP2* has been reported [53].

To the best of our knowledge, no study has previously examined if a GRS for T2D modifies associations between a T2D-specific dietary risk pattern and incidence of T2D. Similar to our findings, no interaction was observed between a GRS for T2D and dietary habits assessed by a Mediterranean diet score [31]. In line with this, an overall healthy diet score associated with lower fasting glucose and fasting insulin independently of genotypes previously associated with glucose homeostasis [45]. However, in US

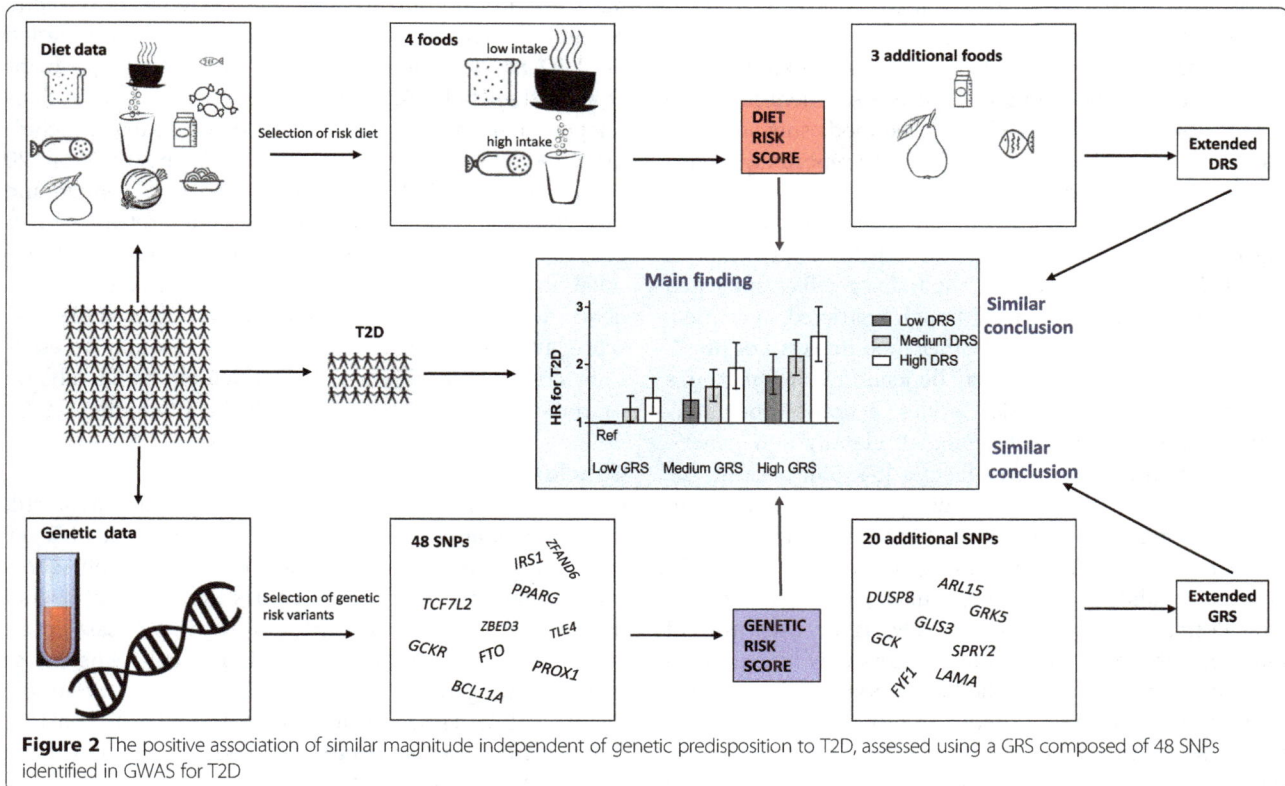

Figure 2 The positive association of similar magnitude independent of genetic predisposition to T2D, assessed using a GRS composed of 48 SNPs identified in GWAS for T2D

The 6% of the individuals in our study, categorized as having both high genetic susceptibility and unfavourable dietary habits, were found to have twice until up to three times as high risk compared to those with low genetic susceptibility and favourable dietary habits. Our findings also show that dietary habits previously associated with T2D are of importance in the prevention of the disease independently of an individual's genetic susceptibility, as the magnitude of our observed relative risk decrease by favourable diet was similar in individuals with high and low GRS. Still, it is important to consider that a 30% risk decrease, as observed at a low compared with a high DRS in our study, would be more important for individuals with higher genetic susceptibility to T2D, as the absolute risk decrease would be greater (i.e. a decrease from about 10 to 7 incident cases per 1000 person-years in the highest GRS tertile, compared with a decrease from 6 to 4 cases in the lowest GRS tertile), meaning that healthy dietary habits should be especially crucial for individuals genetically predisposed to the disease.

Regarding the observed tendencies of interactions between the GRS and whole grain in the gender-specific analyses, we are prone to believe that the inconsistent associations between whole grain and T2D in strata of the GRS may have occurred due to chance, or loss of power when stratifying on both gender and GRS, especially since we observed tendencies of interactions in opposite directions in women and men and since those tendencies disappeared when waist or body fat percent replaced BMI in the statistical models.

We examined interaction between a DRS of known dietary T2D risk factors and a GRS of GWAS-identified T2D SNPs. However, it is possible that the foods showing consistent overall associations with T2D are repeatedly identified as risk factors due to low degree of interaction with other factors, such as genetics. Indeed, our results regarding foods previously showing less consistent associations with T2D, such as intakes of fruit and vegetables, indicated some putative interactions, although restricted to women. It remains to be examined if other food intakes not previously associated with T2D may be identified in subgroups depending on genetic risk. Besides, genome-wide interaction studies could be designed to identify new genetic loci interacting with dietary factors [54, 55], because the genetic variants that are most likely to interact with lifestyle factors may not be identified in conventional GWAS, as such variants may only associate with T2D in subgroups of individuals that are similar with regard to certain lifestyle factors [56, 57]. Finally, as we eat a mix of foods or nutrients and as dietary factors may interact with each other, it is from a public health point of view crucial to examine if overall genetic predisposition to disease modifies the importance of overall dietary patterns. Nevertheless, as different food components and variations in different genetic loci are critical in disease development via various mechanisms, genetic variants and dietary factors involved in the same biological pathways are more likely to interact. Consequently, the fact that most T2D SNPs associate with beta cell dysfunction and thus insulin secretion, while dietary factors may more likely associate with insulin resistance, could partly explain the lack of interaction between the GRS and the DRS. Whether our DRS for T2D and its included components interact with specific T2D loci was out of the scope of the present study. Despite lack of interaction between diet and accumulated genetic risk for T2D, dietary factors may still be more or less important depending on whether we carry single genetic risk variants that interact with those dietary factors, and therefore, our results do not contradict previous studies indicating that interactions between specific loci and individual dietary components exist. However, well-powered studies with good-quality dietary data are needed to replicate findings of both kinds [58].

Our study has several strengths that can be emphasized. Firstly, it is a large study with long follow-up time. Second, due to the population-based prospective design, selection bias and reverse causation should be minor issues. Third, we have extensive information on potential confounders. Fourth, diet data were of high quality [37, 38] and the foods included in the DRS clearly associated with T2D in expected directions. Moreover, we had the possibility to exclude individuals with reported dietary changes in the past. Still, it is a limitation that diet was only measured at baseline. Moreover, we did not have genotype information on T2D SNPs identified after the publication by Morris et al. in the whole study sample. However, our main finding persisted similar in the analysis of a subsample including 17% of the individuals with genotype data on 20 additional T2D SNPs. Our focus on overall genetic and diet risks may also be a limitation, and future studies could aim at constructing scores based on functional annotations. Further, due to lack of sufficient scientific evidence, we were not able to construct a weighted diet risk score, although some of the dietary factors may be especially crucial with regard to T2D development. Finally, we cannot exclude occurrence of residual confounding.

Conclusions

Our findings show that both the dietary and genetic risk factors examined in this study add to the risk of T2D; the highest risk was seen in individuals with high scores for both factors. The study supports the view that overall dietary and genetic risk contribute to the disease in an independent fashion and that all individuals, whether at high or low genetic risk, may benefit from favourable dietary habits. However, it may be essential to consider that a similar relative decrease in risk is of greater value to individuals already at high genetic risk.

Additional files

Additional file 1: Table S1. Single nucleotide polymorphisms included in the GRS as they were reported to associate with type 2 diabetes by Morris et al. **Table S2.** Baseline characteristics in 25,069 cases and non-cases of incident type 2 diabetes from Malmö diet and cancer. **Table S3.** Correlation coefficients[a] between energy-adjusted intakes of components in a diet risk score for type 2 diabetes in 25,069 individuals from Malmö diet and cancer. **Table S4.** Hazard ratios of incident type 2 diabetes according to combinations of a weighted genetic risk score and a diet risk score based on intakes of processed meat, sugar-sweetened beverages (SSB), whole grain and coffee in 15,380 women and 9689 men from Malmö diet and cancer. **Table S5.** HR of incident type 2 diabetes according to combinations of a weighted genetic risk score and components of a diet risk score in 15,380 women and 9689 men from Malmö diet and cancer. **Table S6.** HR[a] of incident type 2 diabetes according to extended dietary risk scores (DRS) for type 2 diabetes and the added dietary components in 15,380 women and 9689 men from Malmö diet and cancer. **Table S7.** HR of incident type 2 diabetes according to tertiles of a genetic risk score and alternative dietary risk scores (DRS) including additional diet components in 15,380 women and 9689 men from Malmö diet and cancer. **Table S8.** HR of incident type 2 diabetes (T2D) according to tertiles of a genetic risk score and intakes of the additional components in the alternative dietary risk scores in 15,380 women and 9689 men from Malmö diet and cancer. **Table S9.** Additional single nucleotide polymorphisms included in the extended GRS and reported to associate with type 2 diabetes by Fuchsberger et al. 2016

Additional file 2: Figure S1. In a subsample ($n = 4193$), with genetic data on 68 T2D SNPs (20 additional SNPs), the findings were similar to those in the whole study sample. No statistical interaction was observed between the extended genetic risk score and the dietary risk scores ($P = 0.34$). Individuals with both high genetic susceptibility and unfavourable dietary habits had more than twice as high risk (HR: 3.82; 95% CI: 2.18, 6.71) of developing T2D compared to those with low genetic susceptibility and favourable dietary habits (reference HR = 1.00).

Abbreviations
DRS: Diet risk score; GRS: Genetic risk score; MDC: Malmö Diet and Cancer; T2D: Type 2 diabetes

Acknowledgements
We thank the staff and participants of the Malmö Diet and Cancer Study. We are also grateful to Malin Svensson at the Department of Clinical Sciences in Malmö for excellent technical assistance.
Of the 28,098 participants in the MDC cohort, 1758 incident diabetes cases and 1758 controls are included in the EPIC InterAct Consortium for the study of genetic factors and gene-lifestyle interactions on incident type 2 diabetes. Being a large cohort study, the MDC represents a different study design, compared to the case-control study design of EPIC InterAct. The dietary data used within EPIC InterAct is harmonized between several study centres, and many details found in the MDC dietary data, used in the current study, are lacking in these harmonized data. That is, different study design, different study size, extensive information on confounding variables, the possibility to exclude individuals with reported dietary change, and uniform dietary data of high relative validity ensure the uniqueness of the present study vs. the pooled analyses that may be performed within the EPIC InterAct.

Funding
This study received funding from the European Research Council ERC-CoG-2014-649021 (for Orho-Melander), the Swedish Research Council, The Swedish Heart and Lung Foundation, the Region Skåne, the Novo Nordic Foundation and the Albert Påhlsson Research Foundation.

Authors' contributions
UE and MOM formulated the research questions and designed the research; UE performed statistical analysis and wrote the paper; UE, GH, ID, CAS, LB, SH, PA and MOM contributed to the interpretation of results and revision of the manuscript; PA gave statistical advice. All authors read and approved the final version.

Competing interests
The authors declare that they have no competing interests.

References
1. Franks PW. The complex interplay of genetic and lifestyle risk factors in type 2 diabetes: an overview. Scientifica. 2012;2012:482186. https://doi.org/10.6064/2012/482186. PubMed PMID: 24278702; PubMed Central PMCID: PMC3820646.
2. Hindy G, Sonestedt E, Ericson U, Jing XJ, Zhou Y, Hansson O, et al. Role of TCF7L2 risk variant and dietary fibre intake on incident type 2 diabetes. Diabetologia. 2012; https://doi.org/10.1007/s00125-012-2634-x. Epub 2012/07/12. PubMed PMID: 22782288.
3. Lamri A, Abi Khalil C, Jaziri R, Velho G, Lantieri O, Vol S, et al. Dietary fat intake and polymorphisms at the PPARG locus modulate BMI and type 2 diabetes risk in the D.E.S.I.R. prospective study. Int J Obes. 2011; https://doi.org/10.1038/ijo.2011.91. Epub 2011/05/05. PubMed PMID: 21540831.
4. McCarthy MI. Genomics, type 2 diabetes, and obesity. N Engl J Med. 2010; 363(24):2339–50. https://doi.org/10.1056/NEJMra0906948. PubMed PMID: 21142536.
5. Morris AP, Voight BF, Teslovich TM, Ferreira T, Segre AV, Steinthorsdottir V, et al. Large-scale association analysis provides insights into the genetic architecture and pathophysiology of type 2 diabetes. Nat Genet. 2012;44(9): 981–90. https://doi.org/10.1038/ng.2383. PubMed PMID: 22885922; PubMed Central PMCID: PMCPMC3442244.
6. Aune D, Ursin G, Veierod MB. Meat consumption and the risk of type 2 diabetes: a systematic review and meta-analysis of cohort studies. Diabetologia. 2009;52(11):2277–87. https://doi.org/10.1007/s00125-009-1481-x. Epub 2009/08/08. PubMed PMID: 19662376.
7. Micha R, Wallace SK, Mozaffarian D. Red and processed meat consumption and risk of incident coronary heart disease, stroke, and diabetes mellitus: a systematic review and meta-analysis. Circulation. 2010;121(21):2271–83. https://doi.org/10.1161/CIRCULATIONAHA.109.924977. Epub 2010/05/19. PubMed PMID: 20479151; PubMed Central PMCID: PMC2885952
8. Pan A, Sun Q, Bernstein AM, Schulze MB, Manson JE, Willett WC, et al. Red meat consumption and risk of type 2 diabetes: 3 cohorts of US adults and an updated meta-analysis. Am J Clin Nutr. 2011; https://doi.org/10.3945/ajcn.111.018978. Epub 2011/08/13. PubMed PMID: 21831992.
9. Greenwood DC, Threapleton DE, Evans CE, Cleghorn CL, Nykjaer C, Woodhead C, et al. Association between sugar-sweetened and artificially sweetened soft drinks and type 2 diabetes: systematic review and dose-response meta-analysis of prospective studies. Br J Nutr. 2014;112(5):725–34. https://doi.org/10.1017/S0007114514001329. PubMed PMID: 24932880.
10. Imamura F, O'Connor L, Ye Z, Mursu J, Hayashino Y, Bhupathiraju SN, et al. Consumption of sugar sweetened beverages, artificially sweetened beverages, and fruit juice and incidence of type 2 diabetes: systematic review, meta-analysis, and estimation of population attributable fraction. BMJ. 2015;351:h3576. https://doi.org/10.1136/bmj.h3576. PubMed PMID: 26199070; PubMed Central PMCID: PMCPMC4510779.
11. Wang M, Yu M, Fang L, Hu RY. Association between sugar-sweetened beverages and type 2 diabetes: a meta-analysis. J Diabetes Investig. 2015; 6(3):360–6. https://doi.org/10.1111/jdi.12309. PubMed PMID: 25969723; PubMed Central PMCID: PMCPMC4420570.
12. Aune D, Norat T, Romundstad P, Vatten LJ. Whole grain and refined grain consumption and the risk of type 2 diabetes: a systematic review and dose-response meta-analysis of cohort studies. Eur J Epidemiol. 2013;28(11):845–58. https://doi.org/10.1007/s10654-013-9852-5. PubMed PMID: 24158434.
13. Chanson-Rolle A, Meynier A, Aubin F, Lappi J, Poutanen K, Vinoy S, et al. Systematic review and meta-analysis of human studies to support a quantitative recommendation for whole grain intake in relation to type 2 diabetes. PLoS One. 2015;10(6):e0131377. https://doi.org/10.1371/journal.pone.0131377. PubMed PMID: 26098118; PubMed Central PMCID: PMCPMC4476805.

14. Ding M, Bhupathiraju SN, Chen M, van Dam RM, Hu FB. Caffeinated and decaffeinated coffee consumption and risk of type 2 diabetes: a systematic review and a dose-response meta-analysis. Diabetes Care. 2014;37(2):569–86. https://doi.org/10.2337/dc13-1203. PubMed PMID: 24459154; PubMed Central PMCID: PMCPMC3898757.

15. Jiang X, Zhang D, Jiang W. Coffee and caffeine intake and incidence of type 2 diabetes mellitus: a meta-analysis of prospective studies. Eur J Nutr. 2014;53(1):25–38. https://doi.org/10.1007/s00394-013-0603-x. PubMed PMID: 24150256.

16. Kim Y, Keogh J, Clifton P. A review of potential metabolic etiologies of the observed association between red meat consumption and development of type 2 diabetes mellitus. Metab Clin Exp. 2015;64(7):768–79. https://doi.org/10.1016/j.metabol.2015.03.008. PubMed PMID: 25838035.

17. Atkinson FS, Foster-Powell K, Brand-Miller JC. International tables of glycemic index and glycemic load values: 2008. Diabetes Care. 2008;31(12):2281–3. https://doi.org/10.2337/dc08-1239. Epub 2008/10/07. PubMed PMID: 18835944; PubMed Central PMCID: PMC2584181.

18. Ye EQ, Chacko SA, Chou EL, Kugizaki M, Liu S. Greater whole-grain intake is associated with lower risk of type 2 diabetes, cardiovascular disease, and weight gain. J Nutr. 2012;142(7):1304–13. https://doi.org/10.3945/jn.111.155325. PubMed PMID: 22649266.

19. Santos RM, Lima DR. Coffee consumption, obesity and type 2 diabetes: a mini-review. Eur J Nutr. 2016;55(4):1345–58. https://doi.org/10.1007/s00394-016-1206-0. PubMed PMID: 27026242.

20. Li M, Fan Y, Zhang X, Hou W, Tang Z. Fruit and vegetable intake and risk of type 2 diabetes mellitus: meta-analysis of prospective cohort studies. BMJ Open. 2014;4(11):e005497. https://doi.org/10.1136/bmjopen-2014-005497. PubMed PMID: 25377009; PubMed Central PMCID: PMCPMC4225228.

21. Cooper AJ, Forouhi NG, Ye Z, Buijsse E, Arriola L, Balkau B, et al. Fruit and vegetable intake and type 2 diabetes: EPIC-InterAct prospective study and meta-analysis. Eur J Clin Nutr. 2012;66(10):1082–92. https://doi.org/10.1038/ejcn.2012.85. PubMed PMID: 22854878; PubMed Central PMCID: PMC3652306.

22. Aune D, Norat T, Romundstad P, Vatten LJ. Dairy products and the risk of type 2 diabetes: a systematic review and dose-response meta-analysis of cohort studies. Am J Clin Nutr. 2013;98(4):1066–83. https://doi.org/10.3945/ajcn.113.059030. PubMed PMID: 23945722.

23. Sluijs I, Forouhi NG, Beulens JW, van der Schouw YT, Agnoli C, Arriola L, et al. The amount and type of dairy product intake and incident type 2 diabetes: results from the EPIC-InterAct Study. Am J Clin Nutr. 2012;96(2):382–90. https://doi.org/10.3945/ajcn.111.021907. PubMed PMID: 22760573.

24. Ericson U, Hellstrand S, Brunkwall L, Schulz CA, Sonestedt E, Wallstrom P, et al. Food sources of fat may clarify the inconsistent role of dietary fat intake for incidence of type 2 diabetes. Am J Clin Nutr. 2015;101(5):1065–80. https://doi.org/10.3945/ajcn.114.103010. PubMed PMID: 25832335.

25. Patel PS, Forouhi NG, Kuijsten A, Schulze MB, van Woudenbergh GJ, Ardanaz E, et al. The prospective association between total and type of fish intake and type 2 diabetes in 8 European countries: EPIC-InterAct study. Am J Clin Nutr. 2012;95(6):1445–53. https://doi.org/10.3945/ajcn.111.029314. PubMed PMID: 22572642; PubMed Central PMCID: PMC3623039.

26. Wu Y, Zhang D, Jiang X, Jiang W. Fruit and vegetable consumption and risk of type 2 diabetes mellitus: a dose-response meta-analysis of prospective cohort studies. Nutr Metab Cardiovasc Dis. 2015;25(2):140–7. https://doi.org/10.1016/j.numecd.2014.10.004. PubMed PMID: 25456152.

27. Djousse L, Gaziano JM, Buring JE, Lee IM. Dietary omega-3 fatty acids and fish consumption and risk of type 2 diabetes. Am J Clin Nutr. 2011;93(1):143–50. https://doi.org/10.3945/ajcn.110.005603. Epub 2010/10/29. PubMed PMID: 20980491; PubMed Central PMCID: PMC3001602.

28. Carter P, Gray LJ, Troughton J, Khunti K, Davies MJ. Fruit and vegetable intake and incidence of type 2 diabetes mellitus: systematic review and meta-analysis. BMJ. 2010;341:c4229. Epub 2010/08/21. PubMed PMID: 20724400; PubMed Central PMCID: PMC2924474.

29. Warensjo E, Nolan D, Tapsell L. Dairy food consumption and obesity-related chronic disease. Adv Food Nutr Res. 2010;59:1–41. https://doi.org/10.1016/S1043-4526(10)59001-6. PubMed PMID: 20610172.

30. Forouhi NG, Koulman A, Sharp SJ, Imamura F, Kroger J, Schulze MB, et al. Differences in the prospective association between individual plasma phospholipid saturated fatty acids and incident type 2 diabetes: the EPIC-InterAct case-cohort study. Lancet Diabetes Endocrino. 2014;2(10):810–8. https://doi.org/10.1016/S2213-8587(14)70146-9. PubMed PMID: 25107467; PubMed Central PMCID: PMC4196248.

31. Langenberg C, Sharp SJ, Franks PW, Scott RA, Deloukas P, Forouhi NG, et al. Gene-lifestyle interaction and type 2 diabetes: the EPIC interact case-cohort study. PLoS Med. 2014;11(5):e1001647. https://doi.org/10.1371/journal.pmed.1001647. PubMed PMID: 24845081; PubMed Central PMCID: PMCPMC4028183.

32. Mandalazi E, Drake I, Wirfalt E, Orho-Melander M, Sonestedt E. A high diet quality based on dietary recommendations is not associated with lower incidence of type 2 diabetes in the Malmo Diet and Cancer cohort. Int J Mol Sci. 2016;17(6) https://doi.org/10.3390/ijms17060901. PubMed PMID: 27338354; PubMed Central PMCID: PMCPMC4926435.

33. Manjer J, Carlsson S, Elmstahl S, Gullberg B, Janzon L, Lindstrom M, et al. The Malmo Diet and Cancer Study: representativity, cancer incidence and mortality in participants and non-participants. Eur J Cancer Prev. 2001;10(6):489–99. PubMed PMID: 11916347.

34. Kong A, Steinthorsdottir V, Masson G, Thorleifsson G, Sulem P, Besenbacher S, et al. Parental origin of sequence variants associated with complex diseases. Nature. 2009;462(7275):868–74. https://doi.org/10.1038/nature08625. PubMed PMID: 20016592; PubMed Central PMCID: PMCPMC3746295.

35. Fuchsberger C, Flannick J, Teslovich TM, Mahajan A, Agarwala V, Gaulton KJ, et al. The genetic architecture of type 2 diabetes. Nature. 2016;536(7614):41–7. https://doi.org/10.1038/nature18642. PubMed PMID: 27398621; PubMed Central PMCID: PMCPMC5034897.

36. Wirfalt E, Mattisson I, Johansson U, Gullberg B, Wallstrom P, Berglund G. A methodological report from the Malmo Diet and Cancer study: development and evaluation of altered routines in dietary data processing. Nutr J. 2002;1:3. Epub 2003/01/23. PubMed PMID: 12537595; PubMed Central PMCID: PMC149436.

37. Elmstahl S, Riboli E, Lindgarde F, Gullberg B, Saracci R. The Malmo Food Study: the relative validity of a modified diet history method and an extensive food frequency questionnaire for measuring food intake. Eur J Clin Nutr. 1996;50(3):143–51. Epub 1996/03/01. PubMed PMID: 8654327.

38. Riboli E, Elmstahl S, Saracci R, Gullberg B, Lindgarde F. The Malmo Food Study: validity of two dietary assessment methods for measuring nutrient intake. Int J Epidemiol. 1997;26(Suppl 1):S161–73. Epub 1997/01/01. PubMed PMID: 9126544.

39. The Swedish National Food Administration SLV. Vikttabeller. 1989:1–49.

40. Ardisson Korat AV, Willett WC, Hu FB. Diet, lifestyle, and genetic risk factors for type 2 diabetes: a review from the Nurses' Health Study, Nurses' Health Study 2, and Health Professionals' Follow-up Study. Curr Nutr Rep. 2014;3(4):345–54. https://doi.org/10.1007/s13668-014-0103-5. PubMed PMID: 25599007; PubMed Central PMCID: PMCPMC4295827.

41. Lindholm E, Agardh E, Tuomi T, Groop L, Agardh CD. Classifying diabetes according to the new WHO clinical stages. Eur J Epidemiol. 2001;17(11):983–9. Epub 2002/10/17. PubMed PMID: 12380709.

42. Cederholm J, Eeg-Olofsson K, Eliasson B, Zethelius B, Nilsson PM, Gudbjornsdottir S. Risk prediction of cardiovascular disease in type 2 diabetes: a risk equation from the Swedish National Diabetes Register. Diabetes Care. 2008;31(10):2038–43. https://doi.org/10.2337/dc08-0662. Epub 2008/07/02. PubMed PMID: 18591403; PubMed Central PMCID: PMC2551651.

43. Hanas R, John G. 2010 consensus statement on the worldwide standardization of the hemoglobin A1C measurement. Diabetes Care. 2010;33(8):1903–4. https://doi.org/10.2337/dc10-0953. Epub 2010/06/04. PubMed PMID: 20519665; PubMed Central PMCID: PMC2909083.

44. Hoelzel W, Weykamp C, Jeppsson JO, Miedema K, Barr JR, Goodall I, et al. IFCC reference system for measurement of hemoglobin A1c in human blood and the national standardization schemes in the United States, Japan, and Sweden: a method-comparison study. Clin Chem. 2004;50(1):166–74. https://doi.org/10.1373/clinchem.2003.024802. Epub 2004/01/08. PubMed PMID: 14709644.

45. Nettleton JA, Hivert MF, Lemaitre RN, McKeown NM, Mozaffarian D, Tanaka T, et al. Meta-analysis investigating associations between healthy diet and fasting glucose and insulin levels and modification by loci associated with glucose homeostasis in data from 15 cohorts. Am J Epidemiol. 2013;177(2):103–15. https://doi.org/10.1093/aje/kws297. Epub 2012/12/21. PubMed PMID: 23255780.

46. Qi L, Cornelis MC, Zhang C, van Dam RM, Hu FB. Genetic predisposition, Western dietary pattern, and the risk of type 2 diabetes in men. Am J Clin Nutr. 2009;89(5):1453–8. https://doi.org/10.3945/ajcn.2008.27249. PubMed PMID: 19279076; PubMed Central PMCID: PMCPMC2676999.

47. Ortega-Azorin C, Sorli JV, Asensio EM, Coltell O, Martinez-Gonzalez MA, Salas-Salvado J, et al. Associations of the FTO rs9939609 and the MC4R rs17782313 polymorphisms with type 2 diabetes are modulated by diet, being higher when adherence to the Mediterranean diet pattern is low. Cardiovasc Diabetol. 2012;11:137. https://doi.org/10.1186/1475-2840-11-137. PubMed PMID: 23130628; PubMed Central PMCID: PMCPMC3495759.

48. Laaksonen DE, Siitonen N, Lindstrom J, Eriksson JG, Reunanen P, Tuomilehto J, et al. Physical activity, diet, and incident diabetes in relation to an ADRA2B polymorphism. Med Sci Sports Exerc. 2007;39(2):227–32. https://doi.org/10.1249/01.mss.0000246998.02095.bf. PubMed PMID: 17277585.

49. Villegas R, Goodloe RJ, BE MC Jr, Boston J, Crawford DC. Gene-carbohydrate and gene-fiber interactions and type 2 diabetes in diverse populations from the National Health and Nutrition Examination Surveys (NHANES) as part of the Epidemiologic Architecture for Genes Linked to Environment (EAGLE) study. BMC Genet. 2014;15:69. https://doi.org/10.1186/1471-2156-15-69. PubMed PMID: 24929251; PubMed Central PMCID: PMCPMC4094781.

50. Fretts AM, Follis JL, Nettleton JA, Lemaitre RN, Ngwa JS, Wojczynski MK, et al. Consumption of meat is associated with higher fasting glucose and insulin concentrations regardless of glucose and insulin genetic risk scores: a meta-analysis of 50,345 Caucasians. Am J Clin Nutr. 2015;102(5):1266–78. https://doi.org/10.3945/ajcn.114.101238. PubMed PMID: 26354543; PubMed Central PMCID: PMCPMC4625584.

51. Fisher E, Boeing H, Fritsche A, Doering F, Joost HG, Schulze MB. Whole-grain consumption and transcription factor-7-like 2 (TCF7L2) rs7903146: gene-diet interaction in modulating type 2 diabetes risk. Br J Nutr. 2009;101(4):478–81. https://doi.org/10.1017/S0007114508020369. PubMed PMID: 19149908.

52. Hindy G, Mollet IG, Rukh G, Ericson U, Orho-Melander M. Several type 2 diabetes-associated variants in genes annotated to WNT signaling interact with dietary fiber in relation to incidence of type 2 diabetes. Genes Nutr. 2016; https://doi.org/10.1186/s12263-016-0524-4. Epub 2016/11/6.

53. Lee JK, Kim K, Ahn Y, Yang M, Lee JE. Habitual coffee intake, genetic polymorphisms, and type 2 diabetes. Eur J Endocrinol. 2015;172(5):595–601. https://doi.org/10.1530/EJE-14-0805. PubMed PMID: 25755232.

54. Patel CJ. Analytical complexity in detection of gene variant-by-environment exposure interactions in high-throughput genomic and exposomic research. Curr Environ Health Rep. 2016;3(1):64–72. https://doi.org/10.1007/s40572-016-0080-5. PubMed PMID: 26809563; PubMed Central PMCID: PMCPMC4789192.

55. Winkler TW, Justice AE, Graff M, Barata L, Feitosa MF, Chu S, et al. The influence of age and sex on genetic associations with adult body size and shape: a large-scale genome-wide interaction study. PLoS Genet. 2015; 11(10):e1005378. https://doi.org/10.1371/journal.pgen.1005378. PubMed PMID: 26426971; PubMed Central PMCID: PMCPMC4591371.

56. Frazier-Wood AC. Dietary patterns, genes, and health: challenges and obstacles to be overcome. Curr Nutr Rep. 2015;4:82–7. https://doi.org/10.1007/s13668-014-0110-6. PubMed PMID: 25664222; PubMed Central PMCID: PMCPMC4315873.

57. Franks PW, Pearson E, Florez JC. Gene-environment and gene-treatment interactions in type 2 diabetes: progress, pitfalls, and prospects. Diabetes Care. 2013;36(5):1413–21. https://doi.org/10.2337/dc12-2211. PubMed PMID: 23613601; PubMed Central PMCID: PMC3631878.

58. InterAct C. Investigation of gene-diet interactions in the incretin system and risk of type 2 diabetes: the EPIC-InterAct study. Diabetologia. 2016;59(12): 2613–21. https://doi.org/10.1007/s00125-016-4090-5. PubMed PMID: 27623947.

18

High nutrient intake during the early postnatal period accelerates skeletal muscle fiber growth and maturity in intrauterine growth-restricted pigs

Liang Hu[†], Fei Han[†], Lin Chen, Xie Peng, Daiwen Chen, De Wu, Lianqiang Che[*]● and Keying Zhang[*]

Abstract

Background: Intrauterine growth-restricted (IUGR) neonates impair postnatal skeletal muscle growth. The aim of this study was to investigate whether high nutrient intake (HNI) during the suckling period could improve muscle growth and metabolic status of IUGR pigs.

Methods: Twelve pairs of IUGR and normal birth weight (NBW) pigs (7 days old) were randomly assigned to adequate nutrient intake and HNI formula milk groups. Psoas major (PM) muscle sample was obtained after 21 days of rearing.

Results: IUGR decreased cross-sectional areas (CSA) and myofiber numbers, activity of lactate dehydrogenase (LDH), and mRNA expression of insulin-like growth factor 1 (IGF-1), IGF-1 receptor (IGF-1R), mammalian target of rapamycin (mTOR), ribosomal protein s6 (RPS6), eukaryotic translation initiation factor 4E (eIF4E), protein expression of phosphorylated mTOR (P-mTOR), and phosphorylated protein kinase B (P-Akt) in the PM muscle of pigs. Irrespective of birth weight, HNI increased muscle weight and CSA, the concentration of RNA, and ratio of RNA to DNA, as well as ratio of LDH to β-hydroxy-acyl-CoA-dehydrogenase in the PM muscle of pigs. Furthermore, HNI increased percentages of MyHC IIb, mRNA expression of IGF-1, IGF-1R, Akt, mTOR, RPS6, and eIF4E, as well as protein expression of P-mTOR, P-Akt, P-RPS6, and P-eIF4E in the PM muscle of pigs.

Conclusion: The present findings suggest that high nutrient intake during the suckling period could improve skeletal muscle growth and maturity, which is associated with increasing the expression of protein deposition-related genes and accelerating the development of glycolytic-type myofiber in pigs.

Keywords: Birth weight, Nutrient intake, Skeletal muscle, Metabolic status, Pigs

Background

Epidemiological studies have demonstrated that intrauterine growth-restricted (IUGR) neonates are associated with the higher morbidity and mortality during the early life period, as well as a greater risk of the metabolic syndrome in adult life [1, 2]. Furthermore, previous studies showed that IUGR had negative impacts on the growth and development of skeletal muscle in pigs, including reduced skeletal muscle mass [3] and total myofiber number [4],

increased cross-sectional area (CSA) [5], and abnormal lipid deposition [6]. Skeletal muscle plays an important role in the metabolic homeostasis [7], and a defect in normal muscle development during the early postnatal period can permanently alter the subsequent muscle growth, contractile performance, and metabolism [8]. Therefore, improving skeletal muscle development of neonates with IUGR would be beneficial.

Postnatal muscle growth is mostly determined by the total myofiber number and fiber CSAs [9], as well as controlled by many signaling pathways in vivo [10]. Among those, the IGF1-Akt-mammalian target of rapamycin (mTOR) pathway acts as a major positive regulator of muscle growth [11]. Our previous study found high

---

* Correspondence: clianqiang@hotmail.com; zkeying@yahoo.com
[†]Liang Hu and Fei Han contributed equally to this work.
Institute of Animal Nutrition, Key Laboratory of Animal Disease-Resistance Nutrition, Sichuan Agricultural University, Ministry of Education, No.211 Huimin Road, Wenjiang District, Chengdu 611130, Sichuan, People's Republic of China

High nutrient intake during the early postnatal period accelerates skeletal muscle fiber growth and maturity...

195

nutrient intake (HNI) could lead to catch-up growth during the suckling period in IUGR pigs [12]; nevertheless, it is not clear whether HNI affects muscle growth and muscle growth-related molecular signal pathway. Since skeletal muscle accounts for about 50% of body mass and approximately 25% of the basal metabolic rate [13], changes in metabolic properties of muscle in the neonatal phase are also correlated with early muscle growth and myofiber maturation [14]. Thus, understanding the effects of HNI during the early postnatal period on the muscular metabolic status may provide new insights into the fiber development of IUGR.

Due to the physiological and genomic similarities between pigs and humans, pigs have been recognized as an excellent experimental model for the study of clinical nutrition [15]. Moreover, pigs exhibit severe naturally occurring IUGR [16]. In the present study, we investigated the effects of HNI on skeletal muscle growth, metabolic status, and the expressions of muscle growth and development-related genes of IUGR pigs.

Methods

The experiment followed the actual law of animal protection and was approved by the Animal Care and Use committee of Sichuan Agricultural University and performed in accordance with the National Research Council's Guide for the Care and Use of Laboratory Animals.

Animals, experimental design, and formula milk

In the current study, we collected the samples from the same animal experiment of our previous study. The experimental pigs and diets were detailed described in our previous study [12]. In brief, 12 pairs of IUGR (~ 0.87 kg) and normal birth weight (NBW, ~ 1.52 kg) pigs (Duroc × (Landrace × Yorkshire)) from 12 healthy sows were selected and all pigs were moved to be individually fed in nursing cages (0.8 m × 0.7 m × 0.4 m) when they were 7 days old (~ 1.68 for IUGR vs. ~ 2.78 kg for NBW). For nutritional treatments, six pairs of NBW and IUGR pigs were allocated to have adequate nutrient intake (ANI), while other six pairs of NBW and IUGR pigs were allocated to have high nutrient intake (HNI). This produced four experimental groups (birth weight/ nutrient intake (NI)): IUGR/ANI, NBW/ANI, IUGR/ HNI, and NBW/HNI ($n = 6$, per group). The ANI formula milk was made by mixing 1 kg of formula powder with 4 l of water, whereas HNI formula milk was made by mixing 1.73 kg of formula powder with 4 l of water, whose nutrient contents were about 1.5-fold of the ANI. The basic formula milk powder was formulated according to our previous study [12], and the composition was shown in Additional file 1: Table S1. One hundred milliliters of ANI formula milk contained 5.06 g protein, 4.64 g lactose,

and 5.20 g lipids, which were similar to that in the same volume of sow milk, containing 5.00 g protein, 5.06 g lactose, and 7.90 g lipids [12]. One hundred milliliters of HNI formula milk contained 7.59 g protein, 6.96 g lactose, and 7.80 g lipids. All pigs were fed with corresponding formula milk at 50 ml/kg body weight (BW) per meal with a feeding bottle seven times per day at 3-h intervals between 06:00 and 24:00. Pigs had free access to water. The ambient temperature and humidity were controlled around 30 °C and 50~60%, respectively. This experiment lasted for 21 days.

Tissue sample collection

At the end of the trial, all pigs were anesthetized with an intravenous injection of pentobarbital sodium (15 mg/kg BW) and killed. A set of morphometric measurements were made: head length (snout to between ears, HL), crow-rump length (between ears to end of tail; CRL), and abdominal circumference (AC), before slaughtering. Body mass index (BMI; BW/CRL^2) was calculated for each pig. The brain and heart of each pig were weighed immediately. The semitendinosus (ST) muscle and psoas major (PM) muscle from the left side of each carcass were completely excised and weighed, and the length and the circumference of the mid belly muscles were recorded. Muscle samples for histological analyses were excised from the central region of PM muscle, and then stored in 4% methanol solution. In addition, other muscle samples of PM muscle were collected, snap-frozen in liquid nitrogen, and stored at − 80 °C.

Muscular morphology

The PM muscle samples stored in 4% methanol solution were prepared after staining with hematoxylin and eosin using standard paraffin-embedding procedures. All sections were photographed using a digital microscope (Nikon), and muscle fibers were counted over five randomly selected fields of known size (1.01 mm², 200–300 fibers) as the myofiber density [17]. Muscle CSA was calculated from the circumference of the mid belly muscle. Then, the estimated total myofiber number was obtained by multiplying the fiber number per unit area by the CSA of PM muscle. The myofiber density was used to estimate the total number of fiber by multiplying with the CSA of PM muscle. The mean muscle fiber diameter in the united area was measured by Image-Pro Plus 6.0 software (Media Cybernetics, Bethesda, MD).

Biochemical analyses

Total RNA of PM muscle samples was extracted using TRIzol reagent (Invitrogen, USA) according to the manufacturer's instruction. RNA concentration and quality were verified by both spectrometry and agarose gel (1.0%) electrophoresis. DNA of muscle samples was extracted using the QIAamp® DNA mini kit (Qiagen) according to the manufacturer's instructions, and DNA quantification was performed using a NanoVue Plus spectrophotometer (GE Lifescience, Piscataway, NJ, USA). Protein concentration, lactate dehydrogenase (LDH), citrate synthase (CS), and β-hydroxy-acyl-CoA-dehydrogenase (HAD) activities of muscular samples were determined by using a commercial kit (Nanjing Jiancheng Bioengineering Institute, Nanjing, China) according to the instruction manuals. Briefly, frozen muscle samples (approximately 50 mg) were homogenized in 450 µl of 0.9% saline and then centrifuged at 3500g for 10 min at 4 °C. The protein content in muscle supernatant was determined based on the method of Coomassie brilliant blue dyeing using bovine serum albumin as the standard. The rate of change of absorbance was monitored at 440, 340, and 412 nm for evaluation of LDH, CS, and HAD activity using a biochemical analyzer (Multiskan Spectrum, Thermo Scientific), respectively. Their activities were expressed as units per gram of protein (U/g protein).

Real-time reverse transcription-PCR (RT-PCR)

Reverse transcription was performed at 37 °C for 15 min, followed by RT inactivation at 85 °C for 5 s using PrimeScript™ RT reagent Kit (Catalog no. RR047A; Takara). A portion of the RT products (1 µl) was used directly for real-time PCR. Real-time PCR assays were performed on complementary DNA samples in 384 well-optical plates on a 7900HT ABI Prism Sequence Detection System (Applied Biosystems, Foster City, CA, USA) using the SYBR green system (Catalog no. RR820A; Takara). Primers for individual genes were designed using Primer Express 3.0 (Applied Biosystems) and given in Table 1. The reaction mixture (10 µl) contained 5 µl of fresh SYBR® Premix Ex TaqII (Tli RNaseH Plus) and 0.2 µl ROX Reference Dye II (50×), 0.8 µl of the primers, 1 µl of RT products, and 3 µl dH$_2$O. The PCR protocol was used as follows: 1 cycle (95 °C 30 s), 40 cycles (95 °C 5 s, 60 °C 31 s), and 1 cycle (95 °C 15 s, 60 °C 1 min and 95 °C 15 s). The standard curve of each gene was run in duplicate and three times for obtaining reliable amplification efficiency values as described previously [18]. The correlation coefficients (r) of all the standard curves were more than 0.99, and the amplification efficiency values were between 90 and 110%. At the end of amplification, dissociation analyses of the PCR product were performed to confirm the specificity of PCR products. The relative mRNA abundance of analyzed genes was calculated using the method of $2^{-\Delta\Delta Ct}$ [19], and 18S rRNA was used as a reference gene in this study. In addition, the percentages of MyHC isoforms was calculated as the ratio of the normalized expression level of each MyHC isoform to the total expression of MyHC [20].

Western blotting

Western blot analysis was performed as previously described [21]. For the preparation of protein lysates, frozen muscle samples were powdered under liquid nitrogen and was homogenized in 1 ml cell lysis buffer (Beyotime Biotechnology, Shanghai, China) supplemented with protease inhibitor cocktail (Roche, Mannheim, Germany) on a homogenizer. The protein lysate was centrifuged at 12,000g and 4 °C for 30 min, and the supernatant was transferred to a new EP tube. The concentration of protein in the supernatant was measured with a BCA Protein Assay Kit (Thermo). One hundred micrograms protein was used to prepare an electrophoresis sample with loading buffer (Bio-Rad, Shanghai, China) in a volume of 30 µl for each sample. Proteins were separated on 12% polyacrylamide gel, and then transferred onto polyvinylidene fluoride membranes (Bio-Rad Laboratories). The membranes were blocked in 1% BSA/1×TBST for 1 h at room temperature, followed by incubation with the appropriate primary antibodies overnight. Total mTOR (1:1000; Santa Cruz), phosphorylated mTOR (Ser[2448], 1:1000 dilution), total eIF4E (1:1000 dilution), and phosphorylated eIF4E (Ser[209], 1:1000 dilution) were obtained from Santa Cruz (Shanghai, China); total RPS6 (1:2000 dilution), phosphorylated RPS6 (Ser[235/236], 1:1000 dilution), total Akt (1:1000 dilution), phosphorylated Akt (Ser[473], 1:1000 dilution), and β-actin (1:500 dilution) were obtained from Cell Signaling Technology (Shanghai, China). The membrane was then washed with 1×TBST for three times at 4 °C. After thorough washing, membranes were incubated with appropriate horseradish peroxidase-linked secondary antibodies (Cell Signaling Technology, Shanghai, China) (1:2000 dilution in 5% milk/1×TBST) for 1 h. After further thorough washing, protein signals were detected by ECL western blotting detection reagent (Bio-Rad, Shanghai, China) on a Molecular Imager ChemiDoc XRS+ System (Bio-Rad Laboratories). Blots were quantified with ImageJ software (National Institutes of Health, Bethesda, MD).

Statistical analysis

Results are presented as means with their standard errors (SEM). Analysis of variance using the General Linear Model (GLM) procedure of SPSS statistical software (Ver.20.0 for Windows, SPSS, Chicago, IL, USA) in the following model: $y_{ijk} = \mu + a_i + b_j + (ab)_{ij} + e_{ijk}$ ($i = 1, 2, j = 1, 2, k = 1, 2,..., n_{ij}$), where y_{ijk} represents the dependent variable, μ is the mean, a_i is the effect of BW (IUGR, NBW), b_j is the effect of NI (ANI, HNI), $(ab)_{ij}$ is the interaction between BW and NI, and e_{ijk} is the error term. The normality and homogeneity of variances were evaluated by Shapiro–Wilk W test and Levene's test respectively. Differences were considered as significant when $P < 0.05$, and a tendency was recognized when $0.05 < P < 0.10$. When

Table 1 Primer sequences of target and reference genes

Gene	Primer sequence (5'–3')	Product size (bp)	Genbank ID
IGF-1	F: GAACTGAAGAGCGTCCACCA	81	NM_214256.1
	R: TGCTTGCTCTCCTTCACCAG		
IGF-1R	F: ATGGATCACAAAGCCCTCGG	148	HQ322390.1
	R: CTGCCGCCACTACTACTACG		
GHR	F: GCTGTATGGATCCAGGGCTC	144	NM_214254.2
	R: TGCAGAGAGTTCATCCAGGC		
Akt	F: TCCAGCTTGAGGTCCCGATA	132	NM_001159776.1
	R: GCTCTTCTTCCACCTGTCCC		
mTOR	F: GGGGTTTGGATCAGGGTCTG	80	XM_003127584.4
	R: GACTCATCCGCCCCTACATG		
RPS6K	F: TTGAACTTCTCCAGCGTCCC	106	XM_003131671.3
	R: GCCTCCCTACCTCACACAAG		
RPS6	F: TACTCAGTAGCAGGCGGACT	92	XM_005660083.1
	R: TACTCAGTAGCAGGCGGACT		
eIF4E	F: ATGGAAGTCACTGTGGCCTG	133	DQ826509.1
	R: TCGTCCCACTAGCTCACAGA		
eIF4EBP1	F: CACAGGTGAGTTCCGACACT	105	NM_001244225.1
	R: GACTACAGCACCACTCCCG		
MyHC I	F: AAGGGCTTGAACGAGGAGTAGA	130	AB053226
	R: TTATTCTGCTTCCTCCAAAGGG		
MyHC IIa	F: GCTGAGCGAGCTGAAATCC	155	AB025260
	R: ACTGAGACACCAGAGCTTCT		
MyHC IIb	F: ATGAAGAGGAACCACATTA	137	AB025261
	R: TTATTGCCTCAGTAGCTTG		
MyHC IIx	F: AGAAGATCAACTGAGTGAACT	113	AB025262
	R: AGAGCTGAGAAACTAACGTG		
18S rRNA	F: GACTCAACACGGGAAACCTCAC	146	AY265350.1
	R: ATCGCTCCACCAACTAAGAACG		

IGF-1 insulin-like growth factor 1, *IGF-1R* insulin-like growth factor 1 receptor, *GHR* growth hormone receptor, *Akt* protein kinase B, *mTOR* mammalian target of rapamycin, *RPS6K* ribosomal protein S6 kinase, *RPS6* ribosomal protein S6, *eIF4E* eukaryotic translation initiation factor 4E, *eIF4EBP1* eukaryotic translation initiation factor 4E binding protein 1, *MyHC* myosin heavy chain

significant main effects or interactive effects were observed, the means were compared using Tukey's multiple comparisons with a $P < 0.05$ indicating significance.

Results
Organ indices
IUGR markedly decreased heart weight, AC, and CRL ($P < 0.05$), but increased the ratio of brain to BW and the ratio of HL to BW ($P < 0.05$) (Table 2). HNI increased heart weight, AC, and BMI ($P < 0.05$), but decreased the ratio of brain to BW and the ratio of HL to BW ($P < 0.05$) regardless of BW. In addition, no interaction between BW and NI was found on organ indices. Furthermore, compared with NBW pigs receiving ANI, the heart weight, AC, and BMI were higher ($P < 0.05$), but the relative brain weight and the ratio of HL to BW were lower ($P < 0.05$) in NBW pigs receiving HNI, respectively.

Muscle weight
IUGR significantly decreased the weight, length, and the relative weight to BW of both ST and PM muscles ($P < 0.05$) (Table 3), while increased the ratio of brain to ST weight and the ratio of brain to PM weight of pigs ($P < 0.05$). HNI increased the weight and length of PM muscle ($P < 0.05$) but decreased the ratio of brain to PM muscle weight ($P < 0.05$). Although not statistically significant, HNI tended to exhibit longer ST ($P = 0.095$) and greater ($P = 0.085$) ratio of PM weight to BW. Compared

Table 2 Effects of the level of nutrient intake on the organ weights, organ to body weight ratios, and morphometry of intrauterine growth-restricted (IUGR) and normal birth weight (NBW) pigs

Items	ANI		HNI		SEM	P value		
	IUGR	NBW	IUGR	NBW		BW	NI	BW × NI
Brain, g	58.0	60.4	63.3	56.7	7.2	0.585	0.837	0.255
Heart, g	31.1[a]	42.3[b]	36.4[a]	50.6[c]	3.8	< 0.001	0.003	0.439
Brain: BW, %	1.05[c]	0.82[b]	0.94[b,c]	0.64[a]	0.11	0.001	0.025	0.573
Heart: BW, %	0.56	0.57	0.54	0.57	0.05	0.406	0.605	0.559
HL, cm	17.8	18.5	18.8	17.0	2.1	0.632	0.801	0.272
AC, cm	35.4[a]	42.1[b]	37.8[a]	45.5[c]	1.9	< 0.001	0.012	0.608
CRL, cm	43.6[a]	48.3[a,b]	46.0[a,b]	51.3[b]	3.4	0.017	0.871	0.161
BMI, kg/m²	29.1[a]	28.2[a]	33.3[a,b]	38.4[b]	4.59	0.431	0.016	0.268
HL:BW, cm/kg	3.2[c]	2.5[b]	2.8[b,c]	1.9[a]	0.36	0.001	0.011	0.723

Data are presented as mean values with their standard errors, $n = 6$ in each group. Mean values within a row with different superscript letters (a, b, c) were significantly different between four groups ($P < 0.05$)
ANI adequate nutrient intake, HNI high nutrient intake, BW body weight, NI nutrient intake, HL head length, AC abdominal circumference, CRL crown-rump length, BMI body mass index

with IUGR pigs receiving ANI, the PM weight and length were higher ($P < 0.05$), but the ratio of brain to PM was lower ($P < 0.05$) in IUGR pigs receiving HNI, respectively.

Muscle characteristics

IUGR decreased the CSA and myofiber number ($P < 0.05$) in the PM muscle of pigs, respectively (Table 4). Although not statistically significant, moreover, IUGR pigs tended to show higher myofiber density of PM ($P = 0.083$) than NBW pigs. HNI increased the CSA ($P < 0.05$) and tended to decrease myofiber density of PM muscle ($P = 0.054$) regardless of BW. BW and NI had a significant interaction effect on the CSA and myofiber density of PM muscle ($P < 0.05$). The CSA of PM was higher ($P < 0.05$) while the myofiber density was lower ($P < 0.05$) in NBW pigs receiving HNI, respectively, compared with NBW pigs receiving ANI.

Biochemical properties

IUGR had no influence on RNA, DNA, and protein concentrations of PM muscle (Table 5). HNI markedly increased the concentrations of RNA and the ratio of RNA to DNA in PM muscles ($P < 0.05$) regardless of BW. Although not statistically significant, HNI tended to increase the concentration of protein in the PM muscle ($P = 0.082$). Compared with NBW pigs receiving ANI, the RNA concentration of PM was higher ($P < 0.05$) in IUGR pigs receiving HNI.

Metabolic enzyme activities

IUGR tended to decrease the LDH activity of PM (Fig. 1, $P = 0.068$) although not statistically significantly. Regardless of BW, HNI increased the ratio of LDH to HAD ($P < 0.05$) but decreased the activity of HAD and the ratio of HAD to CS in the PM muscle ($P < 0.05$). BW and NI had significant interaction effect on the ratio

Table 3 Effects of the level of nutrient intake on the muscle weights and lengths, muscle to body weight ratios, and brain to muscle ratios of intrauterine growth-restricted (IUGR) and normal birth weight (NBW) pigs

Items	ANI		HNI		SEM	P value		
	IUGR	NBW	IUGR	NBW		BW	NI	BW × NI
ST weight, g	16.5[a]	27.3[b]	19.9[a]	30.8[b]	4.52	< 0.001	0.167	0.972
ST length, cm	5.8[a]	6.9[b]	6.7[a,b]	7.3[b]	0.68	0.028	0.095	0.471
ST: BW, %	0.30	0.37	0.29	0.35	0.06	0.048	0.662	0.752
Brain: ST	3.66[b]	2.21[a]	3.31[b]	1.92[a]	0.60	0.001	0.320	0.921
PM weight, g	15.3[a]	23.9[b]	21.5[b]	30.0[c]	2.46	< 0.001	< 0.001	0.995
PM length, cm	7.5[a]	9.5[b]	9.4[b]	10.6[b]	0.93	0.005	0.006	0.416
PM: BW, %	0.28[a]	0.32[a,b]	0.32[a,b]	0.34[b]	0.03	0.048	0.085	0.429
Brain: PM	3.81[c]	2.57[b]	2.97[b]	1.90[a]	0.38	< 0.001	0.002	0.666

Data are presented as mean values with their standard errors, $n = 6$ in each group. Mean values within a row with different superscript letters (a, b, c) were significantly different between four groups ($P < 0.05$)
ANI adequate nutrient intake, HNI high nutrient intake, BW body weight, NI nutrient intake, ST semitendinosus, PM psoas major

Table 4 Effects of the level of nutrient intake on histomorphometry of psoas major muscle of intrauterine growth-restricted (IUGR) and normal birth weight (NBW) pigs

Items	ANI		HNI		SEM	P value		
	IUGR	NBW	IUGR	NBW		BW	NI	BW × NI
CSA, mm^2	156.2^a	209.1^b	176.2^{a,b}	344.8^c	30.7	< 0.001	< 0.001	0.003
Myofiber diameter, um	24.7	23.4	23.3	23.6	2.4	0.720	0.663	0.555
Myofiber density, mm^2	2161^b	2270^b	2227^b	1463^a	338	0.083	0.054	0.027
Myofiber number, thousand	337.2^a	461.6^b	394.6^{a,b}	498.7^b	68.1	0.004	0.178	0.764

Data are presented as mean values with their standard errors, n = 6 in each group. Mean values within a row with different superscript letters (a, b, c) were significantly different between four groups (P < 0.05)
ANI adequate nutrient intake, HNI high nutrient intake, BW body weight, NI nutrient intake, CSA cross-sectional area

LDH to HAD (P < 0.05) in the PM muscle. Compared with IUGR pigs receiving ANI, the HAD activity and the ratio of HAD to CS were lower (P < 0.05), but the ratio of LDH to HAD was higher (P < 0.05) in IUGR pigs receiving HNI, respectively.

Messenger RNA expression
To clarify the mechanism involved in protein synthesis in the PM muscle of pigs, we measured the expression of gene-related protein synthesis. IUGR pigs had significantly decreased the mRNA abundance of IGF1, IGF1R, mTOR, RPS6, and eIF4E (P < 0.05) in the PM muscle relative to NBW pigs (Fig. 2). Regardless of BW, HNI significantly increased the mRNA abundance of IGF1, IGF1R, Akt, mTOR, RPS6, and eIF4E in the PM muscle (P < 0.05). Significant interaction effects were found between BW and NI on the mRNA abundance of GHR and RPS6 (P < 0.05) in the PM muscle. BW and NI had a significant interaction effect on the mRNA abundance of RPS6 (P < 0.05). Compared with IUGR pigs receiving ANI, the mRNA abundance of IGF1, IGF1R, Akt, mTOR, RPS6, and eIF4E were higher in the PM of IUGR pigs receiving HNI (P < 0.05).

The composition of myofiber type
HNI increased the percentage of MyHC IIb in the PM muscle (P < 0.05) of pigs (Fig. 3). No significant changes in the percentages of other MyHC were found between groups (P > 0.05). The percentage of MyHC IIb in the PM muscle was higher (P < 0.05) in IUGR pigs receiving HNI compared with IUGR pigs receiving ANI.

Protein expressions
We measured the protein expression of IGF-1-Akt-mTOR signal pathway in the PM muscle. IUGR pigs had significantly decreased the protein expression of P-mTOR (Fig. 4a) and P-Akt (Fig. 4b) in the PM muscle relative to NBW pigs (P < 0.05). Regardless of BW, HNI significantly increased the protein expressions of P-mTOR (Fig. 4a), P-Akt (Fig. 4b), P-RPS6 (Fig. 4c), and P-eIF4E (Fig. 4d) in the PM muscle of pigs (P < 0.05). Compared with IUGR pigs receiving ANI, the protein expression of P-RPS6 (Fig. 4c) and P-eIF4E (Fig. 4d) were higher (P < 0.05) in IUGR pigs receiving HNI.

Discussion
Previous studies have been shown that neonates with IUGR receiving high-density nutrition intake have high risk of adult onset metabolic diseases, such as type 2 diabetes and cardiovascular disease [22, 23]. Skeletal muscle plays important roles in many physiological activities and is vital for contributing to basal metabolic rate of body [24]. However, little is known about the effects of HNI during the early postnatal period on skeletal muscle

Table 5 Effects of the level of nutrient intake on the concentrations of RNA, DNA, and protein in psoas major muscle of intrauterine growth-restricted (IUGR) and normal birth weight (NBW) pigs

Items	ANI		HNI		SEM	P value		
	IUGR	NBW	IUGR	NBW		BW	NI	BW × NI
RNA, mg/g	1.68^{a,b}	1.63^a	2.05^b	1.79^{a,b}	0.23	0.209	0.039	0.392
DNA, mg/g	1.50	1.40	1.48	1.38	0.20	0.292	0.884	0.987
Protein, mg/g	181.6	173.9	186.0	190.6	12.6	0.725	0.082	0.248
RNA: DNA	1.14	1.18	1.39	1.30	0.19	0.828	0.047	0.478
Protein: DNA	123.3	126.5	139.7	126.4	15.7	0.353	0.350	0.611

Data are presented as mean values with their standard errors, n = 6 in each group. Mean values within a row with different superscript letters (a, b) were significantly different between four groups (P < 0.05)
ANI adequate nutrient intake, HNI high nutrient intake, BW body weight, NI nutrient intake

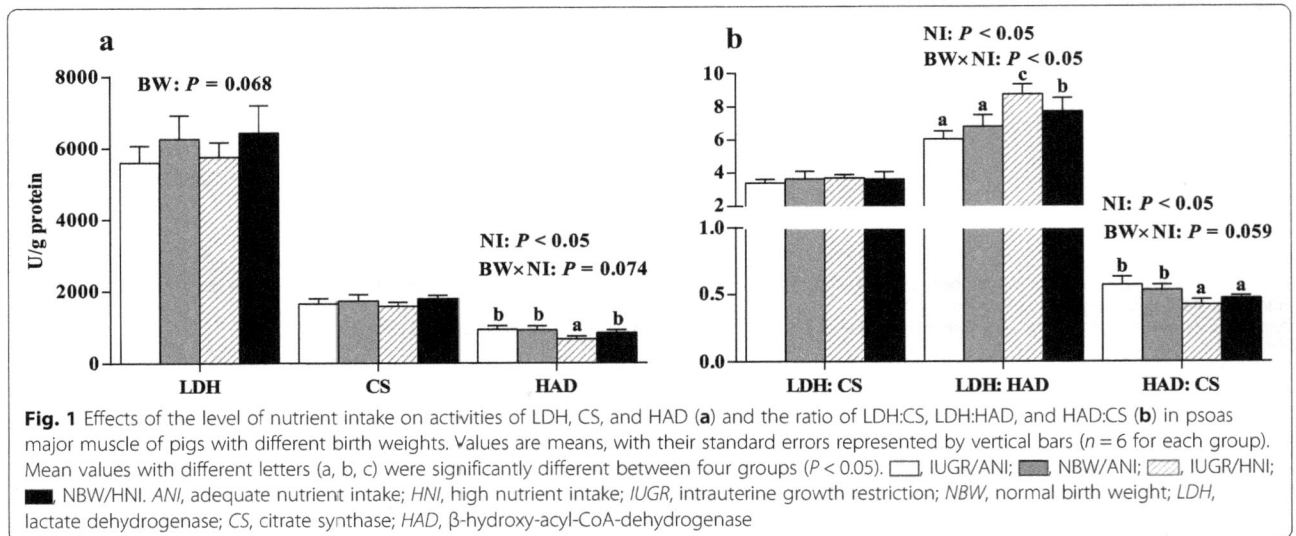

Fig. 1 Effects of the level of nutrient intake on activities of LDH, CS, and HAD (**a**) and the ratio of LDH:CS, LDH:HAD, and HAD:CS (**b**) in psoas major muscle of pigs with different birth weights. Values are means, with their standard errors represented by vertical bars ($n = 6$ for each group). Mean values with different letters (a, b, c) were significantly different between four groups ($P < 0.05$). ☐, IUGR/ANI; ▨, NBW/ANI; ▨, IUGR/HNI; ■, NBW/HNI. *ANI*, adequate nutrient intake; *HNI*, high nutrient intake; *IUGR*, intrauterine growth restriction; *NBW*, normal birth weight; *LDH*, lactate dehydrogenase; *CS*, citrate synthase; *HAD*, β-hydroxy-acyl-CoA-dehydrogenase

growth and metabolic status or its potential mechanism in IUGR neonates. The major finding of this study is that HNI during the early postnatal period improved the skeletal growth through mechanisms stimulating protein synthesis in IUGR pigs. HNI exerted marked differential effects on metabolic status and muscle properties; these changes reflected catch-up development induced by HNI during the early postnatal period. These findings have important implications for long-term muscle development of human infants with IUGR.

Neonates with IUGR had lighter body weight and increased relative internal organ weights [25], which is consistent with the observed shorter AC and CRL of IUGR pigs compared with that of NBW pigs in our study. By contrast, IUGR pigs had a markedly higher relative brain weight than that of NBW pigs, indicating that the maintenance of brain weight is of primary importance for IUGR pigs [26]. This phenotype could be due to the metabolic priority for the growth of key organs when fetus suffering maternal malnutrition in uterus [27]. The increased BMI and heart weight in IUGR

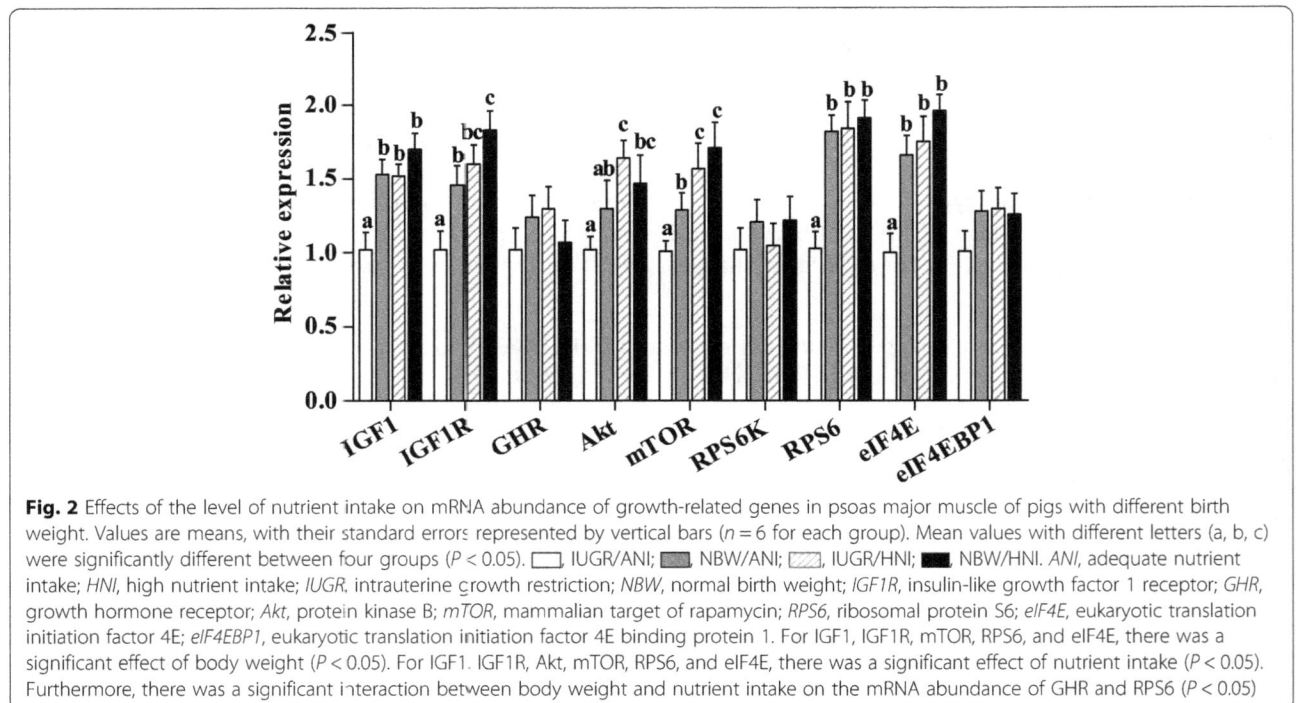

Fig. 2 Effects of the level of nutrient intake on mRNA abundance of growth-related genes in psoas major muscle of pigs with different birth weight. Values are means, with their standard errors represented by vertical bars ($n = 6$ for each group). Mean values with different letters (a, b, c) were significantly different between four groups ($P < 0.05$). ☐, IUGR/ANI; ▨, NBW/ANI; ▨, IUGR/HNI; ■, NBW/HNI. *ANI*, adequate nutrient intake; *HNI*, high nutrient intake; *IUGR*, intrauterine growth restriction; *NBW*, normal birth weight; *IGF1R*, insulin-like growth factor 1 receptor; *GHR*, growth hormone receptor; *Akt*, protein kinase B; *mTOR*, mammalian target of rapamycin; *RPS6*, ribosomal protein S6; *eIF4E*, eukaryotic translation initiation factor 4E; *eIF4EBP1*, eukaryotic translation initiation factor 4E binding protein 1. For IGF1, IGF1R, mTOR, RPS6, and eIF4E, there was a significant effect of body weight ($P < 0.05$). For IGF1. IGF1R, Akt, mTOR, RPS6, and eIF4E, there was a significant effect of nutrient intake ($P < 0.05$). Furthermore, there was a significant interaction between body weight and nutrient intake on the mRNA abundance of GHR and RPS6 ($P < 0.05$)

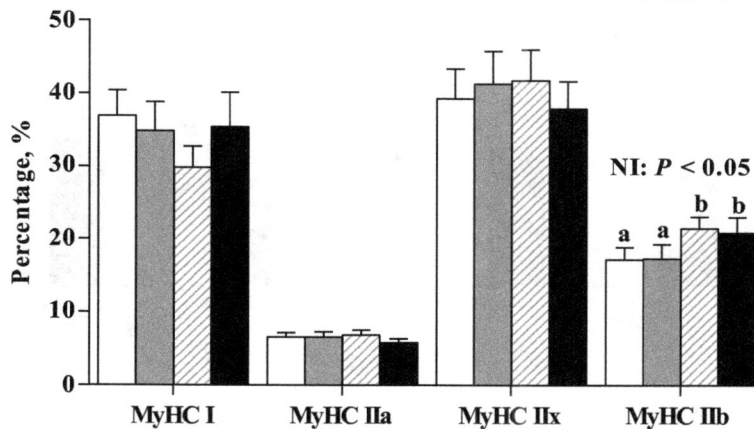

Fig. 3 Effects of the level of nutrient intake on the percentage of MyHC in psoas major muscle of pigs with different birth weights. Values are means, with their standard errors represented by vertical bars ($n = 6$ for each group). Mean values with different letters (a, b) were significantly different between four groups ($P < 0.05$). □, IUGR/ANI; ▨ (grey), NBW/ANI; ▨, IUGR/HNI; ▨ (black), NBW/HNI. *ANI*, adequate nutrient intake. *HNI*, high nutrient intake; *IUGR*, intrauterine growth restriction; *NBW*, normal birth weight; *MyHC*, myosin heavy chain

pigs with HNI may be resulting from the compensatory growth during the early postnatal period, which is in accordance with the report of Greenwood et al., who showed that IUGR sheep with a high postnatal nutrition resulted in a greater internal organ weight [28].

Numerous studies had demonstrated that pigs suffering IUGR had smaller muscle mass [29, 30], reflecting decreased muscle growth prenatally and/or postnatally [6, 31]. In the present study, IUGR decreased the PM and ST muscle weight of pigs, which are in agreement with previous findings [32]. However, we found that there was a comparable PM muscle weight between IUGR pigs with HNI and NBW pigs with ANI. The growth performance found in our previous study showed IUGR pigs receiving HNI were able to exert a similar growth rate and comparable weight gain to NBW pigs with ANI [12].

Neonates suffering IUGR formed a lower myofiber number which will restrict the potential of lean growth after birth [4]. In our study, both the myofiber number and CSA of PM muscle were lower in IUGR pigs than NBW pigs, which are in agreement with previous reports [4, 5, 29]. Consistent with pervious study [32], IUGR pigs had a higher myofiber density than their normal littermate. However, HNI tended to decrease the myofiber density during the suckling period, which may result from increased CSA. The number and CSA of muscle fiber are known to be an important determinant of postnatal muscle growth [33]. Total myofiber number of pigs has been reported to be fixed at birth [34, 35], but most recently, many studies have found that there might be a "third generation" for muscle fiber growth during the early postnatal period [36–38], which are shown by the occurrence of very small-diameter myofibers containing

embryonic and/or neonatal isoforms of myosin heavy chain in porcine muscles [39]. Interestingly, compared with NBW pigs, a comparable myofiber number of PM muscle in IUGR pigs were found when receiving HNI, which suggests that the restricted myofiber of pigs suffering IUGR could be induced by HNI during the early postnatal period. Similarly, Losel et al. reported that L-carnitine supplementation also increased the myofiber number of IUGR pigs during the suckling period [40]. Ratios of protein to DNA and RNA to DNA have been used as indexes of hypertrophy and potential cellular activity respectively [41]. In the current study, the early postnatal fiber formation of IUGR pigs in response to HNI was associated with greater RNA concentrations and the ratio of RNA to DNA, as well as tended to increase the concentration of protein in the PM muscle, which could be explained as a shift to intensified myogenic proliferation [40]. These results provide another line of evidence for the increased myofiber number of IUGR pigs receiving HNI during the suckling period. Taken together, these results indicated the myofiber formation in IUGR pigs has not fully ceased at birth and can be improved by HNI in the early postnatal phase.

Muscle development in postnatal pigs is regulated by gene expression and growth factors [42]. IGF-1 acts as an important mediator to promote cell differentiation and protein synthesis in fetuses [43]. Skeletal muscle growth in response to IGF-1 is precisely mediated by the serine/threonine kinase Akt, the downstream targets of mTOR signal pathway, through regulation of mRNA translation and protein synthesis [11, 44]. Consistent with previous studies [45, 46], the decreased mRNA abundance of IGF1, IGF1R, mTOR, RPS6, and eIF4E

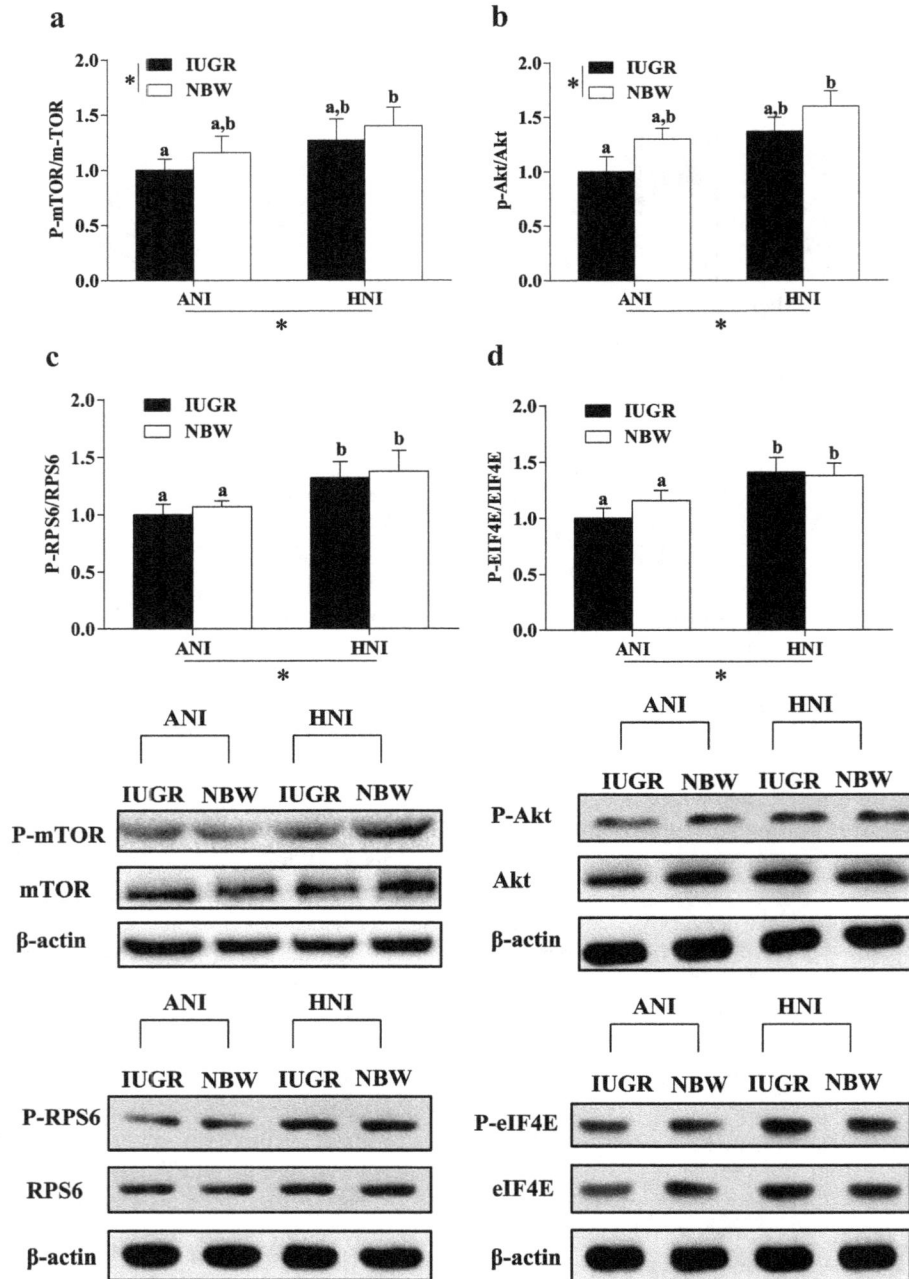

Fig. 4 Effects of the level of nutrient intake on abundance of growth-related proteins in psoas major muscle of pigs with different birth weight. *ANI*, adequate nutrient intake; *HNI*, high nutrient intake; *IUGR*, intrauterine growth restriction; *NBW*, normal birth weight; *mTOR*, mammalian target of rapamycin; *p-mTOR*, phosphorylated mTOR; *Akt*, protein kinase B; *P-Akt*, phosphorylated Akt; *RPS6*, ribosomal protein S6; *P-RPS6*, phosphorylated RPS6; *eIF4E*, eukaryotic translation initiation factor 4E; *P-eIF4E*, phosphorylated eIF4E. Values are means, with their standard errors represented by vertical bars ($n = 6$ for each group). Mean values with different letters (a, b) were significantly different between four groups ($P < 0.05$). *$P < 0.05$ for the respective sources of variation (nutrition intake or body weight)

and protein expression of P-mTOR and P-Akt suggested that the muscle growth is compromised in pigs suffering IUGR. However, our results demonstrated that HNI improved muscle growth via IGF1-Akt-mTOR signal pathway, as indicated by the enhanced expressions at

the transcriptional level. Moreover, Akt activation is reported to stimulate protein synthesis [47]. Therefore, the increased Akt phosphorylation by HNI may be responsible for enhancing the downstream effector. mTOR, as an essential component of the signaling pathway that regulates protein synthesis, is directly activated by the intake of nutrients [48]. Additionally, phosphorylation of mTOR on Ser2448 is positively related to the activity of mTOR [49]. Consistent with this observation, we found that HNI resulted in an increase of the protein expressions of P-mTOR in the PM muscle of pigs, suggesting that HNI during the early postnatal period enhanced the activation of elements involved in the mTOR protein synthesis pathway. Moreover, the increased P-RPS6 and P-eIF4E by HNI (the downstream effector of mTOR) supported this conclusion. eIF4E phosphorylation status was examined because it influences mRNA bindings to the 43S preinitiation complex, resulting in increased protein synthesis in cell culture [50]. Zhu et al. has reported that restricted nutrient intake affected the protein expressions by mTOR-RPS6 pathway in the muscle of sheep [51].

Rapid myofibril protein accretion and changes in MyHC polymorphism of myofibers in the skeletal muscle of pigs have been reported during the neonatal period [52]. In the present study, we found that HNI increased the percentage of MyHC IIb-type muscle fiber in the PM muscle of both IUGR and NBW pigs. Studies have suggested that high muscularity is positively related to a high abundance of MyHC IIb transcript [20]; the MyHC IIb mRNA levels had been shown to be steadily increased from days 7 to 180 after birth. Furthermore, the phenotypic changes in muscle characteristics are often linked to the metabolic and functional alterations [11]; therefore, the activities of related metabolic enzymes were measured in the present study. The activities of CS, HAD, and LDH were used as markers of overall oxidative capacity (tricarboxylic cycle), lipid β-oxidation, and glycolytic potential, respectively [7]. In the present study, we found that IUGR tended to decrease the activity of LDH in the PM muscle of pigs, which suggested that glycolytic muscles might be more susceptible to IUGR. However, the ratio of LDH to HAD in the PM muscle of pigs was enhanced by HNI, which is indicative of increased glycolytic capacity of skeletal muscle when pigs are receiving HNI [14]. Moreover, a shift toward a lower lipid β-oxidation capacity was observed in the PM muscle of pigs receiving HNI, as suggested by the decreased HAD activity and the ratio of HAD to CS. Most importantly, IUGR pigs receiving HNI had a higher ratio of LDH to HAD than those receiving ANI, suggesting that restricted glycolytic capacity could be restored by HNI during the early postnatal period. Similarly, Lefaucheur et al. has shown that high food intake during the early postnatal period enhanced the muscular glycolytic capacity, as indicated by the increased ratio of LDH to HAD in the muscle of pigs [14], the increased glycolytic enzyme activity could be observed in the early postnatal phase during the muscular development [53]. Based on the data of metabolic enzymes and MyHC isoform, HNI during the suckling period may accelerate the muscle maturity of pigs.

Conclusion

In summary, the results of the current study indicate that high nutrient intake during the early postnatal period contributed to skeletal muscle fiber growth and maturity through stimulating protein synthesis-related gene expression and accelerating glycolytic fiber development in IUGR pigs, associated with changing the metabolic status, which indicated the long-term effect of IUGR on muscle development.

Acknowledgements
The present study was supported by the National Key Research and Development Program of China (grant number 2016YFD0501204), the project on commercialization of research findings under funding of government of Sichuan province (grant number 16ZHSF0385) and the National 973 Project (grant number 2012CB124701).

Authors' contributions
LH, FH, L. Chen, and XP carried out the animal experiments and performed the laboratory work. DC and DW performed the statistical analysis. L. Che and KZ designed the study and helped in drafting the manuscript. LH and FH wrote the paper. All authors read and approved the final manuscript.

Competing interests
The authors declare that they have no competing interests.

References
1. Mandruzzato G, Antsaklis A, Botet F, Chervenak FA, Figueras F, Grunebaum A, et al. Intrauterine restriction (IUGR). J Perinat Med. 2008;36:277–81.
2. Ergaz Z, Avgil M, Ornoy A. Intrauterine growth restriction—etiology and consequences: what do we know about the human situation and experimental animal models? Reprod Toxicol. 2005;20:301–22.
3. D'Inca R, Gras-Le Guen C, Che L, Sangild PT, Le Huerou-Luron I. Intrauterine growth restriction delays feeding-induced gut adaptation in term newborn pigs. Neonatol. 2011;99:208–16.
4. Rehfeldt C, Kuhn G. Consequences of birth weight for postnatal growth performance and carcass quality in pigs as related to myogenesis. J Anim Sci. 2006;84(Suppl):E113–23.
5. Gondret F, Lefaucheur L, Louveau I, Lebret B, Pichodo X, Le Cozler Y. Influence of piglet birth weight on postnatal growth performance, tissue lipogenic capacity and muscle histological traits at market weight. Livest Prod Sci. 2005;93:137–46.
6. Karunaratne JF, Ashton CJ, Stickland NC. Fetal programming of fat and collagen in porcine skeletal muscles. J Anat. 2005;207:763–8.
7. Harrison AP, Rowlerson AM, Dauncey MJ. Selective regulation of myofiber differentiation by energy status during postnatal development. Am J Phys. 1996;270:R667–74.
8. Yates DT, Macko AR, Nearing M, Chen X, Rhoads RP, Limesand SW. Developmental programming in response to intrauterine growth restriction impairs myoblast function and skeletal muscle metabolism. J Pregnancy. 2012;2012:631038.
9. Joo ST, Kim GD, Hwang YH, Ryu YC. Control of fresh meat quality through manipulation of muscle fiber characteristics. Meat Sci. 2013;95:828–36.
10. Egerman MA, Glass DJ. Signaling pathways controlling skeletal muscle mass. Crit Rev Biochem Mol Biol. 2014;49:59–68.
11. Schiaffino S, Dyar KA, Ciciliot S, Blaauw B, Sandri M. Mechanisms regulating skeletal muscle growth and atrophy. FEBS J. 2013;280:4294–314.
12. Han F, Hu L, Xuan Y, Ding X, Luo Y, Bai S, et al. Effects of high nutrient intake on the growth performance, intestinal morphology and immune function of neonatal intra-uterine growth-retarded pigs. Br J Nutr. 2013;110:1819–27.

13. Henriksson J. The possible role of skeletal muscle in the adaptation to periods of energy deficiency. Eur J Clin Nutr. 1990;44(Suppl 1):55–64.

14. Lefaucheur L, Ecolan P, Barzic YM, Marion J, Le Dividich J. Early postnatal food intake alters myofiber maturation in pig skeletal muscle. J Nutr. 2003; 133:140–7.

15. Ferenc K, Pietrzak P, Godlewski MM, Piwowarski J, Kilianczyk R, Guilloteau P, et al. Intrauterine growth retarded piglet as a model for humans—studies on the perinatal development of the gut structure and function. Reprod Biol. 2014;14:51–60.

16. Sangild PT. Gut responses to enteral nutrition in preterm infants and animals. Exp Biol Med (Maywood). 2006;231:1695–711.

17. Wan H, Zhu J, Wu C, Zhou P, Shen Y, Lin Y, et al. Transfer of β-hydroxy-β-methylbutyrate from sows to their offspring and its impact on muscle fiber type transformation and performance in pigs. J Anim Sci Biotechnol. 2017;8:2.

18. Hu L, Liu Y, Yan C, Peng X, Xu Q, Xuan Y, et al. Postnatal nutritional restriction affects growth and immune function of piglets with intra-uterine growth restriction. Br J Nutr. 2015;114:53–62.

19. Livak KJ, Schmittgen TD. Analysis of relative gene expression data using real-time quantitative PCR and the 2(−Delta Delta C(T)) method. Methods. 2001;25:402–8.

20. Wimmers K, Ngu NT, Jennen DG, Tesfaye D, Murani E, Schellander K, et al. Relationship between myosin heavy chain isoform expression and muscling in several diverse pig breeds. J Anim Sci. 2008;86:795–803.

21. Zhang Y, Wang P, Lin S, Mercier Y, Yin H, Song Y, et al. mTORC1 signaling-associated protein synthesis in porcine mammary glands was regulated by the local available methionine depending on methionine sources. Amino Acids. 2018;50:105–15.

22. Simmons RA, Templeton LJ, Gertz SJ. Intrauterine growth retardation leads to the development of type 2 diabetes in the rat. Diabetes 2001;50:2279–86.

23. Gluckman PD, Lillycrop KA, Vickers MH, Pleasants AB, Phillips ES, Beedle AS, et al. Metabolic plasticity during mammalian development is directionally dependent on early nutritional status. Proc Natl Acad Sci U S A. 2007;104: 12796–800.

24. Ruiz-Rosado A, Fernandez-Valverde F, Mariscal-Tovar S, Hinojosa-Rodriguez CX, Hernandez-Valencia JA, Anzueto-Rios A, et al. Histoenzymatic and morphometric analysis of muscle fiber type transformation during the postnatal development of the chronically food-deprived rat. J Histochem Cytochem. 2013;61:372–81.

25. Morise A, Seve B, Mace K, Magliola C, Le Huerou-Luron I, Louveau I. Growth, body composition and hormonal status of growing pigs exhibiting a normal or small weight at birth and exposed to a neonatal diet enriched in proteins. Br J Nutr. 2011;105:1471–9.

26. Pardo CE, Berard J, Kreuzer M, Bee G. Intrauterine crowding impairs formation and growth of secondary myofibers in pigs. Animal. 2013;7:430–8.

27. Bauer R, Walter B, Hoppe A, Gaser E, Lampe V, Kauf E, et al. Body weight distribution and organ size in newborn swine (sus scrofa domestica)—a study describing an animal model for asymmetrical intrauterine growth retardation. Exp Toxicol Pathol. 1998;50:59–65.

28. Greenwood PL, Hunt AS, Bell AW. Effects of birth weight and postnatal nutrition on neonatal sheep: IV. Organ growth J Anim Sci. 2004;82:422–8.

29. Gondret F, Lefaucheur L, Juin H, Louveau I, Lebret B. Low birth weight is associated with enlarged muscle fiber area and impaired meat tenderness of the longissimus muscle in pigs. J Anim Sci. 2006;84:93–103.

30. Bauer R, Gedrange T, Bauer K, Walter B. Intrauterine growth restriction induces increased capillary density and accelerated type I fiber maturation in newborn pig skeletal muscles. J Perinat Med. 2006;34:235–42.

31. Bee G. Birth weight of litters as a source of variation in postnatal growth, and carcass and meat quality. Adv Pork Prod. 2007;18:191–6.

32. Alvarenga AL, Chiarini-Garcia H, Cardeal PC, Moreira LP Foxcroft GR, Fontes DO, et al. Intra-uterine growth retardation affects birthweight and postnatal development in pigs, impairing muscle accretion, duodenal mucosa morphology and carcass traits. Reprod Fertil Dev. 2013;25:387–95.

33. Lefaucheur L. A second look into fibre typing—relation to meat quality. Meat Sci. 2010;84:257–70.

34. Staun H. The nutritional and genetic influence on number and size of muscle fibers and their response to carcass quality in pigs. World Rev Anim Prod. 1972;8:8–26.

35. Stickland NC, Goldspink G. Possible indicator muscle for fiber content and growth characteristics of porcine muscle. Anim Prod. 1973;16:135–46.

36. Rehfeldt C, Fiedler I, Dietl G, Ender K. Myogenesis and postnatal skeletal muscle cell growth as influenced by selection. Livest Prod Sci. 2000;66:177–88.

37. Rehfeldt C, Henning M, Fiedler I. Consequences of pig domestication for skeletal muscle growth and cellularity. Livest Sci. 2008;116:30–41.

38. Berard J, Kalbe C, Losel D, Tuchscherer A, Rehfeldt C. Potential sources of early-postnatal increase in myofibre number in pig skeletal muscle. Histochem Cell Biol. 2011;136:217–25.

39. Mascarello F, Stecchini ML, Rowlerson A, Ballocchi E. Tertiary myotubes in postnatal growing pig muscle detected by their myosin isoform composition. J Anim Sci. 1992;70:1806–13.

40. Losel D, Kalbe C, Rehfeldt C. L-carnitine supplementation during suckling intensifies the early postnatal skeletal myofiber formation in piglets of low birth weight. J Anim Sci. 2009;87:2216–26.

41. Scheaffer AN, Caton JS, Redmer DA, Arnold DR, Reynolds LP. Effect of dietary restriction, pregnancy, and fetal type on intestinal cellularity and vascularity in Columbia and Romanov ewes. J Anim Sci. 2004;82:3024–33.

42. Wan H, Zhu J, Su G, Liu Y, Hua L, Hu L, et al. Dietary supplementation with beta-hydroxy-beta-methylbutyrate calcium during the early postnatal period accelerates skeletal muscle fibre growth and maturity in intra-uterine growth-retarded and normal-birth-weight piglets. Br J Nutr. 2016;115:1360–9.

43. Froesch ER, Schmid C, Schwander J, Zapf J. Actions of insulin-like growth factors. Annu Rev Physiol. 1985;47:443–67.

44. Bodine SC, Stitt TN, Gonzalez M, Kline WO, Stover GL, Bauerlein R, et al. Akt/mTOR pathway is a crucial regulator of skeletal muscle hypertrophy and can prevent muscle atrophy in vivo. Nat Cell Biol. 2001;3:1014–9.

45. Lin G, Liu C, Feng C, Fan Z, Dai Z, Lai C, et al. Metabolomic analysis reveals differences in umbilical vein plasma metabolites between normal and growth-restricted fetal pigs during late gestation. J Nutr. 2012;142:990–8.

46. Wang J, Chen L, Li D, Yin Y, Wang X, Li P, et al. Intrauterine growth restriction affects the proteomes of the small intestine, liver, and skeletal muscle in newborn pigs. J Nutr. 2008;138:60–6.

47. Schiaffino S, Mammucari C. Regulation of skeletal muscle growth by the IGF1-Akt/PKB pathway: insights from genetic models. Skelet Muscle. 2011;1:4.

48. Wang X, Proud CG. The mTOR pathway in the control of protein synthesis. Physiology (Bethesda). 2006;21:362–9.

49. Holz MK, Ballif BA, Gygi SP, Blenis J. mTOR and S6K1 mediate assembly of the translation preinitiation complex through dynamic protein interchange and ordered phosphorylation events. Cell. 2005;123:569–80.

50. Minich WB, Balasta ML, Goss DJ, Rhoads RE. Chromatographic resolution of in vivo phosphorylated and nonphosphorylated eukaryotic translation initiation factor eIF-4E: increased cap affinity of the phosphorylated form. Proc Natl Acad Sci U S A. 1994;91:7668–72.

51. Zhu MJ, Ford SP, Nathanielsz PW, Du M. Effect of maternal nutrient restriction in sheep on the development of fetal skeletal muscle. Biol Reprod. 2004;71:1968–73.

52. Picard B, Lefaucheur L, Berri C, Duclos MJ. Muscle fibre ontogenesis in farm animal species. Reprod Nutr Dev. 2002;42:415–31.

53. Lefaucheur L, Ecolan P, Lossec G, Gabillard JC, Butler-Browne GS, Herpin P. Influence of early postnatal cold exposure on myofiber maturation in pig skeletal muscle. J Muscle Res Cell Motil. 2001;22:439–52.

19

Genetic polymorphism in selenoprotein P modifies the response to selenium-rich foods on blood levels of selenium and selenoprotein P

Tine Iskov Kopp[1,2,3,5]* (iD), Malene Outzen[1,2], Anja Olsen[2], Ulla Vogel[4] and Gitte Ravn-Haren[1]

Abstract

Background: Selenium is an essential trace element and is suggested to play a role in the etiology of a number of chronic diseases. Genetic variation in genes encoding selenoproteins, such as selenoprotein P and the glutathione peroxidases, may affect selenium status and, thus, individual susceptibility to some chronic diseases. In the present study, we aimed to (1) investigate the effect of mussel and fish intake on glutathione peroxidase enzyme activity and (2) examine whether single nucleotide polymorphisms in the *GPX1*, *GPX4*, and *SELENOP* genes modify the effect of mussel and fish intake for 26 weeks on whole blood selenium, plasma selenoprotein P concentrations, and erythrocyte GPX enzyme activity in a randomized intervention trial in Denmark.

Results: CC homozygotes of the *SELENOP*/rs3877899 polymorphism who consumed 1000 g fish and mussels per week for 26 consecutive weeks had higher levels of both selenoprotein P (difference between means − 4.68 ng/mL (95% CI − 8.49, − 0.871)) and whole blood selenium (difference between means − 5.76 (95% CI − 12.5, 1.01)) compared to fish and mussel consuming T-allele carriers although the effect in whole blood selenium concentration was not statistically significant.

Conclusions: Our study indicates that genetically determined variation in *SELENOP* leads to different responses in expression of selenoproteins following consumption of selenium-rich foods. This study also emphasizes the importance of taking individual aspects such as genotypes into consideration when assessing risk in public health recommendations.

Keywords: Selenium, Selenoprotein P, Glutathione peroxidase, Dietary intervention, Randomized, Gene-diet interaction, *SELENOP*, *GPX1*, *GPX4*, Single nucleotide polymorphisms

Background

Selenium is an essential trace element and is suggested to play a role in the etiology of a number of chronic diseases [9, 37]. Several factors can affect selenium status; these include exposure to selenium through diet or dietary supplements [32, 33, 35] and lifestyle factors such as body mass index (BMI) and smoking [6]. Furthermore, genetic

variation has been proposed to influence selenium status of the individual [14].

Most of the biological functions of selenium are carried out by selenoproteins [30]. Among the best characterized selenoproteins with essential functions are selenoprotein P and the glutathione peroxidases (GPX), including GPX1 and GPX4 [30]. Besides functioning as storage and transport protein for selenium, some studies suggest that selenoprotein P is involved in the antioxidant defense which also comprises the glutathione peroxidases [40]. These antioxidant selenoenzymes detoxify a range of hydroperoxides, including lipid and phospholipid hydroperoxides,

* Correspondence: tine.iskov.kopp@regionh.dk
[1]National Food Institute, Technical University of Denmark, Kemitorvet, Building 202, 2800 Kgs Lyngby, Denmark
[2]Danish Cancer Society Research Center, Strandboulevarden 49, 2100 Copenhagen Ø, Denmark
Full list of author information is available at the end of the article

thereby ensuring a reducing environment and protecting cell components such as proteins, lipids, and DNA from oxidative damage [36]. Nutritional deficiency in selenium results in decreased selenoprotein concentrations and a compromised enzymatic antioxidant defense. Selenium supplementation is known to affect selenoprotein expression in a hierarchical manner. GPX4 ranks higher in the hierarchy of selenoproteins compared to GPX1 which is much more responsive to both selenium depletion and repletion [2, 4]. Humans differ in their ability to metabolize selenium and respond differently to selenium supplementation. These differences are likely to be due to genetic variation in selenoprotein genes [6, 16]. Specifically, functional single nucleotide polymorphisms (SNPs) in GPX1 (encoding GPX1), GPX4 (encoding GPX4), and SELENOP (encoding SELENOP) have been shown to affect blood selenium or selenoprotein levels in response to supplementation [19, 20, 23]. The GPX1/rs1050450 polymorphism is a Pro to Leu substitution at position 197 [10] which results in reduced enzyme activity [16, 34] and higher DNA damage levels [25]. GPX1/rs1050450 has also been associated with risk of several diseases, including lung [31, 39], breast [8, 21, 34], and prostate cancer [3, 43]; peripheral neuropathy [45]; coronary heart diseases [26, 50]; septic shock [18]; and mortality [42], and correlation between GPX1 activity and serum selenium concentration has been reported for this polymorphism [16]. GPX4/rs713041 affects protein binding to the 3′-untranslated region close to a selenocysteine insertion sequence required for selenoprotein synthesis [20, 48] and has been associated with decreased GPX enzyme activity [21], risk of colorectal cancer [43], and mortality [47]. SELENOP/rs3877899 causes an Ala to Thr amino acid substitution at position 234, and SELENOP/rs7579 is located in the 3′-untranslated region of SELENOP mRNA, where it causes a G to A base change [19]. Both SELENOP polymorphisms lead to alterations in selenium metabolism by changing the proportion of the 60-kDa isoform of selenoprotein P [23]. They have been shown to affect selenium and selenoprotein P blood concentrations after supplementation with selenium [19] and have also been associated with risk of various diseases, including breast [21], prostate [7, 13, 43], and colorectal cancer [22, 23] and aortic aneurisms [44]. Taken together, these results point to a regulatory role of these polymorphisms in the expression of the encoded selenoproteins. However, it is not clear whether this is also the case at selenium intakes that are dietary feasible.

In a previous randomized dietary intervention with fish and mussels in middle-aged Danes, we found increased whole blood selenium and plasma selenoprotein P concentrations among healthy participants after 26 weeks' intervention [28]. We hypothesized that SELENOP gene variations modify the effect of increased dietary selenium intake on markers of selenium status. Thus, in the present

paper, we aimed to (1) investigate the effect of mussel and fish intake on GPX enzyme activity and (2) examine whether SNPs in the GPX1, GPX4, and SELENOP genes modify the effect of the intervention with mussel and fish on whole blood selenium, plasma selenoprotein P concentrations, and erythrocyte GPX enzyme activity in the same study population of healthy middle-aged Danish men and women.

Methods

Study population

This study is based on data from a randomized dietary intervention study with the primary aim of studying the influence of increased intake of fish and mussels on blood selenium levels. The study design and methods are described in details elsewhere [28].

The study took place in the northern part of Jutland, Denmark, from September 2010 to March 2011 as a 26-week randomized dietary intervention study with two parallel groups including healthy middle-aged participants. Eligibility for randomization was determined by potential participants completing a questionnaire 3 months before baseline measurements on lifestyle, diet, and health status.

The goal was to recruit a total of 100 men and women aged 50–74 years with a BMI of 18.5–28 kg/m^2 based on a power calculation where a minimum detectable difference of 10 ng/mL (SD = 10) or 30 ng/mL (SD = 10) in selenium concentration between groups with a statistical power of 87 or 99%, respectively, was allowed [29]. The exclusion criteria included current smoking, intake of dietary supplements containing selenium 3 months before baseline measurements, frequent intake of fish and shellfish (> 300 g/week), excessive intake of alcohol (according to the official Danish guidelines at study recruitment: women > 14 units of alcohol/week, men > 21 units of alcohol/week), strenuous exercise (> 10 h/week), severe chronic disease, and frequent use of specified medication (including diabetic medicine, anticoagulant medicine, and medication for heart disease), or a cancer diagnosis within the past 5 years. Study participants were requested to inform the investigators of any changes regarding disease or medication occurring during the study. Study participants were recruited through local media, including newspaper advertisements. Of the 102 men and women enrolled in the study, 83 completed the intervention. Flow chart of the participants is illustrated in Additional file 1 as previously published [28].

Dietary intervention

Participants in the intervention group were provided with 1000 g raw fish and raw or processed mussels (portion size of 200 g; five portions/week) once a week for 26 weeks. This amount corresponds to an intake of approximately 50.3 µg selenium/day (based on data from the Danish Food Composition Databank) [41]. The participants received four or five different types of fish per week. Diversity in the type of fish provided was prioritized to ensure variation and thereby optimize compliance. The participants were allowed to consume other meals containing fish or shellfish besides the experimental foods. The intervention diet has been described in detail elsewhere [28].

To monitor their compliance, the participants were provided with a self-monitoring record and kitchen scales to weigh the amount of received fish and mussels (prepared or raw) not consumed during the study period. At study initiation, participants were instructed on how to complete the self-monitoring record. Compliance was calculated as total received amount—not ingested amount after preparation)/by total received amount; the median of ingested proportion was 99% of the received fish and mussels [28].

Participants in the control group received no intervention and were advised to maintain their habitual diets.

Data collection

Non-fasting blood samples were collected three times (weeks 0, 13, and 26) from each participant during the study. Blood samples were drawn in K2-EDTA-coated blood drawing tubes as whole blood samples or blood samples that were separated into plasma, erythrocytes, and buffy coat by centrifugation. All samples were stored at −80 °C until analysis.

Biochemical analyses

Whole blood selenium analyses were conducted using an ELAN 6100 DRC inductively coupled plasma-mass spectrometer (ICP-MS) in accordance with a method described in detail in [15]. The concentration of selenoprotein P in plasma was determined using its selective retention by heparin-affinity high-performance liquid chromatography (HPLC) and online detection by ICP-DRC-MS of selenium eluting from the HPLC column. In addition to determining selenoprotein P, the concentration of total selenium in plasma was also quantified by isotope dilution on the basis of the area under the complete chromatogram. However, even though the results seemed accurate (that is, the values obtained from plasma selenium did not deviate from certified values from reference material), the method used to determine plasma selenium in this way was less precise than that used to determine selenium in whole blood. Therefore, the baseline plasma selenium concentration was used only for comparison with other studies measuring plasma selenium in healthy populations. The analysis methods have been described in details previously [28].

GPX enzyme activities were spectrophotometrically assayed in erythrocyte lysates on a Pentra 400 (Horiba ABX, Montpellier, France), using t-butylhydroperoxide as substrate according to the method described by Wheeler et al. [49]. GPX activities were related to the amount of hemoglobin (Hb) in the lysates. Hb content was determined using a commercially available kit (Randox Ardmore, UK, cat. no HG 980). Samples from each individual were run in the same batch in random order to decrease variation, and a control sample was included for every 15th sample. Intra- and inter-day variations were < 5 and $< 10\%$, respectively.

SNP selection and genotyping

The following polymorphisms were selected based on their known functionality and association with disease: *GPX1*/rs1050450, *GPX4*/rs713041, *SELENOP*/rs3877899, and *SELENOP*/rs7579.

DNA from the participants was extracted from frozen lymphocytes as described [24]. Genotypes were determined using RT-PCR and allelic discrimination on ABI 7900HT instruments (Applied Biosystems, Nærum, Denmark). Generally, 40–200 ng/μl DNA was obtained and 10 ng of DNA was genotyped in 5 μl containing 50% $2 \times$ Mastermix (Applied Biosystems, Nærum, Denmark), 100 nM probes, and 900 nM primers.

GPX1/rs1050450: primers: F: 5′-TGT GCC CCC TAC GCA GGT ACA-3′, R: 5′-CCC CCG AGA CAG CAG CA-3′ (TAGCopenhagen, Copenhagen, Denmark), T-allele: 5′-FAM-CTG TCT CAA GGG CTC AGC TGT-MGB-3′, C-allele: 5′-VIC-CTG TCT CAA GGG CCC AGC TGT-MGB-3′ (Applied Biosystems, Nærum, Denmark).

GPX4/rs713041: primers: F: 5′-CCC ACT ATT TCT AG C TCC ACA AGT G-3′, R: 5′-GTC ATG AGT GCC GGT GGA A-3′ (TAGCopenhagen, Copenhagen, Denmark), T-allele: 5′-FAM-ACG CCC TTG GAG C-MGB-3′, C-allele: 5′-VIC-ACG CCC TCG GAG C-MGB-3′ (Applied Biosystems, Nærum, Denmark).

SELENOP/rs3877899 was determined using the TaqMan® Pre-designed SNP genotyping; assay ID C_2 841533_10, respectively (Applied Biosystems, Nærum, Denmark).

SELENOP/rs7579: primers: F: 5′-CAA AAA AGT GA G AAT GAC CTT CAA ACT-3′, R: 5′-ATG CTG GAA ATG AAA TTG TGT CTA GA-3′ (TAGCopenhagen, Copenhagen, Denmark), G-allele: 5′-FAM-AAA ATA G GA CAT ACT CCC C-MGB-3′, A-allele: 5′-VIC-AAA T AG AAC ATA CTC CCC AAT T-MGB-3′ (Applied Biosystems, Nærum, Denmark).

All samples were determined as duplicates with known positive controls (three for each genotype) and three negative controls containing Milli Q water. All duplicates yielded 100% identical genotypes.

Statistical methods

The statistical analysis was based on all available observations. Participants who were randomized into a group, but did not attend the baseline appointment (week 0), were excluded. Baseline characteristics are presented as either number with its percentage and medians with 5th and 95th percentiles for each study group. For the polymorphisms, minor allele frequencies are also presented. Outlying observations were identified from visual inspection of the data (correlation plots of week 0 vs. week 13 and week 0 vs. week 26). Deviation from Hardy–Weinberg equilibrium was assessed using a chi-square test.

Linear multiple regression analysis was applied to evaluate the intervention effect on erythrocyte GPX enzyme activity. Within the two groups, mean changes (weeks 0–13, weeks 0–26) and the difference between the groups' mean changes (weeks 0–26) were calculated from the linear multiple regression. All values of GPX enzyme activity were log-transformed to correct for right-skewed distribution.

To examine the association between mean concentrations of whole blood selenium, plasma selenoprotein P or erythrocyte GPX enzyme activity according to genotype at baseline, week 13 and week 26, respectively, a linear multiple regression analysis was applied using least square means adjusted for baseline concentrations of whole blood selenium, plasma selenoprotein P, or erythrocyte GPX enzyme activity, respectively. Adjustment for baseline level was done to eliminate baseline levels' influence on the effect of the SNPs. In order to increase the statistical power, heterozygote variant allele and homozygote variant allele carriers were pooled in the analyses.

Moreover, we examined whether sex, BMI, and age modified the relationship between intervention outcomes and the polymorphisms. An interaction term between sex, BMI, and age, respectively, and the studied polymorphisms was therefore included in the model.

A mixed-model, repeated-measures analysis of variance (ANOVA) was used to determine the within-subject effect between genotype and erythrocyte GPX enzyme activity, whole blood selenium, or plasma selenoprotein P concentrations during the entire intervention period.

The statistical analyses were carried out using SAS (release 9.4, SAS Institute, Inc., Cary, NC, USA) and the procedure general linear model (GLM).

For all tests, a P value less than 0.05 was considered statistically significant.

Results

We evaluated the effect of four functional polymorphisms in *GPX1*, *GPX4*, and *SELENOP* on erythrocyte GPX enzyme activity, whole blood selenium, and plasma selenoprotein P concentrations after consumption of 1000 g fish and mussels per week for 26 consecutive weeks (~ 50 μg selenium/day) in volunteer participants [28]. Furthermore, we evaluated the effect of the intervention on erythrocyte GPX enzyme activity.

Baseline characteristics of all participants including the control group are presented in Table 1 as published previously [28], except for GPX enzyme activity measurements, which have not been published previously. None of the baseline variables differed between the two groups (Table 1) or according to genotype (results not shown). The genotype distributions of the studied polymorphisms were in Hardy–Weinberg equilibrium (results not shown).

In Table 2, changes in erythrocyte GPX enzyme activity measurements within groups (intervention and control) and differences between group changes are illustrated. There were no statistically significant differences in erythrocyte GPX enzyme activity changes between the intervention and control groups after, neither 13 nor 26 weeks (Table 2).

In Table 3, the associations between mean erythrocyte GPX enzyme activity, concentrations of whole blood selenium and plasma selenoprotein P, and the studied polymorphisms, and within-subject effects between genotype and time for the intervention group, are shown. A difference in mean GPX enzyme activity at baseline was found for the *GPX1*/rs1050450 polymorphism among participants who were randomized to the intervention ($P = 0.044$). This difference in enzyme activity persisted after 13 and 26 weeks' intervention, resulting in no statistically significant difference in response to the increased selenium intake between genotypes. Mean GPX enzyme activity at baseline among CC homozygotes was 104.1 and 84.0 U/g Hb among variant T-allele carriers (intervention group only—results not shown). There was no interaction between any of the studied polymorphisms and whole blood selenium or plasma selenoprotein P concentrations (Table 3). However, there was a statistically significant difference of -4.68 ng/mL (95% CI -8.49, -0.871) between mean concentration of plasma selenoprotein P at week 26 for variant T-allele and CC homozygotes of the *SELENOP*/rs3877899 polymorphism (Table 3). A mean difference in whole blood selenium for the *SELENOP*/rs3877899 polymorphism was also seen; however, this association was not statistically significant (difference between means -5.76 (95% CI -12.5, 1.01). Results for the control group are presented in Additional file 2. None of the polymorphisms among participants in the control group differed for either of the outcome measures as expected.

In order to elucidate whether these differences in selenoprotein P and whole blood selenium concentrations were due to chance or an effect of the intervention, we examined the association between the *SELENOP*/rs3877899 polymorphism and whole blood selenium and selenoprotein P concentrations, respectively, with the control group included in the model (Figs. 1 and 2). After 26 weeks, the

Table 1 Baseline characteristics of the participants presented as either number (%) or median value (5th–95th percentiles)

Variable	MAF (%)	Intervention group (n = 49)	Control group (n = 45)
Women		21 (43%)	19 (42%)
Men		28 (57%)	26 (58%)
Age, years		61 (51–72)	59 (51–73)
BMI, kg/m^2		26.3 (21.0–31.1)	25.2 (20.3–32.5)
Whole blood selenium, ng/mL		113.5 (91.3–147.4)	114.6 (96.6–136.0)[1]
Plasma selenoprotein P, ng selenium/mL		51.4 (35.0–63.9)[2]	51.4 (35.4–65.7)[3]
Plasma selenium, ng/mL		84.7 (67.8–106.5)[2]	86.4 (70.5–103.3)[3]
Erythrocyte GPX enzyme activity, U/g Hb		86 (57–153)[4]	84 (54–156)[5]
GPX1/rs1050450	29.8		
CC		23 (47%)	22 (49%)
CT		22 (45%)	20 (44%)
TT		4 (8%)	3 (7%)
GPX4/rs713041	37.8		
CC		16 (33%)	17 (38%)
CT		25 (51%)	26 (58%)
TT		8 (16%)	2 (4%)
SELENOP/rs3877899	19.1		
CC		30 (61%)	30 (67%)
CT		18 (37%)	14 (31%)
TT		1 (2%)	1 (2%)
SELENOP/rs7579	30.3		
GG		24 (49%)	19 (42%)
GA		22 (45%)	23 (51%)
AA		3 (6%)	3 (7%)

Part of this table has been published in [28]. MAF, minor allele frequency for the studied population (n = 94). [1]n = 44 due to exclusion of outlying values (n = 1), all whole blood and plasma selenium and selenoprotein P concentrations for this person were excluded; [2]n = 46 due to errors in the laboratory measures (n = 3), all plasma selenoprotein P concentrations and the plasma selenium concentration analyzed only at baseline were excluded for these persons; [3]n = 42 due to errors in the laboratory measures (n = 2), all plasma selenoprotein P concentrations and the plasma selenium concentration analyzed only at baseline were excluded for these persons, and due to exclusion of outlying values (n = 1). [4]n = 44 since GPX activity was not analyzed on persons having only baseline levels measured (n = 1). [5]n = 41 since GPX activity was not analyzed on persons having only baseline levels measured (n = 8)

difference in whole blood selenium mean concentrations between CC homozygotes and T-allele carriers was only borderline statistically significant ($P = 0.088$) (Fig. 1), whereas the mean difference in selenoprotein P concentrations between CC homozygotes and T-allele carriers of the SELENOP/rs3877899 polymorphism was still statistically significant ($P = 0.048$) (Fig. 2).

We also tested whether sex, age, or BMI modified the effect on the intervention for the studied polymorphisms, but we did not find any sign of such effect modification (results not shown).

Discussion

The present study showed that CC homozygotes of the SELENOP/rs3877899 polymorphism who consumed 1000 g fish and mussels per week for 26 consecutive weeks had higher levels of both selenoprotein P and whole blood selenium compared to fish and mussel consuming variant T-allele carriers and the control group although the effect in whole blood selenium concentration was not statistically significant.

To our knowledge, this is the first study investigating the effect of SELENOP and GPX polymorphisms after ingestion of high selenium content foods in a controlled randomized trial. The SELGEN study [19] examined the effect on plasma selenium and selenoprotein P concentrations of the same SELENOP polymorphisms as in the present study before and after selenium supplementation in a UK population also known to be low in selenium status. Mean baseline plasma selenium concentrations in the two studies were comparable (1.15 μmol/l corresponding to 90.8 ng/mL in the SELGEN study and 85.8 ng/mL in the present study). The two investigated SELENOP polymorphisms significantly affected plasma selenium concentration after 6 weeks of supplementation with 100 μg selenium/day as sodium selenite [19]. The authors noted that the effect was strongest among participants with a BMI exceeding 30 where SELENOP/rs3877899 CC homozygotes (referred to as GG in [19]) and variant A-allele carriers of SELENOP/rs7579 responded better to selenium supplementation compared to carriers of the variant T-allele (referred to as A-allele in [19]) and GG homozygotes, respectively. The same study reported a statistically significant increase in plasma selenoprotein P concentration following selenium supplementation and gender-specific differences in

Table 2 Changes within groups and differences between group changes in erythrocyte GPX enzyme activities

	Mean change within group, log (U/g Hb) (95% CI)[a]				Difference between group mean change, log (U/g Hb) (95% CI)*	
	N	Weeks 0–13	n	Weeks 0–26	N	Weeks 0–26
Intervention	41	0.0332 (0.0160, 0.0503)	41	0.0461 (0.0239, 0.0684)	85	0.0263 (− 0.00498, 0.0577)
Control	44	0.0169 (0.000278, 0.0334)	44	0.0198 (− 0.00221, 0.0418)		

[a]Adjusted for baseline levels of GPX enzyme activity

Table 3 Association between mean concentrations of erythrocyte GPX enzyme activity, whole blood selenium, and selenoprotein P in relation to the studied polymorphisms, and within-subject effects between genotype and time in the intervention group

Erythrocyte GPX enzyme activity, log (U/g Hb)

SNP	n	Baseline		13 weeks[c]		26 weeks[c]		P value for interaction between genotype and time
		Difference between means (95% CI)	P value	Difference between means (95% CI)	P value	Difference between means (95% CI)	P value	
GPX1/rs1050450								
CC	20	− 0.224 (− 0.442, − 0.00638)	0.044	0.0299 (− 0.00981, 0.0696)	0.14	− 0.00585 (− 0.06278, 0.0511)	0.84	0.085
CT + TT	21							
GPX4/rs713041								
CC	15	0.129 (− 0.105, 0.364)	0.27	− 0.00532 (− 0.0462, 0.0355)	0.79	− 0.0143 (− 0.0711, 0.0424)	0.61	0.79
CT + TT	26							
SELENOP/rs3877899								
CC	25	− 0.0228 (− 0.258, 0.212)	0.85	− 0.00617 (− 0.0459, 0.0335)	0.75	0.0145 (− 0.0407, 0.0697)	0.60	0.70
CT + TT	16							
SELENOP/rs7579								
GG	22	− 0.0278 (− 0.258, 0.202)	0.81	− 0.0134 (− 0.0521, 0.0252)	0.49	− 0.0143 (− 0.0683, 0.0397)	0.60	0.81
GA + AA	19							

Whole blood selenium, ng/mL

SNP	n*	Baseline		13 weeks[d]		26 weeks[d]		P value for interaction between genotype and time
		Difference between means (95% CI)	P value	Difference between means (95% CI)	P value	Difference between means (95% CI)	P value	
GPX1/rs1050450								
CC	23	3.20 (− 5.46, 11.9)	0.46	− 0.989 (− 7.89, 5.91)	0.77	− 1.24 (− 8.11, 5.63)	0.72	0.83
CT + TT	26							
GPX4/rs713041								
CC	16	4.85 (− 4.32, 14.0)	0.29	− 2.76 (− 9.91, 4.38)	0.44	− 1.77 (− 8.93, 5.39)	0.62	0.54
CT + TT	33							
SELENOP/rs3877899								
CC	30	0.989 (− 7.93, 9.91)	0.82	0.675 (− 6.37, 7.72)	0.85	− 5.76 (− 12.5, 1.01)	0.093	0.13
CT + TT	19							
SELENOP/rs7579								
GG	24	4.44 (− 4.16, 13.0)	0.30	− 4.04 (− 10.9, 2.80)	0.24	1.60 (− 5.32, 8.53)	0.64	0.23
GA + AA	25							

Selenoprotein P, ng/mL

SNP	n[b]	Baseline		13 weeks[e]		26 weeks[e]		P value for interaction between genotype and time
		Difference between means (95% CI)	P value	Difference between means (95% CI)	P value	Difference between means (95% CI)	P value	
GPX1/rs1050450								
CC	21	4.17 (− 0.51, 8.85)	0.080	− 1.17 (− 5.38, 3.04)	0.58	− 2.56 (− 6.60, 1.47)	0.21	0.071
CT + TT	25							
GPX4/rs713041								

Table 3 Association between mean concentrations of erythrocyte GPX enzyme activity, whole blood selenium, and selenoprotein P in relation to the studied polymorphisms, and within-subject effects between genotype and time in the intervention group (Continued)

Erythrocyte GPX enzyme activity, log (U/g Hb)								
CC	16	3.49 (− 1.47, 8.45)	0.16	0.801 (− 3.41, 5.01)	0.70	− 1.17 (− 5.32, 2.97)	0.57	0.48
CT + TT	30							
SELENOP/rs3877899								
CC	28	− 2.33 (− 7.23, 2.57)	0.34	− 2.43 (− 6.53, 1.67)	0.24	− 4.68 (− 8.49, − 0.871)	0.018	0.33
CT + TT	18							
SELENOP/rs7579								
GG	23	2.16 (− 2.63, 6.94)	0.37	1.72 (− 2.35, 5.79)	0.40	− 0.630 (− 4.66, 3.40)	0.75	0.79
GA + AA	23							

[a]13 and 26 weeks' measurements only included 41 participants due to discontinuation of intervention
[b]13 and 26 weeks' measurements only included 38 participants due to discontinuation of intervention
[c]Adjusted for baseline levels of erythrocyte GPX enzyme activity
[d]Adjusted for baseline levels of whole blood selenium
[e]Adjusted for baseline levels of selenoprotein P

baseline concentrations and post-supplementation with SELENOP/rs3877899 and SELENOP/rs7579, respectively. Lower baseline concentration of plasma selenoprotein P was measured in women who were heterozygous T-allele carriers of the SELENOP/rs3877899 polymorphism compared to men with corresponding genotype, while the opposite applied for CC homozygotes. Among carriers of the SELENOP/rs7579 variant A-allele, men had higher plasma selenoprotein P concentrations post-supplementation compared to women. We were not able to reproduce the findings on gender and BMI which could be due to a lack of power to study gene-environment interactions in the present study given the relatively small sample size. Our study differs from the SELGEN intervention in several ways which might contribute to the different findings.

Besides a longer study period (26 weeks compared to 6 weeks in the SELGEN study), different sources of selenium and dosage levels were used in the interventions. We supplemented with a dietary source of selenium, while selenite was used in the SELGEN study, and at a dosage level that was half the one given by Méplan et al. [19]. Compared to inorganic selenium, organic selenium compounds, such as selenomethionine present in fish and mussels, are non-specifically incorporated into the general protein pool, leaving a smaller part of the absorbed selenium readily available for biosynthesis of selenoproteins. However, it is not clear whether this had an impact on the results, given the long supplementation period and the relatively high bioavailability of selenium from fish which has been reported to be between 56 and 90% [11, 12, 38].

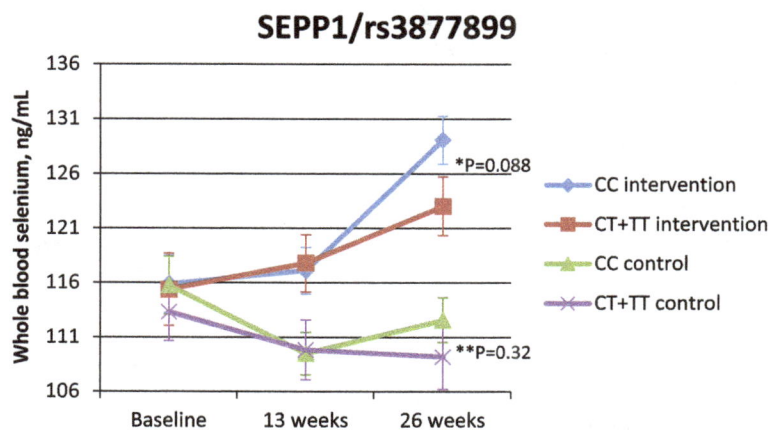

Fig. 1 Association between mean concentrations of whole blood selenium and the SELENOP/rs3877899 polymorphism. Mean concentrations of whole blood selenium ± SD for the intervention and control group estimated by linear multiple regression adjusted for baseline level of whole blood selenium. P values for difference in mean whole blood selenium concentrations at week 26 for genotype effect within the intervention group (*) and within the control group (**), respectively, are illustrated

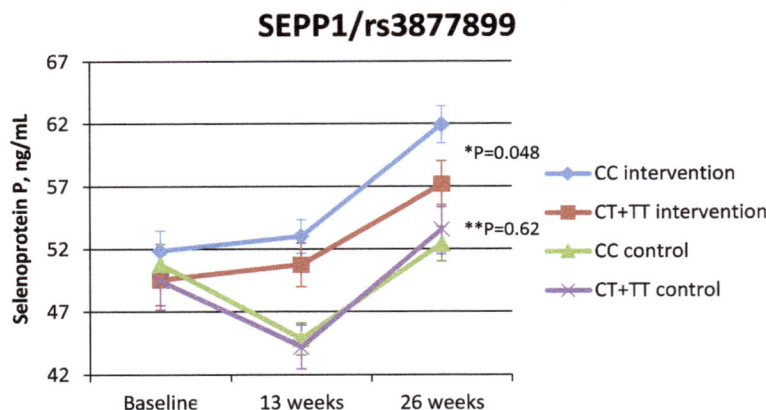

Fig. 2 Association between mean concentrations of selenoprotein P and the *SELENOP*/rs3877899 polymorphism. Mean concentrations of selenoprotein P ± SD for the intervention and control group estimated by linear multiple regression adjusted for baseline level of selenoprotein P. *P* values for difference in mean selenoprotein P concentrations at week 26 for genotype effect within the intervention group (*) and within the control group (**), respectively, are illustrated

Increasing the intake of selenium with fish and mussels did not affect erythrocyte GPX enzyme activity, suggesting that this selenoprotein was maximally expressed prior to supplementation. This is consistent with previous results, showing that the antioxidant enzyme GPX is saturated at blood selenium concentrations around 100 ng/mL [27, 46]. When stratifying the data according to genotype, in line with previous findings [34], carriers of the variant *GPX1* allele had significantly lower erythrocyte GPX activity compared to CC homocygotes. A compromised antioxidant defense may lead to increased susceptibility to oxidative stress and DNA damage [25].

The increase in selenoprotein P concentration in the control group from week 13 to week 26 is unexpected and is difficult to explain (Fig. 2). This has been discussed in more detail in the main paper that evaluated the intervention effect on blood selenium status [28].

Strengths and limitations of the overall study design were thoroughly described by Outzen et al. [28]. Shortly, the strengths of the study are the design with the randomization procedure, which ensure evenly distribution of confounders, the restrictive inclusion and exclusion criteria, and the long-term duration of the intervention combined with the high compliance. Limitations include lack of blinding and that participants were non-fasting at blood sampling. However, we based our results on whole blood which has been shown to reflect the long-term selenium status [1, 17] as opposed to plasma selenium, which has a short half-life [5]. With regard to the lack of blinding, this is not expected to influence on this study since we mainly studied the effect of genetic variation in the intervention group. We are well aware of the present study being underpowered due to the small sample size. Nevertheless, our study is in accordance with the SELGEN study, and we are therefore

able to support the notion that variation in the *SELENOP* gene affects selenium biomarker concentration after intake of both a selenium dietary supplement and food with a high content of selenium.

Conclusion

Taken together, our study indicates that genetically determined variation in *SELENOP* leads to different responses in expression of selenoproteins following consumption of selenium-rich foods. This emphasizes the importance of taking individual aspects such as genotypes into consideration when assessing risk in public health recommendations, since they may affect selenium metabolism and response to selenium intake and thereby enable a more personalized approach to micronutrient requirements.

Abbreviations

BMI: Body mass index; GPX: Glutathione peroxidases; SNP: Single nucleotide polymorphism

Acknowledgements

The authors thank Lene Svensson and Annette Landin (Technical University of Denmark, National Food Institute) for technical assistance with determining GPX enzyme activity and DNA extraction and Erik Huusfeldt Larsen for performing plasma selenoprotein P, plasma selenium, and whole blood selenium measurements.

Funding

The dietary intervention study was supported by funds from the Bjarne Saxhof Foundation. The Foundation had no influence on the design and conduct of the study, management, analysis, and interpretation of the data or preparation of the manuscript.

Authors' contributions

TIK, MO, GRH, and UV conceived the study. TIK extracted DNA, genotyped the participants, analyzed the data, and wrote the first draft of the manuscript. MO and AO designed and conducted the randomized intervention study. GRH analyzed GPX enzyme activities and participated in writing the first draft of the manuscript. All authors have contributed to the interpretation of data, critically revised the manuscript for important intellectual content, and approved the final manuscript.

Competing interests
The authors declare that they have no competing interests.

Author details
[1]National Food Institute, Technical University of Denmark, Kemitorvet, Building 202, 2800 Kgs Lyngby, Denmark. [2]Danish Cancer Society Research Center, Strandboulevarden 49, 2100 Copenhagen Ø, Denmark. [3]The Danish Multiple Sclerosis Registry, Copenhagen University Hospital, Rigshospitalet, Blegdamsvej 9, 2100 Copenhagen Ø, Denmark. [4]National Research Centre for the Working Environment, Lersø Parkallé 105, 2100 Copenhagen Ø, Denmark. [5]The Danish Multiple Sclerosis Center, Department of Neurology, The Danish Multiple Sclerosis Registry, Section 7801, Rigshospitalet, Blegdamsvej 9, 2100 Copenhagen Ø, Denmark.

References
1. Ashton K, Hooper L, Harvey LJ, et al. Methods of assessment of selenium status in humans: a systematic review. Am J Clin Nutr. 2009;89:2025S–39S. https://doi.org/10.3945/ajcn.2009.27230F.
2. Bermano G, Arthur JR, Hesketh JE. Role of the 3′ untranslated region in the regulation of cytosolic glutathione peroxidase and phospholipid-hydroperoxide glutathione peroxidase gene expression by selenium supply. Biochem J. 1996;320(3):891–5.
3. Blein S, Berndt S, Joshi AD, et al. Factors associated with oxidative stress and cancer risk in the Breast and Prostate Cancer Cohort Consortium. Free Radic Res. 2014;48:380–6. https://doi.org/10.3109/10715762.2013.875168.
4. Brigelius-Flohé R, Müller C, Menard J, et al. Functions of GI-GPx: lessons from selenium-dependent expression and intracellular localization. BioFactors. 2001;14:101–6. https://doi.org/10.1002/biof.5520140114.
5. Bügel S, Larsen EH, Sloth JJ, et al. Absorption, excretion, and retention of selenium from a high selenium yeast in men with a high intake of selenium. Food Nutr Res. 2008;52:1642. https://doi.org/10.3402/fnr.v52i0.1642.
6. Combs GF Jr, Watts JC, Jackson MI, et al. Determinants of selenium status in healthy adults. Nutr J. 2011;10:75. https://doi.org/10.1186/1475-2891-10-75.
7. Cooper ML, Adami H-O, Grönberg H, et al. Interaction between single nucleotide polymorphisms in selenoprotein P and mitochondrial superoxide dismutase determines prostate cancer risk. Cancer Res. 2008;68:10171–7. https://doi.org/10.1158/0008-5472.CAN-08-1827.
8. Cox DG, Tamimi RM, Hunter DJ. Gene x Gene interaction between MnSOD and GPX-1 and breast cancer risk: a nested case-control study. BMC Cancer. 2006;6:217. https://doi.org/10.1186/1471-2407-6-217.
9. Fairweather-Tait SJ, Bao Y, Broadley MR, et al. Selenium in human health and disease. Antioxid redox signal. 2011;14:1337–83. https://doi.org/10.1089/ars.2010.3275.
10. Forsberg L, De Faire U, Morgenstern R. Low yield of polymorphisms from EST blast searching: analysis of genes related to oxidative stress and verification of the P197L polymorphism in GPX1. Hum Mutat. 1999;13:294–300. https://doi.org/10.1002/(SICI)1098-1004(1999)13:4<294::AID-HUMU6>3.0.CO;2-5.
11. Fox TE, Atherton C, Dainty JR, et al. Absorption of selenium from wheat, garlic, and cod intrinsically labeled with Se-77 and Se-82 stable isotopes. Int J Vitam Nutr Res. 2005;75:179–86. https://doi.org/10.1024/0300-9831.75.3.179.
12. Fox TE, Van den Heuvel EGHM, Atherton CA, et al. Bioavailability of selenium from fish, yeast and selenate: a comparative study in humans using stable isotopes. Eur J Clin Nutr. 2004;58:343–9. https://doi.org/10.1038/sj.ejcn.1601787
13. Geybels MS, van den Brandt PA, Schouten LJ, et al. Selenoprotein gene variants, toenail selenium levels, and risk for advanced prostate cancer. J Natl Cancer Inst. 2014;106:dju003. https://doi.org/10.1093/jnci/dju003.
14. Hurst R, Collings R, Harvey LJ, et al. EURRECA—estimating selenium requirements for deriving dietary reference values. Crit Rev Food Sci Nutr. 2013;53:1077–96. https://doi.org/10.1080/10408398.2012.742861.
15. J a N, Batista BL, Rodrigues JL, et al. A simple method based on Icp-Ms for estimation of background levels of arsenic, cadmium, copper, manganese, nickel, lead, and selenium in blood of the Brazilian population. J Toxicol Environ Heal Part A. 2010;73:878–87. https://doi.org/10.1080/15287391003744807.
16. Karunasinghe N, Han DY, Zhu S, et al. Serum selenium and single-nucleotide polymorphisms in genes for selenoproteins: relationship to markers of oxidative stress in men from Auckland, New Zealand. Genes Nutr. 2012;7:179–90. https://doi.org/10.1007/s12263-011-0259-1.
17. Longnecker MP, Stram DO, Taylor PR, et al. Use of selenium concentration in whole blood, serum, toenails, or urine as a surrogate measure of selenium intake. Epidemiology. 1996;7:384–90. https://doi.org/10.1097/00001648-199607000-00008.
18. Majolo F, de Oliveira Paludo FJ, Ponzoni A, et al. Effect of 593C> T GPx1 SNP alone and in synergy with 47C> T SOD2 SNP on the outcome of critically ill patients. Cytokine. 2015;71:312–7. https://doi.org/10.1016/j.cyto.2014.10.020.
19. Méplan C, Crosley LK, Nicol F, et al. Genetic polymorphisms in the human selenoprotein P gene determine the response of selenoprotein markers to selenium supplementation in a gender-specific manner (the SELGEN study). FASEB J. 2007;21:3063–74.
20. Meplan C, Crosley LK, Nicol F, et al. Functional effects of a common single-nucleotide polymorphism (GPX4c718t) in the glutathione peroxidase 4 gene: interaction with sex. Am J Clin Nutr. 2008;87:1019–27.
21. Méplan C, Dragsted LO, Ravn-Haren G, et al. Association between polymorphisms in glutathione peroxidase and selenoprotein P genes, glutathione peroxidase activity, HRT use and breast cancer risk. PLoS One. 2013;8:e73316. https://doi.org/10.1371/journal.pone.0073316.
22. Meplan C, Hughes DJ, Pardini B, et al. Genetic variants in selenoprotein genes increase risk of colorectal cancer. Carcinogenesis. 2010;31:1074–9. https://doi.org/10.1093/carcin/bgq076.
23. Méplan C, Nicol F, Burtle BT, et al. Relative abundance of selenoprotein P isoforms in human plasma depends on genotype, se intake, and cancer status. Antioxid Redox Signal. 2009;11:2631–40. https://doi.org/10.1089/ars.2009.2533.
24. Miller SA, Dykes DD, Polesky HF. A simple salting out procedure for extracting DNA from human nucleated cells. Nucleic Acids Res. 1988;16:1215.
25. Miranda-Vilela AL, Alves PC, Akimoto AK, et al. Gene polymorphisms against DNA damage induced by hydrogen peroxide in leukocytes of healthy humans through comet assay: a quasi-experimental study. Environ Health. 2010;9:21. https://doi.org/10.1186/1476-069X-9-21.
26. Nemoto M, Nishimura R, Sasaki T, et al. Genetic association of glutathione peroxidase-1 with coronary artery calcification in type 2 diabetes: a case control study with multi-slice computed tomography. Cardiovasc Diabetol. 2007;6:23. https://doi.org/10.1186/1475-2840-6-23.
27. Nève J. Methods in determination of selenium states. J Trace Elem Electrolytes Health Dis. 1991;5:1–17.
28. Outzen M, Tjønneland A, Larsen EH, et al. The effect on selenium concentrations of a randomized intervention with fish and mussels in a population with relatively low habitual dietary selenium intake. Nutrients. 2015a;7:608–24. https://doi.org/10.3390/nu7010608.
29. Outzen M, Tjønneland A, Larsen EH, et al. Effect of increased intake of fish and mussels on exposure to toxic trace elements in a healthy, middle-aged population. Food Addit Contam Part A. 2015b;32:1858–66. https://doi.org/10.1080/19440049.2015.1072878.
30. Papp LV, Lu J, Holmgren A, Khanna KK. From selenium to selenoproteins: synthesis, identity, and their role in human health. Antioxid Redox Signal. 2007;9:775–806. https://doi.org/10.1089/ars.2007.1528.
31. Raaschou-Nielsen O, Soerensen M, Hansen RDRD, et al. GPX1 Pro198Leu polymorphism, interactions with smoking and alcohol consumption, and risk for lung cancer. Cancer Lett. 2007;247:293–300. https://doi.org/10.1016/j.canlet.2006.05.006
32. Ravn-Haren G, Bügel S, Krath BN, et al. A short-term intervention trial with selenate, selenium-enriched yeast and selenium-enriched milk: effects on oxidative defence regulation. Br J Nutr. 2008a;99(4):883–92. https://doi.org/10.1017/S0007114507825153
33. Ravn-Haren G, Krath BN, Overvad K, et al. Effect of long-term selenium yeast intervention on activity and gene expression of antioxidant and xenobiotic metabolising enzymes in healthy elderly volunteers from the Danish

Prevention of Cancer by Intervention by Selenium (PRECISE) pilot study. Br J Nutr. 2008b;99:1190–8. https://doi.org/10.1017/S0007114507882948.

34. Ravn-Haren G, Olsen A, Tjonneland A, et al. Associations between GPX1 Pro198Leu polymorphism, erythrocyte GPX activity, alcohol consumption and breast cancer risk in a prospective cohort study. Carcinogenesis. 2006;27:820–5.

35. Rayman MP. Food-chain selenium and human health: emphasis on intake. Br J Nutr. 2008;100(2):254–68. https://doi.org/10.1017/S0007114508939830.

36. Rayman MP. Selenoproteins and human health: insights from epidemiological data. Biochim Biophys Acta - Gen Subj. 2009;1790:1533–40.

37. Rayman MP. Selenium and human health. Lancet. 2012;379:1256–68.

38. Robinson MF, Rea HM, Friend GM, et al. On supplementing the selenium intake of New Zealanders. 2. Prolonged metabolic experiments with daily supplements of selenomethionine, selenite and fish. Er J Nutr. 1978;39:589–600.

39. Rosenberger A, Illig T, Korb K, et al. Do genetic factors protect for early onset lung cancer? A case control study before the age of 50 years. BMC Cancer. 2008;8:60. https://doi.org/10.1186/1471-2407-8-60.

40. Saito Y, Sato N, Hirashima M, et al. Domain structure of bi-functional selenoprotein P. Biochem J. 2004;381:341–6. https://doi.org/10.1042/BJ20040328.

41. Saxholt E, Christensen AT, Møller A, et al (2008) Danish Food Composition Databank, revision 7. In: Dep. Nutr. Natl. Food Institute, Tech. Univ. Denmark. http://www.foodcomp.dk/

42. Soerensen M, Christensen K, Stevnsner T, Christiansen L. The Mn-superoxide dismutase single nucleotide polymorphism rs4880 and the glutathione peroxidase 1 single nucleotide polymorphism rs1050450 are associated with aging and longevity in the oldest old Mech Ageing Dev. 2009;130:308–14. https://doi.org/10.1016/j.mad.2009.01.005.

43. Steinbrecher A, Méplan C, Hesketh J, et al. Effects of selenium status and polymorphisms in selenoprotein genes on prostate cancer risk in a prospective study of European men. Cancer Epidemiol Biomark Prev. 2010; 19:2958–68. https://doi.org/10.1158/1055-9965.EPI-10-0364.

44. Strauss E, Oszkinis G, Staniszewski R. SEPP1 gene variants and abdominal aortic aneurysm: gene association in relation to metabolic risk factors and peripheral arterial disease coexistence. Sci Rep. 2014;4:7061. https://doi.org/10.1038/srep07061.

45. Tang TS, Prior SL, Li KW, et al. Association between the rs1050450 glutathione peroxidase-1 (C > T) gene variant and peripheral neuropathy in two independent samples of subjects with diabetes mellitus. Nutr Metab Cardiovasc Dis. 2012;22:417–25. https://doi.org/10.1016/j.numecd.2010.08.001.

46. Thomson CD. Assessment of requirements for selenium and adequacy of selenium status: a review. Eur J Clin Nutr. 2004;58:391–402. https://doi.org/10.1038/sj.ejcn.1601800.

47. Udler M, Maia AT, Cebrian A, et al. Common germline genetic variation in antioxidant defense genes and survival after diagnosis of breast cancer. J Clin Oncol. 2007;25:3015–23.

48. Villette S, Kyle JAM, Brown KM, et al. A novel single nucleotide polymorphism in the 3′ untranslated region of human glutathione peroxidase 4 influences lipoxygenase metabolism. Blood Cells Mol Dis. 2002; 29:174–8. https://doi.org/10.1006/bcmd.2002.0556.

49. Wheeler CR, Salzman JA, Elsayed NM, et al. Automated assays for superoxide dismutase, catalase, glutathione peroxidase, and glutathione reductase activity. Anal Biochem. 1990;184:193–9.

50. Ye H, Li X, Wang L, et al. Genetic associations with coronary heart disease: meta-analyses of 12 candidate genetic variants. Gene. 2013;531:71–7. https://doi.org/10.1016/j.gene.2013.07.029.

Permissions

List of Contributors

Anne Leiteritz, Benjamin Dilberger, Uwe Wenzel and Elena Fitzenberger
Molecular Nutrition Research, Interdisciplinary Research Center, Justus-Liebig-University of Giessen, Heinrich-Buff-Ring 26-32, 35392 Giessen, Germany

Mitsuru Tanaka
Nissin Global Innovation Center, Nissin Foods Holdings, 2100 Tobukimachi, Hachioji-shi, Tokyo 192-0001, Japan

Akihito Yasuoka
Project on Health and Anti-Aging, Kanagawa Academy of Science and Technology, Life Science and Environment Research Center (LiSE) 4F C-4, 3-25-13 Tonomachi, Kawasaki-ku, Kawasaki, Kanagawa 210-0821, Japan

Manae Shimizu, Kei Kumakura and Toshitada Nagai
Department of Health and Nutrition, Takasaki University of Health and Welfare, 37-1 Nakaorui-machi, Takasaki, Gunma 370-0033, Japan

Yoshikazu Saito and Tomiko Asakura
Department of Applied Biological Chemistry, Graduate School of Agricultural and Life Sciences, The University of Tokyo, 1-1-1 Yayoi, Bunkyo-ku, Tokyo 113-8657, Japan

Sophie Hellstrand, Ulrika Ericson, Christina-Alexandra Schulz, Isabel Drake, Marju Orho-Melander and Emily Sonestedt
Diabetes and Cardiovascular Disease—Genetic Epidemiology, Department of Clinical Sciences Malmö, Lund University, Jan Waldenströms gata 35, SE-20502 Malmö, Sweden

Bo Gullberg
Nutritional Epidemiology, Department of Clinical Sciences Malmö, Lund University, Jan Waldenströms gata 35, SE-20502 Malmö, Sweden

Bo Hedblad and Gunnar Engström
Cardiovascular Epidemiology, Department of Clinical Sciences Malmö, Lund University, Jan Waldenströms gata 35, SE-20502 Malmö, Sweden

L. Della Casa, E. Rossi, C. Romanelli and A. Iannone
"ProteoWork Lab", Dipartimento di Medicina Diagnostica, Clinica e di Sanità
Pubblica, Università di Modena e Reggio Emilia, via Campi 287, 41125 Modena, Italy

L. Gibellini
Dipartimento Chirurgico, Medico, Odontoiatrico e di Scienze Morfologiche con Interesse Trapiantologico, Oncologico e di Medicina Rigenerativa, Università di Modena e Reggio Emilia, via Campi 287, 41125 Modena, Italy

B. Allam-Ndoul, F. Guénard and M-C Vohl
Institute of Nutrition and Functional Foods (INAF), Laval University, Pavillon
des Services, 2440 Hochelaga Blvd, Québec, Québec, Canada

O. Barbier
Laboratory of Molecular Pharmacology, CHU de Québec Research Center, 2705 Laurier
Blvd, Québec, Québec G1V 4G2, Canada

Mari C. W. Myhrstad
Department of Health, Nutrition and Management, Faculty of Health Sciences, Oslo and Akershus University College of Applied Sciences, St. Olavs plass, 0130 Oslo, Norway

Stine M. Ulven
Department of Health, Nutrition and Management, Faculty of Health Sciences, Oslo and Akershus University College of Applied Sciences, St. Olavs plass, 0130 Oslo, Norway
Department of Nutrition, Institute for Basic Medical Sciences, University of Oslo, Blindern, 0317 Oslo, Norway

Inger Ottestad
Department of Nutrition, Institute for Basic Medical Sciences, University of Oslo, Blindern, 0317 Oslo, Norway
Department of Health, Nutrition and Management, Faculty of Health Sciences, Oslo and Akershus University College of Applied Sciences, St. Olavs plass, 0130 Oslo, Norway

Kirsten B. Holven
Department of Nutrition, Institute for Basic Medical Sciences, University of Oslo, Blindern, 0317 Oslo, Norway
Norwegian National Advisory Unit on Familial Hypercholesterolemia, Department of Endocrinology, Morbid Obesity and Preventive Medicine, Oslo University Hospital Rikshospitalet, Nydalen, Oslo, Norway

Clara-Cecilie Günther
Norwegian Computing Center, 0314 Oslo, Norway

Einar Ryeng
Department of Cancer Research and Molecular Medicine, Norwegian University of Science and Technology, 7489 Trondheim, Norway

Astrid Nilsson and Grethe I. A. Borge
Nofima AS, Norwegian Institute of Food, Fisheries and Aquaculture Research, PB 210, Aas N-1431, Norway

Achim Kohler
Nofima AS, Norwegian Institute of Food, Fisheries and Aquaculture Research, PB 210, Aas N-1431, Norway
Department of Mathematical Sciences and Technology (IMT), Norwegian University of Life Sciences, 1432 Ås, Norway

Kirsti W. Brønner
TINE SA, Centre for Research and Development, Kalbakken, 0902 Oslo, Norway

Jian Yang, Cecilia Primo and Ismail Elbaz-Younes
USDA/ARS Children's Nutrition Research Center, Baylor College of Medicine, 1100 Bates Street, Houston, TX 77030, USA

Kendal D. Hirschi
USDA/ARS Children's Nutrition Research Center, Baylor College of Medicine, 1100 Bates Street, Houston, TX 77030, USA
Vegetable and Fruit Improvement Center, Texas AandM University, College Station, TX 77845, USA

Soon-Sen Leow and Ravigadevi Sambanthamurthi
Malaysian Palm Oil Board, No. 6, Persiaran Institusi, Bandar Baru Bangi, 43000 Kajang, Selangor, Malaysia

Julia Bolsinger, Andrzej Pronczuk and K. C. Hayes
Brandeis University, 415 South Street, Waltham, MA 02454, USA

Silvia Parolo, Sébastien Lacroix and Marie-Pier Scott-Boyer
The Microsoft Research, University of Trento Centre for Computational
Systems Biology (COSBI), piazza Manifattura 1, 38068 Rovereto, TN, Italy

Jim Kaput
Vydiant, Inc, Gold River, CA, USA

Aneta A.Koronowicz, Paula Banks, Dominik Domagała, Teresa Leszczyńska, Ewelina Piasna and Mariola Marynowska
Department of Human Nutrition, Faculty of Food Technology, University of Agriculture, Krakow, Poland

Adam Master
Department of Biochemistry and Molecular Biology, Medical Centre for Postgraduate Education, Warsaw, Poland

Piotr Laidler
Department of Medical Biochemistry, Jagiellonian University Medical College, Krakow, Poland

I. P. G. Van Bussel, A. Jolink-Stoppelenburg and C. P. G. M. De Groot
Division of Human Nutrition, Wageningen University, Bomenweg 2, 6703 HD Wageningen, The Netherlands

M. R. Müller
Division of Human Nutrition, Wageningen University, Bomenweg 2, 6703 HD Wageningen, The Netherlands
Current Address: Norwich Medical School, University of East Anglia, Norwich NR4 7TJ, UK

L. A. Afman
Division of Human Nutrition, Wageningen University, Bomenweg 2, 6703 HD Wageningen, The Netherlands
Division of Human Nutrition, Wageningen University and Research centre, NL-6700 EV Wageningen, The Netherlands

T. J. van den Broek, G. C. M. Bakker, C. M. Rubingh, S. Bijlsma, J. H. M. Stroeve, B. van Ommen, M. J. van Erk and S.Wopereis
TNO, Utrechtseweg 48, 3704 HE Zeist, The Netherlands

Zoe Daniel, Angelina Swali and Simon C Langley-Evans
School of Biosciences, University of Nottingham, Sutton Bonington, Loughborough LE12 5RD, UK

Richard Emes
School of Veterinary Medicine and Science, University of Nottingham, Sutton Bonington, Loughborough, UK
Advanced Data Analysis Centre, University of Nottingham, Sutton Bonington, Loughborough, UK

Xianyong Ma, Wei Fang, Zongyong Jiang, Li Wang, Xuefen Yang and Kaiguo Gao
Institute of Animal Science, Guangdong Academy of Agricultural Sciences, 510640 Guangzhou, China
The Key Laboratory of Animal Nutrition and Feed Science (South China) of Ministry of Agriculture, 510640 Guangzhou, China
State Key Laboratory of Livestock and Poultry Breeding, 510640 Guangzhou, China
Guangdong Public Laboratory of Animal Breeding and Nutrition, 510640 Guangzhou, China
Guangdong Key Laboratory of Animal Breeding and Nutrition, 510640 Guangzhou, China

Emily S. Mohn
Jean Mayer United States Department of Agriculture
Human Nutrition Research Center on Aging, Tufts
University, Boston, MA, USA

Elizabeth J. Johnson
Jean Mayer United States Department of Agriculture
Human Nutrition Research Center on Aging, Tufts
University, Boston, MA, USA
Antioxidants Research Laboratory, 711 Washington
Street, Boston, MA 02111, USA

John W. Erdman Jr
Department of Food Science and Human Nutrition,
University of Illinois at Urbana-Champaign, Urbana,
IL, USA

Martha Neuringer
Division of Neuroscience, Oregon National Primate
Research Center, Oregon Health and Science University,
Beaverton, Oregon, USA

Matthew J. Kuchan
Abbott Nutrition, Columbus, Ohio, USA

**Sylwia Szrok, Ewa Stelmanska, Jacek Turyn and
Julian Swierczynski**
Department of Biochemistry, Medical University of
Gdansk, Debinki 1, 80-211 Gdansk, Poland

Aleksandra Bielicka-Gieldon
Department of Environmental Technology, University
of Gdansk, Wita Stwosza 63, 80-952 Gdansk, Poland

Tomasz Sledzinski
Department of Pharmaceutical Biochemistry, Medical
University of Gdansk, Debinki 1,
80-211 Gdansk, Poland

**George Hindy, Isabel Drake, Christina-Alexandra
Schulz, Louise Brunkwall, Sophie Hellstrand, Peter
Almgren and Marju Orho-Melander**
Diabetes and Cardiovascular Disease, Genetic
Epidemiology, Department of Clinical Sciences,
Malmö, Lund University, Malmö, Sweden

Ulrika Ericson
Diabetes and Cardiovascular Disease, Genetic
Epidemiology, Department of Clinical Sciences,
Malmö, Lund University, Malmö, Sweden

Clinical Research Centre, Building 60, floor 13, SUS in
Malmö, entrance 72, Jan Waldenströms gata 35, SE-205
02 Malmö, Sweden

**Liang Hu, Fei Han, Lin Chen, Xie Peng, Daiwen
Chen, De Wu, Lianqiang Che and Keying Zhang**
Institute of Animal Nutrition, Key Laboratory of Animal
Disease-Resistance Nutrition, Sichuan Agricultural
University, Ministry of Education, No.211 Huimin
Road, Wenjiang District, Chengdu 611130, Sichuan,
People's Republic of China

Gitte Ravn-Haren
National Food Institute, Technical University of
Denmark, Kemitorvet, Building 202, 2800 Kgs Lyngby,
Denmark

Malene Outzen
National Food Institute, Technical University of
Denmark, Kemitorvet, Building 202, 2800 Kgs Lyngby,
Denmark
Danish Cancer Society Research Center,
Strandboulevarden 49, 2100 Copenhagen Ø, Denmark

Tine Iskov Kopp
National Food Institute, Technical University of
Denmark, Kemitorvet, Building 202, 2800 Kgs Lyngby,
Denmark
Danish Cancer Society Research Center,
Strandboulevarden 49, 2100 Copenhagen Ø, Denmark
The Danish Multiple Sclerosis Registry, Copenhagen
University Hospital, Rigshospitalet, Blegdamsvej 9,
2100 Copenhagen Ø, Denmark
The Danish Multiple Sclerosis Center, Department of
Neurology, The Danish Multiple Sclerosis Registry,
Section 7801, Rigshospitalet, Blegdamsvej 9, 2100
Copenhagen Ø, Denmark

Anja Olsen
Danish Cancer Society Research Center,
Strandboulevarden 49, 2100 Copenhagen Ø, Denmark

Ulla Vogel
National Research Centre for the Working Environment,
Lersø Parkallé 105, 2100 Copenhagen Ø, Denmark

Index

www.ingramcontent.com/pod-product-compliance
Lightning Source LLC
Chambersburg PA
CBHW080627200326
41458CB00013B/4541